Essential Ultrasound Anatomy

Second Edition

Essential Ultrasound Anatomy

Second Edition

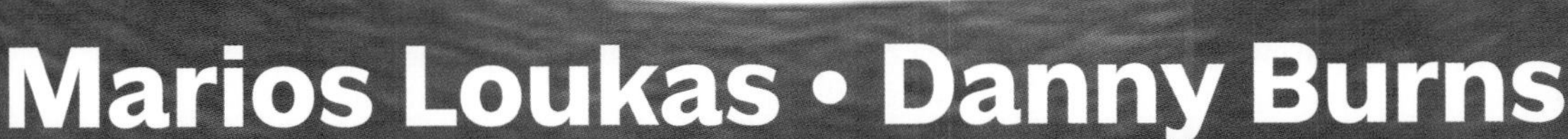

Marios Loukas
Dean School of Medicine
Professor Department of Anatomical Sciences
Professor Department of Pathology
St. George's University
Grenada West Indies
Dean, College of Medicine
Nicolaus Copernicus Superior School
Olsztyn, Poland

Danny Burns
Professor Department of Anatomical Sciences
St. George's University
Grenada, West Indies

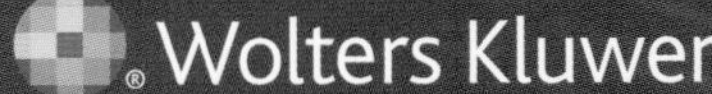

Philadelphia • Baltimore • New York • London
Buenos Aires • Hong Kong • Sydney • Tokyo

Senior Acquisitions Editor: Crystal Taylor
Development Editor: Amy Millholen
Editorial Coordinator: Erin E. Hernandez
Editorial Assistant: Parisa Saranj
Marketing Manager: Danielle Klahr
Production Project Manager: Frances Gunning
Manager, Graphic Arts & Design: Stephen Druding
Manufacturing Coordinator: Margie Orzech-Zeranko
Prepress Vendor: TNQ Tech

Throughout this book, a portion of the cadaveric images were made possible by using the NLM Visible Human Project®: http://www.nlm.nih.gov/research/visible/visible_human.html.

9 8 7 6 5 4 3 2 1

Printed in Mexico

Library of Congress Cataloging-in-Publication Data

ISBN-13: 978-1-975216-88-7

Cataloging in Publication data available on request from publisher.

shop.lww.com

QUADM0924

Dedications

To Marti, my spouse and best friend for her patience and support throughout the years. To my mentors in medical and graduate school, and to the many students and junior colleagues whose excitement about learning has made this journey so much fun. **–D.B**

To my daughter Nikol, my son Chris, and my wife Joanna for their patience and support putting up with my early mornings and late nights *during the creation* of this book. Love you so much. **–M.L**

Acknowledgments

We would like to thank all the donors and their families for their ultimate donation for the benefit of future generations of physicians and scientists. This book could have never materialized without their immeasurable contributions.

The production of the cadaveric materials is a huge team effort that has involved several faculty, laboratory technicians, and administrative staff.

We would also like to thank the following colleagues for their technical expertise in dissections and their enormous help with this project including 1st and 2nd editions:

Nelson Davis, Damion Richards, Rodon Marrast, Shiva Mathurin, Romeo Cox, Seikou Phillip, Marlon Joseph, Travis Joseph, Simone Francis, Charlon Charles, Arnelle Gibbs, Sheryce Fraser, Chad Phillip, Ryan Jacobs, Nadica Thomas-Dominique, Tracy Shabazz, and Yvonne James of the Department of Anatomical Sciences, St. George's University, School of Medicine, Grenada, West Indies, for their technical, laboratory, and administrative assistance.

The following faculty also assisted with this project: Drs. Theofanis Kollias, Maira DuPlessis, Yusuf Oladimeji Alimi, Seid Eid, Sasha Lake, Ahmed Mahgoub, Michael Montalbano, Fawwaz R. Safi, Yuvedha Senthil, Kadesha Ferguson, Sanyukta Dudhat, Shanado Williams, Ali Walji, Rabjot Rai, Ramesh Rao, Asad Rizvi, Wallisa Roberts, Sonja Salandi, and Deepak Sharma from the Department of Anatomical Sciences, St. George's University, School of Medicine, Grenada, West Indies.

Special thanks to Jennifer Kelly, RDMS, RTNM, who was excited about this project from the very beginning and who spent countless hours obtaining many of the ultrasound images and videos used in this book and working with the St. George's University illustration team documenting patient positioning and probe placement.

We thank the following instructors of the Department of Anatomical Sciences, St. George's University, School of Medicine, Grenada, West Indies, for their contributions in illustrations: David Nahabedian, Sue Simon, Claudia Cárceles Román, Sarah Gluschitz, Farihah Khan, Linden Pederson, Jack Nelson, Jessica Holland, Brandon Holt, Luz Ortiz Nieto, Charles Price, Xochitl Vinaja, and Katie Yost. We are grateful for their hard work, talent, ideas, patience, and creativity and feel fortunate that they are our colleagues and friends.

Lastly, we express our gratitude to the students and faculty who have utilized this book and shared the valuable feedback to enhance its content, effectiveness, and learning experience. Their contributions have been instrumental in refining the material and ensuring its relevance and impact on education.

Preface

For physicians, ultrasound is a valuable tool for real-time visualization of certain parts of the human body, but it requires significant training. To address this, we started teaching medical students at St. George's University hands-on ultrasound anatomy during their basic sciences education. We believe that the increasing use of ultrasound in various medical specialties in the past decade calls for a strong foundation in ultrasound technique, anatomy, and physiology from the beginning of medical training. Point-of-care ultrasound is now widely available in clinics and hospitals, making ultrasound examination skills as crucial as using a stethoscope. For many, ultrasound is the stethoscope of the future.

One of the challenges we faced at the early stages of ultrasound implementation in the curriculum was how to optimize the time students spent with standardized patients during hands-on sessions. We realized that too much time was spent explaining patient positioning, probe placement, and the appearance of ultrasound images. To address this, we wanted students to come prepared to the sessions with a basic understanding of optimal patient positioning, probe placement, and how to identify key landmarks in real-time ultrasound images. We aimed to provide reference materials that would allow students to arrive at the laboratory ready to start practicing with the ultrasound probe while instructors guided and assisted them.

Existing resources on ultrasound techniques primarily target physicians already using ultrasound in their clinical practice. These resources mainly focus on technical aspects of clinical applications. However, our book aims to bridge this gap by offering a foundation in regional ultrasound anatomy accessible to students early in their medical education and detailed enough to interest practicing physicians incorporating ultrasound into their daily practice. The book is organized by anatomical regions, and each section follows a similar structure. It begins with an overview of the relevant anatomy, followed by a section on technique. Both sections provide textual explanations and illustrations of the technical details and skills required to obtain specific ultrasound images from that region. Each figure in the book includes an unlabeled and labeled ultrasound image, a representation of tissue texture, a drawing illustrating patient positioning and probe placement, and a labeled cadaver slice corresponding to the ultrasound images. The technique text is accompanied by quick reference tabs that identify ultrasound image orientation, content, and refer to the specific figure where the image is found.

The book can be read chapter by chapter or section by section to gain an overview of the ultrasound images and important structures encountered in each anatomical region. Alternatively, readers can easily locate specific ultrasound images along with illustrations and descriptions of how to obtain those images and identify structures and landmarks within them. Instructors can select two or three images from an anatomical region and assign corresponding readings to prepare students for laboratory sessions where they will practice proper patient positioning, probe placement, and identification of landmarks and structures.

In this second edition, we have made significant improvements to enhance the usefulness of the book for future clinical practice. Almost every chapter has been expanded with additional content. Additionally, the cadaveric dissections have been improved to provide a clearer view of the entire dissected area, replacing the unclear visuals from previous editions.

We have also expanded the USMLE multiple-choice questions, which are now included in every chapter. These questions are designed to help the reader assess their clinical knowledge and provide valuable feedback to students, instructors, and physicians.

A special chapter has been dedicated to describing and illustrating normal and abnormal findings in the FAST examination, which is a commonly used clinical application of ultrasound. This chapter allows readers to apply their ultrasound anatomy knowledge to real-life scenarios involving the heart, upper abdomen, and pelvis.

Our aim is for this book to serve as a resource for anyone interested in exploring the use of ultrasound, providing a solid anatomical basis for locating and identifying important structures throughout the body.

Table of Contents

1 Introduction 1

Ultrasound Basics 2
Different Probes for Different Applications 2
Using US Probes 3
Appearance of Tissues in US Images 5
Basic "Knobology" and Image Optimization 7

2 Basic Ultrasound Physics 9

Sound Waves 10
Attenuation 13
US Probes 15
Producing an Image 18
Specular and Diffuse Reflection 20
Bioeffects of US Energy 24

3 Back 25

Lumbar Spine 26
Review of the Anatomy 26
Technique 27

Cervical Spine and Greater Occipital Nerve 32
Review of the Anatomy 32
Technique 33

4 Upper Limb 37

Shoulder 38
Review of the Anatomy 38
Technique 40

Brachial Plexus 48
Review of the Anatomy 48
Technique 49

Arm 53
Review of the Anatomy 53
Technique 55

Elbow 61
Review of Anatomy 61
Technique 63

Forearm, Wrist, and Hand 72
Review of the Anatomy 72
Technique 74

5 Lower Limb 91

Proximal Thigh and Inguinal Region 92
Review of the Anatomy 92
Technique 95

Gluteal Region 103
Review of the Anatomy 103
Technique 105

Thigh 110
Review of the Anatomy 110
Technique 112

Knee 123
Review of the Anatomy 123
Technique 126

Leg 136
Review of the Anatomy 136
Technique 139

Ankle and Foot 147
Review of the Anatomy 147
Technique 151

6 Thorax: Chest Wall and Pleura; Breast 165

Chest Wall and Pleura 166
Review of the Anatomy 166
Technique 168

Breast 173
Review of the Anatomy 173
Technique 174

7 Heart 179

Review of the Anatomy 180
Technique 184

8 Abdomen 193

Abdominal Wall 194
Review of the Anatomy 194
Technique 196

Peritoneum, Gastrointestinal Tract, and Liver 199
Review of the Anatomy 199
Technique 203

Gallbladder 212
Review of the Anatomy 212
Technique 213

Spleen and Kidneys 216
Review of the Anatomy 216
Technique 218

Pancreas 222
Review of the Anatomy 222
Technique 223

Abdominal Vessels 225
Review of the Anatomy 225
Technique 228

9 Female Pelvis 237

Review of the Anatomy 238
Technique 240

10 Male Pelvis 245

Review of the Anatomy 246
Erection and Ejaculation 249
Technique 250

11 Neck, Face and Eye 257

Neck 258
Review of the Anatomy 258
Technique 264

Viscera of the Neck 271
Review of the Anatomy 271
Technique 273

Face 278
Review of the Anatomy 278
Technique 282

Eye and Orbit 283
Review of the Anatomy 283
Technique 284

12 Focused Assessment with Sonography for Trauma (FAST) 291

Overview of Focused Assessment With Sonography for Trauma 292
Review of the Anatomy 293

Right Upper Quadrant 294

Table of Contents

Technique 294

Left Upper Quadrant 297

Technique 297

Suprapubic Views of Abdomen/Pelvis 299

Technique 299

Heart and Pericardial Space 303

13 Clinical Applications 307

Central Venous Catheterization 308

Lumbar Puncture 311

Pericardiocentesis 314

Procedure (Parasternal Approach) 316

Alternative Method: Subxiphoid and Apical Approach 317

Knee Joint Aspiration 318

Shoulder Aspiration 320

Elbow Joint Aspiration 323

Answers to Multiple Choice Questions 327

GLOSSARY 329

INDEX 351

1 Introduction

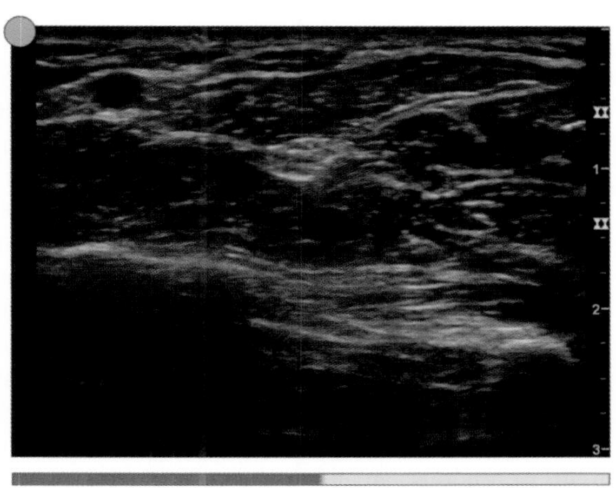

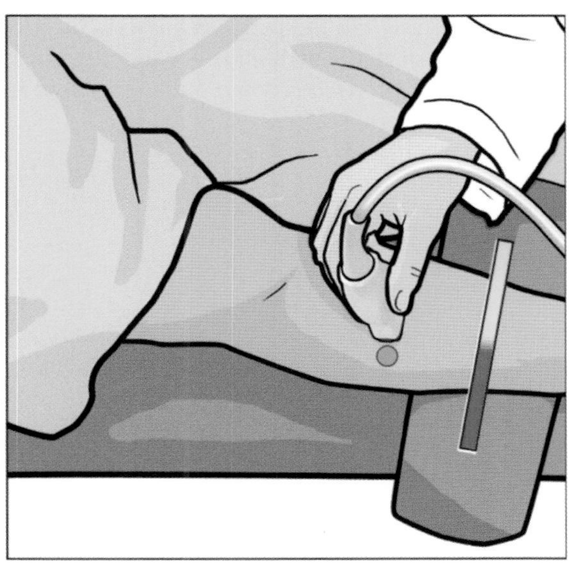

Ultrasound Basics

Ultrasound (US) is an imaging technology widely used across multiple medical specialties. The devices are portable and free of ionizing radiation, with low risk of harm even in the most vulnerable populations. The portability, safety, and relatively low cost of US imaging have increasingly made it widely available for bed-side and other point-of-care imaging as an extension of the physical examination (eg, examination of the peritoneal spaces for the presence of free fluid when intraperitoneal bleeding is suspected) or for guiding interventional procedures, such as central line placement, nerve blocks, joint injections, and biopsies.

Typical US images display 2-dimensional slices of internal structures. Depending on the placement and orientation of the probe on the body surface, the image may be transverse, sagittal/parasagittal, coronal, or oblique. The images are acquired in real time, such that respiratory movements, ventricular contractions, arterial pulsations, phasic changes in venous blood flow, muscle/tendon/joint movements, or the effects of provocative stresses on ligaments or tendons can all be easily observed by experienced operators.

From a transducer housed in the US probe, short pulses of extremely high frequency sound are transmitted across the body surface into the patient's body. As the US pulses propagate through the body and encounter tissues with different acoustic properties, some sound energy is reflected back to the transducer (echo) and some continues to penetrate into deeper tissues (through-transmission). The echo signals that return to the probe are processed and combined to generate an image of the slice being scanned.

Different Probes for Different Applications

IMAGE SHAPE AND DEPTH OF DIFFERENT PROBES
FIG. 1.1

There are three commonly used surface probe types for most general-purpose US imaging applications: **abdominal probes**, **cardiac probes**, and **high-frequency linear probes**.

Abdominal (Convex or Curved Array) Probes

These are low- to intermediate-frequency (2-5 MHz) probes with a curved face and a "footprint" of typically 4 to 6 cm (the side-to-side dimension of the probe face). As the name implies, these probes are commonly used for general-purpose abdominal imaging, but they are also used for other applications such as transabdominal pelvic imaging, obstetrical imaging, and certain musculoskeletal imaging, such as spine and hip joints. The relatively low frequencies available with these probes allow for imaging up to depths of 20 cm or so, and the sector image produced is the width

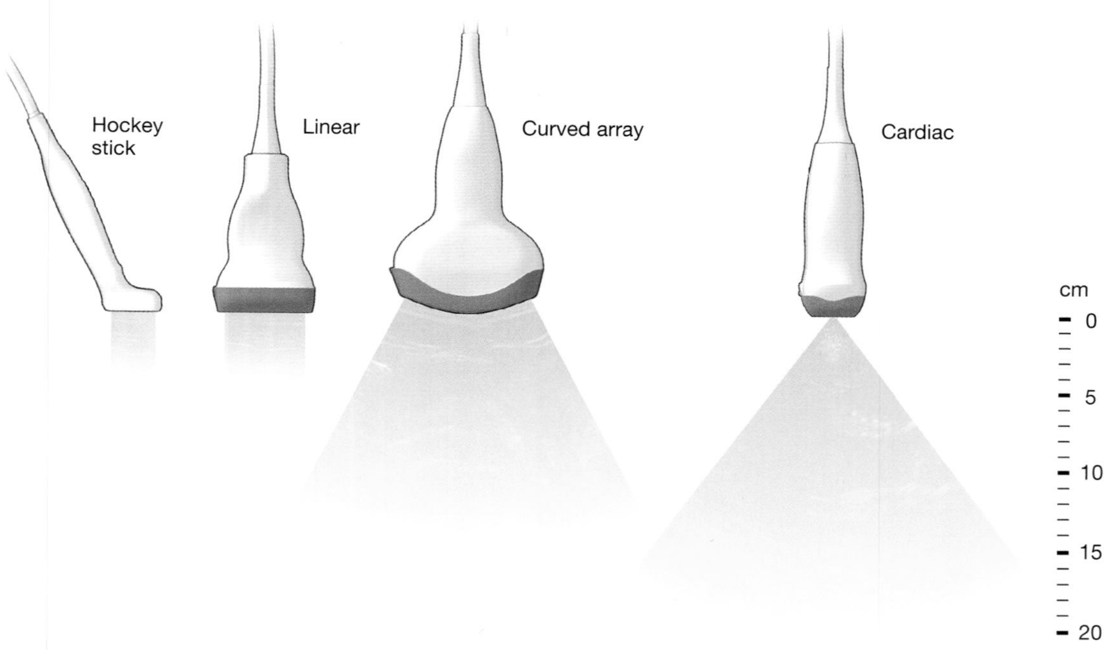

Figure 1.1 Linear, hockey stick, abdominal, and cardiac probes. The shape of the image produced by each probe type is depicted with blue shading.

of the probe footprint at the skin surface, becoming progressively wider as the depth increases. This allows for a wide-angle field of view for imaging large deeper structures (eg, kidneys) and landmarks, but owing to the width of the footprint, it is also possible to image structures nearer to the skin surface with a reasonably wide field of view.

Cardiac (Sector Array) Probes

These probes are used extensively in heart US imaging (echocardiography), but are well-suited for imaging any relatively large, nonsuperficial structures through narrow sonographic windows (such as intercostal spaces). They produce a sector image that resembles a triangular shape, an extremely small (essentially a point source) surface footprint that becomes progressively wider with increasing depth. The resonant frequency is low (1.5-4.5 MHz), allowing for substantial depth penetration (similar to abdominal probes). Because the image is narrow at the surface, these probes are not useful for imaging superficial structures, but can be adapted to most abdominal US imaging purposes if necessary.

Linear (Linear Array) Probes

Because of their high resonant frequencies (8-15 MHz), these probes offer the best image details but poor depth penetration. Consequently, they are used for musculoskeletal, peripheral nerves, thyroid gland, breast, superficial blood vessels, and other imaging applications that require high-resolution images from relatively superficial tissues (approximately 5-6 cm maximum depth from the skin surface). The images they produce are rectangular in shape. The image width remains the same from the probe face at the surface to the deepest part of the image (the width of the probe footprint, commonly 4-5 cm). A subset of linear probes is the hockey stick ultrasound probe. This ultrasound probe is used to examine fingers, toes, and peripheral nerves, among other small superficial structures.

Using US Probes

US Gel

ULTRASOUND GEL ACOUSTICALLY COUPLES PROBES TO SKIN
FIG. 1.2

The probe face must be coupled to the skin surface by using a water-based gel that has sound transmission properties similar to skin. The gel also excludes air pockets between the probe face and the skin (or skin folds and irregularities), which would interfere with the transmission of US pulses into the skin and on to deeper tissues.

Controlling and Manipulating the Probe

To obtain quality images, US users must learn to control and manipulate the probe in terms of exerting an appropriate amount of pressure; stabilizing the probe face on uneven and slippery surfaces; and making fine adjustments in the angle, rotation, and tilt of the probe face relative to structures of interest.

Most of the time, moderate, evenly applied pressure across the probe face is needed. The screen image drops out from areas of the probe face that does not make sufficient contact with the skin surface. Some US imaging tasks require greater pressures, whereas others need minimal pressures.

Proper rotation and tilting (**fanning** or **toggling**) of the probe face are critical to view structures of interest in their true longitudinal or transverse axis (and to change a view from longitudinal to transverse or vice versa) and to produce accurate images of structures that are not parallel to the skin surface. Some structures, including tendons and nerves, appear much brighter when the US beam is perpendicular to their course.

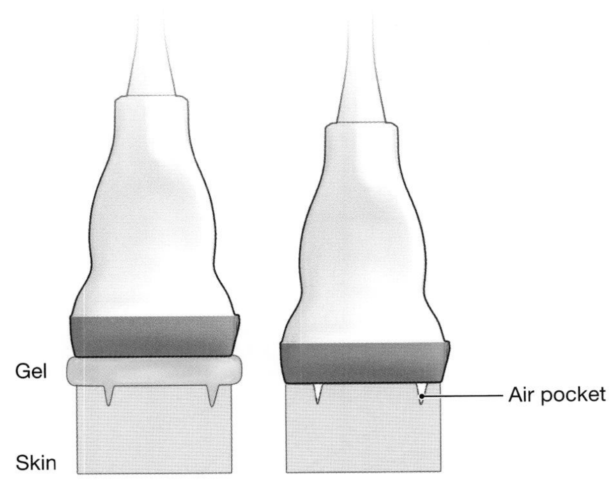

Figure 1.2 Ultrasound gel acoustically couples the outermost layer of the probe face to skin.

Because of probe pressure, probe movement across tender areas, and/or patient positioning, US scanning can occasionally be uncomfortable for patients, but it should never be unnecessarily uncomfortable or painful. Communicating with patients and paying careful attention to their comfort and safety are always a high priority during US scanning.

Probe and Display Orientation Markers

To understand the positions and relationships between structures in US images, you should be able to orient images in terms of superficial to deep and superior to inferior or left to right (lateral to medial). All US probes have an orientation marker on one side near the probe face, usually a raised dot or ridge along the side of the probe, and sometimes a small LED light. The probe orientation marker corresponds to an orientation marker on the display image, usually a colored dot or the manufacturer's logo. Conventionally, for most US imaging, the display orientation marker is placed on the upper left corner of the image. For historical reasons (not just to confuse medical students), the orientation marker is typically placed on the right side of the display for cardiac US. Also, by convention, the orientation marker on the probe should be directed superiorly (cephalad) while performing a scan along the longitudinal axis of the body and directed toward the right side of the patient when performing a scan transverse to the longitudinal axis of the body.

ORIENTING TO SCANS ACQUIRED ALONG THE LONGITUDINAL AXIS
FIG. 1.3

When these conventions are followed, structures closer to the left side (marker side) of the image are more superior and those nearer to the right side (nonmarker side) of the image are more inferior in longitudinal scans. The image in Figure 1.3 was acquired along the longitudinal axis, with the probe face on the skin of the cubital fossa and the probe orientation marker directed superiorly. Knowing this, we can understand the orientation of the image and begin to identify structures and landmarks.

ORIENTING TO SCANS ACQUIRED ALONG THE TRANSVERSE AXIS
FIG. 1.4

Similarly, following the conventions described earlier for longitudinal scans, structures on the marker side of the image are toward the patient's right and those on the nonmarker side toward the patient's left. The image in Figure 1.4 was acquired transverse to the longitudinal axis of the body (which is also transverse to the limb), with the probe face on the skin of the cubital fossa of the patient's right upper limb and the probe orientation marker directed to the right.

In all scans, structures nearer the top of the display image are more superficial and structures nearer the bottom of the image are deeper. The numbers and hash marks located along the side of the image indicate depth in centimeters.

> **QUICK TIP:** Touching or tapping one edge of the probe face with your index finger while observing the screen image for a corresponding flicker is a quick and easy way to determine the probe orientation in relation to the display image.

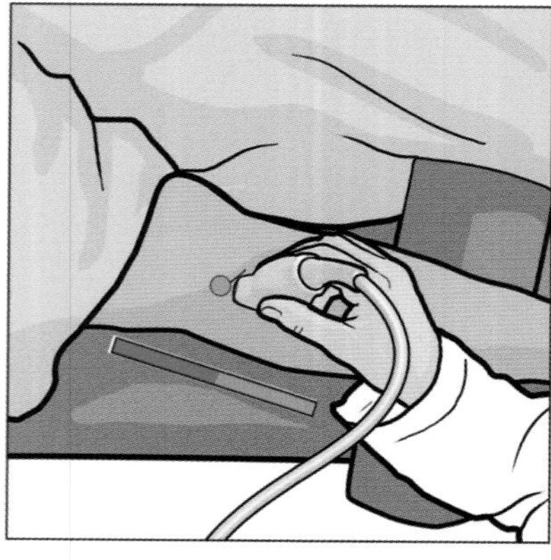

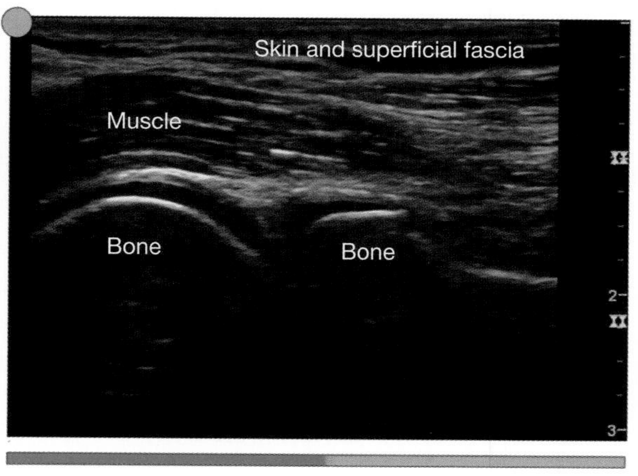

Figure 1.3 Use of the probe marker and display marker to orient to images acquired in the longitudinal axis.

Appearance of Tissues in US Images

ECHOGENICITY: GRAY-SCALE IMAGE DISPLAY
FIG. 1.5

Echogenicity refers to the amount of US reflection by a tissue relative to the surrounding tissues. Whenever there is an interface between tissues with different echogenicities, a visible difference in brightness is seen on the US display. Based on the degree of echogenicity, tissues or structures are described as hyperechoic (white on the display), hypoechoic (gray on the display), or anechoic (black on the display).

APPEARANCE OF COMMONLY ENCOUNTERED TISSUES
FIG. 1.6

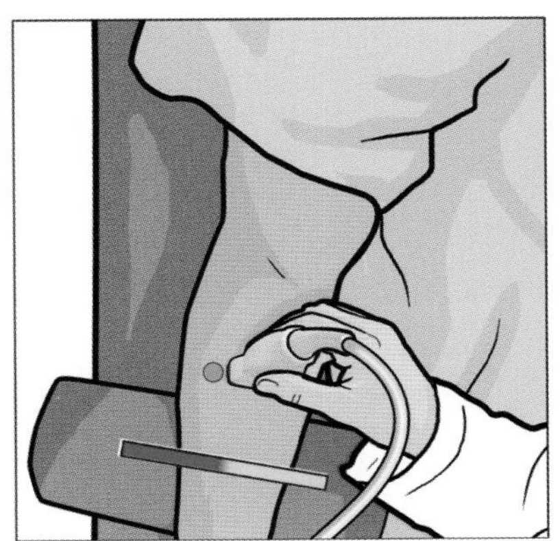

Figure 1.4 Use of the probe marker and display marker to orient to images acquired in the transverse axis.

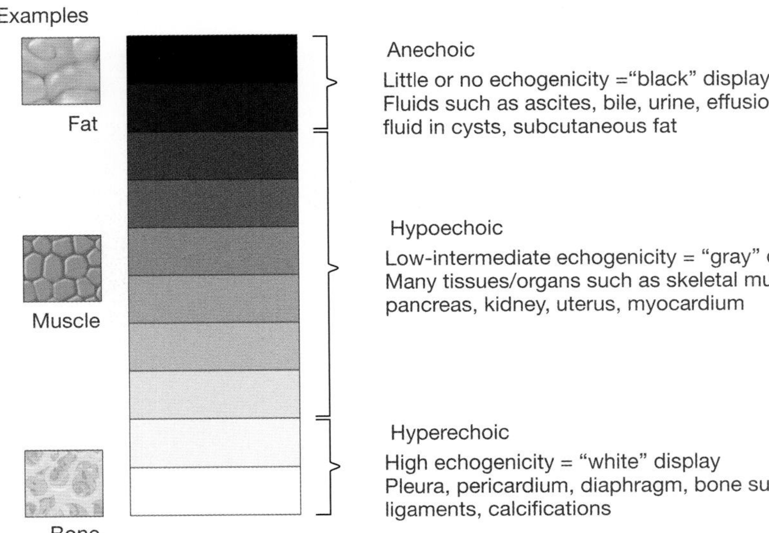

Figure 1.5 Echogenicity and gray-scale image display.

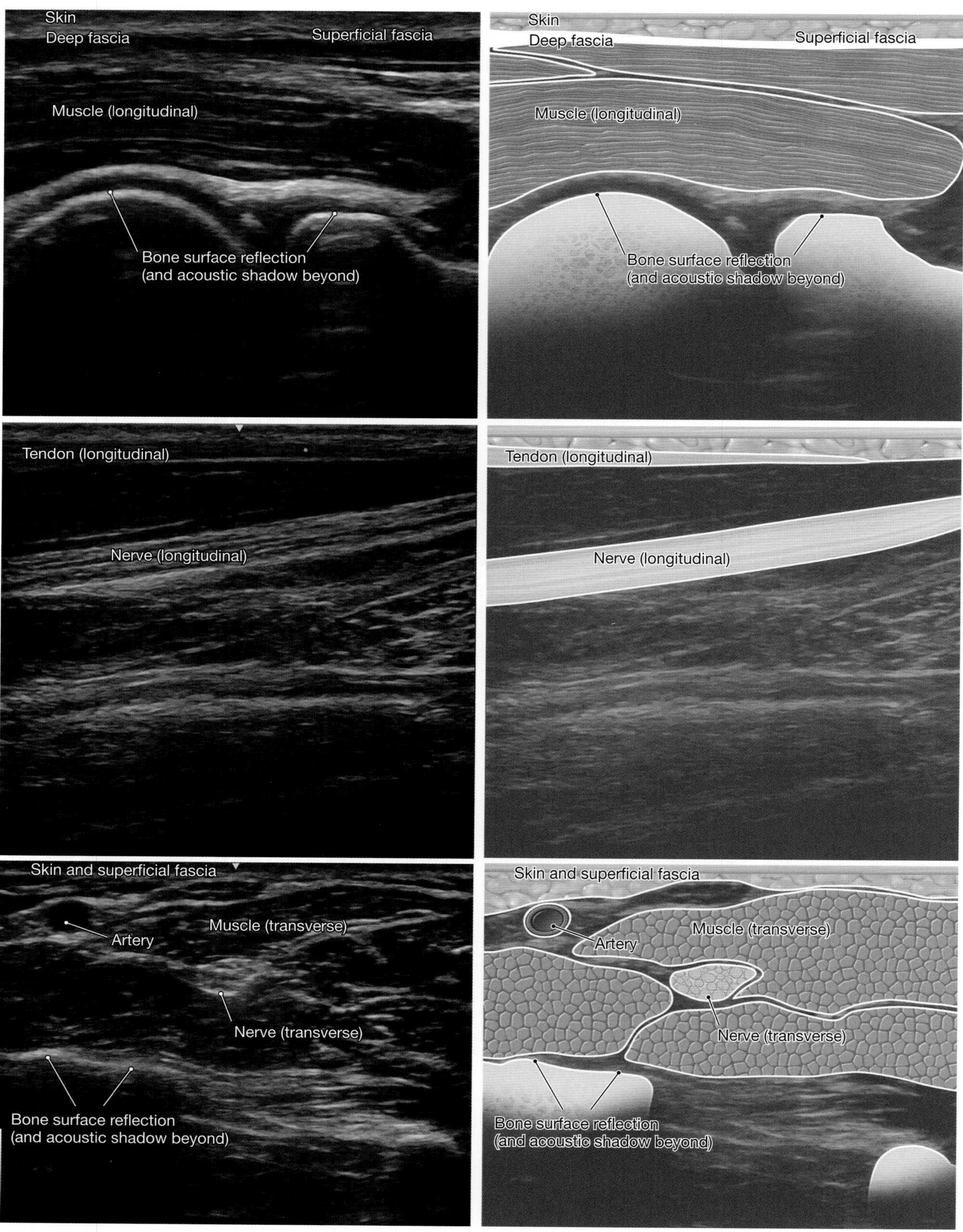

Figure 1.6 Appearance of commonly encountered tissues in ultrasound images.

Skin

The skin appears smooth and bright (**hyperechoic**). The epidermis and dermis can be differentiated only with specialized high-resolution US. There is a very thin and bright epidermal entry echo followed by a slightly-less-hyperechoic band representing the epidermis and dermis. Immediately deeper to the dermis, the subcutaneous fatty/fibrous layer appears generally hypoechoic (dark) in US images, with two components, **anechoic/hypoechoic** fat, interspersed with thin hyperechoic lines representing connective tissue septa.

Skeletal Muscle

Skeletal muscle has a distinct appearance, which varies between transverse views (across the longitudinal axis of the muscle) and longitudinal views (parallel to the muscle's longitudinal axis). In the transverse view, muscle tissue is largely anechoic-hypoechoic speckled with multiple short, thin, hyperechoic lines representing reflections from connective tissue of the perimysium. This is commonly referred to as the *starry sky* appearance.

In the longitudinal view, most of the muscle tissue remains anechoic/hypoechoic, but the hyperechoic lines of perimysium are elongated, revealing the fascicular architecture of the muscle. Most surfaces/boundaries of muscles are readily visible owing to the hyperechoic lines produced by the epimysium and the connective tissue of deep fascia.

Tendons

Tendons have a distinct appearance owing to the highly ordered, parallel bundles of collagen fibers that make up most of the tendon interior. As a result, multiple thin, hyperechoic lines fill in the tendon interior when viewed in the long axis of the tendon (commonly referred to as the *fibrillar* appearance) and there is a hyperechoic border (epitendineum investing the tendon) at the tendon surface.

In the transverse view, tendon interiors are filled in with many small, clustered, hyperechoic dots (commonly referred to as the *bristle-brush* appearance), again with a distinct hyperechoic surface (see Figure 1.6).

Nerves

Nerves have a largely hyperechoic surface and background (owing to reflectivity of connective tissue of the epineurium and perineurium) that is dotted with multiple hypoechoic nerve fascicles (the *honeycomb* appearance), when viewed in their transverse axis.

When viewed in the longitudinal axis, the nerve fascicles appear as multiple, thin, hypoechoic stripes parallel to the longitudinal axis of the nerve, against the hyperechoic background of the perineurium and surrounding epineurium (the *bundle of straws* appearance) (see Figure 1.6).

Bone

Bone surfaces appear as hyperechoic lines with a clean, dark, acoustic shadowing deep to the bone surface. For very small bony projections, acoustic shadowing is often the most obvious visual clue to their presence. Because bone surface is so reflective, artifacts (reverberations and *mirror images*) may appear within the acoustic shadow (see Figure 1.6).

Fluids

Fluids, such as blood, bile, and urine, are anechoic. In addition, sound energy propagates through fluids with minimal energy loss compared with soft tissues. This produces noticeably increased echogenicity in the tissues deep to fluid collections, because more sound energy reaches these tissues compared with the nonfluid sound path on either side of the fluid collection.

Blood Vessels

The blood (a fluid) flowing through the lumens of arteries and veins is anechoic (unless clots are present), whereas the connective tissue in vessel walls is hyperechoic. Arteries tend to have a more circular profile in transverse view than veins (which tend to be more oval), and artery walls are thicker than comparably sized veins (see Figure 1.6). Arterial and venous pulsations can be easily seen in real-time images (this can be confusing at times). However, normal veins are readily compressible by exerting minimal pressure on the probe, whereas arteries are only compressed with substantial pressure.

Basic "Knobology" and Image Optimization

During every US examination, US machine settings should be changed *as needed* to optimize the image quality. Understanding what just a few of the machine's knobs do is sufficient for optimizing most routine scans.

Depth

SCAN DEPTH AND FOCAL POINT INDICATORS
FIG. 1.7

The scan depth is indicated in centimeters on the right side of the image. In general, it is a good idea to start with greater depth to visualize more structures and landmarks in the field in addition to the structure/region of interest. After orienting yourself to the structures in the image and identifying the region of interest, readjust the depth so that the region of interest is located near the center of the display.

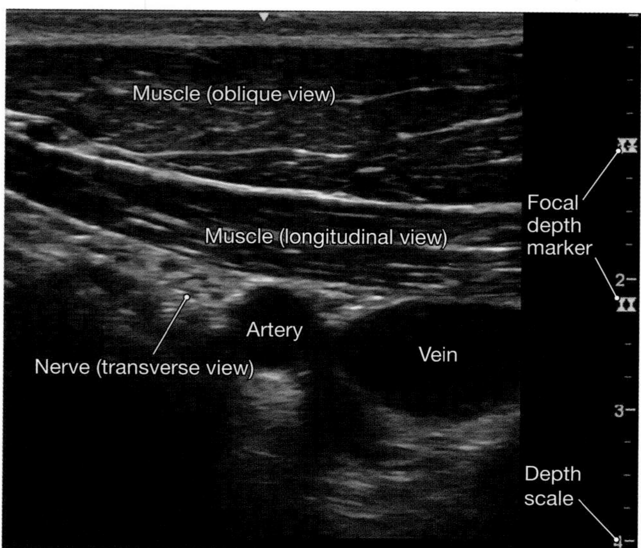

Figure 1.7 Scan depth and focal depth markers.

Focal Points

Most contemporary US units allow the user to set one or more focal depths. Focal depths are indicated alongside the depth markers. For example, the image in Figure 1.7 shows a scan depth of 4 cm, and there are two focal points selected (the yellow *hourglass* icons), set at 1.0 cm and at 2.25 cm.

In general, two or three focal points should be chosen and distributed near the depth(s) that correspond to the region of interest. This provides the best image detail for structures near the focal depth(s).

Gain

Turning the gain knob increases or decreases the amount of amplification of echoes throughout the image, thus increasing or decreasing the overall brightness of the displayed image. Images that are neither too bright nor too dark are best for overall identification of structures (inexperienced examiners tend to choose too much gain).

Tissue Harmonics Imaging

US pulses are produced in the probe transducer at certain fundamental frequency (eg, 12 MHz for a typical high-frequency linear array transducer). As the pulse travels through tissues, the tissues themselves vibrate at multiples of the fundamental frequency (2X = first harmonic, 4X = second harmonic, etc.). The tissue harmonics button on the US device toggles between listening for echoes at the fundamental frequency and listening for echoes only at harmonic frequencies. Tissue harmonics imaging frequently results in improved image quality, in terms of decreases in some artifacts (reverberations), decreased noise throughout the image, fewer internal echoes in fluid-filled spaces (cyst clearing), and improved image detail (spatial resolution).

2

Basic Ultrasound Physics

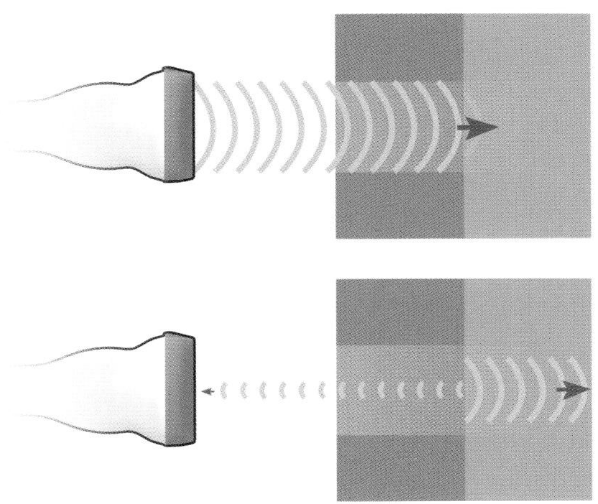

Sound Waves

SOUND WAVE PROPAGATION
FIG. 2.1

Sound is a mechanical wave of alternating pressures that propagates through media (such as tissues) as a series of compressions as the wave pressure rises, and rarefactions as the wave pressure falls of the molecules in the medium. Sound cannot travel through a vacuum.

Sound can be characterized by many different parameters, but one important characteristic of sound is its frequency (number of cycles per unit time, most commonly cycles per second, or Hertz).

One cycle per second = 1 Hertz (Hz)
One thousand cycles per second = 1 kilohertz (kHz)
One million cycles per second = 1 megahertz (MHz)

Therefore, a 12-MHz transducer in a medical ultrasound (US) probe (a "12-MHz probe") transmits pulses with a fundamental frequency of 12,000,000 cycles per second.

Another feature of sound is its velocity. Sound velocity in a given material is constant (at constant temperature), but it varies in different materials. Sound velocity through most soft tissues is fairly similar, although there are some extremes such as lungs (600 m/s) and dense bones (4000 m/s). For image forming, US devices assume that the velocity of sound through tissues is 1540 m/s, the soft-tissue average.

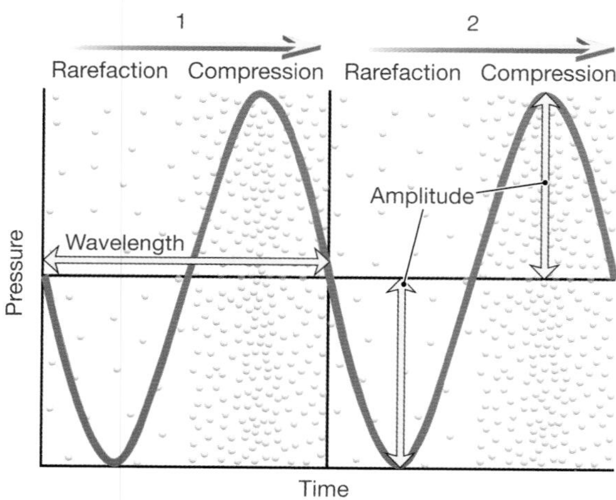

Figure 2.1 Two cycles of sound propagating through a medium.

US PULSE: REFLECTION AND THROUGH-TRANSMISSION
FIG. 2.2

FORMING AN IMAGE: REFLECTION (ECHO) AND THROUGH-TRANSMISSION
FIG. 2.3

In US image forming, an important characteristic of the media (tissues) through which sound energy propagates is **acoustic impedance**, the product of sound velocity through a tissue and the tissue density. Most soft tissues have similar acoustic impedance values, but there are some extremes such as bone, lungs, and collections of air/gas (eg, alveolar air, bowel gas). When sound passes from one tissue (with some value of acoustic impedance) to another (with a different acoustic impedance), some of the sound is reflected at the interface between the two tissues, and some continues to be transmitted to the deeper layers—the greater the difference in impedance, the greater the amount of sound reflection.

Because the impedance values are similar for most tissues, only a small amount of the sound pulse energy is reflected at tissue interfaces. This acoustic matching is good for imaging purposes, as a small amount of energy is reflected back to the probe as echoes for image forming, whereas most of the energy is transmitted deeper onto the next interface to be reflected to form an image there, and so on through the depth of the area being scanned (see Figure 2.3).

BARRIERS TO US IMAGING: BONE AND AIR
FIG. 2.4

With the same logic, imaging problems arise when US pulses encounter an interface between tissues with large differences in acoustic impedance, such as soft tissue to bone or soft tissue to air.

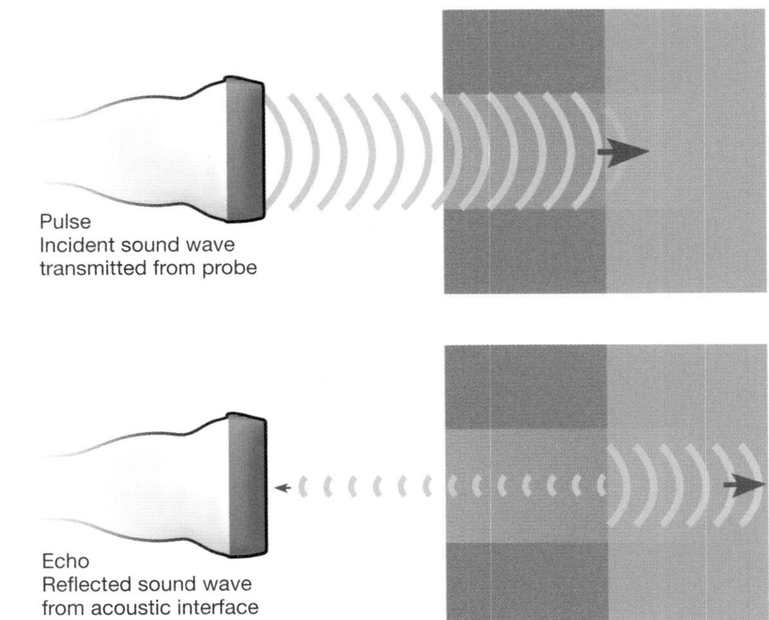

Figure 2.2 Some sound is reflected (echoed) when the ultrasound (US) pulse encounters an interface between tissues with different values of acoustic impedance. The remaining unreflected sound energy continues on (through-transmission).

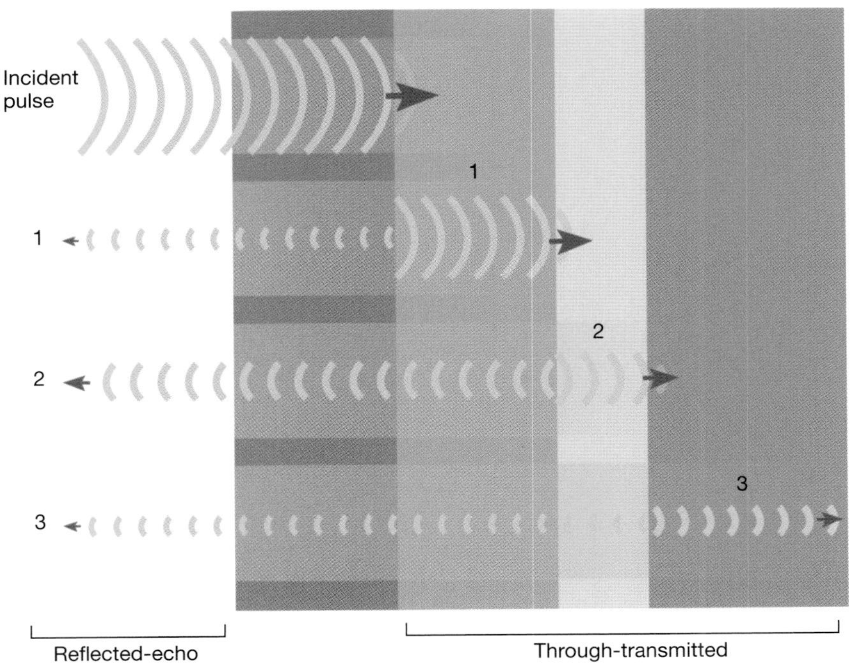

Figure 2.3 Reflection and through-transmission at sequential acoustic interfaces. The greater the difference in acoustic impedance, the greater the amplitude of the reflection.

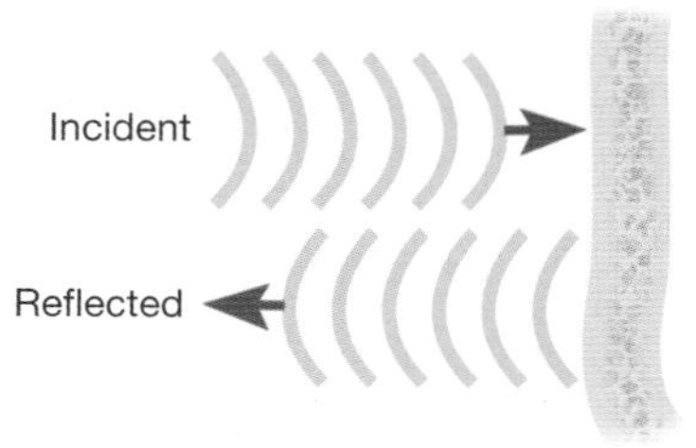

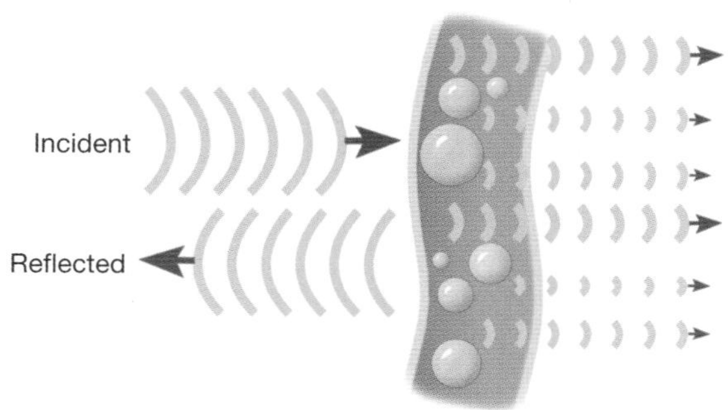

Figure 2.4 Large difference in acoustic impedance at an interface results in a bright reflection and much reduced through-transmission, making it difficult (or impossible) to image tissues beyond the interface.

Attenuation

As US pulses propagate through tissues there is progressive loss of energy, referred to as attenuation. **Attenuation** is mainly due to tissue absorption of sound energy (converted to heat) plus additional energy loss due to reflection and scattering. The absolute amount of attenuation varies in different tissues and is directly proportional to frequency: as frequency increases, attenuation increases. This means that higher-frequency US pulses are limited to imaging relatively superficial structures, whereas lower frequencies must be used for imaging deeper structures (eg, general abdominal imaging).

Fluids

Fluids such as blood, bile, and urine produce an extremely small amount of attenuation compared with other tissues. For this reason, a full urinary bladder provides a useful insonation window for suprapubic transabdominal imaging of pelvic structures, such as the uterus, ovaries, and rectouterine pouch in females or the seminal vesicles and prostate gland in males.

ACOUSTIC SHADOWING AND INCREASED THROUGH-TRANSMISSION
FIG. 2.5

Because sound energy propagates through fluid with minimal attenuation compared with soft tissues, more sound energy is transmitted to the tissues deep to a fluid collection (compared with the nonfluid sound path on either side of the fluid collection). As a result, there is noticeably increased **echogenicity** in the tissues deep to fluid collections, referred to as increased through-transmission (see Figure 2.5C). The presence of increased through-transmission helps confirm that an anechoic space is indeed fluid-filled.

Bone

Bone presents a substantial barrier to US transmission because of attenuation due to reflection and absorption of sound energy by compact bone. As a result, there is a bright echo from bone surfaces with a clean-edged dark acoustic shadow in the US image field beyond (see Figure 2.5A).

Air

Air presents a virtually impenetrable barrier to US imaging because of reflection, reverberation, and scattering. Normally, aerated lungs cannot be imaged with US, which can produce images only up to the depth of the pleura unless pathological fluid fills the alveolar spaces (see Figure 2.6). Gas in the gastrointestinal (GI) tract presents a major barrier in abdominal ultrasonography. In elective abdominal US imaging, patients are instructed to fast for 6 to 12 hours before their appointments to minimize GI gas. For nonelective abdominal US, a variety of tricks and techniques must be learned to obtain useful images when gas present in the bowel obscures the region of interest. Gas (GI gas or pathological gas collections, such as tissue emphysema, pneumobilia, and necrotizing fasciitis) produces a bright reflection and hazy gray-to-black shadowing with indistinct edges (*dirty* shadowing) beyond the reflection (see Figure 2.5B).

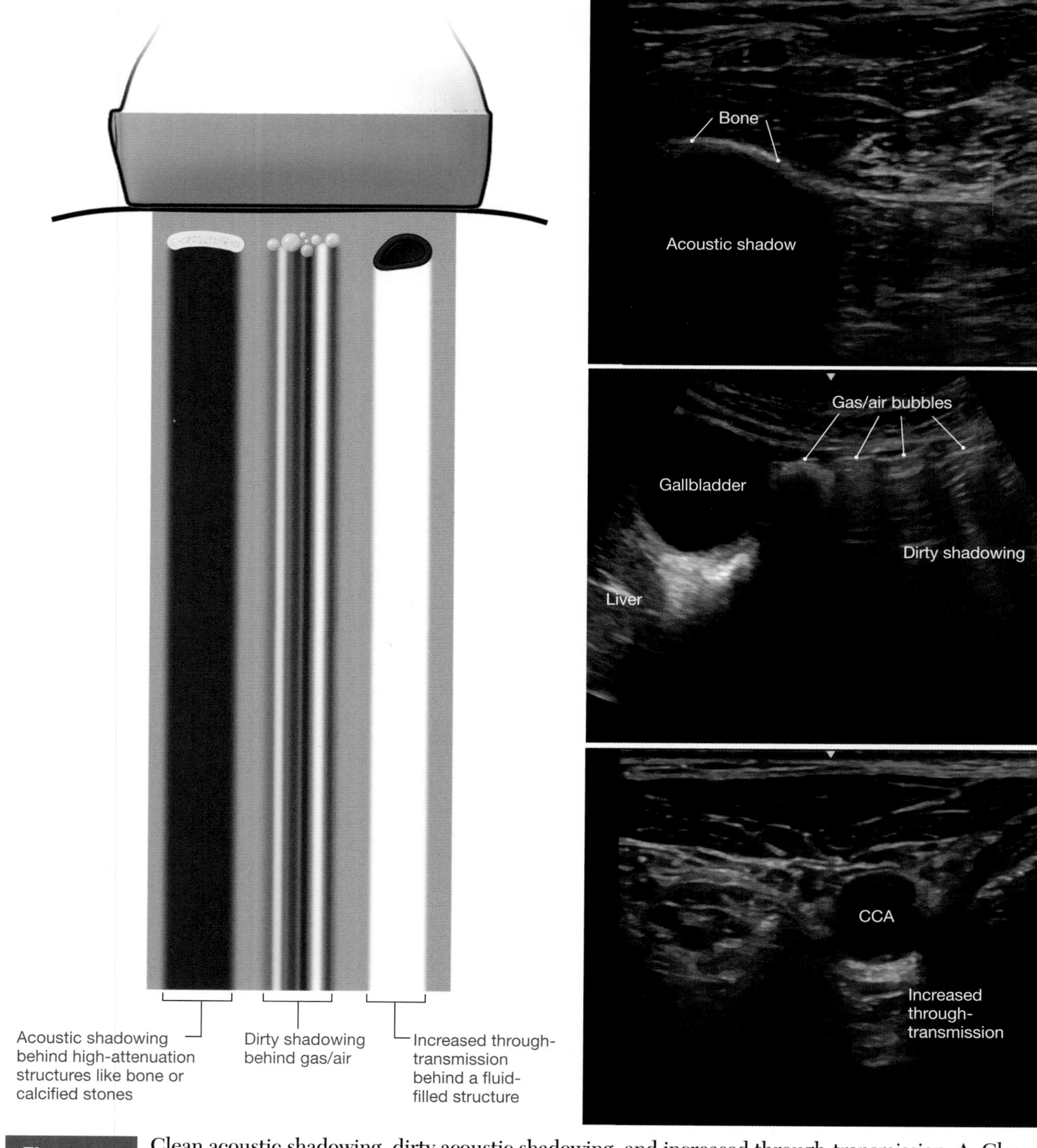

Figure 2.5 Clean acoustic shadowing, dirty acoustic shadowing, and increased through-transmission. A, Clean acoustic shadowing behind bone. B, Dirty shadowing behind gas/air bubbles in the gastrointestinal tract. C, Increased through-transmission behind a fluid path, in which case the fluid is blood flowing through the common carotid artery (CCA).

US Probes

Piezoelectric Effect

PLEURAL LINE AND NORMALLY AERATED LUNG
FIG. 2.6

Piezoelectric effect is the conversion (**transduction**) of a mechanical force (such as sound) to electricity by deforming a piezoelectric crystal. Deformation of piezoelectric crystals results in a net charge across the crystal. As sound wave pressures compress and expand the crystal, the charge magnitude and polarity alternates.

PIEZOELECTRIC EFFECT
FIG. 2.7

The piezoelectric effect also works in reverse, by converting electrical energy into sound energy, through alternating compression and rarefaction (ie, vibration) when an alternating voltage is applied across a piezoelectric crystal.

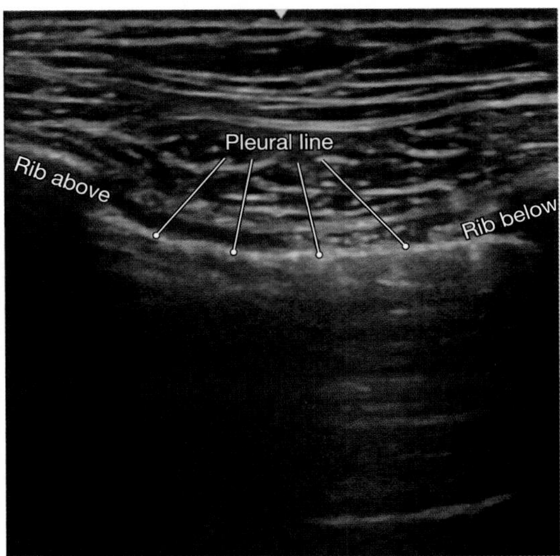

Figure 2.6 The pleural line, consisting of both visceral and parietal pleura, is seen in a longitudinal (parasagittal) view. In this image normally aerated lung is deep to the pleural line. Therefore, any display beyond the pleural line represents air artifacts such as scattering and reverberation. See Chapter 6 for additional information about the pleural line.

Probe Transducers and Crystal Arrays

US transducers are made up of multiple piezoelectric crystals arranged in groups called arrays, housed within the US probe. US **probe transducers** both convert electricity into sound, thereby producing the pulse that is directed into tissues, and convert sound (echoes reflected back to the probe from the tissues) into electrical signals that are then filtered and amplified to form an anatomical image of the slice being examined.

Because of the direct relationship between frequency and attenuation, higher-frequency probes (which produce better image details) cannot be used for US applications that require deeper penetration into tissues such as cardiac and general abdominal imaging. Thus, different US applications require probes with different fundamental frequencies and configurations of crystal arrays.

"REVERSE" PIEZOELECTRIC EFFECT AND US PULSE PRODUCTION
FIG. 2.8

Essentially, all contemporary US probes for medical imaging contain arrays of lead-zirconate-titanate crystals, which are electronically activated sequentially to steer and focus the US beam. This is a complex topic, but, briefly, each individual crystal in an array produces a point source wave (Huygen wavelet) when excited by an electrical pulse.

US PROBE CRYSTAL ARRAYS: INTERACTING SOUND WAVELETS
FIG. 2.9

The wavelets interact with each other constructively and destructively—peaks add up with peaks, troughs subtract from peaks, and troughs subtract from troughs—to produce a wave front with a size, shape, and direction. When crystals in an array are excited simultaneously, the wavelet interference patterns result in a wave front parallel to the array or probe face. When the array elements are excited with a sequential delay from one side to the other, the wavelets and their resulting interference patterns result in a wave-front steering. When the array elements are excited with a peripheral to central delay, the wavelet interference patterns result in a wave-front focusing: the resulting pulse is the narrowest at certain depth (focal depth) and wider before and beyond the focal depth.

STEERING AND FOCUSING US "BEAMS"
FIG. 2.10

Each pulse transmitted by the transducer crystal array (many thousands of pulses are transmitted each second to form the display image) is both steered and focused. The display image is formed one scan line at a time, and a pulse is transmitted along one of a thousand or so sequential scan lines from one side of the image to the other. The next pulse along the next scan line is not transmitted until all the echoes from the previous pulse have had time to return to the transducer. The listening time is calculated from the depth setting using the average soft-tissue sound velocity (0.154 cm/μs). When echoes from the last scan line on the far side of the image return to the transducer, the process begins again. This is repeated 30 to 40 times every second (screen refresh rate or frame rate) for real-time motion to appear undelayed and natural in the screen image. The transducer is in pulse mode less than 1% of the time and in listening mode more than 99% of the time in a typical scan. Some probe arrays produce sector (pie-shaped) images, whereas others produce linear or rectangular images. Sector images become progressively wider with depth, whereas linear images are the same width from the surface to the deepest part of the image.

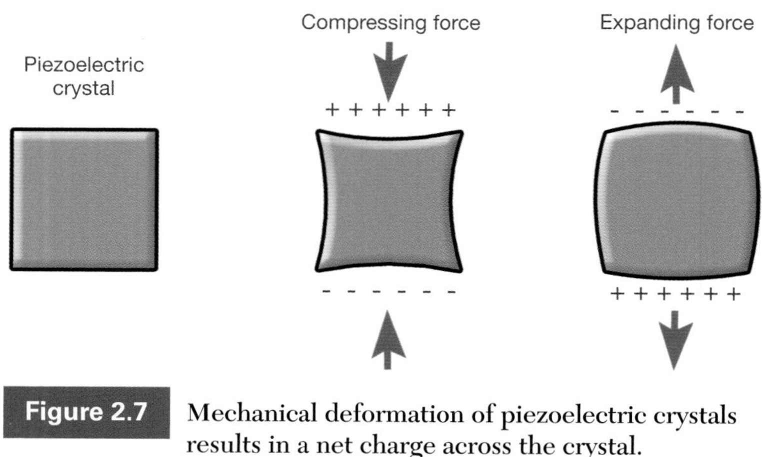

Figure 2.7 Mechanical deformation of piezoelectric crystals results in a net charge across the crystal.

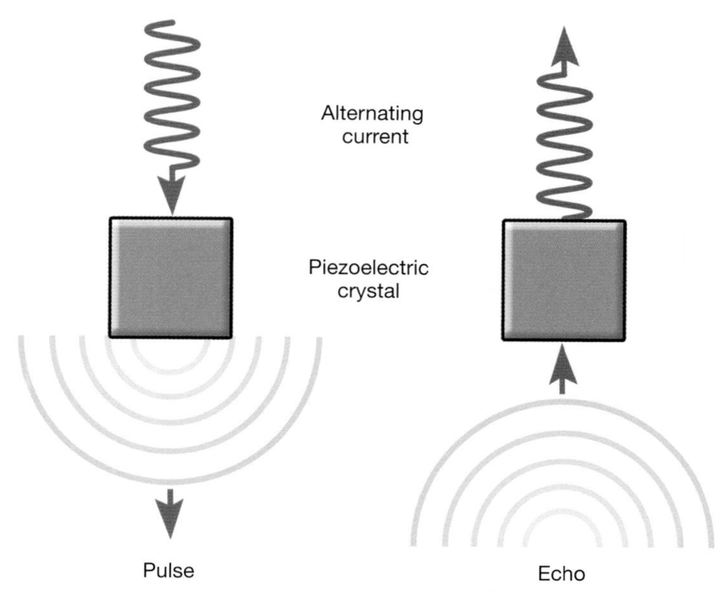

Figure 2.8 Alternating voltage applied across piezoelectric crystals produces the ultrasound pulse. Echoes returning to the probe mechanically deform the crystals producing electrical current, which is analyzed for image forming.

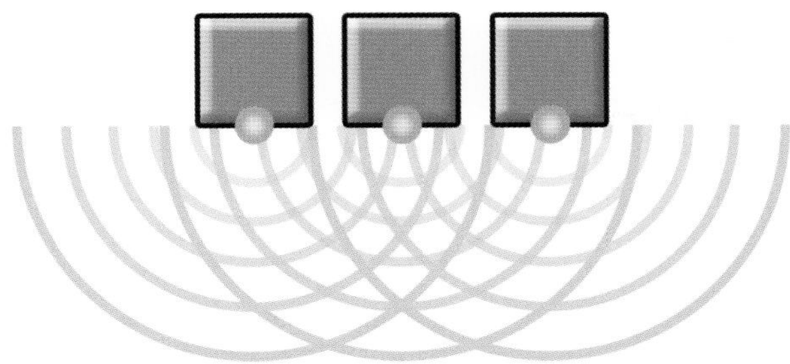

Figure 2.9 Point-source sound waves (Huygen wavelets) interacting.

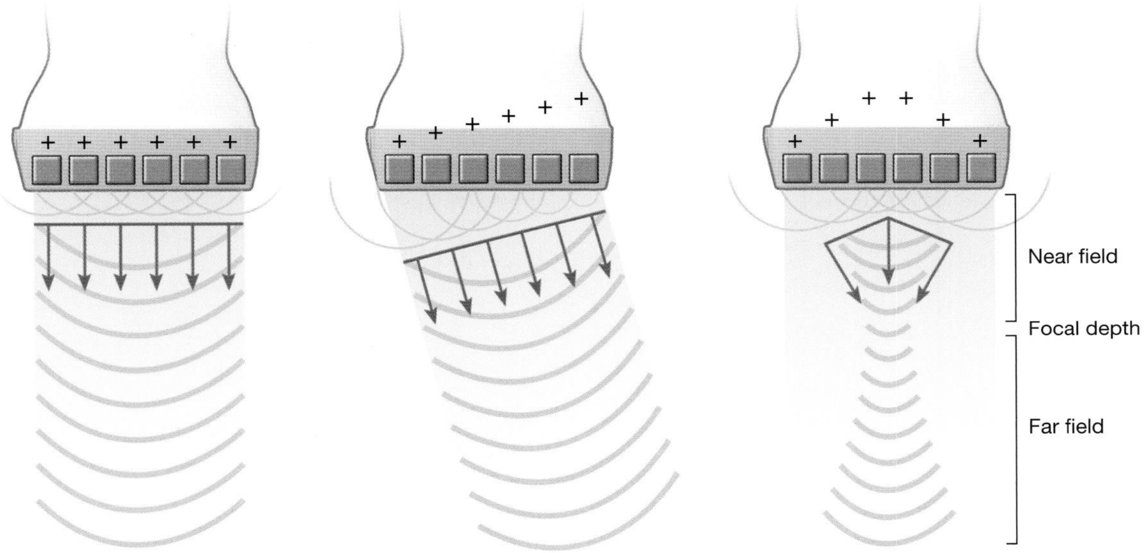

Figure 2.10 Phased excitation of array crystals steers and focuses the ultrasound beam.

Producing an Image

The speed of sound in soft tissue is assumed to be a constant of 1540 m/s (0.154 cm/µs). If, for example, the scan depth is set to 5 cm, the time required for each scan line is 65 µs. The total path length is 10 cm (5 cm from the probe to the depth setting and 5 cm back for returning echoes), so time = 10 cm/0.154 cm/µs = 65 µs. If there is a tissue reflector in the image at a depth of 2 cm, the total path length would be 4 cm (2 cm from the probe to the reflector and 2 cm back to the probe), and the echo from that reflector would return to the transducer at 26 µs (4 cm/0.154 cm/µs = 26 µs). Stated from the point of view of the US unit, any echo from a scan line reaching the transducer at 26 µs is displayed in the image at a depth of 2 cm.

PULSE/ECHO
SCAN LINES
FIG. 2.11

Putting it together, each tissue reflector in the image is displayed (1) in a side-to-side position based on the line being scanned when the echo reaches the transducer, (2) at some depth determined by the time when the echo returns, and (3) at some gray-scale value from black to white based on the intensity (**amplitude**) of the echo.

FORMING IMAGES:
SCAN LINES
ECHO RETURN TIME
AND AMPLITUDE
FIG. 2.12

Last, **spatial resolution** is the ability to distinguish and display small objects that are close together as separate in space. Small objects are displayed as the width of the beam at the depth they are located (lateral smearing artifact). Lateral (side-to-side) resolution, for example, is the ability to distinguish and display two small reflectors that are close together perpendicular to the direction of the US pulse as separate objects. Lateral resolution varies with the beam width, increasing as the width decreases. The beam width is largely determined by the frequency and focal depth. Higher-frequency probes produce narrower beams and, therefore, have better lateral resolution. Lateral resolution is always best at the focal depth, where the beam is the narrowest.

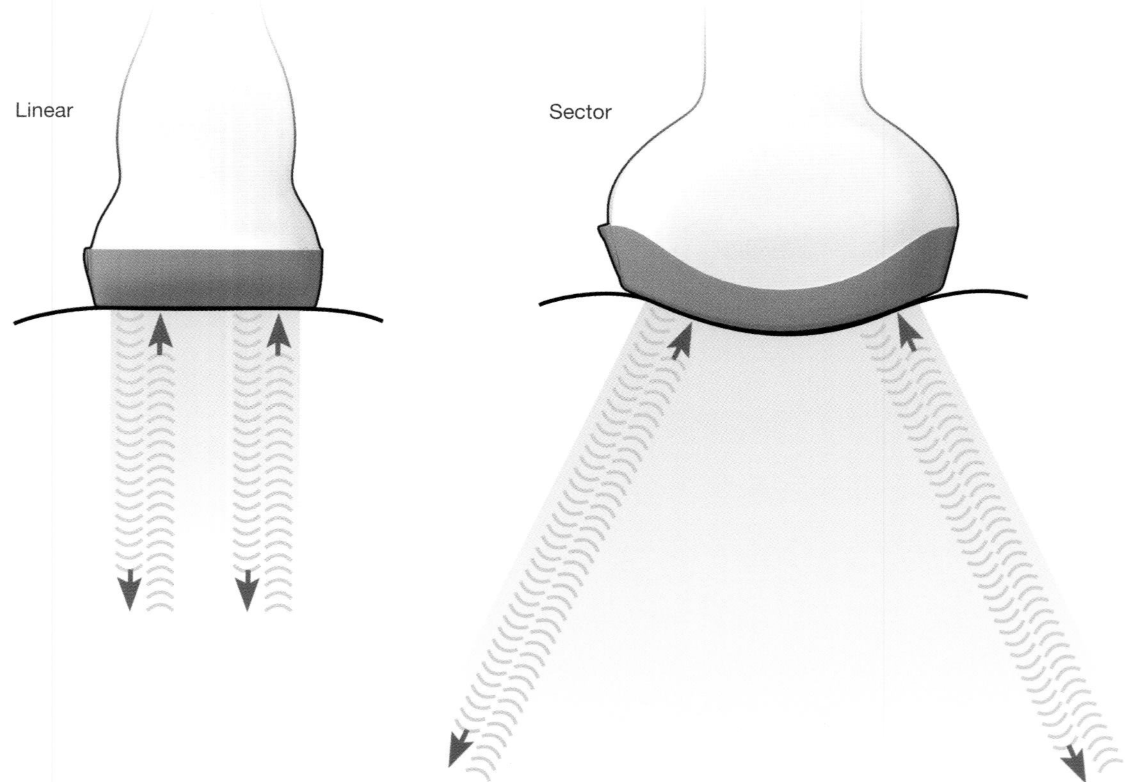

Figure 2.11 Images are formed one scan line at a time, proceeding sequentially from one side of the probe face to the other, repeated many times per second.

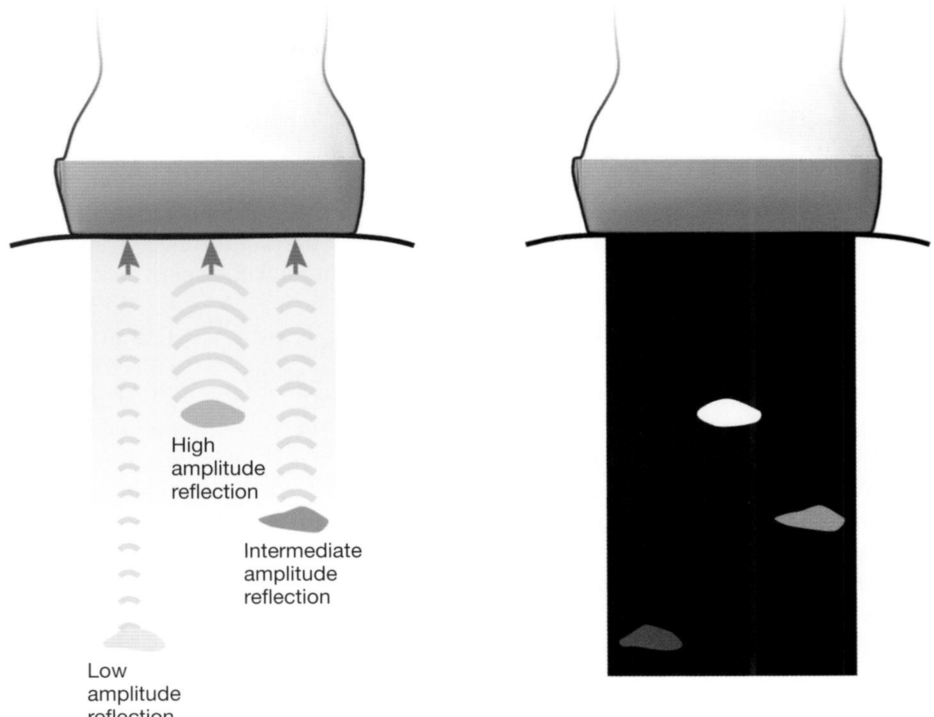

Figure 2.12 Objects are displayed based on the line being scanned when the echo returns, the time when the echo returns, and the amplitude of the echo.

Specular and Diffuse Reflection

In considering how various tissues/structures appear in US images, it is useful to think of two broad categories of sound wave reflection, specular reflection and diffuse reflection (scattering).

BEAM WIDTH: DISPLAY OF SMALL REFLECTORS AND SPATIAL RESOLUTION
FIG. 2.13

Specular reflection occurs when sound waves encounter a smooth surface or a smooth interface between two tissues with different acoustic properties. This type of reflection is responsible for the hyperechoic edges/interfaces seen in US images and for the bright appearance of fibrous structures such as tendons, ligaments, and organ capsules. Specular reflection is best for image forming when the surface or interface is perpendicular to the path of the sound pulses. When sound pulses encounter a specular reflector, its appearance changes as its angle changes relative to the sound path. When the path is perpendicular to a specular reflector, most of the echoed energy returns to the probe to be detected for image forming, so the reflector appears as a bright white (hyperechoic) line in the US display. When sound pulses encounter the same reflector at an angle sufficiently different from 90°, the sound energy is reflected such that none (or only a small proportion) of the echoes return to the probe transducer to form an image—the same reflector appears dark (hypoechoic/anechoic) in the US display.

ANISOTROPY: CHANGING SOUND PATH ANGLE CHANGES US APPEARANCE OF SOME OBJECTS
FIG. 2.14

This artifact, in which the same reflector appears as bright when the angle of insonation is close to perpendicular and appears dark when imaged from a different angle is referred to as anisotropy. In the US image shown in Figure 2.15, fascicles of collagen in the tendon of the infraspinatus muscle act as specular reflectors, giving the characteristic fibrillar appearance of multiple thin bright lines for the region of the tendon that is roughly perpendicular to the probe face. As the tendon curves over the humeral head (and away from the angle perpendicular to the US beam), the bright fibrillar lines darken and disappear owing to anisotropy.

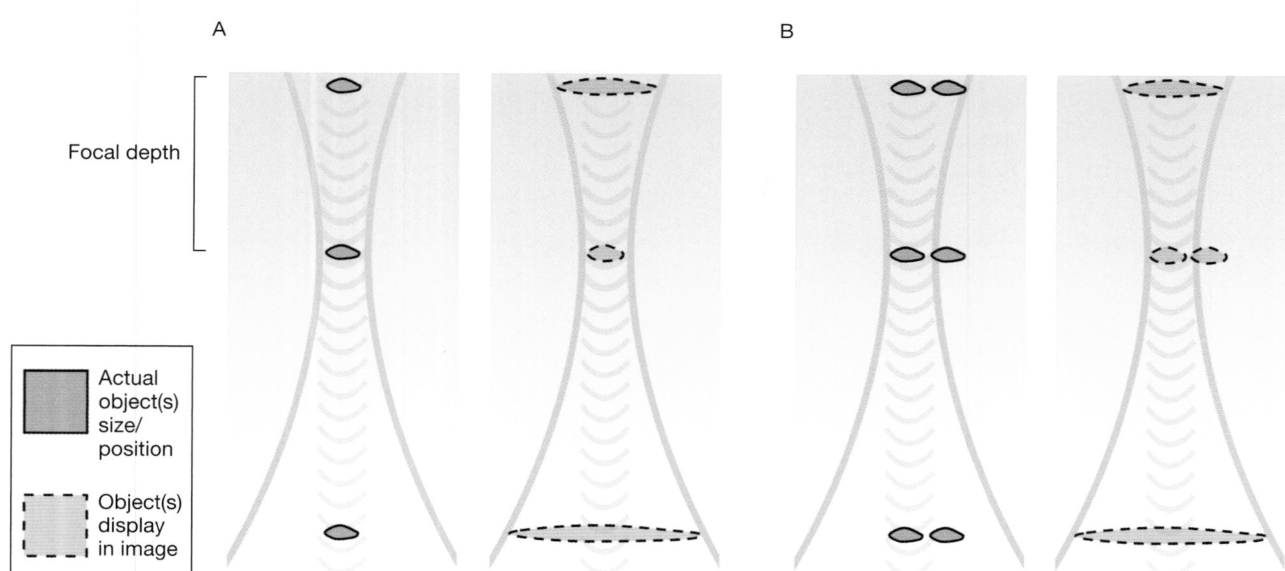

Figure 2.13 Relationship between beam width and how small reflectors are displayed. A, Small reflectors are displayed as the width of the beam at the depth they are located (lateral smearing artifact). B, Lateral resolution (the ability to distinguish the side-by-side small reflectors) is best near the focal depth, where the beam is the narrowest.

ANISOTROPY DEMONSTRATED IN A CURVING TENDON
FIG. 2.15

When sound waves encounter irregular or "bumpy" elements within tissues (irregularities that are smaller than the wavelength of the US), **diffuse reflection** or the scattered sound waves interfere with one another in complex patterns, giving rise to the speckled echo-texture of tissues such as liver, spleen, kidney, and myocardium. Because the

SCATTERING AND "SPECKLED" APPEARANCE OF MANY TISSUES
FIG. 2.16

scattered reflections (and resulting interference patterns) occur in multiple directions, the US appearance of these tissues is relatively unchanging, regardless of the angle of insonation.

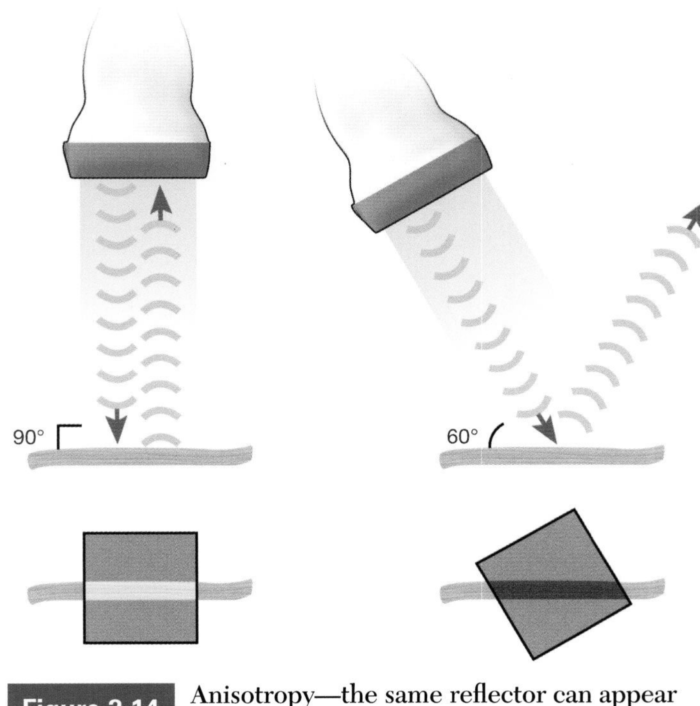

Figure 2.14 Anisotropy—the same reflector can appear as hyperechoic or hypoechoic/anechoic, depending on the angle of the ultrasound beam.

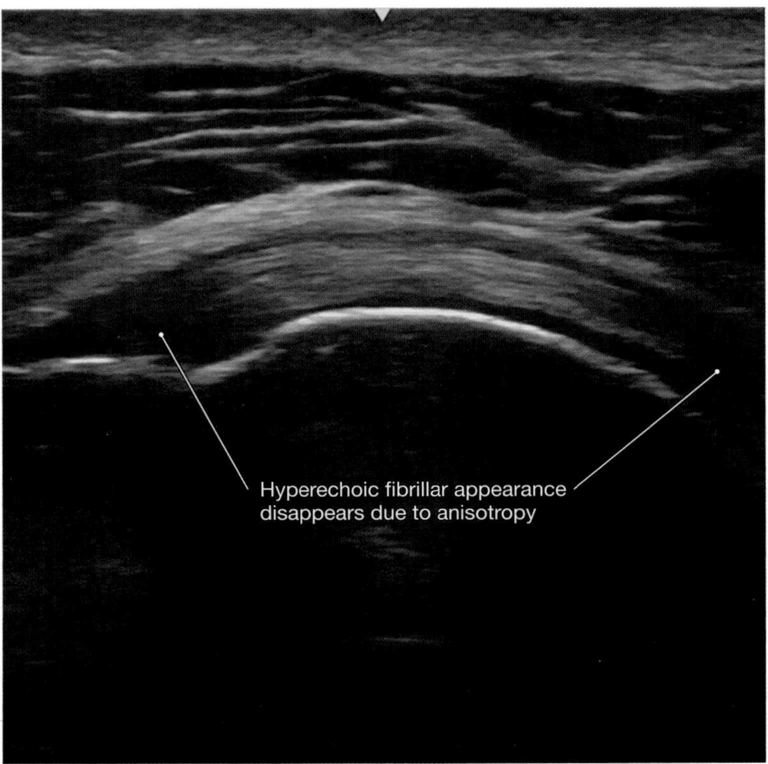
Hyperechoic fibrillar appearance
disappears due to anisotropy

Figure 2.15 Ultrasound image of a tendon demonstrating anisotropy artifact.

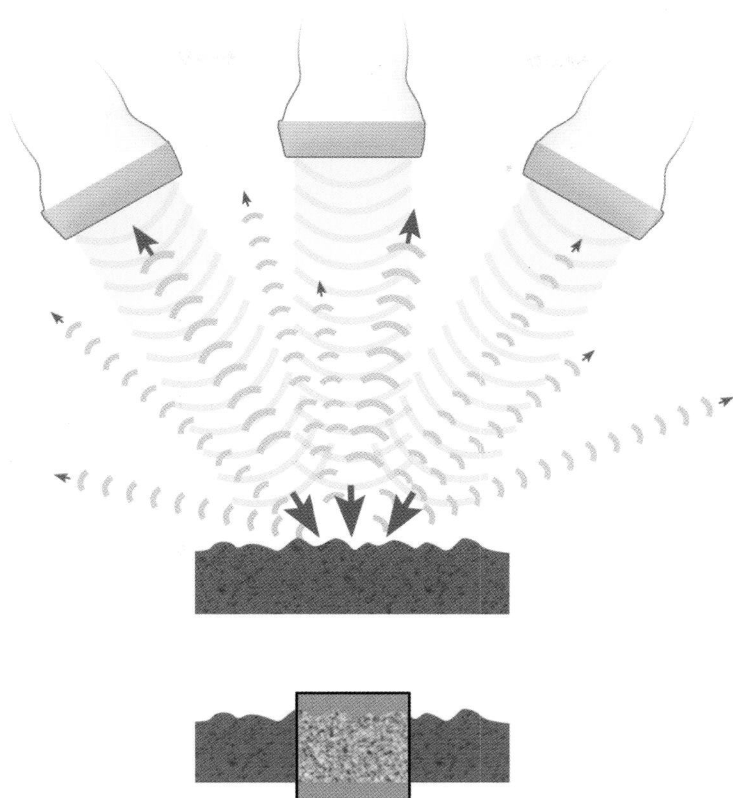

Figure 2.16 Diffuse reflection (scattering) results in interference patterns that produce the speckled echo appearance of many organs. The appearance of these tissues is largely unaffected by the angle of the ultrasound beam.

Bioeffects of US Energy

Because tissue absorption of sound energy is the most important source of attenuation, it also has implications for the health/safety of US imaging. Absorbed sound energy is converted into heat, so there are potential thermal **bioeffects** on tissues. The potential for bioeffects vary with the duration of exposure to sound energy (total scanning time); specific amount of tissue attenuation (more attenuation = more thermal effect, so tissues such as bone are more susceptible); location in the scan field (tissues that are superficial and nearer to the focal zone have the highest exposure); frequency (higher frequencies = more attenuation = greater thermal effect); pulse transmission power; and pulse duration/pulse repetition frequency (some scan modes, such as Doppler , require higher pulse repetition frequencies and therefore result in higher exposure).

3

Back

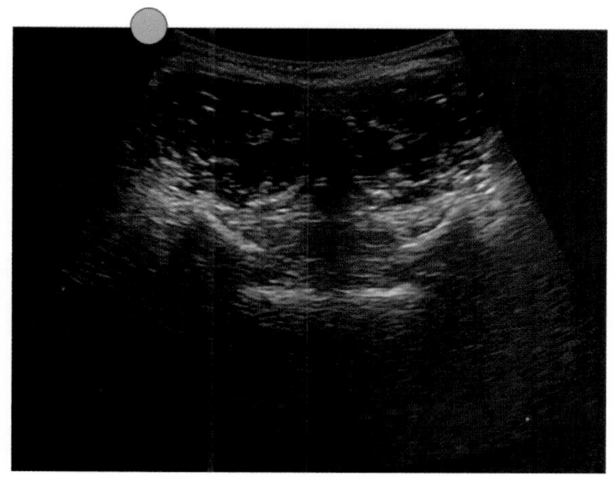

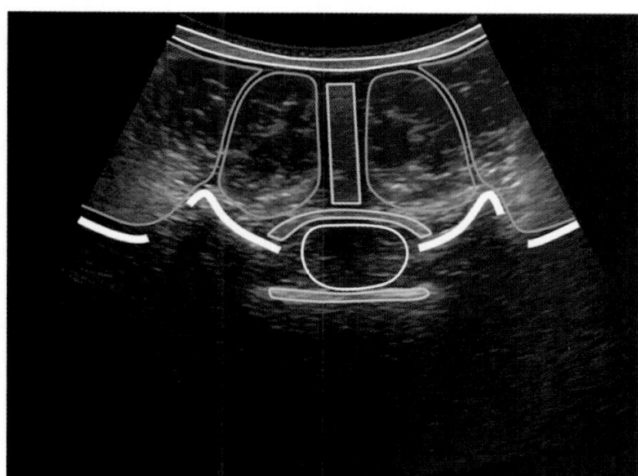

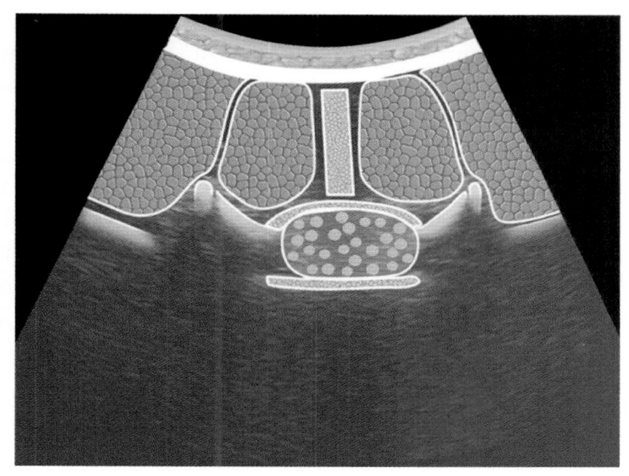

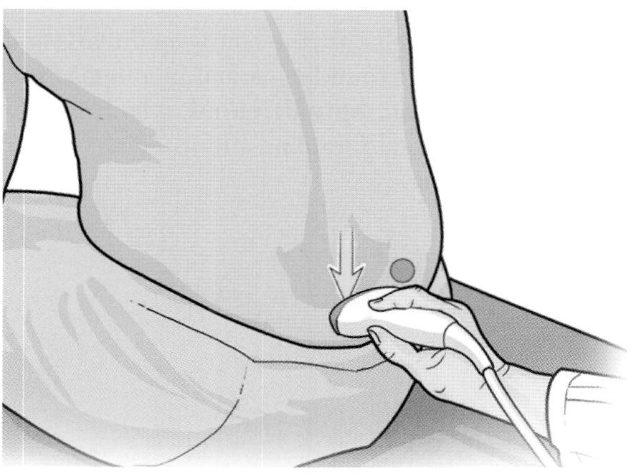

Lumbar Spine

Review of the Anatomy

Lumbar Vertebrae

The five lumbar **vertebrae**, similar to all typical vertebrae, consist of a body anteriorly and a vertebral arch posteriorly. The vertebral arch consists of right and left pedicles that attach the arch to the vertebral body and right and left laminae that fuse in the midline and form the bony roof of the vertebral canal. The transverse processes project laterally from the junction of the pedicles and laminae, and immediately posterior to this point, articular processes project superiorly and inferiorly. The articular surfaces of the superior articular processes face posteromedially, and those of the inferior articular processes face anterolaterally. Zygapophyseal (facet) joints are formed between the inferior articular process of the vertebra above and the superior articular process of the vertebra below. Because of the orientation of lumbar articular processes, the joint space itself is oriented obliquely about halfway between the frontal and sagittal planes. The spinous process projects posteriorly (and slightly inferiorly) in the midline from the junction of the right and left laminae. The posterior surface of the vertebral body, the pedicles, and the laminae form the borders of a bony vertebral foramen in each vertebra.

Adjacent vertebral bodies are joined by intervertebral disks as well as anterior and posterior longitudinal ligaments. Ligamenta flava join the laminae of adjacent vertebrae. The interspinous and supraspinous ligaments join the spinous processes. Zygapophyseal joints between the inferior and superior articular processes are the only synovial joints between adjacent vertebrae.

Spinal Canal

The spinal cord, including the conus medullaris and cauda equina, plus the surrounding spinal meninges are housed within the vertebral **(spinal) canal**, which is formed by the aligned vertebral foramina and associated soft tissues, including the ligamenta flava, intervertebral disks, and the posterior longitudinal ligament. The spinal dura mater is separated from the interior of the canal by a variable amount of extradural fat and venous plexus. The meningeal and neural contents of the lumbar spinal canal include the dural sac, conus medullaris, cauda equina, filum terminale (externum and internum), and lumbar cistern of the subarachnoid space.

Throughout most of the vertebral column, the laminae and spinous processes of adjacent vertebrae overlap to the extent that there is a more or less continuous bony covering of the spinal canal posteriorly. In the lumbar region, however, relatively large spaces between adjacent vertebral arches appear, such that there are gaps (**interlaminar spaces**) in the bony covering of the spinal canal, which are filled by the ligamenta flava. The size of these gaps increases with flexion, and they provide soft-tissue windows for ultrasound imaging of the lumbar spinal canal and its contents.

Deep Back Muscles

The deep fascia of the back and back muscles related to the lumbar vertebrae include the thoracolumbar fascia (fused to the aponeurotic tendon of origin of latissimus dorsi), erector spinae, multifidus, and psoas major muscles. The erector spinae muscle is covered by the thoracolumbar fascia (posterior layer), and most of its muscle mass in the lumbar region is seen overlying (posterior to) the transverse processes of the lumbar vertebrae. The multifidus muscle is well developed in the lumbar region and occupies the space adjacent to the spinous processes and posterior surfaces of the laminae and articular processes/zygapophyseal joints of the lumbar vertebrae. The psoas major muscle is a muscle of the posterior abdominal wall that occupies the space adjacent to the bodies and anterior surfaces of transverse processes of the lumbar vertebrae.

Technique

SPINOUS PROCESS LAMINAE
Transverse
FIG. 3.1

For all of the views described in detail as follows, the patient should be positioned either (1) sitting sideways on the examination table leaning forward (flexing the lumbar region as much as possible to increase the size of the interlaminar spaces) with the forearms resting on the thighs or (2) lying prone on the examination table with a pillow/bolster placed under the lower part of the abdomen (positioned to flex the lumbar region as much as possible). Care should be taken to ensure that the spinous processes are aligned in the sagittal plane with as little tilt/rotation to one side or the other as possible. In clinical settings (eg, for lumbar puncture or epidural anesthesia), the lateral decubitus position with the patient curled into a "fetal position" is also commonly used, but this position tends to be difficult for inexperienced examiners. For orientation purposes, palpate and mark the spinous process of L4 in the midline at the intercristal line (a line interconnecting the highest points on the iliac crests).

INTERLAMINAR SPACE THECAL SAC
Transverse
FIG. 3.2

Using a low-frequency (2-5 MHz) curved array probe, place the probe face transversely over the L4 spinous process. Identify the reflection and acoustic shadow of the spinous process, and position it in the center of the image. Carefully adjust the probe position until the spinous process and laminae can be seen. Look for the thin anechoic/hypoechoic lines representing the zygapophyseal

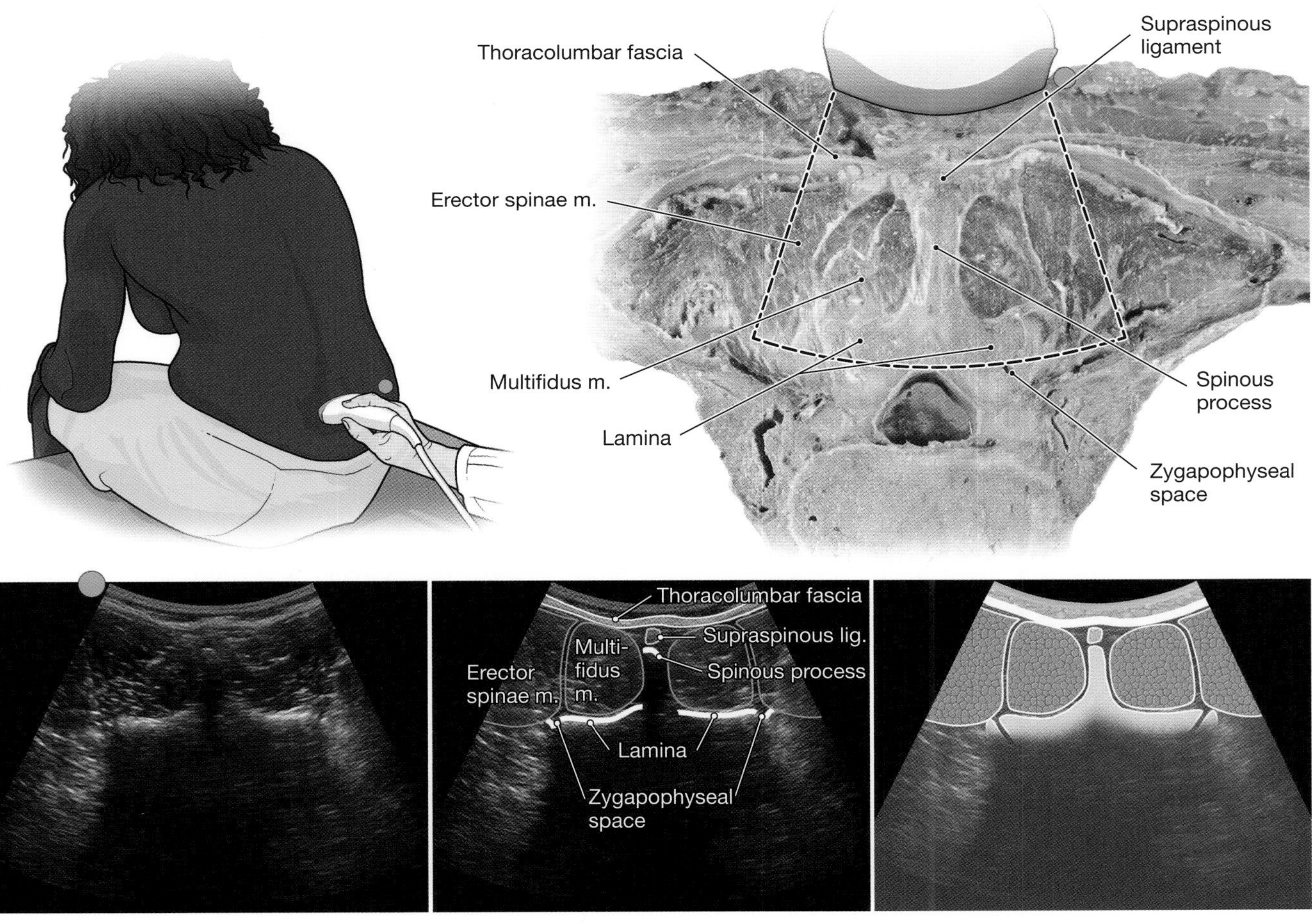

Figure 3.1 Transverse view of spinous process and laminae with overlying deep back muscles.

joint spaces at the lateral extent of the laminae on both sides. Identify the skin and superficial fascia, the hyperechoic thoracolumbar fascia, and the "starry sky" appearance of the multifidus and erector spinae muscles.

TRANSVERSE PROCESSES
Longitudinal
FIG. 3.3

Carefully slide the probe slightly inferiorly until the reflection/acoustic shadow of the spinous process disappears, replaced with the hypoechoic interspinous ligament. The laminae also fall away as the articular processes come into view, 1 to 2 cm deeper in the image. The interlaminar space can be identified as the gap between the medial edges of the articular processes. Two hyperechoic bands, the posterior and anterior complexes, should then be identified. The posterior complex, which spans the interlaminar space immediately superficial to the articular processes, represents the combined reflections of the ligamentum flavum, the extradural space, and the posterior aspect of the dura mater. The anterior complex, the hyperechoic band that is seen 1 to 2 cm deep to the posterior complex, represents the combined reflections of the anterior aspect of the dura mater, the extradural space, and the posterior longitudinal ligament. The anterior complex is visible only when the probe is over the interlaminar space (otherwise hidden in acoustic shadow of the bony vertebral arch structures). Between the posterior and anterior complexes, the contents of the thecal sac (lumbar cistern and cauda equina) can be visualized as an oval-shaped anechoic/hypoechoic space.

ARTICULAR PROCESSES
Longitudinal
FIG. 3.4

Remaining at the L4/L5 level, place the probe along the long axis of the spine a short distance (3-4 cm) lateral to the midline, with the probe marker facing superiorly. Adjust the probe position until two or three transverse processes can be identified as the short curved

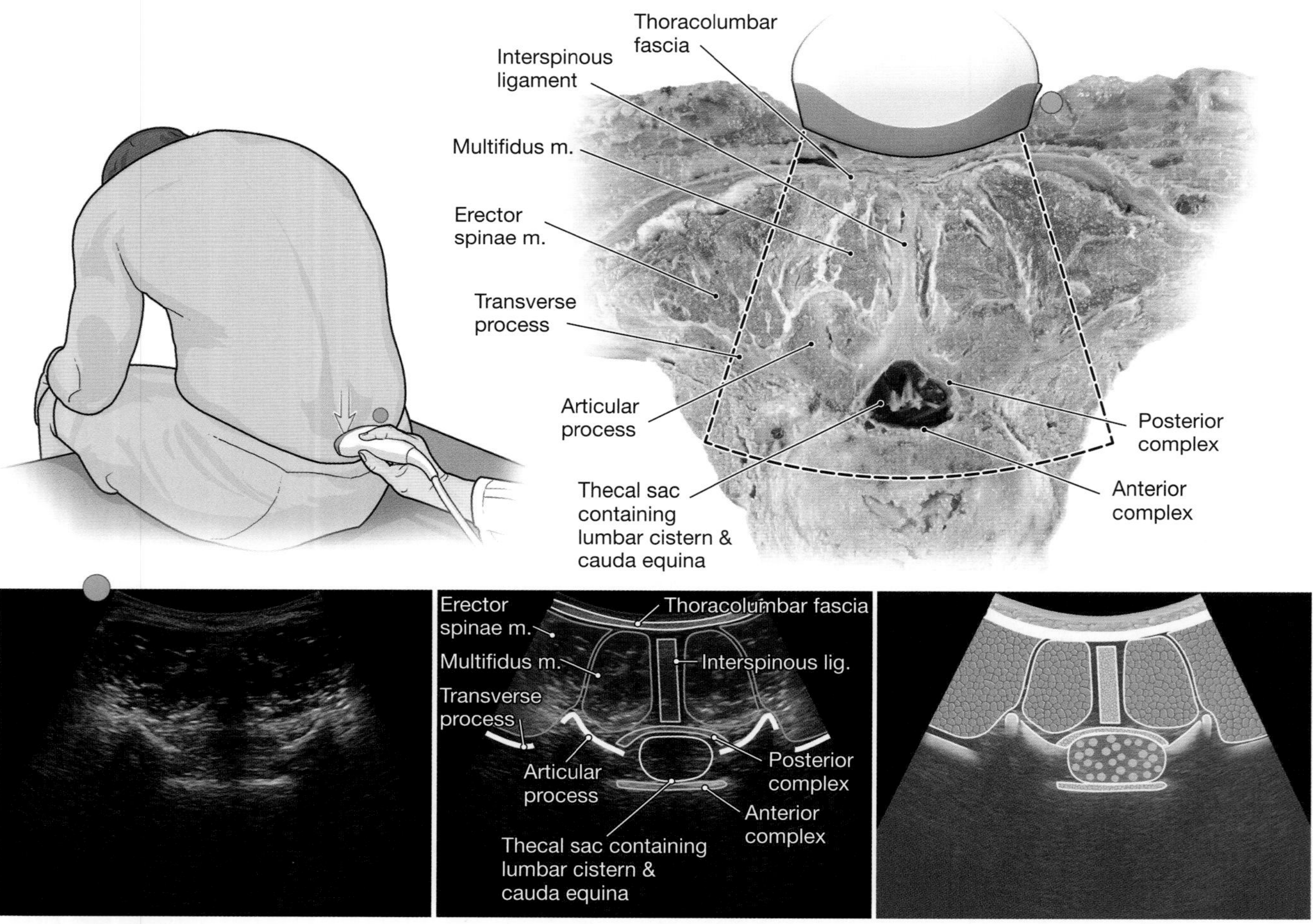

Figure 3.2 Transverse view of interlaminar space and thecal sac containing lumbar cistern and cauda equina. Posterior complex: ligamentum flavum, extradural fat, and posterior aspect of dura mater. Anterior complex: anterior aspect of dura mater, extradural fat, and posterior longitudinal ligament.

hyperechoic lines deep to erector spinae muscle, with their characteristic "finger-like" acoustic shadows. Between the acoustic shadows of successive transverse processes, the psoas major muscle can be seen with its prominent hyperechoic striations. The parietal peritoneum can be identified as the hyperechoic line at the deep surface of psoas major. Respiratory movement of intraperitoneal structures deep to this line can usually be seen.

LAMINAE INTERLAMINAR SPACES
Longitudinal
FIG. 3.5

Next, slide the probe a short distance medially until a continuous line of short bony humps appears, deep to muscle. These are the overlapping articular processes of successive vertebrae, commonly referred to as the "articular column" in ultrasound (US) imaging. The multifidus is the main muscle mass overlying the articular column in the lumbar region.

After identifying the articular column, tilt the probe face slightly medially (so that the US beam is traveling from lateral to medial, from the skin surface to deeper structures) until the laminae and interlaminar spaces of successive vertebrae come into view. The laminae are seen as hyperechoic lines that are tilted relative to the skin surface such that their superior edges are deeper than their inferior edges, giving an overall sawtooth appearance. Between successive laminae and their acoustic shadows, the posterior complex, contents of the thecal sac, and the anterior complex can be seen.

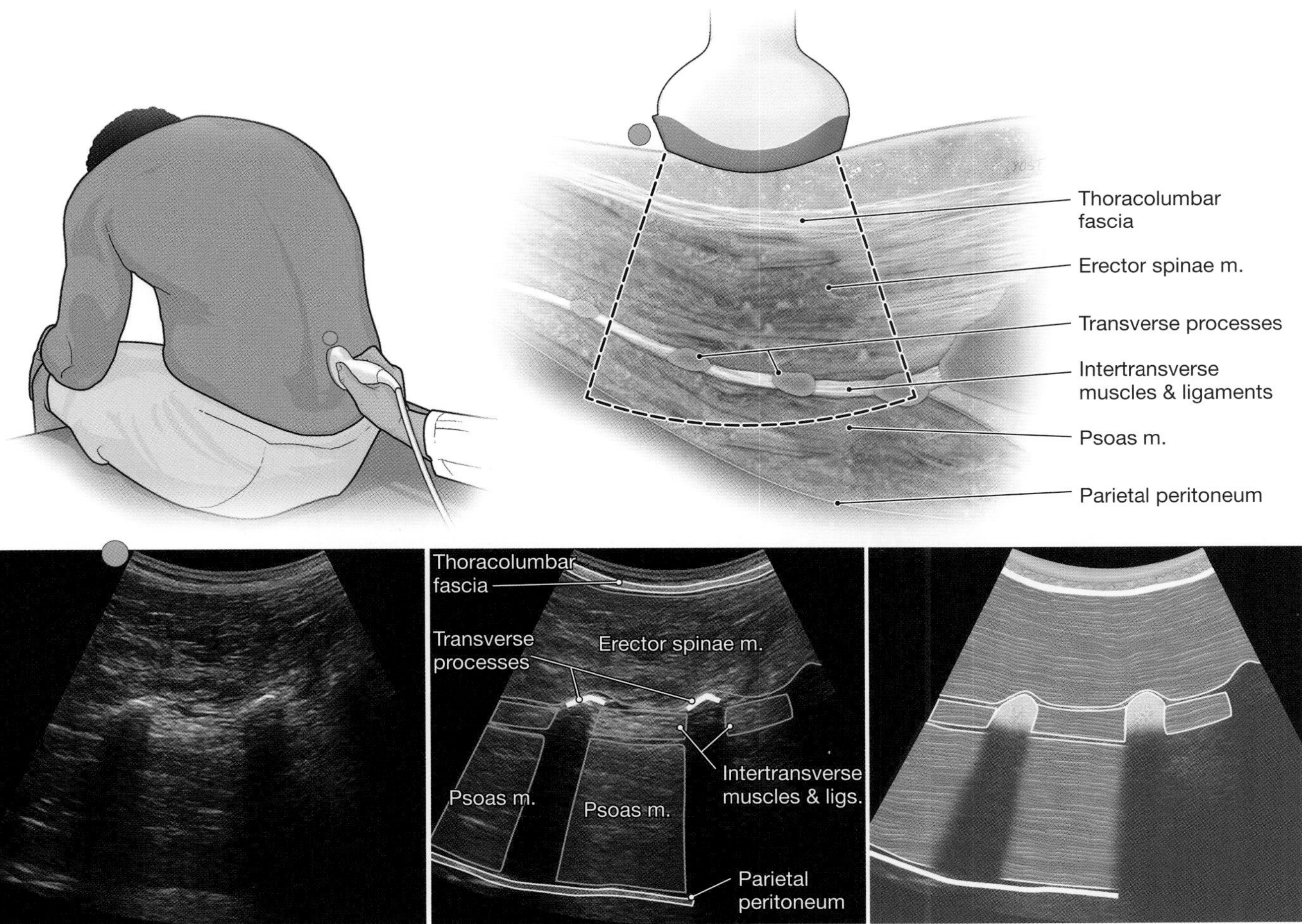

Figure 3.3 Longitudinal (parasagittal) view of erector spinae muscle, transverse processes, and psoas major muscle.

CLINICAL APPLICATIONS

These techniques can be used for evaluating and accurately measuring the anatomy of the lumbar spine and associated ligaments, extradural space, and lumbar cistern before diagnostic lumbar puncture or administration of spinal or epidural anesthesia. For example, the depth from the skin surface to the ligamentum flavum, epidural space, dura mater, and intrathecal space can be accurately measured using the caliper function of the US equipment, and vertebral levels can be ascertained and marked on the skin surface in patients with confusing or difficult anatomy. These techniques can also be used for US-guided needle advancement and insertion during lumbar puncture and/or administration of spinal/epidural anesthesia or zygapophyseal joint injection.

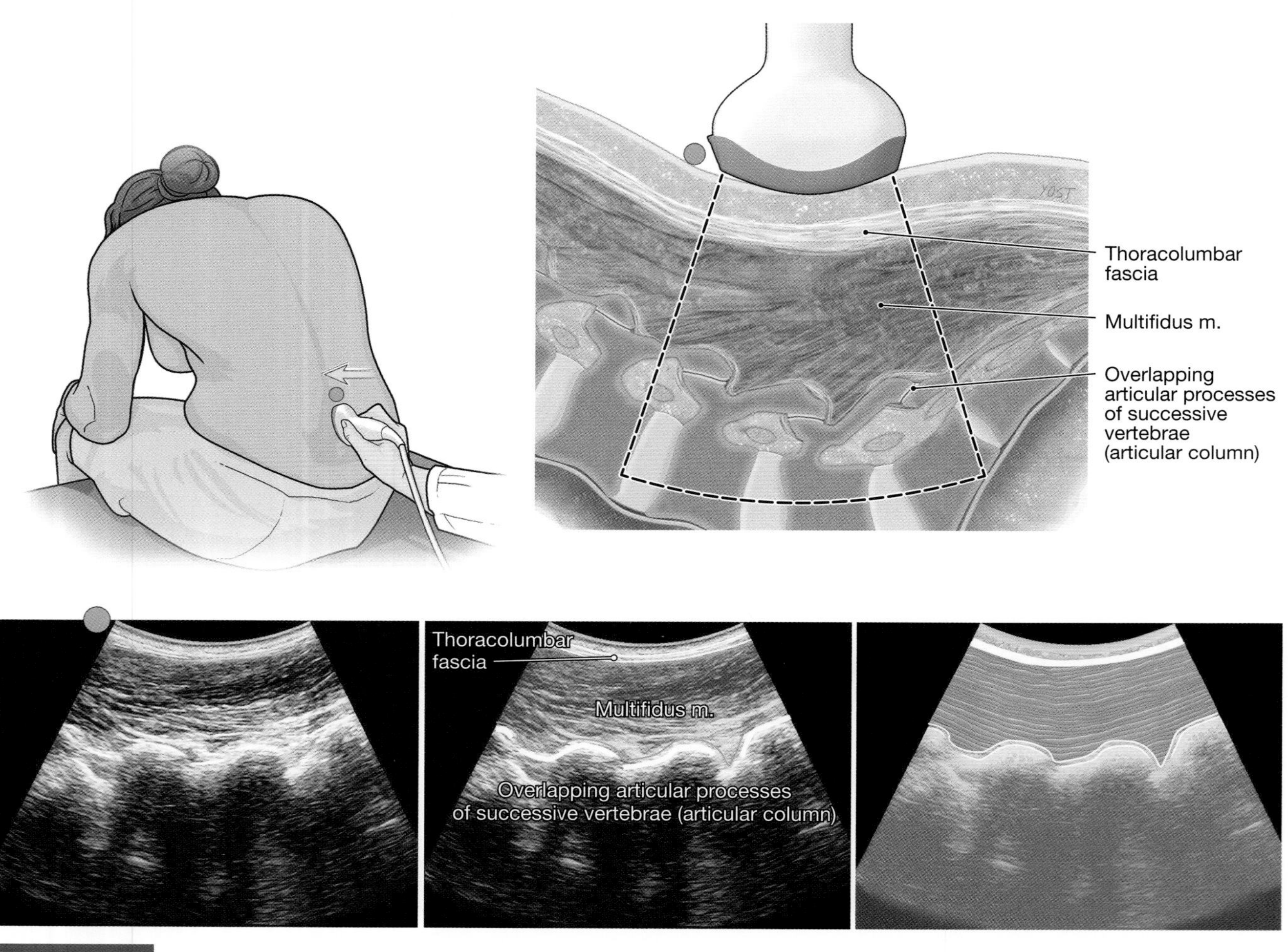

Figure 3.4 Longitudinal (parasagittal) view of articular processes with overlying multifidus muscle.

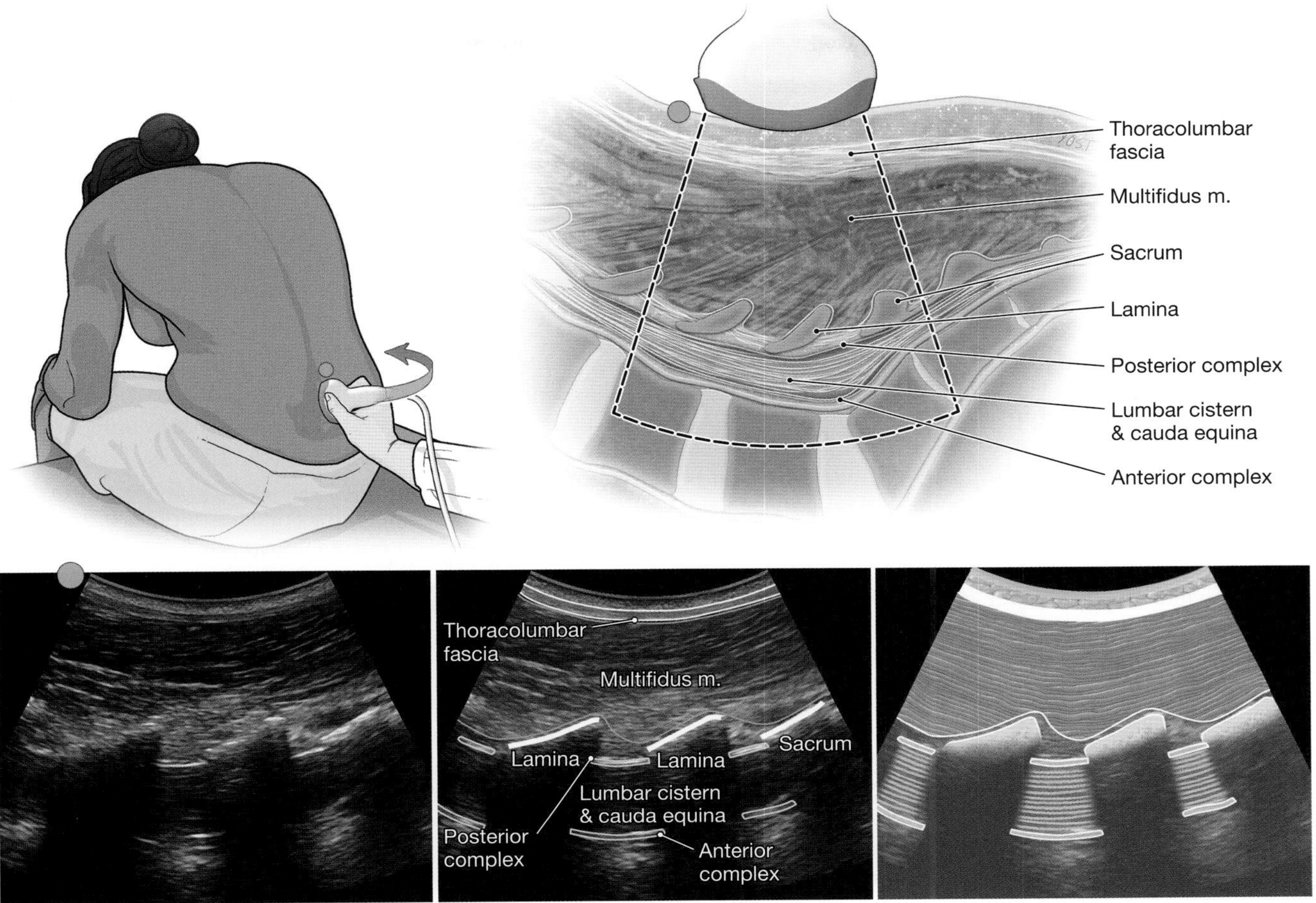

Figure 3.5 Longitudinal (parasagittal oblique) view of laminae, interlaminar spaces, and thecal sac with overlying multifidus muscle. Posterior complex: ligamentum flavum, extradural fat, and posterior aspect of dura mater. Anterior complex: anterior aspect of dura mater, extradural fat, and posterior longitudinal ligament.

Cervical Spine and Greater Occipital Nerve

Review of the Anatomy

Cervical Vertebrae

The neck's skeletal structure consists of seven cervical vertebrae. The cervical vertebrae from C3 to C7 are known as typical cervical vertebrae and possess distinct characteristics. These vertebrae have small vertebral bodies, split spinous processes, and include bilateral transverse processes housing a transverse foramen (foramen transversarium) through which the vertebral artery and vein pass. The transverse processes also feature anterior and posterior tubercles for muscle attachment. On the other hand, the first two cervical vertebrae, C1 (atlas) and C2 (axis), are referred to as atypical cervical vertebrae.

The atlas is a ring-shaped vertebra that articulates with the head and has no spinous process, body, nor intervertebral disk. It is composed of two lateral masses connected by anterior and posterior arches. Each lateral mass articulates superiorly with an occipital condyle. Its superior articular facets (surface) create atlanto-occipital joints with the occipital condyles. Its inferior facets articulate with the C2 vertebra (axis) to create lateral atlanto-axial joints. The axis is the strongest cervical vertebra and contains the dens, a structure that projects superiorly from its body to articulate with the atlas. The axis articulates with the atlas with its anterior arch anteriorly and its transverse ligament posteriorly. The transverse ligament holds the dens in position and allows the atlas and head to rotate on its axis.

Deep Back Muscles, Cervical Region

The deep muscles of the back are the splenius capitis and cervicis (spinotransversales muscles), the erector spinae, transversospinales, interspinales, and intertransversarii. More specifically, the splenius capitis is attached to the occipital bone and mastoid process. The splenius cervicis attaches to the transverse process of the upper cervical vertebrae. The erector spinae is the largest group of deep muscles of the back and is further subdivided into iliocostalis composing its lateral side. It middle portion is made up by the longissimus and the most medial component of the erector spinae is made up by the spinalis. The primary function of the erector spinae is to extend the vertebral column and head. The transversospinales muscles are further subdivided into the semispinalis, multifidus, and rotatores muscles. A small group of the deep muscles of the cervical region are the suboccipital muscles forming the suboccipital triangle; specifically, rectus capitis posterior major (medial border), rectus capitis posterior minor, obliquus capitis superior (lateral border), and obliquus capitis inferior (inferior border). These small muscles extend the head at the atlanto-occipital joint and rotate the head at the atlanto-axial joint. The suboccipital triangle contains the vertebral artery and vein, as well as the posterior ramus of C1.

Greater Occipital Nerve and Third Occipital Nerve

The area of suboccipital triangle receives sensory innervation from the greater occipital nerve, the medial branch of the posterior (dorsal) ramus of the C2 spinal nerve, as well as from the third occipital nerve, a branch of the posterior ramus of the C3 spinal nerve. The greater occipital nerve is located between the first and the second vertebrae and ascends between the inferior border of the obliquus capitis inferior muscle; it then pierces the semispinalis capitis and the aponeurosis of the trapezius muscles inferolateral to the external occipital protuberance. It innervates the area of the skin of the suboccipital triangle and the posterior part of the scalp. The third occipital nerve, similar to the greater occipital nerve, also pierces the semispinalis capitis and trapezius muscles and supplies portions of the lower part of the scalp.

Technique

GREATER OCCIPITAL NERVE
Transverse
FIG. 3.6

In order to obtain this view of the greater occipital nerve, the patient should be sitting up with the neck slightly flexed. Alternatively, the patient can be lying prone with a pillow under the chest. Begin by palpating the external occipital protuberance. Then slide the palpating finger inferiorly approximately 2 cm until the prominent spinous process of the axis, the second cervical vertebra, can be identified (the first cervical vertebra, the atlas, has no spinous process projecting from its posterior arch). Finally palpate the inferior tip of the mastoid process on the side of interest.

Using a high-frequency linear probe, begin by centering the probe face over the external occipital protuberance. From there slide the probe inferiorly (as above, approximately 2 cm) until both tubercles of the spinous process of the axis are seen and identified. Then position the probe such that the nonmarker side is over the tubercle of the spinous process of the side of interest and the marker side is directed toward a point just below the tip of the mastoid process (approximating the position of the transverse process of the atlas). Keeping the tubercle of the spinous process and lamina of the axis in view, identify the obliquus capitis inferior muscle, which is often described as looking like a canoe with its bow resting against the spinous process/lamina of the axis. The muscle which can be seen immediately superficial to obliquus capitis inferior is the semispinalis capitis muscle. The greater occipital nerve can nearly always be readily identified as a slightly hypoechoic oval in the fascial plane between semispinalis capitis muscle and obliquus capitis inferior muscle.

CLINICAL APPLICATIONS

This technique is used almost exclusively to guide needle placement for injecting local anesthetic solution around the greater occipital nerve in the diagnosis and treatment of occipital neuralgia and related conditions.

Occipital neuralgia is a common cause of headache and is characterized by paroxysmal stabbing pain, continuous unilateral pain (bilateral during severe attacks) throughout the occipital and parietal scalp. Furthermore, hyperalgesia, dysesthesia, and paroxysmal vertigo are conditions that are often associated with occipital neuralgia and are similar to symptoms that arise during migraines. Patients experiencing occipital neuralgia describe pain and tenderness along the topographic locations of the greater occipital nerve.

Since entrapment of the greater occipital nerve causes occipital neuralgia, neurolysis of the greater occipital nerve in the nuchal musculature, particularly in regard to the trapezius aponeurosis, has been performed. However, studies have shown this procedure to be ineffective in eliminating recurrence of pain. Therefore, other methods have been implemented for the treatment of occipital neuralgia. Local anesthetic nerve block of the greater occipital nerve has been shown to be the most efficient diagnostic and therapeutic tool in treating this disorder.

According to the International Headache Society, occipital neuralgia is defined as pain that can be alleviated through the administration of local anesthetic block of the greater occipital nerve. Local anesthetic block will confirm diagnosis and will lead to the impairment of nociception conduction of the greater occipital nerve.

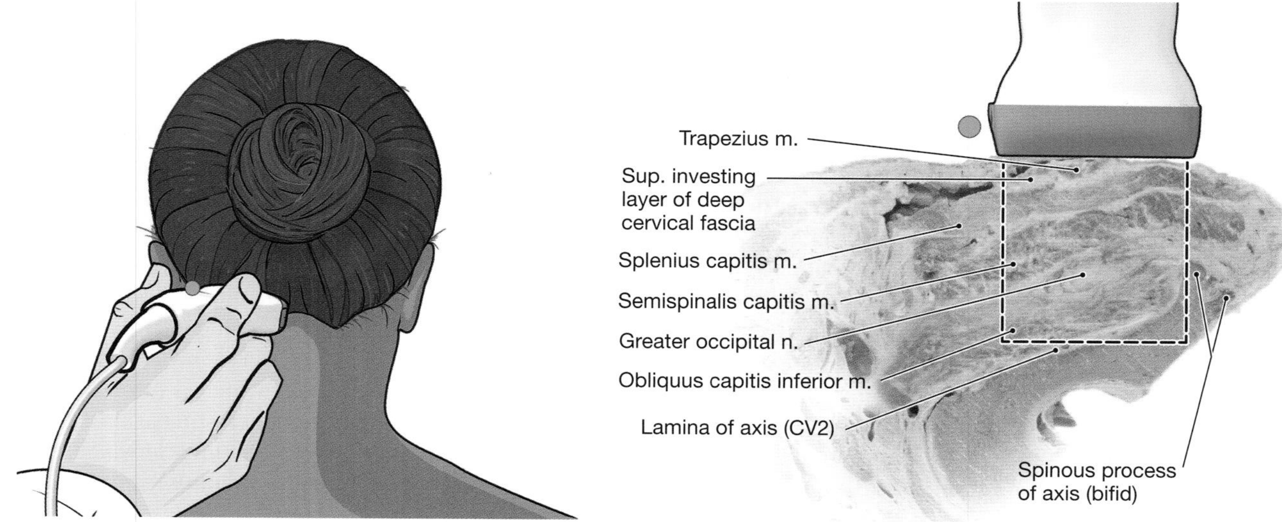

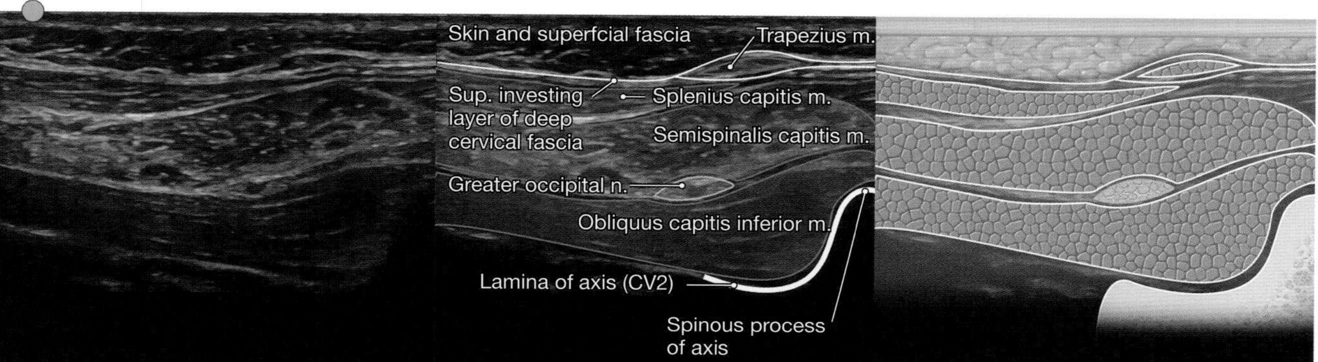

Figure 3.6 Transverse view of the greater occipital nerve in the fascial plane between obliquus capitis inferior and semispinalis capitis muscles.

Multiple Choice Questions

1. A 50-year-old woman is brought to the emergency department because of a 5-day history of high fever and severe headaches. She is HIV positive for the past 10 years and under retroviral treatment. Physical examination shows change in mental status and nuchal rigidity and subacute course of malaise. Cryptococcal meningitis is suspected and she undergoes an ultrasound-guided lumbar puncture. Which of the following structures or spaces will be penetrated/traversed just before the needle enters the lumbar cistern?

   A. Arachnoid mater
   B. Dura mater
   C. Epidural space
   D. Ligamentum flavum
   E. Posterior longitudinal ligament

2. A 29-year-old woman, gravida 1, para 1, is undergoing an ultrasound-guided placement of a catheter for epidural anesthesia during labor. Which of the following structures will be penetrated just before the catheter enters the epidural space?

   A. Anterior longitudinal ligament
   B. Interspinous ligament
   C. Ligamentum flavum
   D. Multifidus muscle
   E. Thoracolumbar fascia

3. A 44-year-old woman was brought to the emergency department by her husband because of a 3-day history of high fever and severe stiffness of her neck. Her temperature is 39 °C (102.2 °F), respirations are 20/min, pulse is 96/min, and blood pressure is 134/85 mm Hg. Meningitis is suspected and an ultrasound-guided lumbar puncture is performed. Microscopic examination of the cerebrospinal fluid shows a large number of red blood cells, white blood cells, and platelets. Which of the following ligaments is most likely penetrated by the needle?

   A. Nuchal
   B. Anterior longitudinal
   C. Posterior longitudinal
   D. Denticulate
   E. Supraspinous

4. A 45-year-old woman comes to the physician because of a 3-month history of intermittent shocking or shooting pain that starts at the base of the head and radiates to the scalp unilaterally. She has been a professional gymnast and now she is a professional dancer. Her vital signs are within normal limits. Physical examination shows point tenderness and elicits pain at the area of suboccipital triangle. An ultrasound examination of the suboccipital triangle is performed to identify the greater occipital nerve. Which of the following landmarks will most likely be used to locate this nerve?

   A. Between semispinalis capitis and obliquus capitis inferior, 2 cm medial to the mastoid process
   B. Between semispinalis capitis and obliquus capitis inferior, 2 cm lateral to the mastoid process
   C. Between semispinalis capitis and trapezius, 2 cm lateral to the mastoid process
   D. Between obliquus capitis inferior and obliquus capitis superior, 2 cm medial to the mastoid process
   E. Between obliquus capitis inferior and rectus capitis posterior major, 2 cm medial to the mastoid process

4

Upper Limb

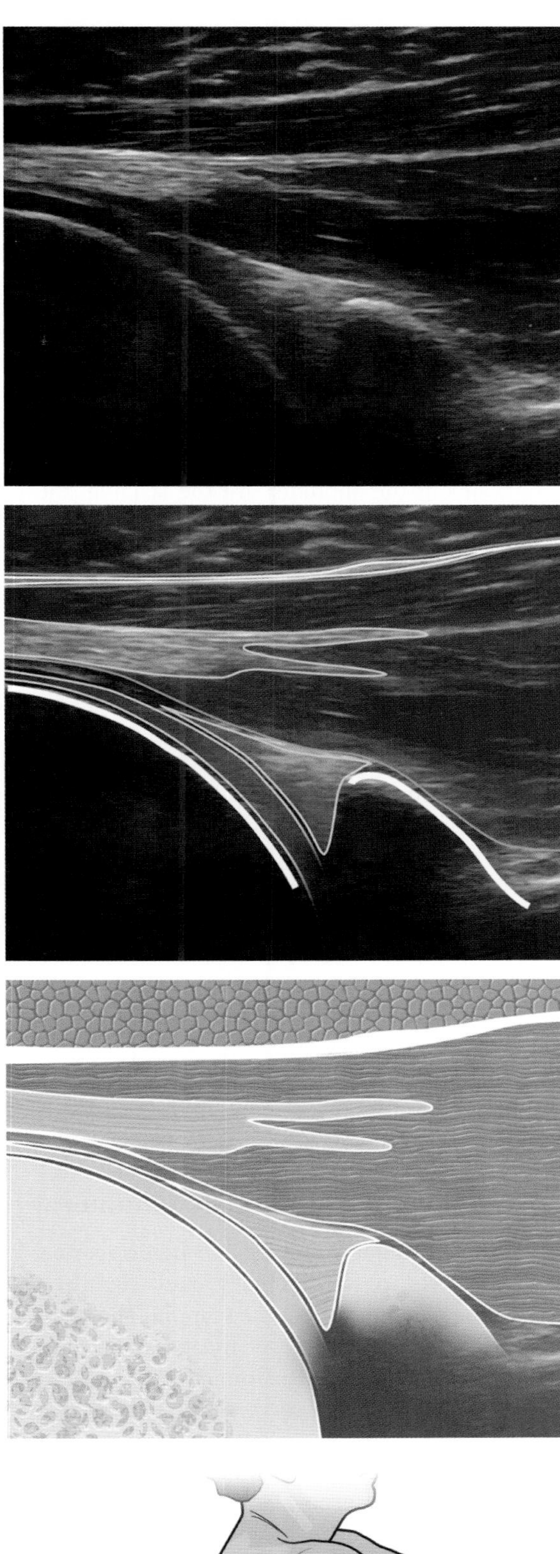

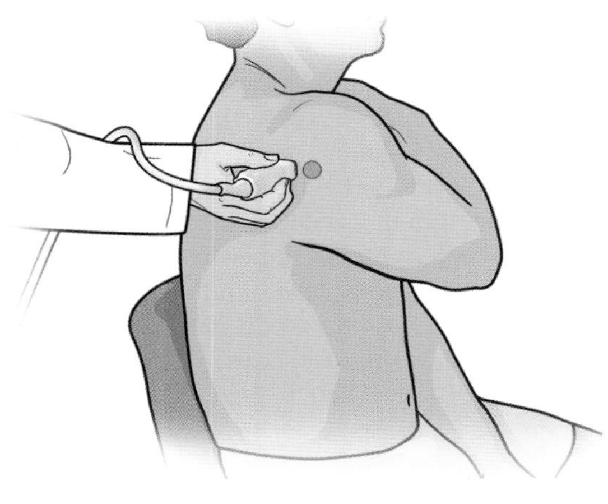

Shoulder

Review of the Anatomy

Bones

The bones of the shoulder are the scapula, the proximal humerus, and the clavicle.

Scapula

The scapula is a large, flat, triangular bone. The scapular spine projects from its posterior surface, dividing the posterior scapula into a supraspinous and an infraspinous fossa. The spine expands at its lateral end into the acromion process, which forms much of the bony roof over the glenohumeral joint; the synovial ball and socket joint between the head of the humerus; and the relatively small, shallow, glenoid cavity at the lateral angle of the scapula. The depth and circumference of the glenoid cavity are increased by a fibrocartilaginous collar, the glenoid labrum. The fingerlike coracoid process that projects anteriorly and laterally from the superior margin of the scapula, together with the acromion and the intervening coracoacromial ligament, makes up the coracoacromial arch, which roofs over the humeral head and glenohumeral joint. The space between the deep surface of the arch and the humeral head is the subacromial space.

Proximal Humerus and Glenohumeral Joint

From the proximal humerus, the hemispherical humeral head projects posteromedially and slightly superiorly toward the glenoid fossa of the scapula. The head is demarcated from the remainder of the proximal humerus by a narrow constriction, the anatomical neck. The greater and lesser tubercles, which serve as attachment sites for the tendons of the rotator cuff muscles, are situated at the anterior aspect of the proximal humerus, separated by the intertubercular groove.

The greater tubercle has a rounded surface that projects anterolaterally, with three facets (superior, middle, and inferior) for attachment of the tendons of the supraspinatus, infraspinatus, and teres minor (the rotator cuff muscles originating from the posterior scapula). The lesser tubercle, projecting anteriorly and somewhat medially, has a flattened to slightly concave surface for attachment of the tendon of subscapularis (the rotator cuff muscle originating from the anterior [costal or thoracic] surface of the scapula).

The tendon of the long head of biceps brachii occupies the intertubercular groove and is stabilized in that position by the transverse humeral ligament. Superiorly, the tendon curves over the humeral head and passes through a small interval (rotator cuff interval) between the tendons of the supraspinatus and subscapularis to enter the glenohumeral joint space. The rotator cuff tendons course superficially over the fibrous capsule of the glenohumeral joint to reach their insertion sites on the greater and lesser tubercles. The fibrous capsule is attached along the anatomical neck of the humerus and along the margin of the glenoid fossa, just outside the glenoid labrum.

Clavicle and Acromioclavicular Joint

The clavicle is subcutaneous throughout its length. Its medial end is attached to the sternum at the sternoclavicular joint, and its lateral end is attached to the acromion of the scapula at the acromioclavicular (AC) joint. The AC joint is a small synovial joint between the anteromedial surface of the acromion and the lateral end of the clavicle. The joint is enclosed by a capsule, which is reinforced by a thickening along its subcutaneous superior surface, the AC ligament.

Muscles

Deltoid

The deltoid muscle, which forms the normal rounded contour of the shoulder, is immediately superficial to the rotator cuff tendons and the tendon of the long head of biceps brachii. The deltoid muscle has a wide U-shaped origin from the scapular spine, acromion, and lateral third of the clavicle and tapers to its insertion on the deltoid tubercle at the lateral lip of the intertubercular groove near the mid-diaphysis of the humerus.

Supraspinatus

The supraspinatus muscle originates from the supraspinous fossa, and its tendon passes through the subacromial space to insert on the superior facet of the greater tubercle. The subacromial bursa separates the tendon from the deep surface of the acromion and coracoacromial arch. Beyond the subacromial space, the tendon is separated from the deep surface of the deltoid muscle by a continuation of the subdeltoid bursa (continuous with the subacromial bursa) and a thin plane of subdeltoid/peribursal fat.

Infraspinatus and Teres Minor

The infraspinatus and teres minor muscles originate from the infraspinous fossa. Their tendons pass beneath the posterior edge of the acromion and over the posterior aspect of the glenohumeral joint and humeral head to insert on the middle and inferior facets of the greater tubercle. These muscles and their tendons are separated from the overlying deltoid muscle by a thin layer of subdeltoid fat and fascia.

Subscapularis

The subscapularis muscle originates from the anterior surface of the scapula, and its tendon passes through the subcoracoid space inferior to the coracoid process and deep to the coracobrachialis and short head of the biceps brachii muscles, then over the anteromedial aspect of the glenohumeral joint and the humeral head to insert on the lesser tubercle. Beyond the subcoracoid space, the tendon is immediately deep to the deltoid muscle and subdeltoid fat and fascia.

Technique

Tendon of the Long Head of Biceps Brachii

INTERTUBERCULAR GROOVE BICEPS BRACHII LONG HEAD TENDON
Transverse
FIG. 4.1

The patient should be seated with the elbow flexed to 90° and the supinated forearm resting on the thigh. While standing behind the patient, position the probe (linear high frequency) transverse to the anterior surface of the proximal humerus with the probe marker pointed laterally. Deep to the deltoid muscle, identify the greater and lesser tubercles and the intervening intertubercular groove. The tendon of the long head of biceps brachii should appear as a hyperechoic oval within the groove. Although a tendon sheath extends along the tendon for a short distance from the glenohumeral joint, it is not normally seen unless there are inflammatory changes such as tenosynovitis or joint effusion. Tilting/fanning the probe alters the appearance of the tendon from hyperechoic to hypoechoic/anechoic (because of anisotropy). A thin hyperechoic band of dense connective tissue, the transverse humeral ligament, should be seen spanning the groove just anterior to the tendon and blending with the connective tissue along the surfaces of the tubercles.

INTERTUBERCULAR GROOVE BICEPS BRACHII LONG HEAD TENDON
Longitudinal
FIG. 4.2

Keeping the tendon in view at the center of the image, rotate the probe by 90° (probe marker facing superiorly) to obtain a longitudinal view. Owing to anisotropy, the tendon "disappears" superiorly as it curves over the humerus into the joint space.

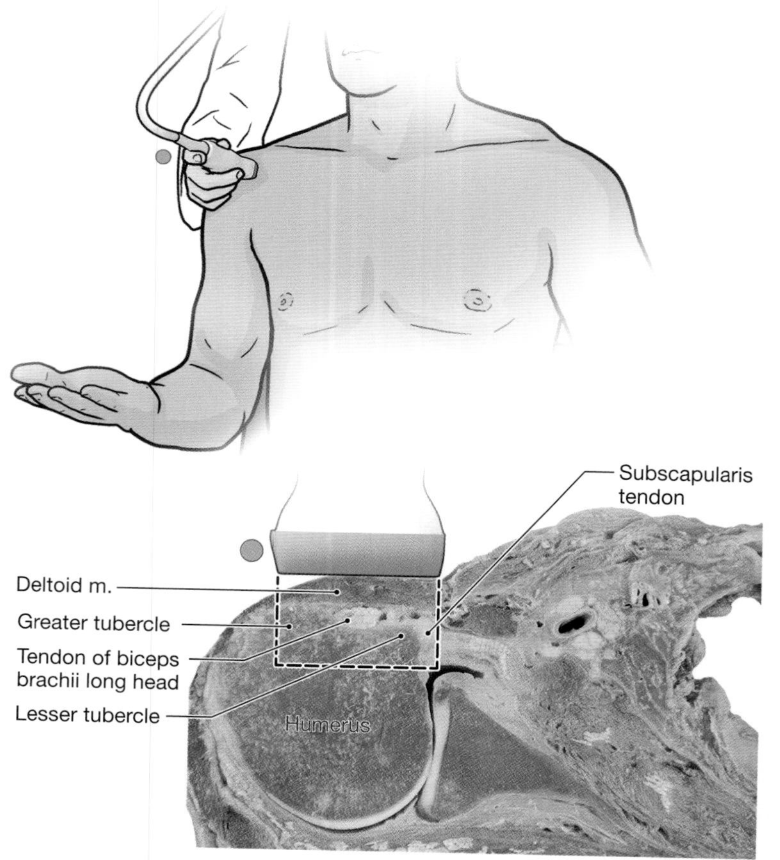

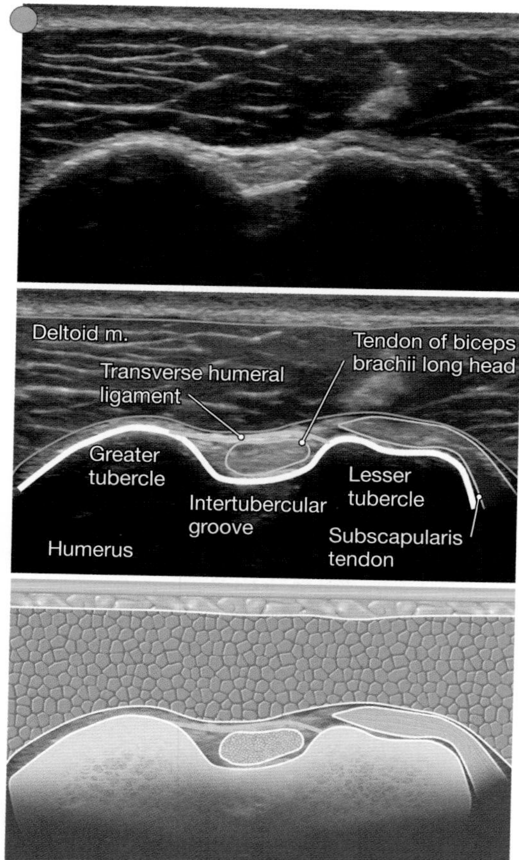

Figure 4.1 Transverse view of the tendon of the long head of biceps brachii in the intertubercular groove of the humerus.

Subscapularis

SUBSCAPULARIS TENDON
Longitudinal
FIG. 4.3

The patient should be seated with the elbow flexed to 90° and the forearm supinated as before. Placing the probe transverse to the anterior aspect of the proximal humerus, once again identify the lesser tubercle and rotate the patient's arm externally. Deep to the deltoid muscle and subdeltoid fat and fascia, the tendon of subscapularis can be viewed (in the longitudinal axis of the tendon). Identify the tendon as it curves over the humeral head from the subcoracoid space to its tapered lateral end, where it inserts into the lesser tubercle.

SUBSCAPULARIS TENDON
Transverse
FIG. 4.4

From the same patient and probe position described above, rotate the probe by 90° (probe marker facing superiorly) to view the tendon transverse to its long axis. Slide the probe medially along a short distance until several hyperechoic tendon bundles interspersed with hypoechoic muscle tissue (myotendinous junctions) can be identified.

Supraspinatus Tendon

GREATER TUBERCLE SUPRASPINATUS TENDON
Longitudinal
FIG. 4.5

The patient's limb should be in the "hand in the back pocket" (modified Crass) position with the palm over the lower back and the elbow pointing posteriorly. This position extends/hyperextends and rotates the humerus externally, bringing the supraspinatus tendon out of the subacromial space. Place the probe over the anterolateral corner of the shoulder just distal to the acromion, angled approximately midway between the sagittal and coronal planes (probe marker pointing anterolaterally) to obtain a longitudinal "bird's beak" view of the tendon. Adjust the position of the probe until the fibrillar appearance of the tendon is clearly seen, and the tapered end of the tendon at its insertion on the greater tubercle is viewed. Identify from superficial to deep: the deltoid muscle, hyperechoic subdeltoid fat and fascia, thin anechoic subdeltoid bursa, supraspinatus tendon, superior facet of the greater tubercle, anatomical neck of the humerus, and humeral head.

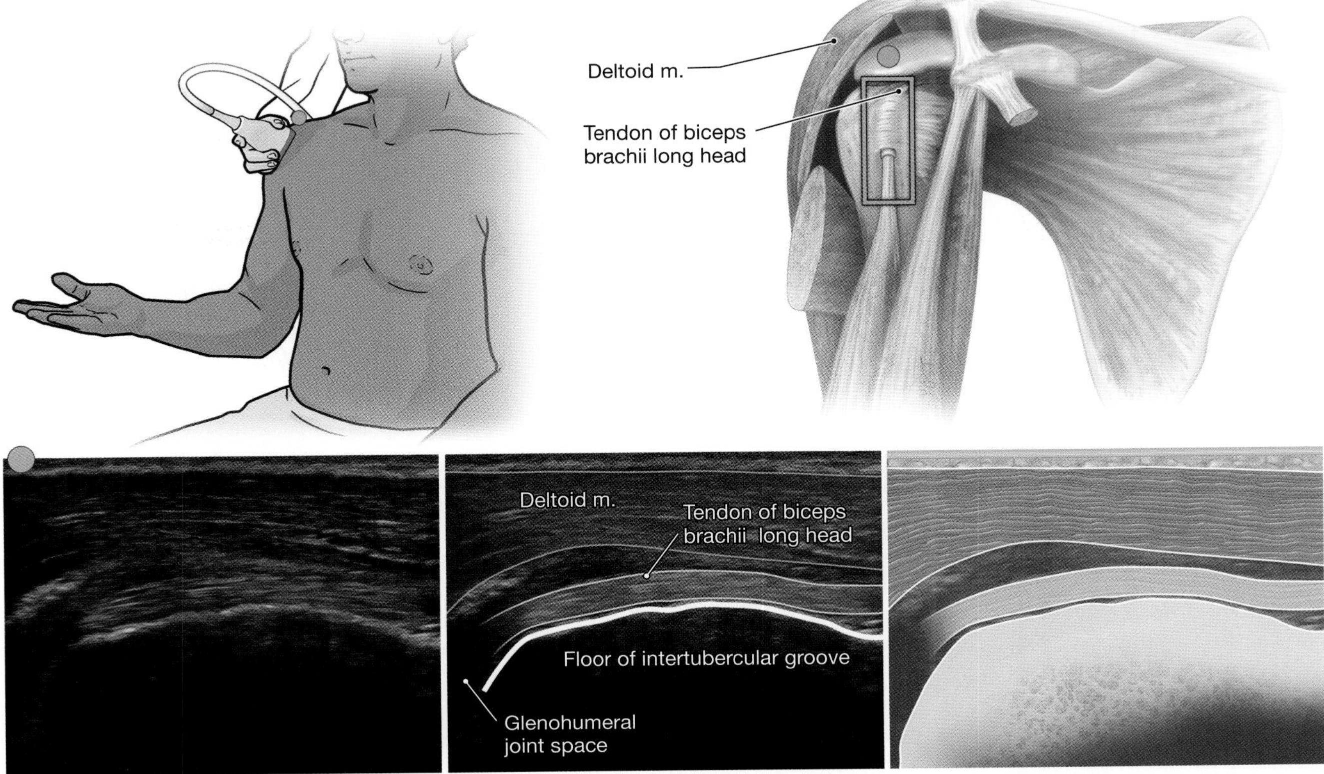

Figure 4.2 Longitudinal view of the tendon of the long head of biceps brachii in the intertubercular groove of the humerus.

SUPRASPINATUS MYOTENDINOUS JUNCTION
Longitudinal
FIG. 4.6

Slide the probe anteriorly and posteriorly in the same orientation to view the tendon from side to side. Slide the probe along the tendon proximally (toward the patient's ear) in the same orientation until the hyperechoic surface of the acromion (and its acoustic shadow) is viewed. The myotendinous junction of the supraspinatus is often visible as it emerges from the subacromial space.

ROTATOR CUFF INTERVAL SUPRASPINATUS TENDON
Transverse
FIG. 4.7

Slide the probe back distally until the tendon and its insertion are visible again. Rotate the probe by 90° (probe marker pointing to the right) to obtain a transverse "tire on the rim" view of the tendon. Slide the probe medially (simultaneously adjusting the tilt/angle) until the hyperechoic oval profile of the tendon of the long head of biceps brachii in the rotator cuff interval can be identified.

Infraspinatus Tendon

INFRASPINATUS TENDON
Longitudinal
FIG. 4.8

The patient's limb should be across the chest with the fingers and palm resting on the contralateral shoulder. Place the probe on the posterior surface of the shoulder just inferior to the posterior corner of the acromion, parallel to the scapular spine. Adjust the probe position anteriorly/posteriorly in this orientation until the fibrillar appearance of the tendon is clearly seen and the tapered end at its insertion on the greater tubercle is viewed. From superficial to deep, identify the deltoid muscle, subdeltoid fat and fascia, infraspinatus tendon, greater tubercle, and head of humerus.

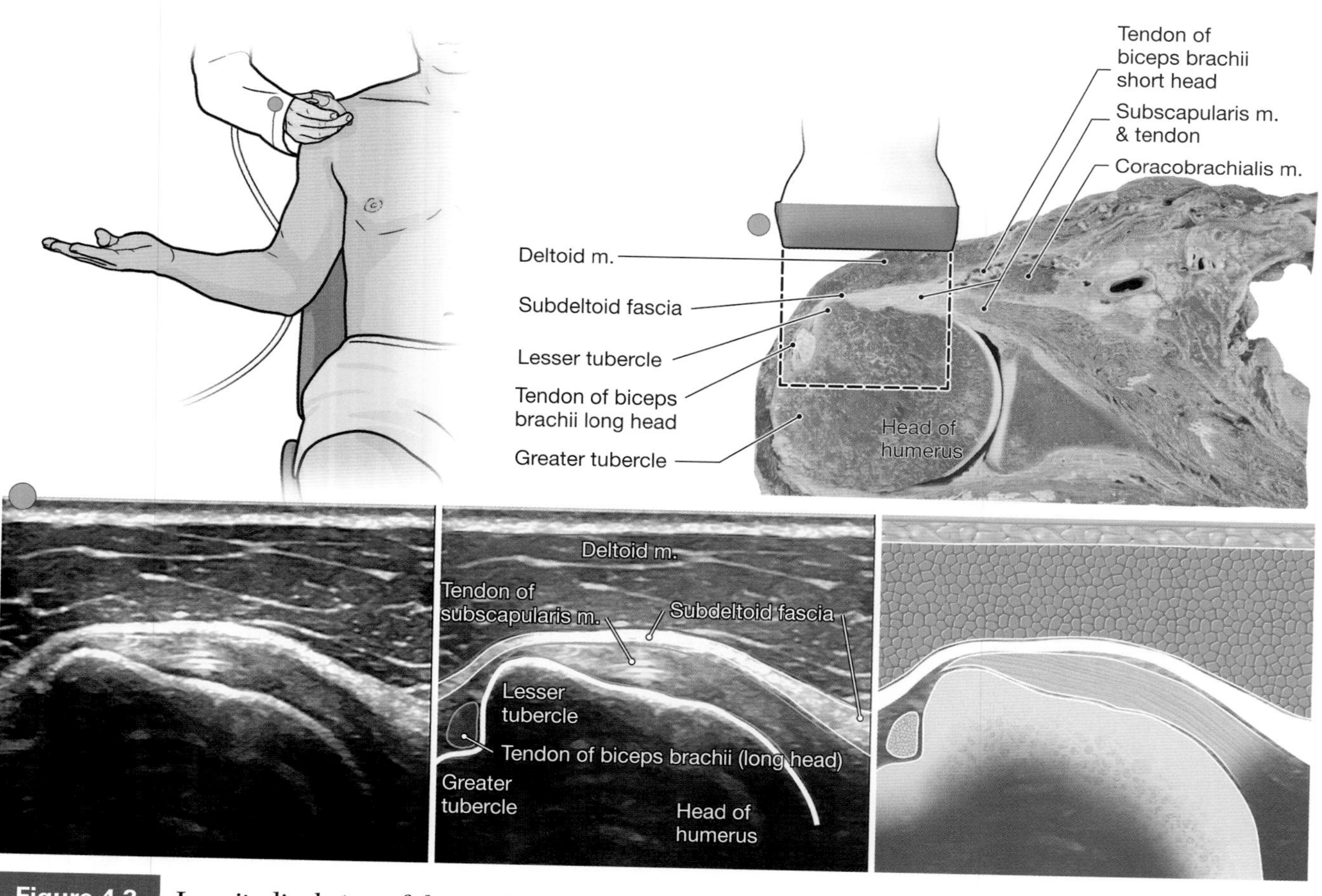

Figure 4.3 Longitudinal view of the tendon of subscapularis at the lesser tubercle of the humerus.

Glenohumeral Joint and Glenoid Labrum

GLENOHUMERAL JOINT GLENOID LABRUM
Transverse
FIG. 4.9

Maintaining the same patient position and probe orientation, slide the probe posteriorly (toward the midline) keeping the supraspinatus tendon in view as it becomes continuous with the muscle tissue (myotendinous junction). Observe the head of the humerus as it curves toward the glenoid fossa, and look for the small bright reflection (and acoustic shadow) of the posterior rim of the glenoid process. At the glenoid rim, look for the hyperechoic triangular profile of the posterior aspect of the glenoid labrum between the articular surface of the humeral head and the infraspinatus tendon and myotendinous junction. The apex of the glenoid labrum is directed anterolaterally. Gently rotate the patient's arm externally and internally to observe the movement of the infraspinatus muscle and tendon over the posterior aspect of the glenohumeral joint and humeral head. At the posteromedial (nonmarker) edge of the image, the spinoglenoid notch (inferior scapular notch) can be seen adjacent to the glenoid process.

AC Joint

ACROMIOCLAVICULAR JOINT
Coronal
FIG. 4.10

With the patient seated and the forearm resting on the thigh, palpate along the distal clavicle to locate the small "step-off" at the AC joint. Center the probe over the joint in a coronal orientation (probe marker pointing to the right). Identify the acromion, AC joint space, lateral end of the clavicle, and AC ligament.

CLINICAL APPLICATIONS

Ultrasound examination is commonly used in the evaluation of musculoskeletal injuries or degenerative disorders resulting in "painful shoulder," such as rotator cuff tendon tears or impingement (eg, subacromial supraspinatus tendon impingement), subacromial/subdeltoid bursitis, biceps tendonitis/tenosynovitis, glenoid labrum tears and cysts, glenohumeral joint effusions, and AC joint separations. These techniques are also used to guide needles into the glenohumeral joint, AC joint, or inflamed bursae for injection of local anesthetic agents and anti-inflammatory steroids.

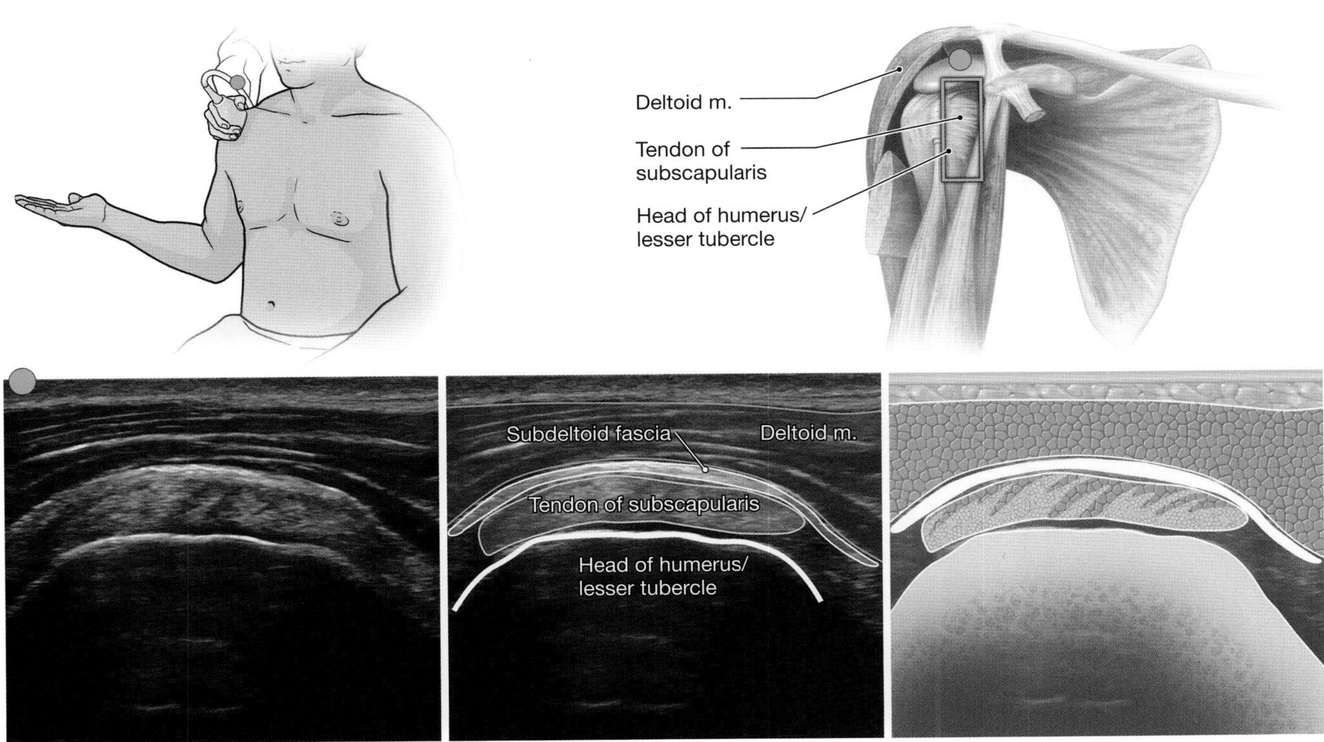

Figure 4.4 Transverse view of the tendon of subscapularis with several myotendinous junctions (multipennate appearance).

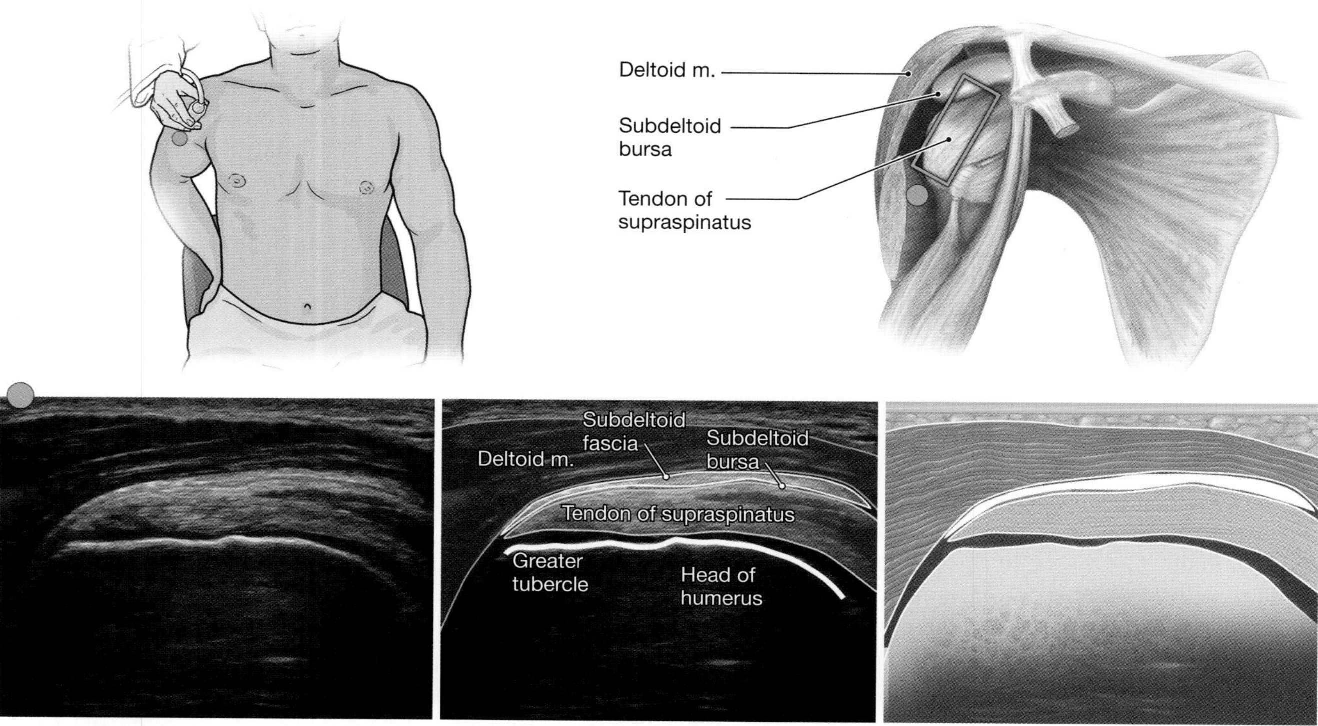

Figure 4.5 Longitudinal view of the supraspinatus tendon and its insertion at the superior facet of the greater tubercle of the humerus.

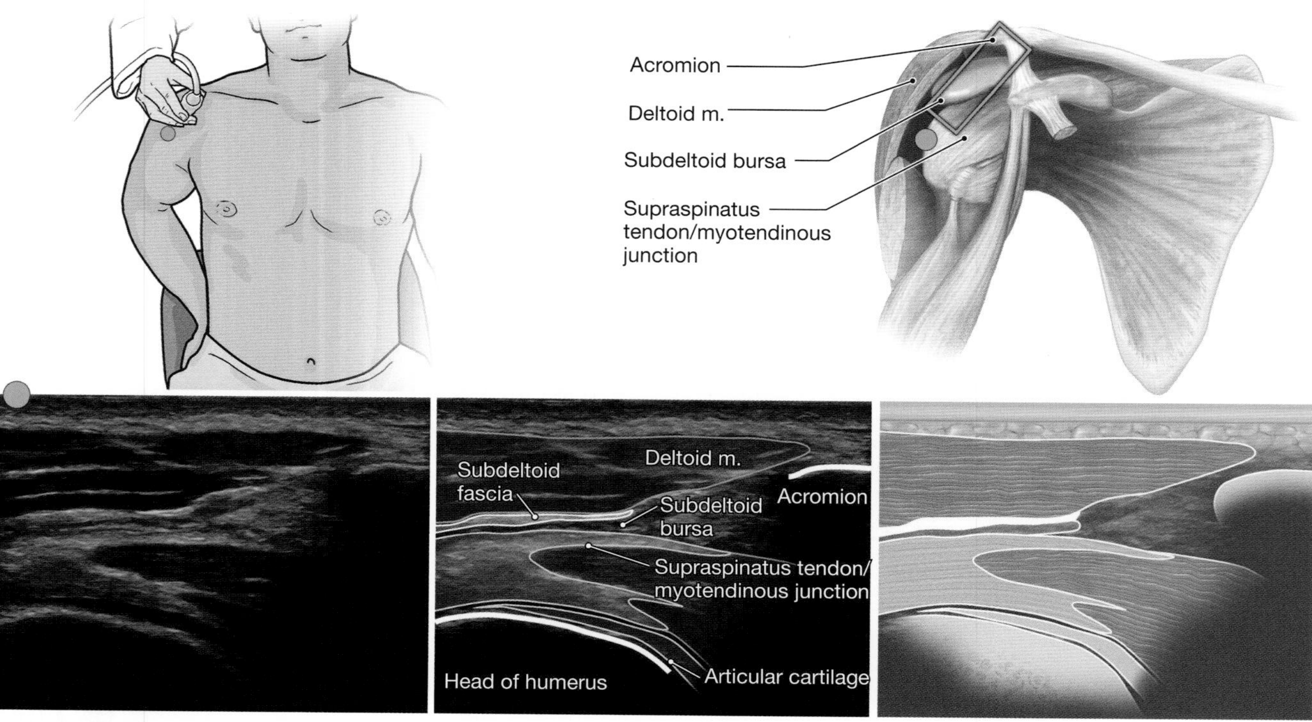

Figure 4.6 Longitudinal view of the supraspinatus myotendinous junction just emerging from the subacromial space.

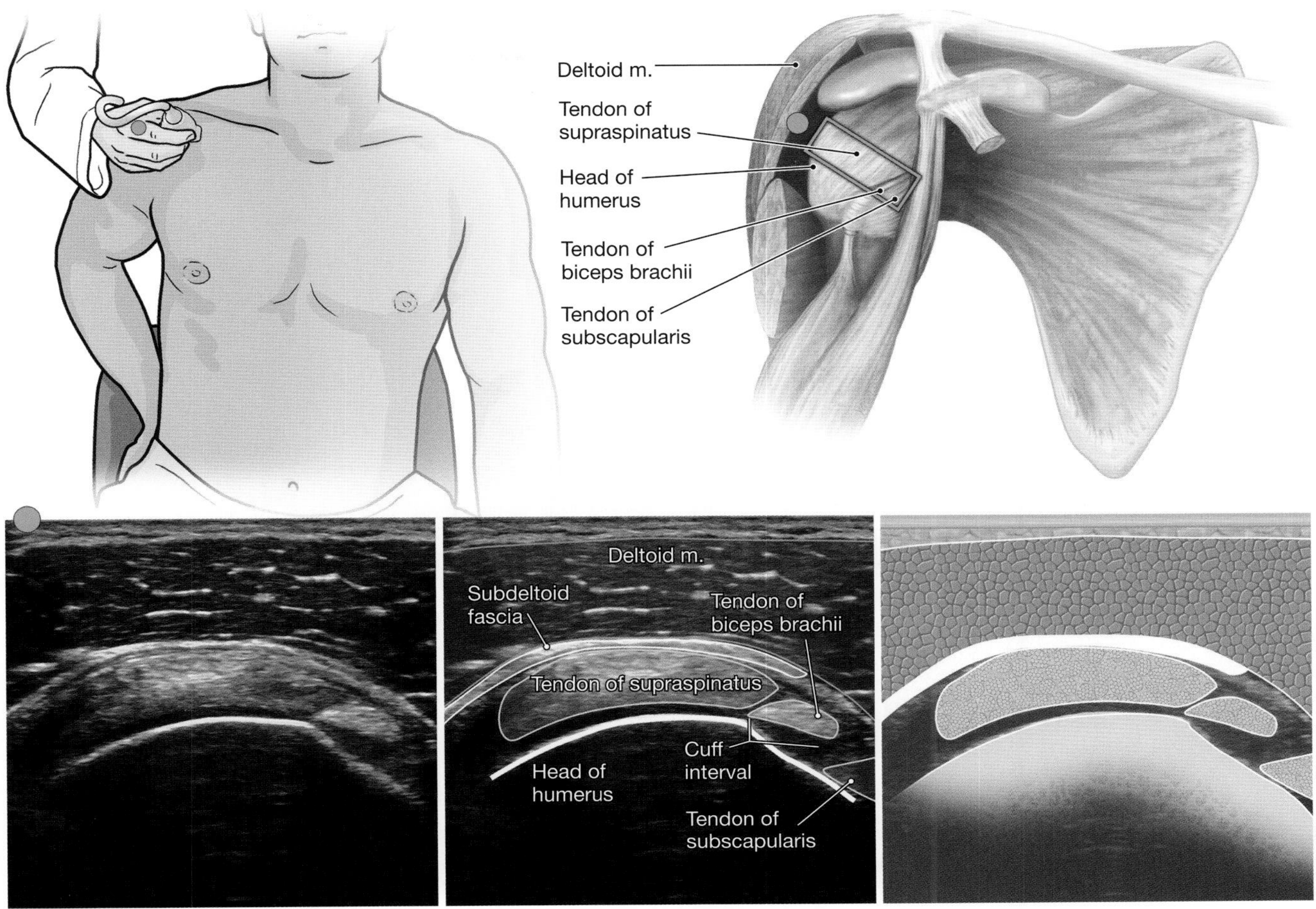

Figure 4.7 Transverse view of the supraspinatus tendon along with the tendon of the long head of biceps brachii in the rotator cuff interval.

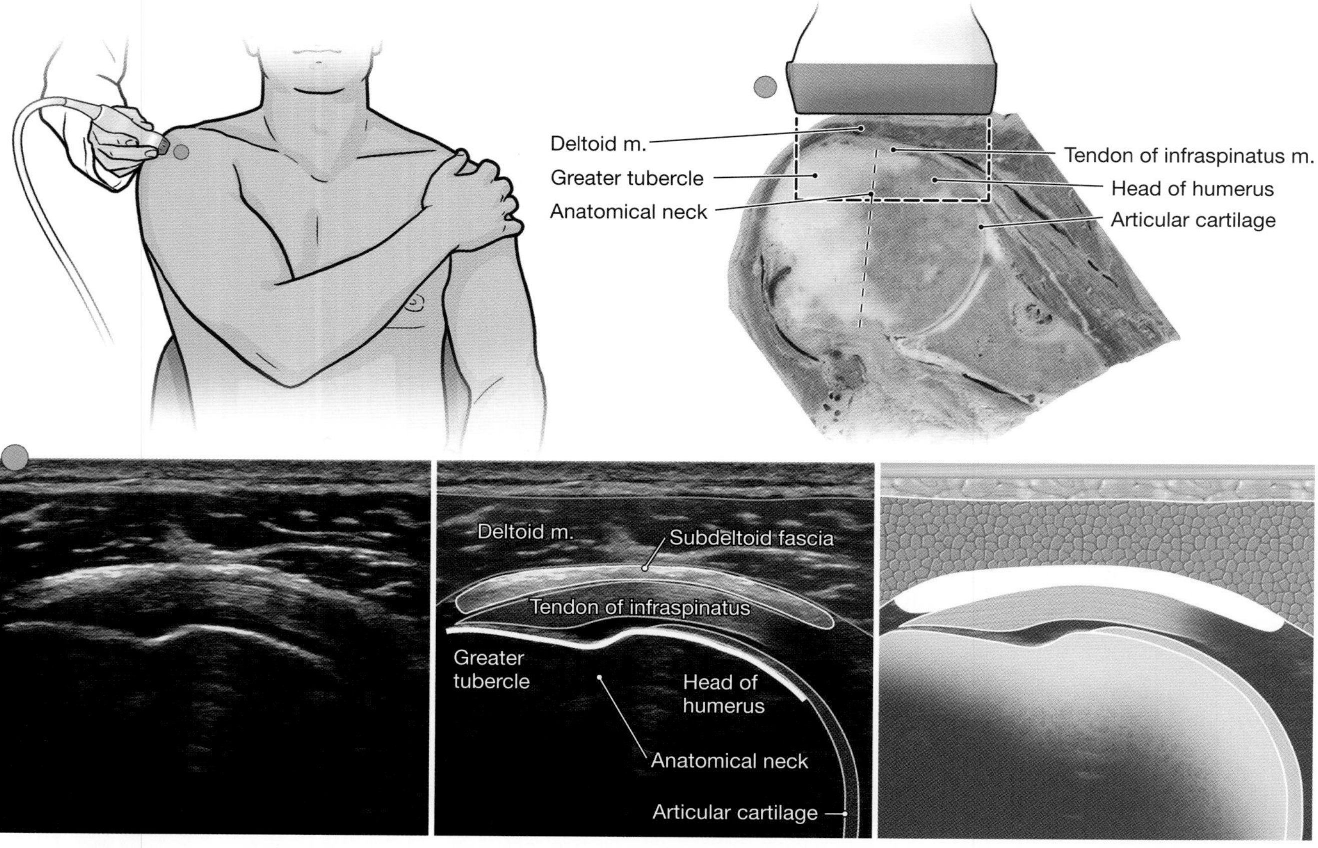

Figure 4.8 Longitudinal view of the tendon of infraspinatus and its insertion onto the middle facet of the greater tubercle of the humerus.

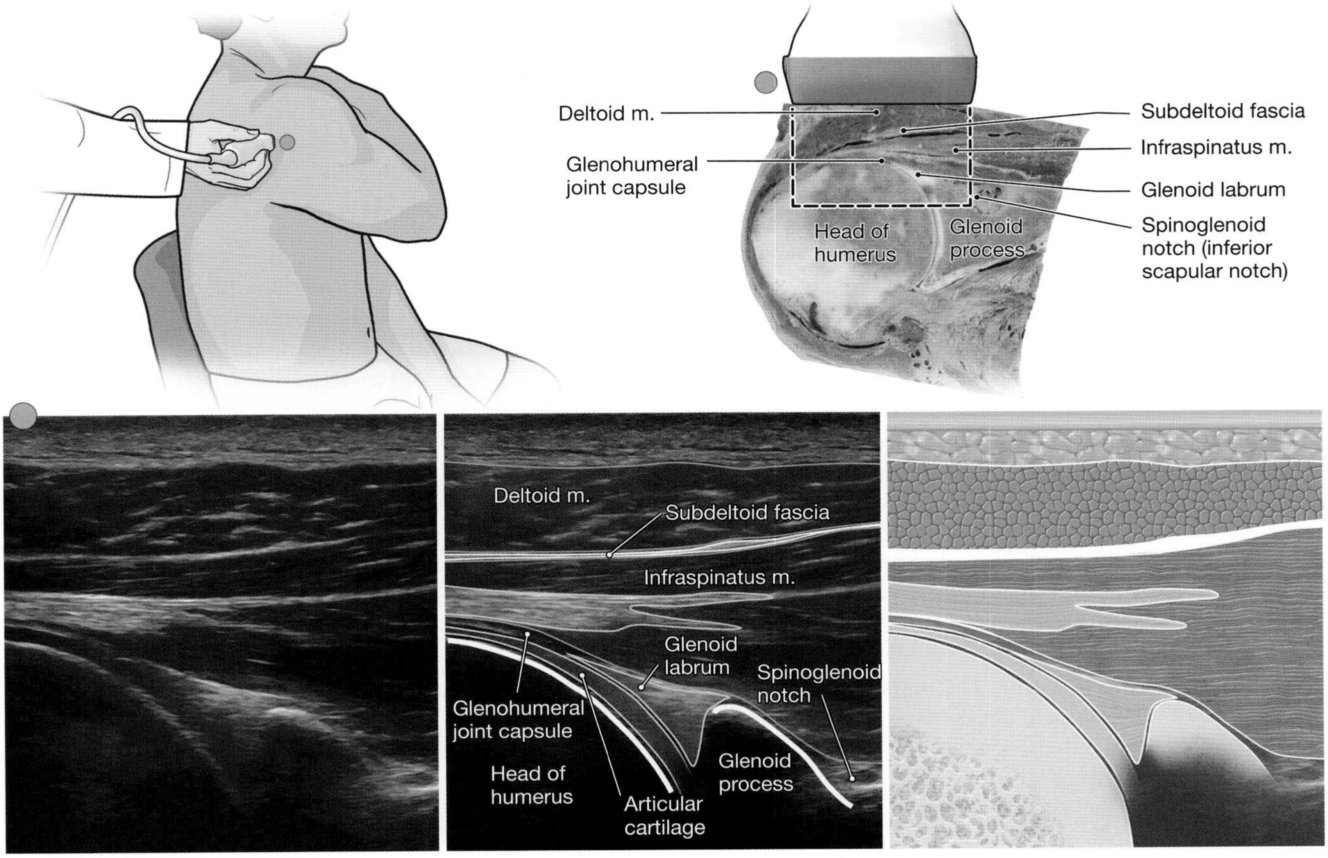

Figure 4.9 Transverse view of the posterior aspect of the glenohumeral joint and glenoid labrum deep to the deltoid and infraspinatus muscles.

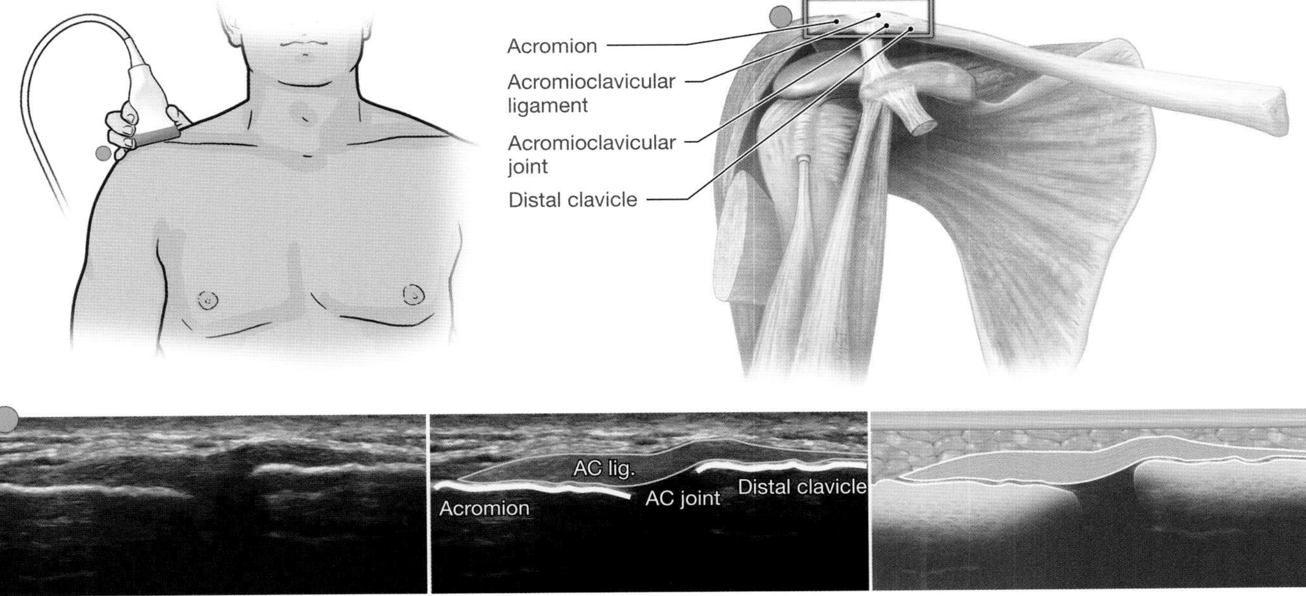

Figure 4.10 Coronal view of the acromioclavicular joint and ligament.

Brachial Plexus

Review of the Anatomy

The brachial plexus is the source of innervation for the upper limb. The plexus forms in the neck from the primary ventral rami of spinal nerves C5 through T1, referred to as the roots of the plexus. The roots emerge from their respective intervertebral foramina into the scalene interval, a narrow space between anterior and middle scalene muscles. Typically, C5 and C6 roots combine to form the upper trunk, C7 root continues as the middle trunk, and the C8 and T1 roots combine to form the lower trunk. The trunks continue toward the root of the neck, where each divides into an anterior and a posterior division. The divisions then cross the first rib just lateral to the subclavian artery, between the anterior and middle scalene tendons (which insert on the first rib). The anterior and posterior divisions recombine to form the cords of the plexus as they pass through the space between the first rib, which is clavicle, and superior margin of the scapula (axillary inlet or cervicoaxillary canal) into the axilla. As it passes beyond the lateral margin of the first rib, the subclavian artery becomes the axillary artery. The axillary vein is medial/inferior to the artery and crosses the first rib on the medial side of the anterior scalene tendon (ie, not through the scalene interval). In their course through the axilla, the divisions, cords, and branches of the plexus, and the axillary vessels are deep to the pectoralis muscles. The axillary artery is described as having 3 parts: the first part is superior/medial to the pectoralis minor muscle, the second is posterior/deep to the pectoralis minor muscle, and the third is inferior/lateral to pectoralis minor. As the cords form from the divisions, they come to surround the second part of the artery and are named for their relationship to the artery in this position: The lateral cord is lateral/superior to the artery, the medial cord is medial/inferior to the artery (between the artery and vein), and the posterior cord is posterior/deep to the artery.

Pectoralis Muscles

Pectoralis major is a large fan-shaped muscle that originates along the medial third of the clavicle, the surface of the sternum, and the first seven costal cartilages. It inserts through a ribbonlike tendon onto the lateral lip of the intertubercular groove. The pectoralis minor muscle, deep to pectoralis major, is a small triangular muscle originating from the surfaces of the ribs 3 to 5 and inserting on the medial aspect of the coracoid process of the scapula.

Technique

Roots, Trunks, and Divisions

SCALENE INTERVAL ROOTS AND TRUNKS
Transverse
FIG. 4.11.

The patient should be supine on the examination table with the head rotated slightly to the contralateral side. Position the probe transversely a few centimeters above the medial third of the clavicle, over the lower part of the sternocleidomastoid muscle. Adjust the probe position as needed to identify the following structures deep to sternocleidomastoid (for additional information, see Chapter 9 Neck and Face), from medial to lateral: the common carotid artery, the internal jugular vein, and the anterior scalene muscle. Slide the probe laterally until the internal jugular vein is just visible at the medial aspect of the image. In this position, identify the anterior and middle scalene muscles and the thin space between them, the scalene interval. Slide the probe superiorly and inferiorly over the scalene interval while adjusting the probe tilt/angle until two or three large bundles of nerve tissue can be identified in the interval (in many patients, because of the oblique course of the roots/trunks relative to the surface of the neck and resulting anisotropy/artifact, the roots/trunks can only be seen as discrete hypoechoic ovals, sometimes referred to as the "traffic-light" sign). The C5, C6, and C7 roots are the most anterior nerve bundles in the interval, and the lower parts of the plexus (C8 and T1 roots) are difficult to definitively image in this location.

ROOT OF THE NECK TRUNKS AND DIVISIONS
Transverse
FIG. 4.12

From the interscalene view of the brachial plexus, simultaneously slide the probe inferiorly toward the supraclavicular fossa while tilting the probe face inferiorly until the view is nearly coronal. While repositioning/tilting the probe, keep the bundles of the

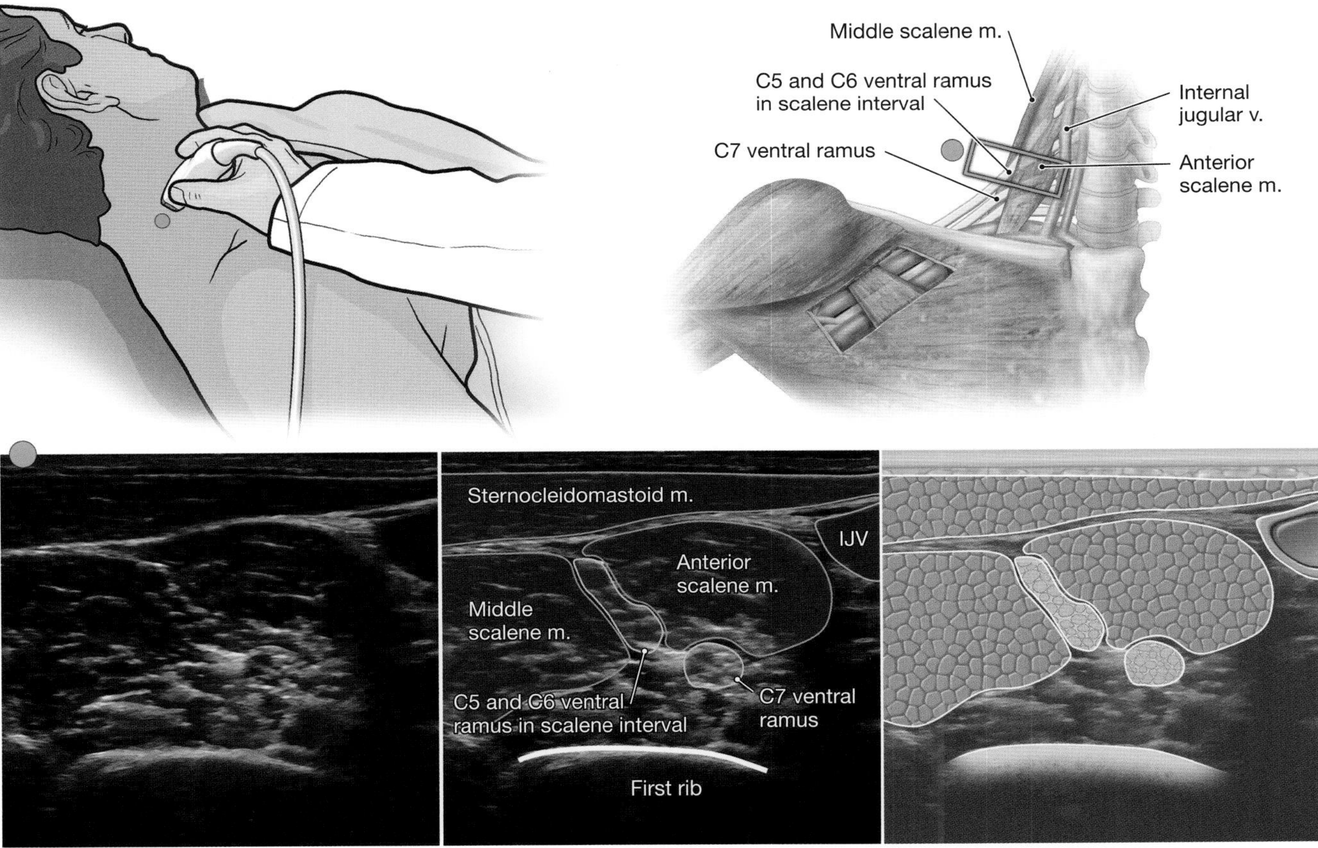

Figure 4.11 Transverse view of the roots and trunks of the brachial plexus in the scalene interval. IJV, internal jugular vein.

nerve tissue of the plexus near the center of the image and look for the appearance of the pulsating subclavian artery and the hyperechoic reflection (and acoustic shadow) of the first rib. The trunks/divisions of the plexus appear as a very large stack of nerve tissue bundles draped over the first rib in contact with the lateral surface of the subclavian artery. The lower trunk (combined C8 and T1 roots) is inferiorly positioned, in contact with the first rib between the middle scalene muscle/tendon and the subclavian artery.

Cords

AXILLA CORDS
Transverse
FIG. 4.13

The patient should be supine on the examination table with the arm resting along the side. In some patients, it may be helpful to ask them to place their hand palm up behind their head, which moves the scapula anteriorly and brings the axillary vessels into a more superficial position. By palpation, locate the positions of the coracoid process and the xiphisternal junction. Place the probe along the diagonal line connecting these landmarks, just below the tip of the coracoid process (probe orientation marker toward the coracoid). Identify the pectoralis major muscle in oblique/transverse view and the pectoralis minor muscle viewed in its longitudinal axis. Deep to the pectoralis minor, identify the pulsating axillary artery (second part) and adjust the probe position, pressure, and tilt as necessary to identify the axillary vein immediately medial/inferior to the artery and to obtain a true transverse view (circular

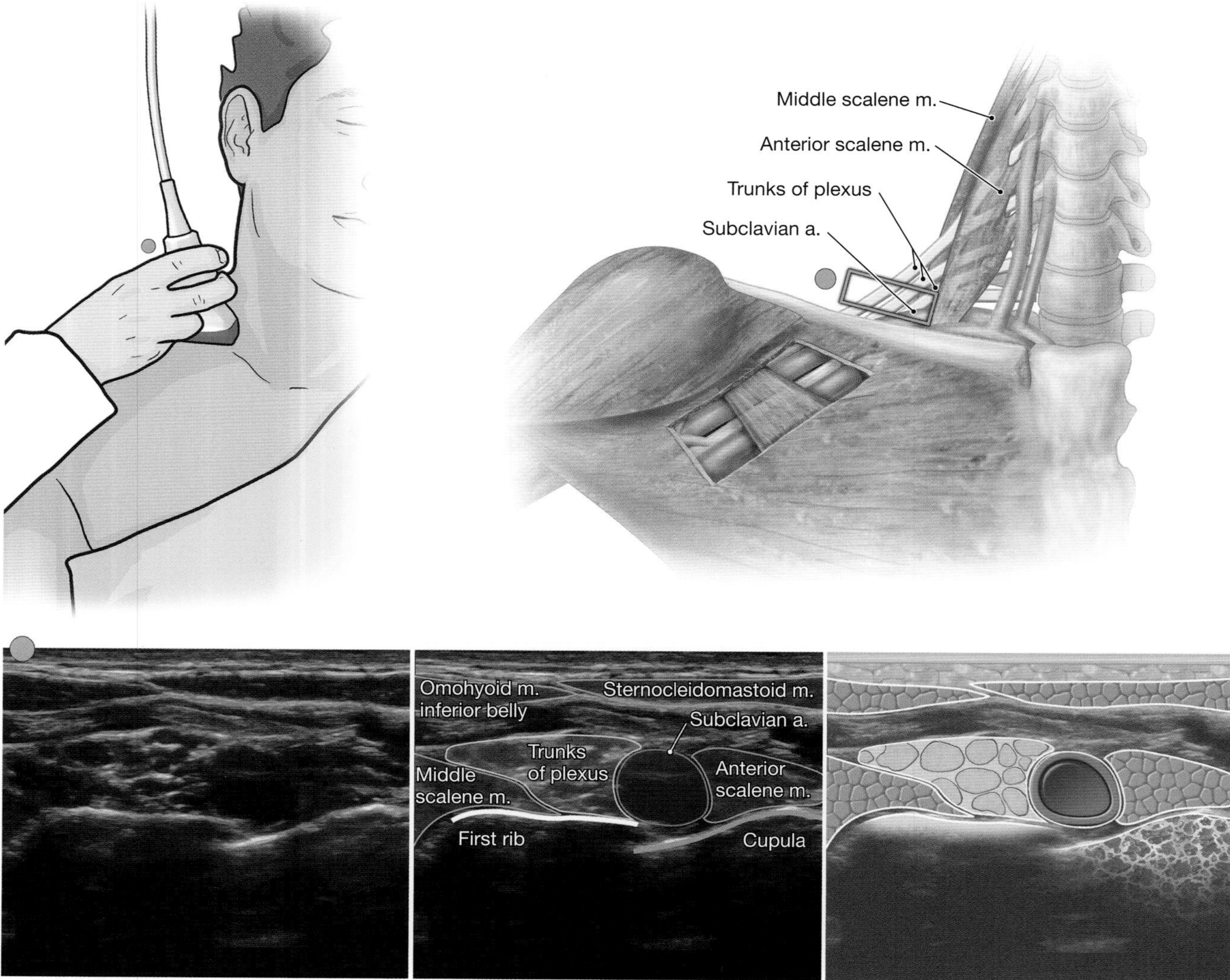

Figure 4.12 Transverse view of the trunks and divisions of the brachial plexus alongside the subclavian artery in the root of the neck.

rather than oval profile) of the artery. Three hyperechoic nerve bundles should be visible near the artery. The lateral cord is seen just lateral/superior to the artery. The posterior cord is immediately deep to the artery. The medial cord is medial/inferior to the artery, situated between the artery and the vein.

CLINICAL APPLICATIONS

These techniques are most commonly used for guiding needles (or catheters) safely into position for infiltration of local anesthetic agents around the components of the brachial plexus to establish regional anesthesia during upper limb surgery and/or for pain control in the postoperative period.

Plexus blocks in the scalene interval are referred to as interscalene blocks. Blocks in the root of the neck are referred to as supraclavicular blocks. Blocks of the cords in the axilla are called infraclavicular blocks.

Each of these sites carries its own set of advantages, disadvantages, and indications for use.

- Interscalene blocks reliably anesthetize the upper arm and shoulder but often miss the C8 and T1 roots, thereby failing to anesthetize the ulnar side of the arm, forearm, and hand.
- Because the nerve trunks/divisions are packed closely together in the root of the neck, supraclavicular blocks reliably produce virtually complete upper limb anesthesia. However, because of the proximity of the lung apex and subclavian artery to the trunks of the plexus in this location, there is risk of puncturing the lung and producing a pneumothorax or arterial puncture and intravascular injection of a local anesthetic.

Infraclavicular blocks (plexus cords) produce reliable anesthesia of the distal two-thirds of the arm, forearm, wrist, and hand. These blocks are often used for surgeries of the upper limb distal to and including the elbow. In addition, there is little risk of puncturing the lung and producing a pneumothorax as compared with supraclavicular blocks.

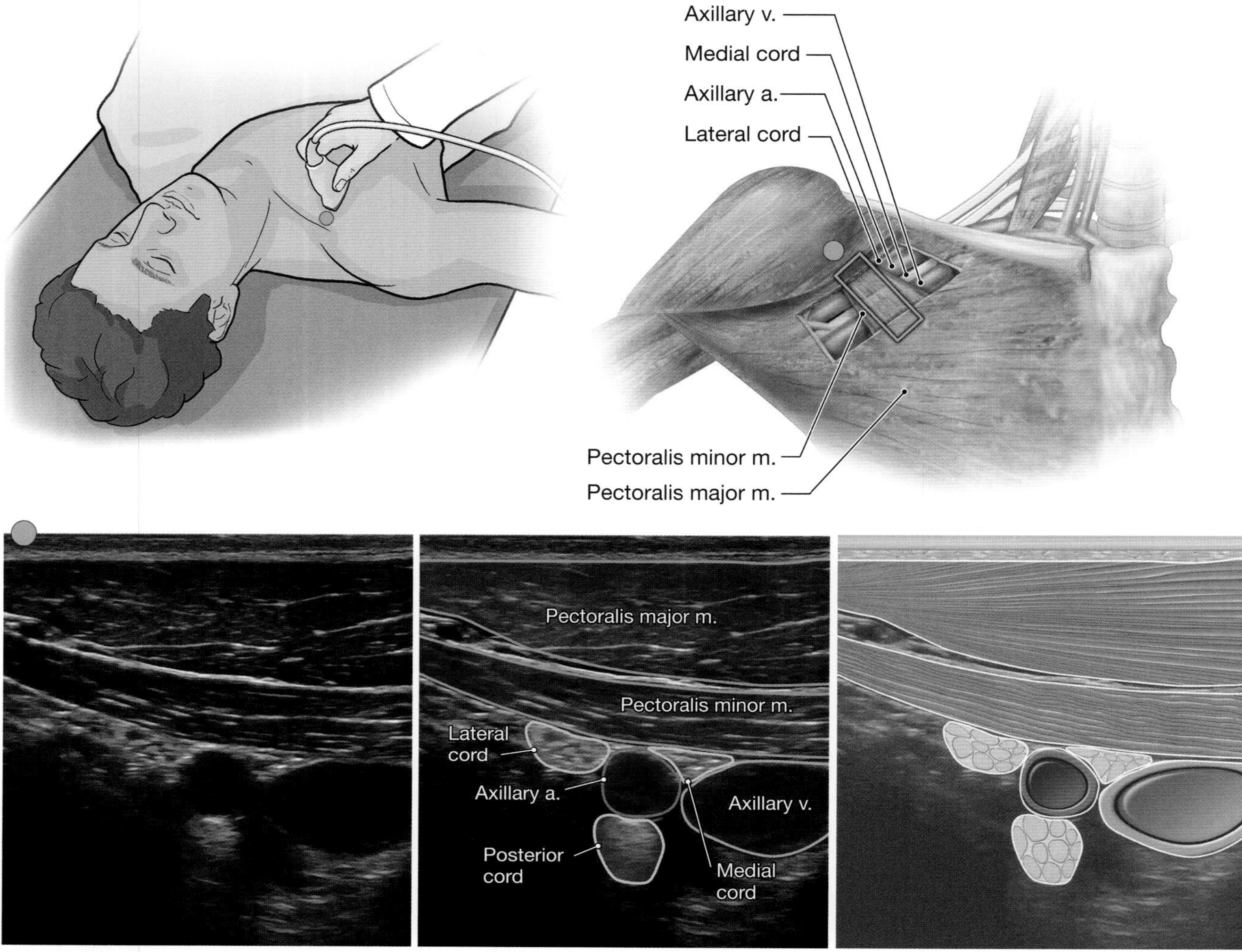

Figure 4.13 Transverse view of the cords of the brachial plexus surrounding the axillary artery, deep to the pectoralis major and minor muscles.

Arm

Review of the Anatomy

Muscles

Posterior Compartment

The main muscle of the posterior compartment of the arm is the triceps brachii. The triceps brachii is formed from three heads: the longhead, medial head, and lateral head. The three heads join and form the triceps tendon, which crosses the elbow to insert on the olecranon process of the ulna.

Anterior Compartment

There are three muscles in the anterior compartment: coracobrachialis, brachialis, and biceps brachii. Biceps brachii is superficial to coracobrachialis in the proximal half of the arm and superficial to brachialis in the distal half. The two heads of the biceps muscle (long and short) join and form the biceps tendon, which crosses the elbow through the antecubital fossa and inserts on the proximal radius. The tendon of brachialis crosses the elbow through the floor of the antecubital fossa to insert on the proximal ulna.

Nerves

Radial Nerve

The radial nerve begins in the axilla as the largest branch of the posterior cord of the brachial plexus. Along with the deep brachial artery, the nerve leaves the axilla and enters the posterior compartment of the arm by passing under the teres major muscle and between the long head of the triceps brachii and the medial aspect of the humerus. The nerve then courses diagonally in the radial groove of the humerus between the medial and lateral heads of the triceps brachii. In its course through the radial groove, the nerve is first accompanied by the deep brachial artery and then by the radial collateral artery, a terminal branch of the deep brachial. While in the radial groove, the nerve gives off muscular branches to the triceps brachii muscle and two cutaneous branches, the inferior lateral cutaneous nerve of the arm and the posterior cutaneous nerve of the forearm. The spiral course of the radial groove brings the nerve across the posterior surface of the humerus to its lateral aspect, where the nerve leaves the groove and courses for a short distance between the lateral head of the triceps brachii and brachialis muscles. The nerve then pierces the lateral intermuscular septum to enter the anterior compartment near the position where the brachioradialis muscle begins to appear at its superior-most point of origin from the humerus. The brachioradialis muscle separates the nerve from the lateral head of the triceps brachii, and the nerve comes to lie for the remainder of its course in the fascial plane between the brachioradialis and brachialis muscles. The radial nerve crosses the elbow adjacent to the cubital fossa in this fascial plane and ends near the elbow joint by dividing into its terminal branches, the deep and superficial radial nerves.

Median Nerve

The median nerve arises in the axilla from its medial and lateral roots, branches of the medial and lateral cords of the brachial plexus. The nerve leaves the axilla along the anterior surface of the axillary artery and subsequently courses through the anterior compartment of the arm immediately adjacent to the brachial artery. In the distal half of the arm, the artery and nerve lie in a groove adjacent to the biceps brachii, brachialis, and medial head of triceps brachii muscles, with the nerve at the medial surface of the artery. The median nerve has no branches in the arm. The nerve crosses the elbow joint through the cubital fossa in the fascial plane between brachialis and pronator teres to course distally through the anterior compartment of the forearm.

Ulnar Nerve

The ulnar nerve arises in the axilla from the medial cord of the brachial plexus and leaves the axilla posteromedial to the axillary artery. For the first part of its course in the arm, the nerve lies posteromedial to the brachial artery in the anterior compartment. In the middle third of the arm, the nerve pierces the medial intermuscular septum and comes to lie along the medial surface of triceps brachii. The ulnar nerve has no branches in the arm. The nerve crosses the elbow joint posteriorly through the cubital tunnel near the ulnar groove of the medial epicondyle of the humerus to continue its course in the anterior compartment of the forearm.

Musculocutaneous Nerve

The musculocutaneous nerve arises from the lateral cord of the brachial plexus and leaves the axilla by entering the substance of the coracobrachialis muscle a few centimeters proximal to its insertion on the anterior surface of the humerus. The nerve passes through coracobrachialis to emerge into the fascial plane first between coracobrachialis and biceps brachii and then between brachialis and biceps brachii. The nerve provides motor innervation to coracobrachialis, biceps brachii, and brachialis muscles, then emerges from between biceps brachii and brachialis laterally just above the elbow, where it pierces the lateral intermuscular septum and continues distally into the forearm as the lateral cutaneous nerve of the forearm.

Technique

Axillary Artery, Median Nerve, Ulnar Nerve, Radial Nerve, and Musculocutaneous Nerve

AXILLARY ARTERY
MEDIAN NERVE
ULNAR NERVE
RADIAL NERVE
MUSCULOCUTANEOUS NERVE
Transverse
FIG. 4.14

The patient should be in the supine position with the arm abducted to 90° and the elbow flexed with the back of the head resting on the palm. Palpate the inferior edge of pectoralis major muscle. Place the probe transverse to the medial surface of the arm immediately distal to the edge of pectoralis major, with the probe marker directed superiorly (laterally with respect to the anatomical position). Identify the pulsating axillary artery (3rd part), and reduce probe pressure momentarily to visualize the nearby axillary veins. Adjust the probe position as needed until the teres major muscle with the hyperechoic conjoined tendon of latissimus dorsi and teres major covering its surface can be well seen occupying half or more of the field deep to the axillary vessels and surrounding branches of the brachial plexus. The median nerve can be identified in the 9 to 12 o'clock position lateral/superficial to the axillary artery. The ulnar nerve is commonly more medial, in the 12 to 3 o'clock position relative to the artery. The large radial nerve is typically deep to the axillary artery, in the 5 to 7 o'clock position and commonly in contact with the conjoined tendon. The musculocutaneous nerve can be seen more laterally within the substance of the coracobrachialis muscle.

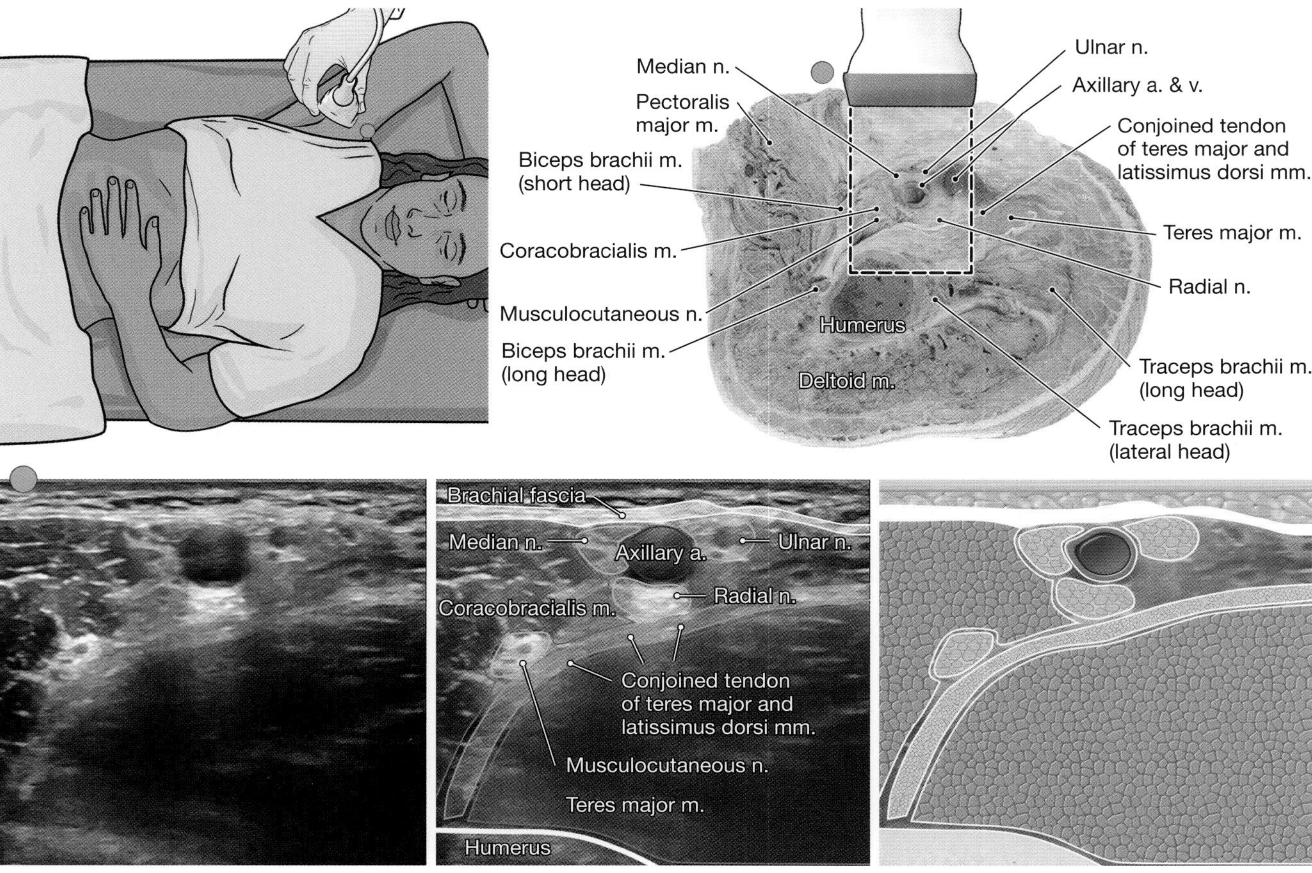

Figure 4.14 Transverse view of the 3rd part of the axillary artery, median nerve, ulnar nerve, radial nerve, and musculocutaneous nerve.

Brachial Artery, Median Nerve, Ulnar Nerve, Radial Nerve, and Musculocutaneous Nerve

BRACHIAL ARTERY
MEDIAN NERVE
ULNAR NERVE
RADIAL NERVE
MUSCULOCUTANEOUS NERVE
Transverse
FIG. 4.15

Starting from the patient and probe position described before and illustrated in Figure 4.14, slide the probe a short distance distally until the probe is just beyond the inferior margin of the teres major muscle and the long head of triceps brachii muscle can be seen in the medial aspect of the image. At the inferior margin of teres major, the artery name changes from axillary to brachial. The median and ulnar nerves maintain their relative positions superficial and medial to the brachial artery. The radial nerve moves posteriorly under teres major into a position between the humeral diaphysis and the long head of triceps brachii, accompanied by the deep brachial artery, approaching the radial groove of the humerus. The musculocutaneous nerve can be seen as it passes through the substance of coracobrachialis muscle and into the fascial plane between the coracobrachialis and biceps brachii muscle, short head.

Brachial Artery

BRACHIAL ARTERY
Longitudinal
FIG. 4.16

The patient should be in the supine position with the arm abducted to 90° and the elbow flexed with the back of the head resting on the palm, as described hereinbefore and illustrated in Figures 4.14 and 4.15. Begin by placing the probe transverse to the medial surface of the arm a short distance above the midhumerus. Position the probe such that the brachial artery is centered in the image, and then rotate the probe 90° into a longitudinal view of the artery with the probe marker directed proximally/superiorly. Adjust the probe position and tilt until the artery can be well seen across the image from superior to inferior. Reduce probe pressure as much as possible while still maintaining good

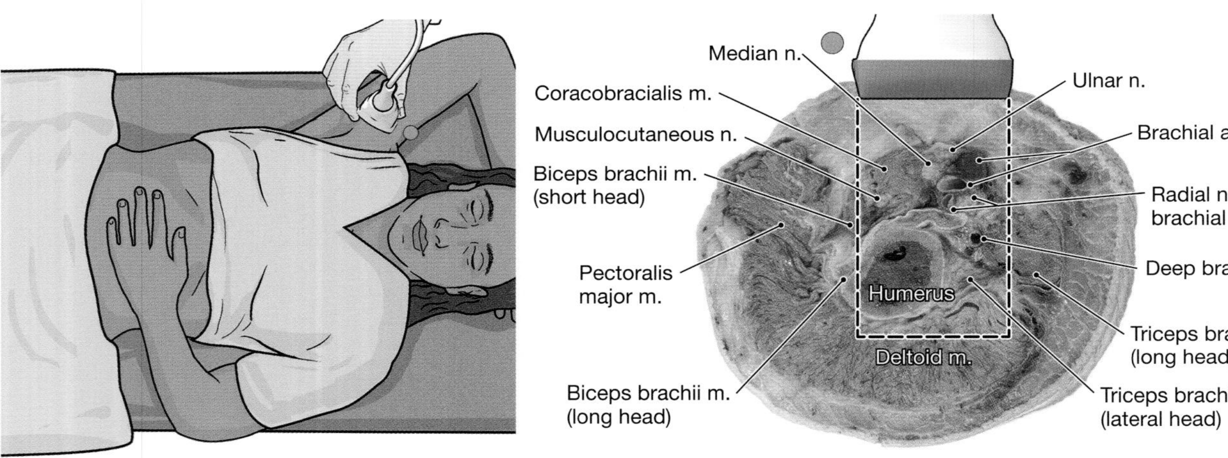

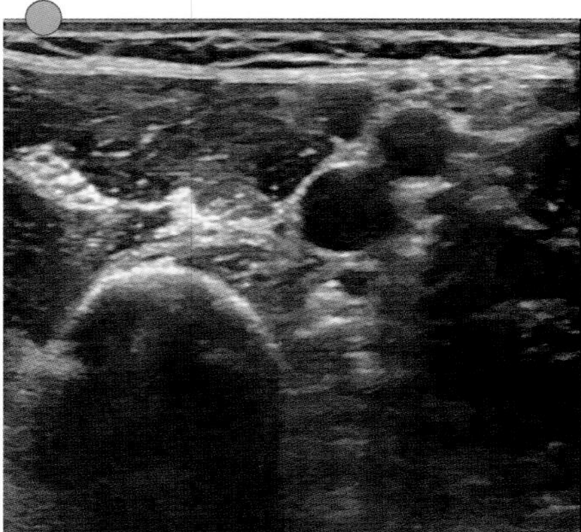

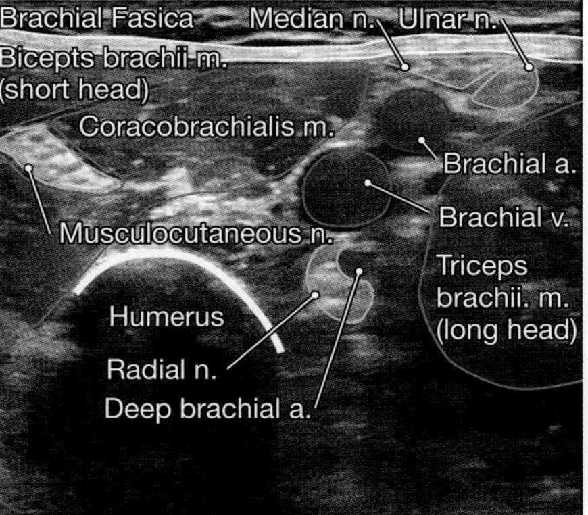

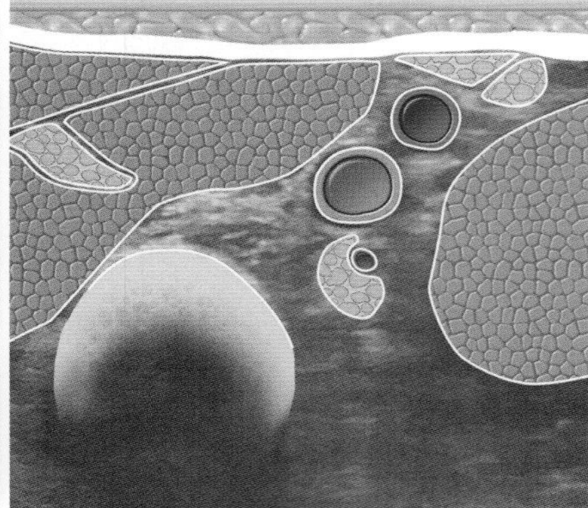

Figure 4.15 Transverse view of the brachial artery, median nerve, ulnar nerve, radial nerve, and musculocutaneous nerve.

skin contact to attempt to observe a brachial vein near the artery. Frequently, the median nerve is located superficial to the artery and can be seen along with the artery in its long axis.

Median and Ulnar Nerves Midhumerus

MID-HUMERUS
MEDIAN NERVE
ULNAR NERVE
Transverse
FIG. 4.17

The patient should be in the supine position with the arm abducted and externally rotated and the forearm supinated and slightly flexed. Position the probe transverse to the medial aspect of the arm a few centimeters distal to the mid-humerus level, with the probe marker facing anteriorly. Identify the hyperechoic cortex of the humerus, biceps brachii, brachialis, and medial head of triceps brachii. Look for the pulsations of the brachial artery and identify the large hyperechoic median nerve at the medial surface of the artery. Identify the ulnar nerve 1 to 2 cm posterior to the brachial artery/median nerve, between the surface of the medial head of triceps and the overlying subcutaneous fat. In the subcutaneous fat between the positions of the median and ulnar nerves, the small hyperechoic medial cutaneous nerve of the forearm can usually be identified. By exerting the least pressure possible on the probe face while still maintaining good skin contact, the brachial veins alongside the brachial artery and the basilic vein in subcutaneous fat should become visible.

Radial Nerve

MID-HUMERUS RADIAL NERVE
Transverse
FIG. 4.18

Begin with the patient in the supine position with the limb adducted, the elbow slightly flexed, and the forearm supinated. Position the probe transverse to the lateral aspect of the arm at about the mid-humerus level. Direct the probe marker such that as you follow the nerve distally and the probe moves toward the anterior surface of the limb, the marker ends up directed toward the patient's right side (for the right

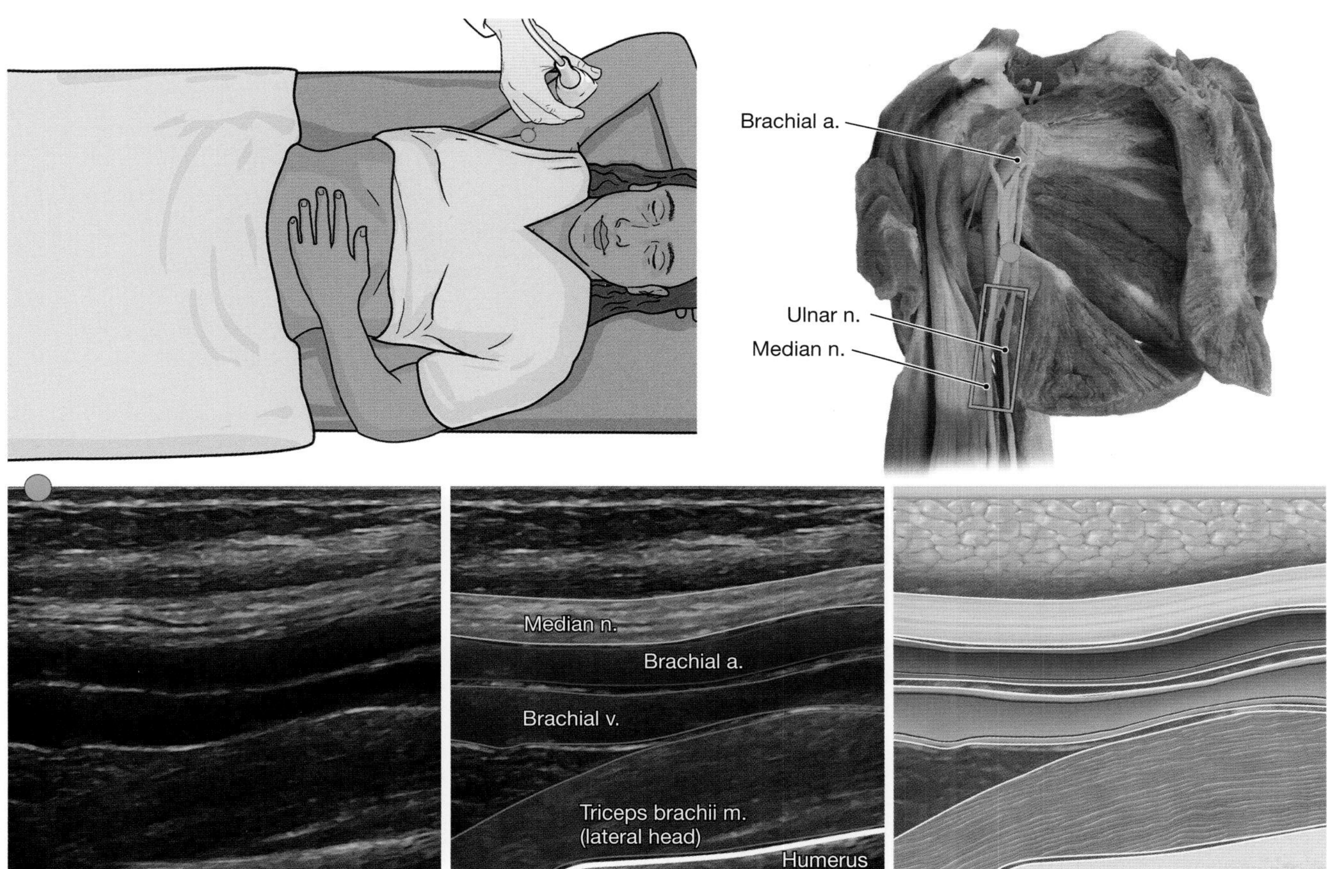

Figure 4.16 Longitudinal view of the brachial artery, brachial vein, and the median nerve.

limb, this means that initially, the probe marker should be directed posteriorly). Identify the hyperechoic cortex of the humerus, the triceps brachii muscle posteriorly, and the brachialis muscle at the anterolateral aspect of the humeral shaft. From this starting position, move the probe superiorly and inferiorly along the lateral aspect of the arm until you can identify the hyperechoic oval profile of the radial nerve as it emerges from the radial groove. The nerve becomes more readily visible as it moves away from the hyperechoic surface of the humerus into the fascial plane between the lateral head of triceps brachii and brachialis, accompanied by the radial collateral artery. The lateral intermuscular septum is seen as a thin hyperechoic fascial band between triceps brachii and brachialis.

PROXIMAL TO ELBOW JOINT RADIAL NERVE
Transverse
FIG. 4.19

Keeping the radial nerve centered in the image, continue scanning a short distance distally and observe that the brachioradialis muscle, as it originates from the lateral supracondylar ridge of the humerus, begins to appear between the lateral head of the triceps brachii and brachialis muscles. At this point, the radial nerve is separated from the lateral head of triceps brachii and comes to lie between the brachioradialis and brachialis muscles. One of the two cutaneous branches of the nerve that arise along its course in the radial groove, the posterior cutaneous nerve of the forearm, may commonly be seen (along with the radial collateral artery) as it diverges from the main trunk of the radial nerve near the brachioradialis muscle. As the brachioradialis muscle appears, the lateral head of the triceps brachii and the posterior cutaneous nerve of the forearm end up on the superficial (posterolateral) aspect of the brachioradialis muscle, whereas the radial nerve and brachialis muscle end up on its deep (anteromedial) aspect. The radial nerve can be followed distally in the fascial plane between the brachioradialis and brachialis for the remainder of its course, until it ends by dividing into its terminal branches anterior to the elbow joint.

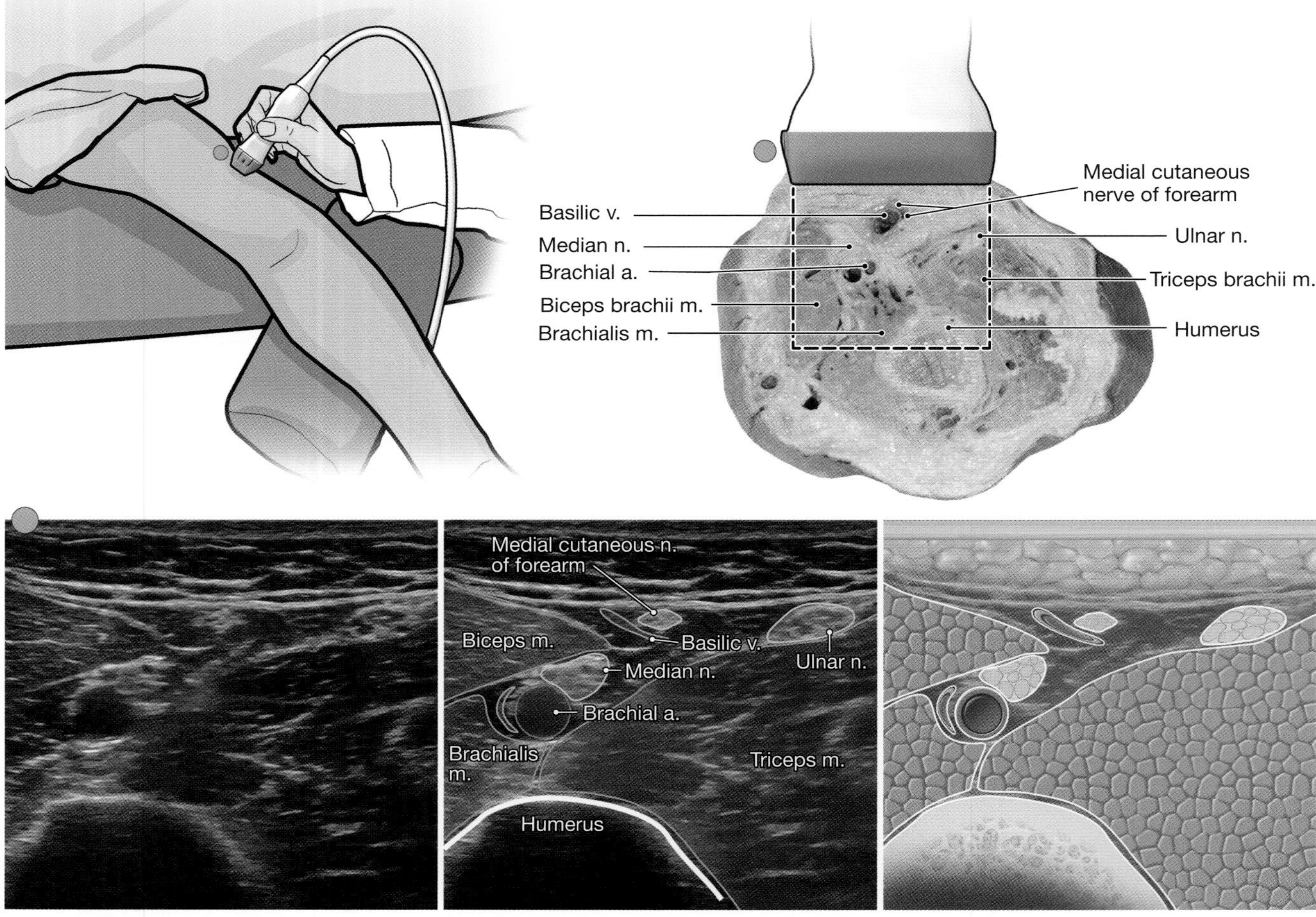

Figure 4.17 Transverse view of the median nerve alongside the brachial artery and the ulnar nerve at the superficial surface of triceps brachii muscle, just distal to the midhumerus.

CLINICAL APPLICATION

In the axilla and proximal arm, ultrasound guidance is commonly used for infiltration of local anesthetic agents around the median, ulnar, radial, and musculocutaneous nerves for regional anesthesia and postoperative pain control in limb surgeries from the mid-arm distally.

Ultrasound examination of the median and ulnar nerves in the mid-arm and distally is used for evaluation of possible nerve entrapment and compressive neuropathy in the distal half of the arm involving osteophytes and/or ligamentous bands. These techniques can also be used for needle guidance and infiltration of local anesthetic agents for regional anesthesia, although more distal sites (ie, near the wrist) are more commonly utilized for median and ulnar blocks.

These techniques can be used for guiding a needle alongside the radial nerve for infiltration of a local anesthetic agent to produce a radial nerve block. Radial nerve blocks may be used in upper limb surgeries distal to the elbow (commonly as an add-on regional anesthesia in addition to the brachial plexus block), for postoperative pain control, or in the differential diagnosis of pain distal to the elbow. Ultrasound examination of the radial nerve may also be used for evaluation of possible nerve entrapment such as those that may occur in the presence of fractures involving the mid-diaphysis or lateral epicondyle of the humerus.

Ultrasound examination of peripheral arteries is used for assessing stenosis/occlusion such as that in peripheral artery disease or thrombosis, and for detecting, measuring and following arterial aneurysms/dissections. Peripheral veins are most commonly assessed with ultrasound for detection of deep vein thrombosis or venous insufficiency.

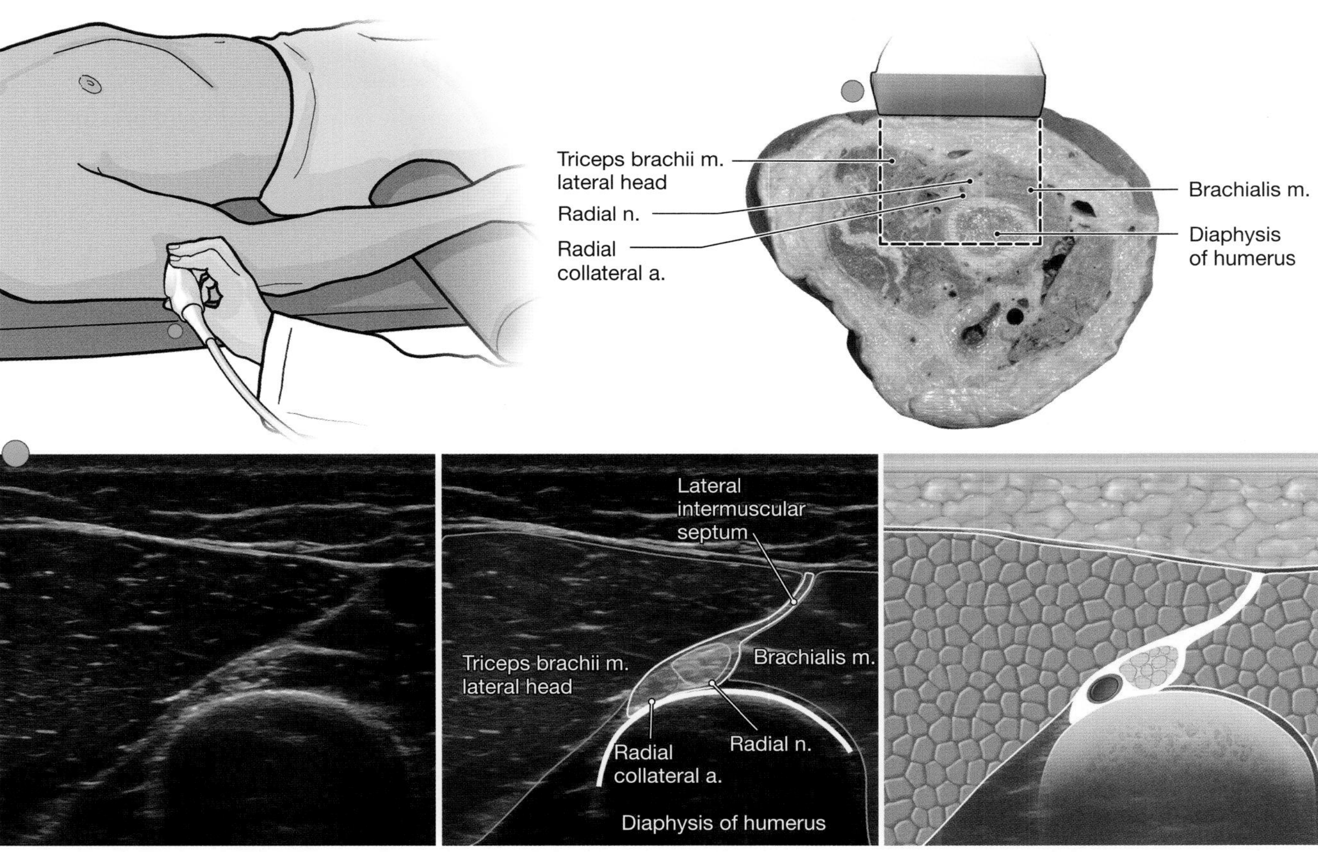

Figure 4.18 Transverse view of the radial nerve in the plane between the lateral head of triceps brachii and brachialis muscles, accompanied by the radial collateral artery.

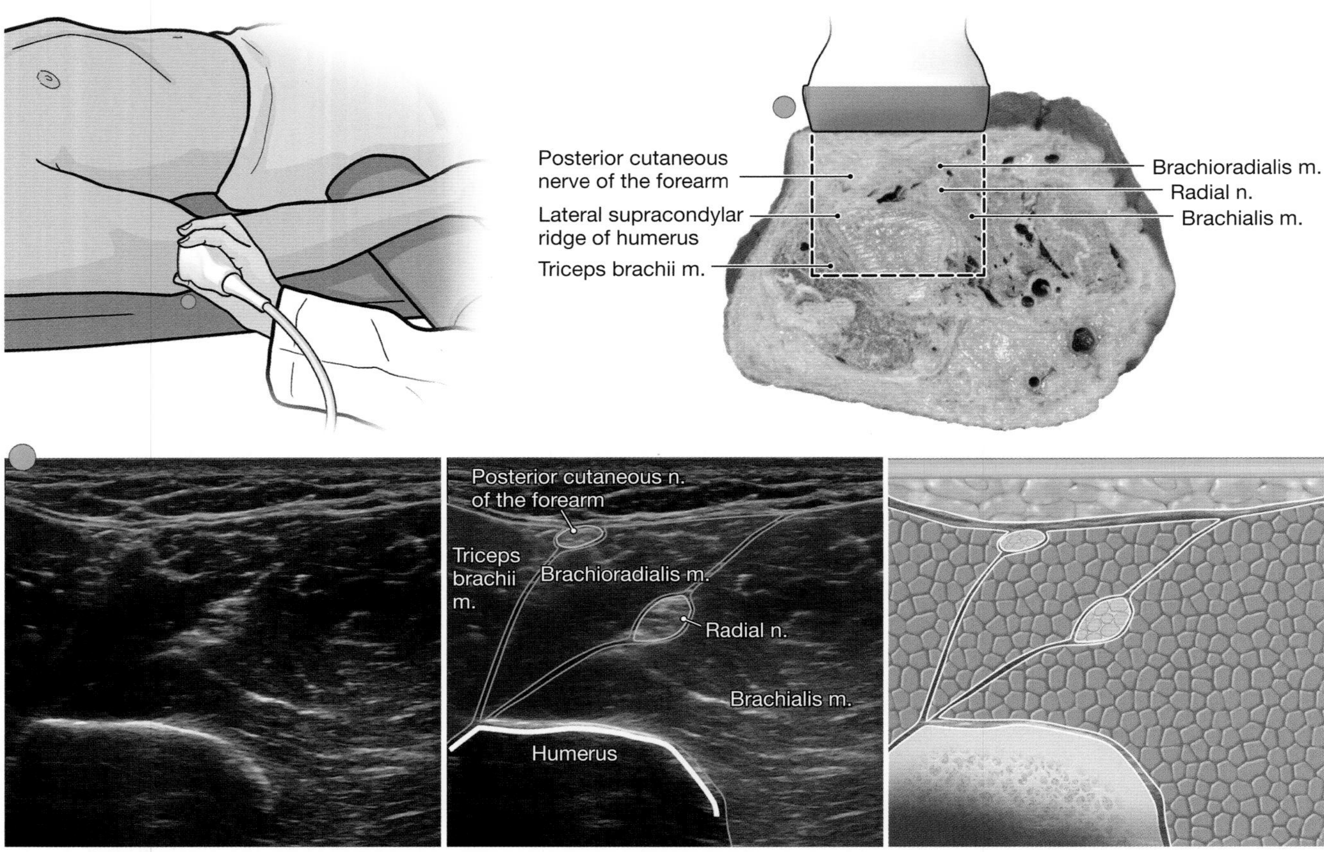

Figure 4.19 Transverse view of the radial nerve in the fascial plane between the brachioradialis and brachialis muscles, a few centimeters proximal to the elbow joint.

Elbow

Review of Anatomy

Elbow Joint

The elbow joint consists of three articulations between the humerus, radius, and ulna, all within a common joint capsule and synovial space. The articular surface of the humerus consists of the capitulum, which articulates with the head of the radius and the trochlea, which articulates with the trochlear notch of the ulna. The radial notch of the ulna articulates with the radial head. There are two anterior fossae on the humerus just above the articular surface: the radial fossa, which accommodates the radial head in flexion, and the coronoid fossa, which accommodates the coronoid process of the ulna in flexion. The olecranon fossa on the posterior surface of the humerus accommodates the olecranon process of the ulna in extension. Fat pads that separate the fibrous joint capsule from the synovial lining in these fossae are clinically referred to as the anterior fat pad (in the coronoid and radial fossae) and the posterior fat pad (in the olecranon fossa). The joint capsule is thickened to form the ulnar and radial collateral ligaments, and there is a thickened ring at the radial head, the annular ligament.

Muscles

The tendon of triceps brachii passes over the posterior fat pad and crosses the elbow joint to insert on the olecranon process of the ulna. Pronator teres and muscles arising from the common flexor tendon cross from the medial epicondyle to enter the anterior forearm compartment. Extensor muscles cross the elbow from the lateral epicondyle and supracondylar ridge to enter the posterior compartment of the forearm. The tendon of biceps brachii crosses the elbow joint through the cubital fossa to insert on the radial tuberosity. A tendinous sheet, the bicipital aponeurosis, extends from the medial side of the biceps tendon and attaches over the pronator teres muscle and proximal muscle mass of the common flexor tendon. The brachialis tendon crosses from the floor of the cubital fossa to insert on the ulnar tuberosity.

Cubital Fossa

The cubital fossa is a triangular depression at the anterior elbow formed by the brachioradialis muscle laterally, the pronator teres muscle medially, and a line interconnecting the humeral epicondyles superiorly. The brachialis muscle forms the bed of the fossa. Contents of the fossa include the biceps tendon, the brachial artery and accompanying veins, and the median nerve. The median cubital vein lies in the roof of the fossa, which is formed by skin and superficial fascia. The brachial artery normally bifurcates into the radial and ulnar arteries in the cubital fossa, although this division sometimes occurs more proximally in the axilla or arm.

Nerves

Radial Nerve

The radial nerve crosses the elbow joint just lateral to the cubital fossa in the fascial plane between brachioradialis and brachialis. The radial nerve continues distally, crossing anterior to the elbow joint at the part between the radius and the capitulum of the humerus where it divides into its terminal branches, the deep and the superficial radial nerves. The deep radial nerve courses posteriorly and enters the substance of the supinator muscle, traveling between two layers of the muscle into the posterior compartment of the forearm, emerging as the posterior interosseous nerve of the forearm. The superficial radial nerve joins the radial artery and continues distally in the anterior compartment under the brachioradialis muscle, winding across its distal tendon to supply the skin over the anatomical "snuffbox," dorsal aspect of the hand, thumb, and proximal index and middle fingers.

Median Nerve

The median nerve crosses the elbow joint through the cubital fossa in the fascial plane between the brachialis and pronator teres, just medial to the brachial artery. The bicipital aponeurosis forms a protective layer over the contents of this fascial plane. The nerve enters the anterior compartment of the forearm by passing between the humeral and ulnar heads of pronator teres to continue its course in the forearm between the flexor digitorum superficialis and flexor digitorum profundus muscles and then crosses the wrist through the carpal tunnel into the hand.

Ulnar Nerve

The ulnar nerve leaves the posterior compartment of the arm by crossing the elbow joint posteriorly through the cubital tunnel near the ulnar groove of the medial epicondyle of the humerus. The arcuate ligament, which spans between the humeral and ulnar heads of flexor carpi ulnaris near their origins, forms the roof of the cubital tunnel, and the posterior layer of the ulnar collateral ligament of the elbow forms the floor (over the elbow joint capsule and ulnar groove of the humerus). The nerve enters the anterior compartment of the forearm between the two heads of the flexor carpi ulnaris and courses through the forearm between the flexor carpi ulnaris and flexor digitorum profundus and then crosses the wrist into the hand.

Technique

Cubital Fossa

CUBITAL FOSSA LATERAL CONTENTS
Transverse
FIG. 4.20

The patient should be supine with the forearm supinated. A small pillow/bolster should be placed under the wrist to help maintain slight flexion at the elbow joint. Place the probe transversely over the elbow crease (probe marker toward the right), and adjust the position until you can clearly identify the hyperechoic profile of the capitulum and trochlea of the humerus. Identify the hyperechoic radial nerve in the fascial plane between the brachioradialis and brachialis muscles. The radial nerve typically divides into its deep and superficial branches near this position, giving it a bilobar appearance, and parts of one or both branches may appear hypoechoic because of anisotropy. By applying as little pressure as possible, identify the median cubital vein in the superficial fascia. Identify the biceps tendon at the surface of the brachialis muscle. The bicipital aponeurosis extends medially from the biceps tendon over the fascial plane between the brachialis and pronator teres.

CUBITAL FOSSA MEDIAL CONTENTS
Transverse
FIG. 4.21

Keeping the humeral trochlea in view, slide the probe medially until the pronator teres and the fascial plane between the brachialis and pronator teres can be identified. In the superficial part of the fascial plane, locate the brachial artery and median nerve, and once again identify the bicipital aponeurosis bridging over the space between the two muscles.

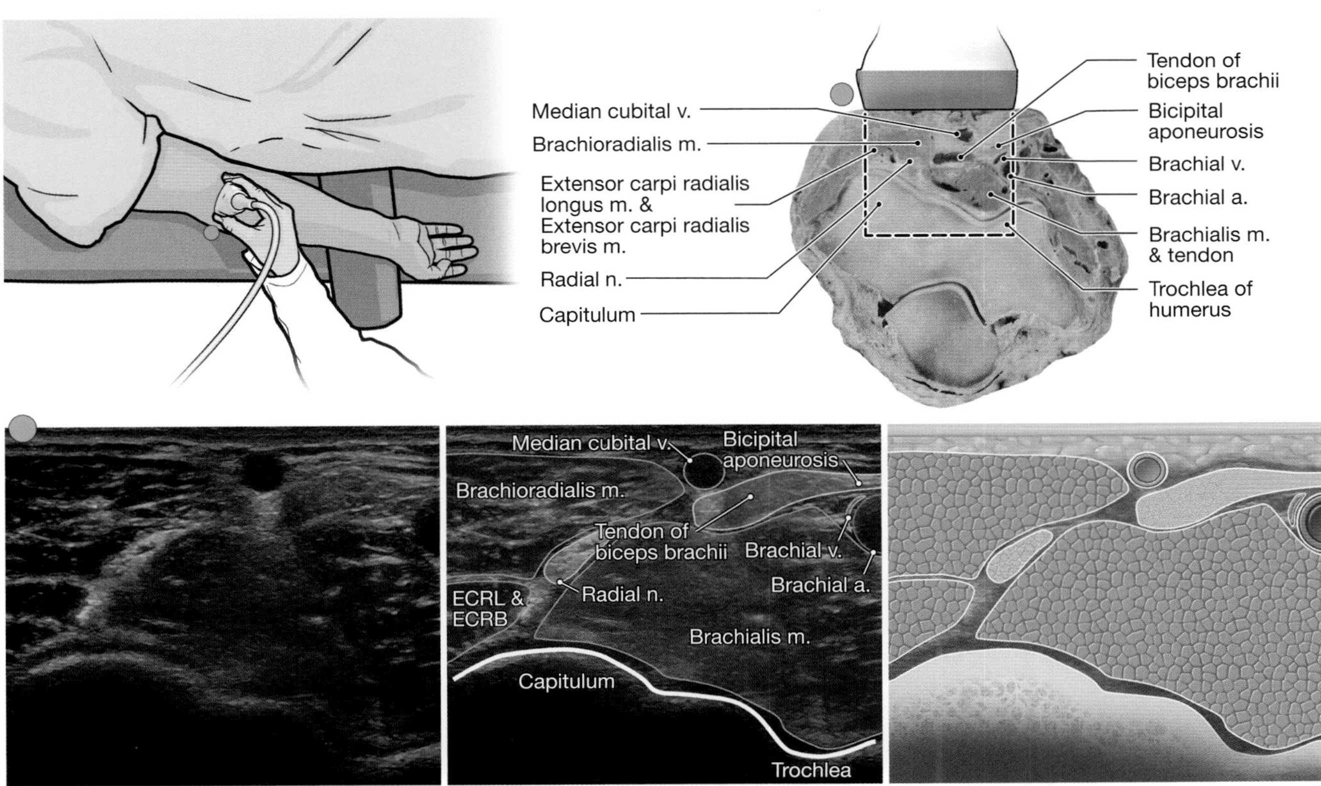

Figure 4.20 Transverse view of the lateral aspect of the cubital fossa and its contents. ECRB, extensor carpi radialis brevis; ECRL, extensor carpi radialis longus.

Superficial and Deep Radial Nerves

SUPERFICIAL RADIAL NERVE DEEP RADIAL NERVE
Transverse
FIG. 4.22

Slide the probe laterally until the radial nerve is once again centered over the humeral capitulum. Slowly move the probe distally, following the radial nerve branches over the radial head and then over the supinator muscle surrounding the radial neck. With careful observation, the superficial and deep branches can be seen to diverge, with the deep radial nerve moving laterally/deeply into the substance of the supinator muscle and the superficial radial nerve moving medially just underneath the brachioradialis. Because of its oblique course, the deep radial nerve is more difficult to follow. The superficial radial nerve can be followed distally under the brachioradialis muscle until it moves alongside the radial artery.

Elbow Joint

ELBOW JOINT HUMEROULNAR COMPONENT
Longitudinal
FIG. 4.23

Slide the probe medially until it is centered over the humeral trochlea. Rotate the probe 90° (marker directed superiorly) into the longitudinal axis of the humeroulnar joint. Adjust the position until the hyperechoic profile of the trochlea and coronoid fossa of the humerus and coronoid process of the ulna can be identified. The articular cartilage over the joint surfaces appears anechoic/hypoechoic. The fibrous joint capsule appears hyperechoic, and the anterior fat pad can be seen occupying the coronoid fossa inside the joint capsule. Identify the brachialis and pronator teres muscles overlying the joint.

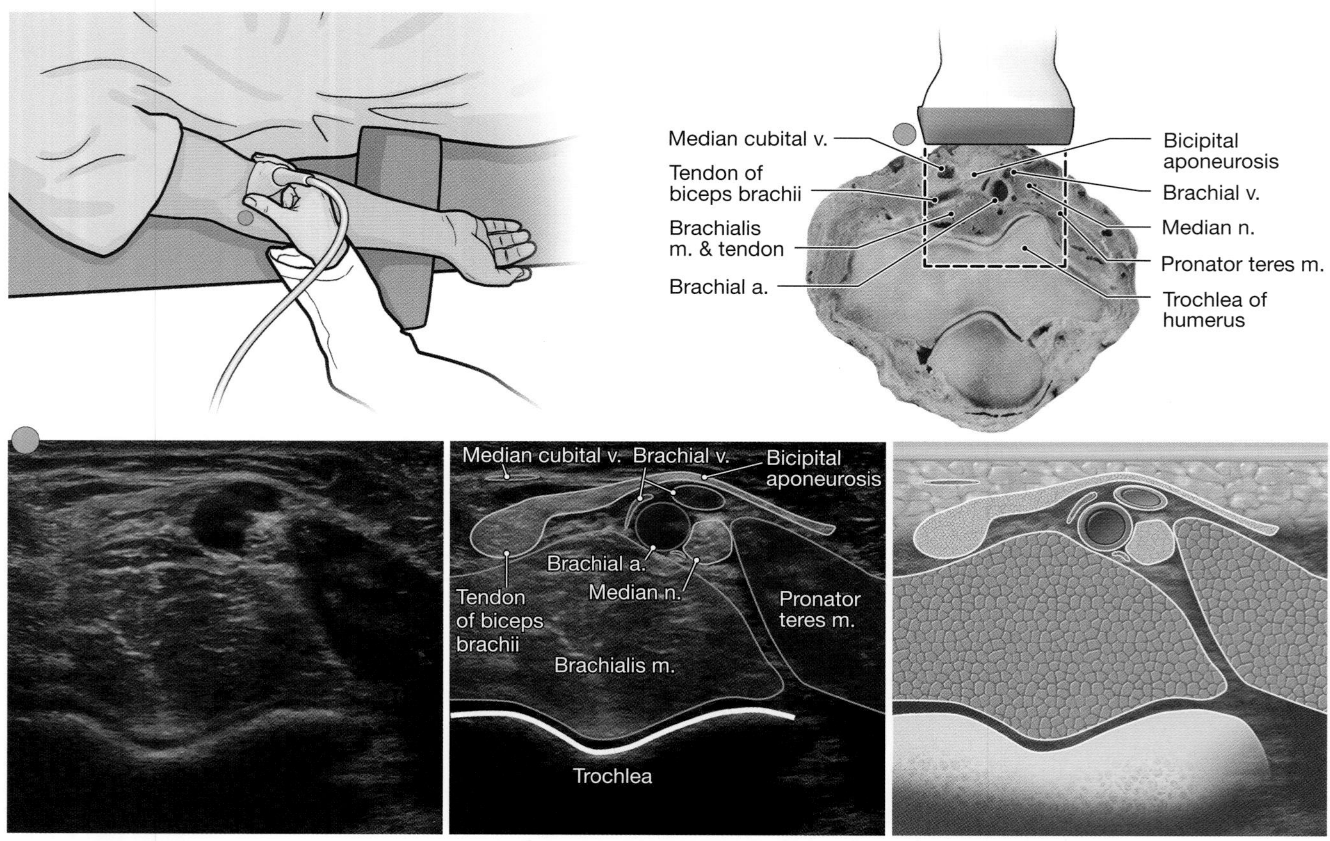

Figure 4.21 Transverse view of the medial aspect of the cubital fossa and its contents.

ELBOW JOINT
HUMERORADIAL (RADIOCAPITELLAR) COMPONENT
Longitudinal
FIG. 4.24

Center the probe transversely over the capitulum and rotate the probe 90° into the longitudinal axis of the humeroradial joint (radiocapitellar joint). Adjust the position until the profile of the capitulum of the humerus, radial head, and proximal part of the radial neck can be identified. Identify the joint capsule and articular cartilage of the humeroradial joint. Locate the annular ligament, a thickening of the joint capsule ringing the head of the radius. The radial fossa can be seen just superior to the capitulum. The lateral aspect of the brachialis muscle can be seen overlying the joint, and the supinator muscle surrounds the neck of the radius just over the distal attachment of the joint capsule.

Ulnar Nerve in the Cubital Tunnel

CUBITAL TUNNEL
ULNAR NERVE
Transverse
FIG. 4.25

The patient should be supine with the arm abducted and externally rotated and the elbow slightly flexed. By palpation, identify the medial epicondyle of the humerus and the tip of the olecranon process of the ulna. Place the probe across these bony landmarks with the marker side over the olecranon process. Identify the hyperechoic profile of the olecranon process, the humeroulnar joint space, and the ulnar groove and prominence of the medial epicondyle of the humerus. The ulnar nerve commonly appears as a hypoechoic/anechoic oval (because of anisotropy), but by tilting/fanning the probe its honeycomb appearance can usually be accentuated. Identify the hyperechoic band of

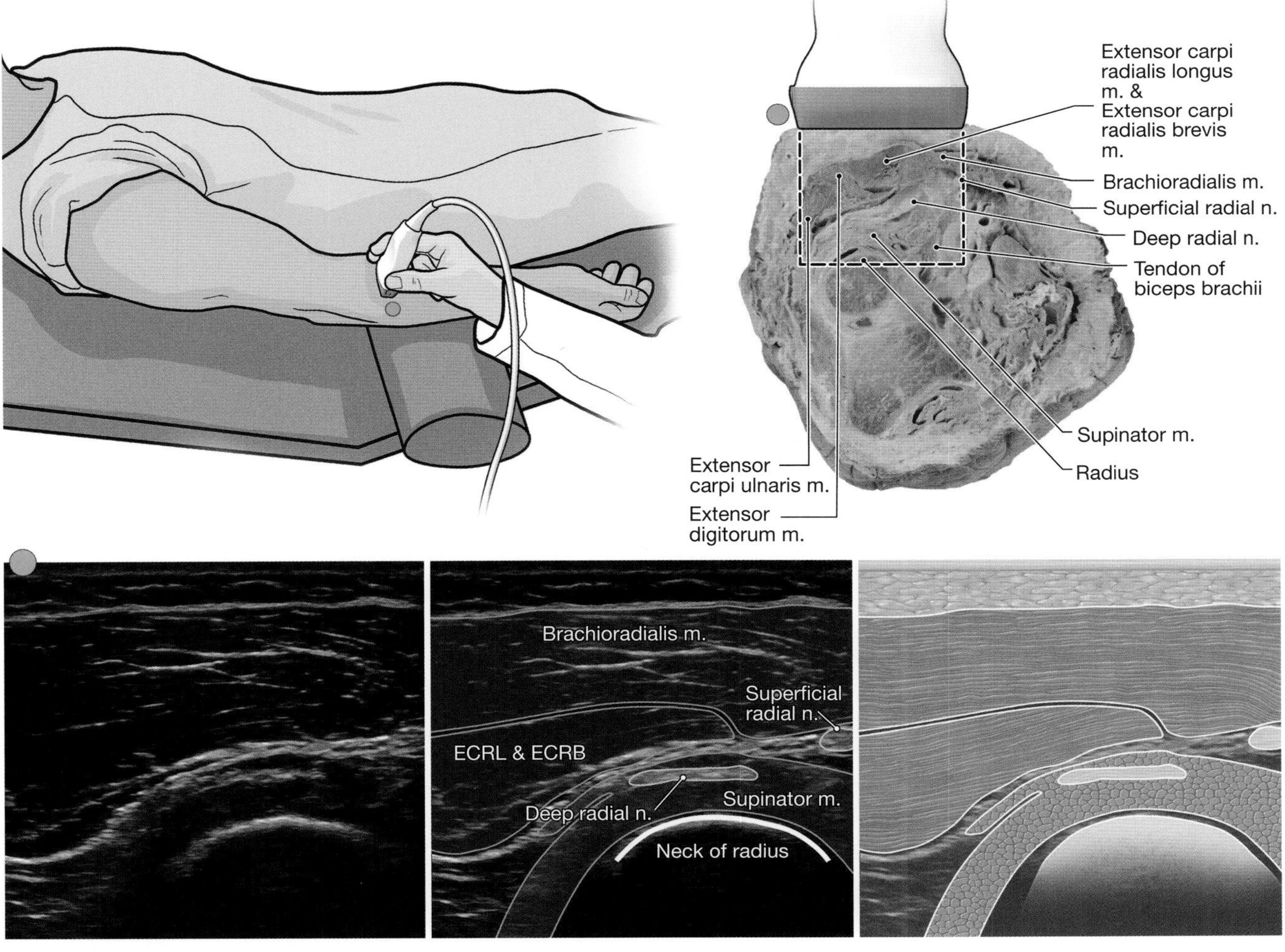

Figure 4.22 Transverse view of the superficial and deep branches of the radial nerve at the lateral aspect of the forearm just distal to the elbow joint.

aponeurosis of the flexor carpi ulnaris (arcuate ligament) immediately superficial to the nerve spanning over and between the humeral and ulnar heads of the flexor carpi ulnaris (you may need to slide the probe distally beyond the ulnar groove to visualize and identify the two heads of the muscle). Immediately deep to the nerve, identify the hyperechoic fibrillar appearance of the posterior layer of the ulnar collateral ligament.

Keeping the nerve and the two heads of the flexor carpi ulnaris in view, slide the probe distally a short distance beyond the cubital tunnel and observe as the two heads join together over the nerve (the hyperechoic honeycomb appearance of the nerve is more readily apparent in this position).

Triceps Brachii Muscle and Tendon

TRICEPS BRACHII MYOTENDINOUS JUNCTION
Longitudinal
FIG. 4.26

The patient should be seated alongside the examination table. The arm should be abducted and the elbow flexed to about 90°, and the forearm fully pronated with the palm on the table surface (the "crab" position). Place the probe over the olecranon process and the distal triceps brachii muscle in the longitudinal axis of the arm (marker directed toward the shoulder). Adjust the probe position until the bony profile of the olecranon process of the ulna and the olecranon fossa of the humerus can be identified. The posterior fat pad can be seen in the olecranon fossa deep to the fibrous joint capsule. The distal triceps brachii muscle, myotendinous junction, and hyperechoic fibrillar triceps brachii tendon can be seen crossing over the olecranon fossa and joint space to the olecranon process.

TENDON OF TRICEPS BRACHII
Longitudinal
FIG. 4.27

Slide the probe distally along the triceps brachii tendon until the tapering beak of the tendon insertion onto the olecranon process can be identified.

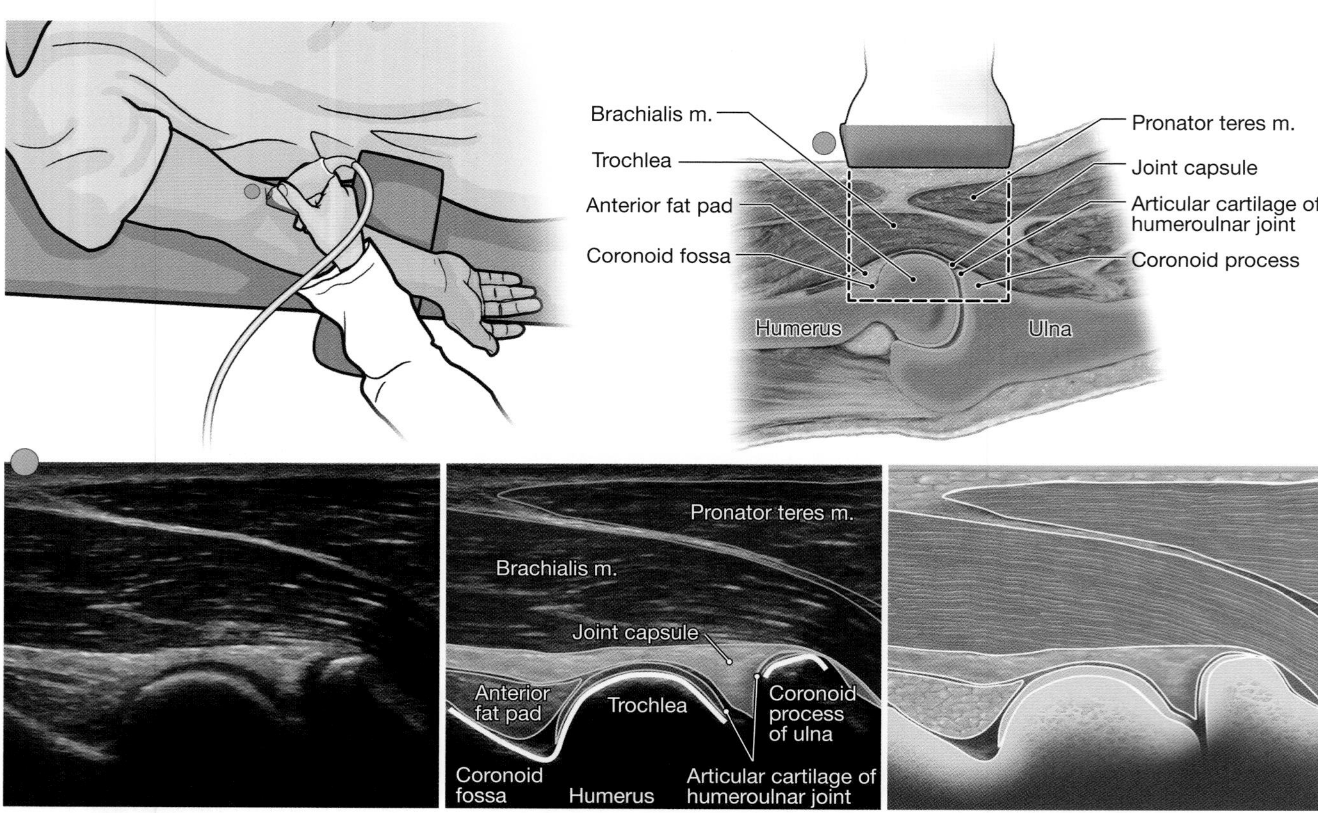

Figure 4.23 Longitudinal view of the humeroulnar component of the elbow joint.

Common Flexor Tendon and Ulnar Collateral Ligament

COMMON FLEXOR TENDON ULNAR COLLATERAL LIGAMENT
Longitudinal
FIG. 4.28

The patient should be supine with the arm abducted and externally rotated and the elbow flexed to approximately 90°. Place the marker end of the probe over the anterior surface of the medial epicondyle along the longitudinal axis of the forearm. The probe should be tilted such that the ultrasound beam is directed from anterior to posterior (not across the elbow from medial to lateral). Adjust the position and tilt until the prominence of the medial epicondyle, the concavity between the epicondyle and the margin of the trochlea, the humeroulnar joint space, and the margin of the trochlear notch of the ulna can be seen. Identify the normally short hyperechoic common flexor tendon and the myotendinous junction of the common flexor muscle mass. The anterior layer of the ulnar collateral ligament can be seen spanning the joint space immediately deep to the common flexor tendon and muscle.

Common Extensor Tendon and Radial Collateral Ligament

COMMON EXTENSOR TENDON RADIAL COLLATERAL LIGAMENT
FIG. 4.29

The patient should be supine with the arm adducted, the elbow slightly flexed, and the forearm in mid-pronation with the ulnar border of the hand resting on the upper thigh. Position the probe along the longitudinal axis of the forearm with the marker end of the probe over the lateral epicondyle. Adjust the probe position until the hyperechoic profile of the lateral epicondyle of the humerus and the head of the radius can be identified. Locate the tapering beak of the common extensor origin from the lateral epicondyle and identify the annular ligament at the radial head (tilting/fanning the probe as needed to accentuate its echogenicity). Identify the radial collateral ligament at the deep surface of the common extensor tendon, spanning from the slight concavity along lateral epicondyle across the humeroradial joint and fusing with the annular ligament.

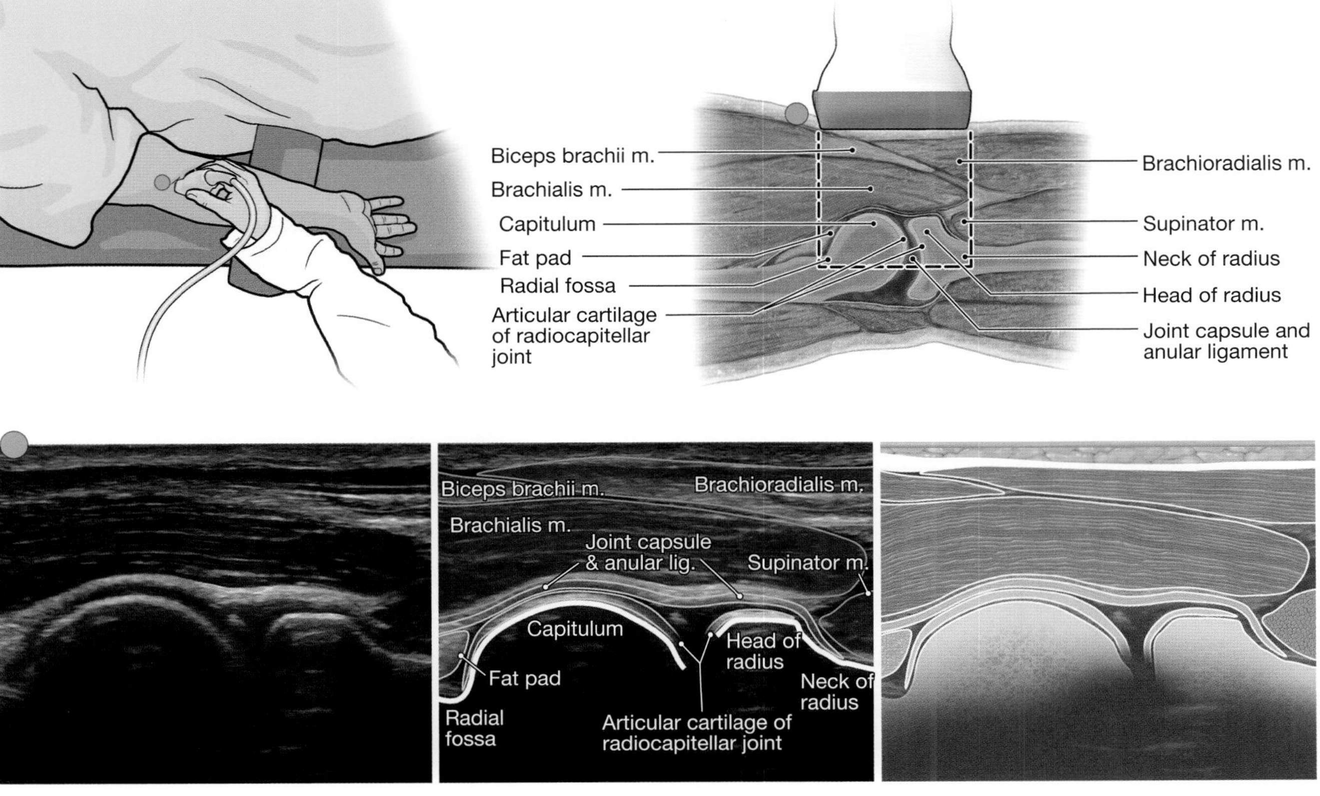

Figure 4.24 Longitudinal view of the humeroradial (radiocapitellar) component of the elbow joint.

CLINICAL APPLICATION

These techniques can be used for guiding needles alongside the radial, median, or ulnar nerves for infiltration of local anesthetic agents to produce nerve blocks. Radial nerve blocks may be used in upper limb surgeries distal to the elbow (commonly as add-on regional anesthesia in addition to brachial plexus block), for postoperative pain control, or in the differential diagnosis of pain distal to the elbow. With ultrasound guidance, the median nerve can be blocked in the cubital fossa alongside the brachial artery and accompanying veins. Ulnar nerve blocks at the elbow should be proximal to the cubital tunnel to avoid possible nerve compression resulting from injection of an anesthetic fluid around the nerve within the relatively limited space of the tunnel. The forearm and wrist are more common sites for median and ulnar blocks.

Ultrasound examination of these nerves may also be used for evaluation of possible nerve entrapment. The posterior interosseous branch nerve can be entrapped in its course through the supinator muscle. The median nerve can be entrapped in its course between the heads of pronator teres, and the cubital tunnel is a common site of ulnar nerve entrapment and compression. The ulnar nerve can also subluxate/dislocate from the cubital tunnel over the anterior surface of the medial epicondyle with flexion/extension.

Ultrasound examination can be used for cannulating veins (eg, median cubital, cephalic, and basilic) and for evaluation of brachial artery aneurysm or stenosis.

Ultrasound examination can be used for evaluation of possible biceps, common flexor, or common extensor tendonitis/tendinosis or ligamentous strains and tears (eg, ulnar collateral and radial collateral ligaments of the elbow). The anterior and posterior fat pads are displaced from their fossae when fluid accumulates within the joint space (joint effusion or bleeding into the joint space in the presence of intra-articular fractures), and these techniques can be used for needle guidance into the elbow joint space for aspiration or injection.

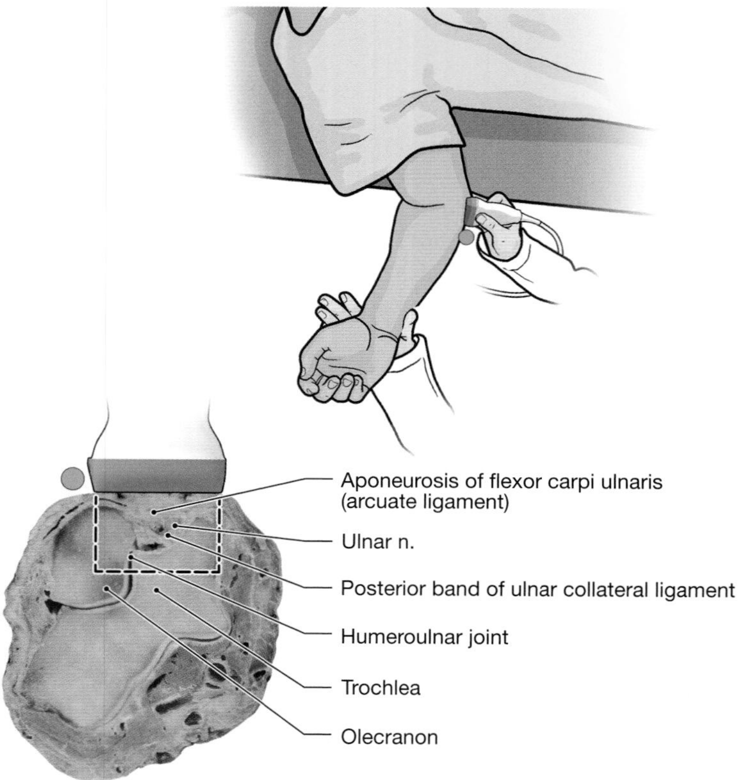

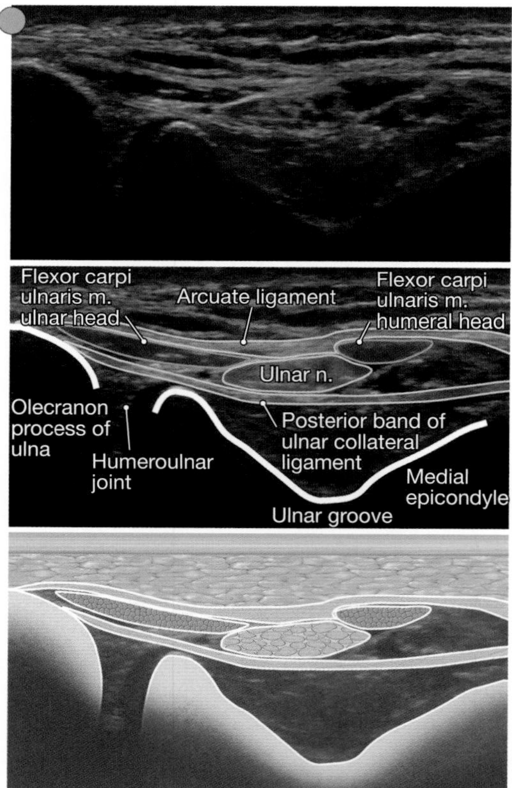

Figure 4.25 Transverse view of the ulnar nerve in the cubital tunnel.

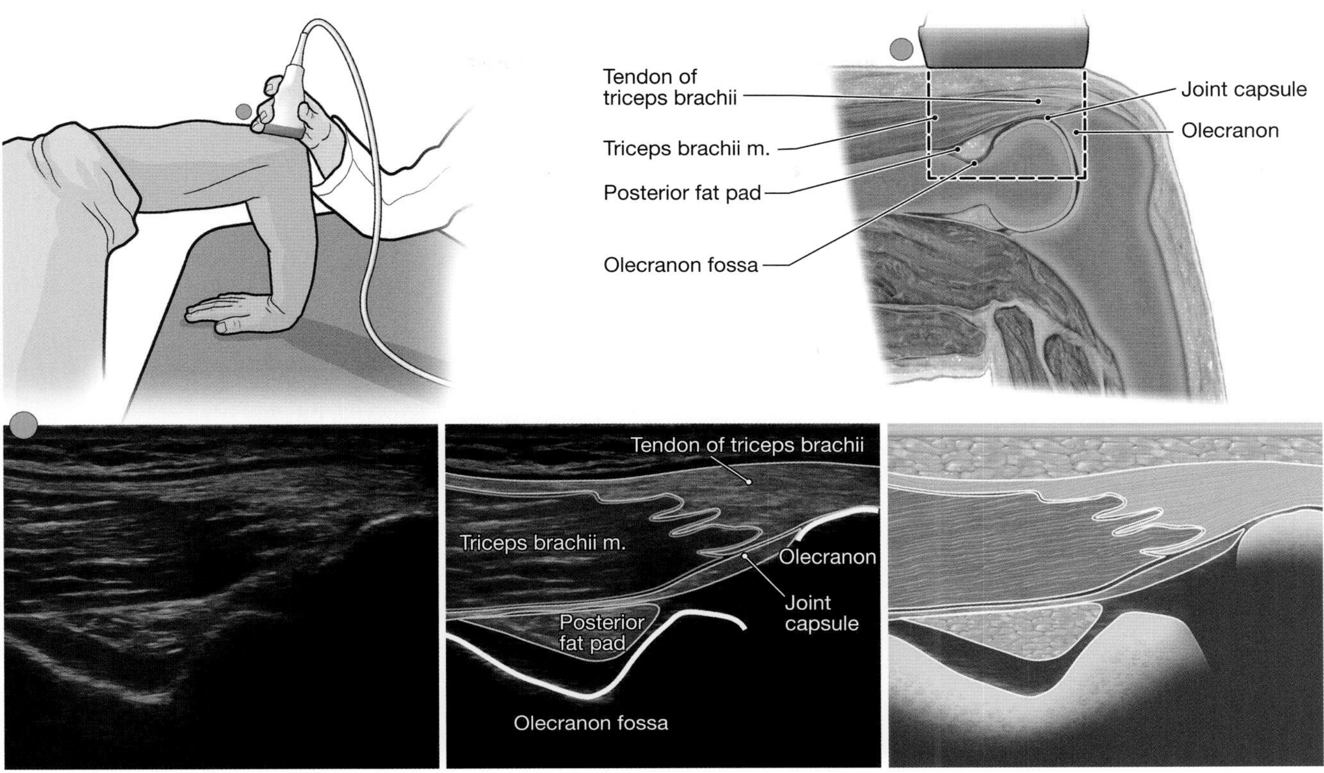

Figure 4.26 Longitudinal view of the triceps brachii muscle, myotendinous junction, and tendon at the posterior aspect of the elbow joint.

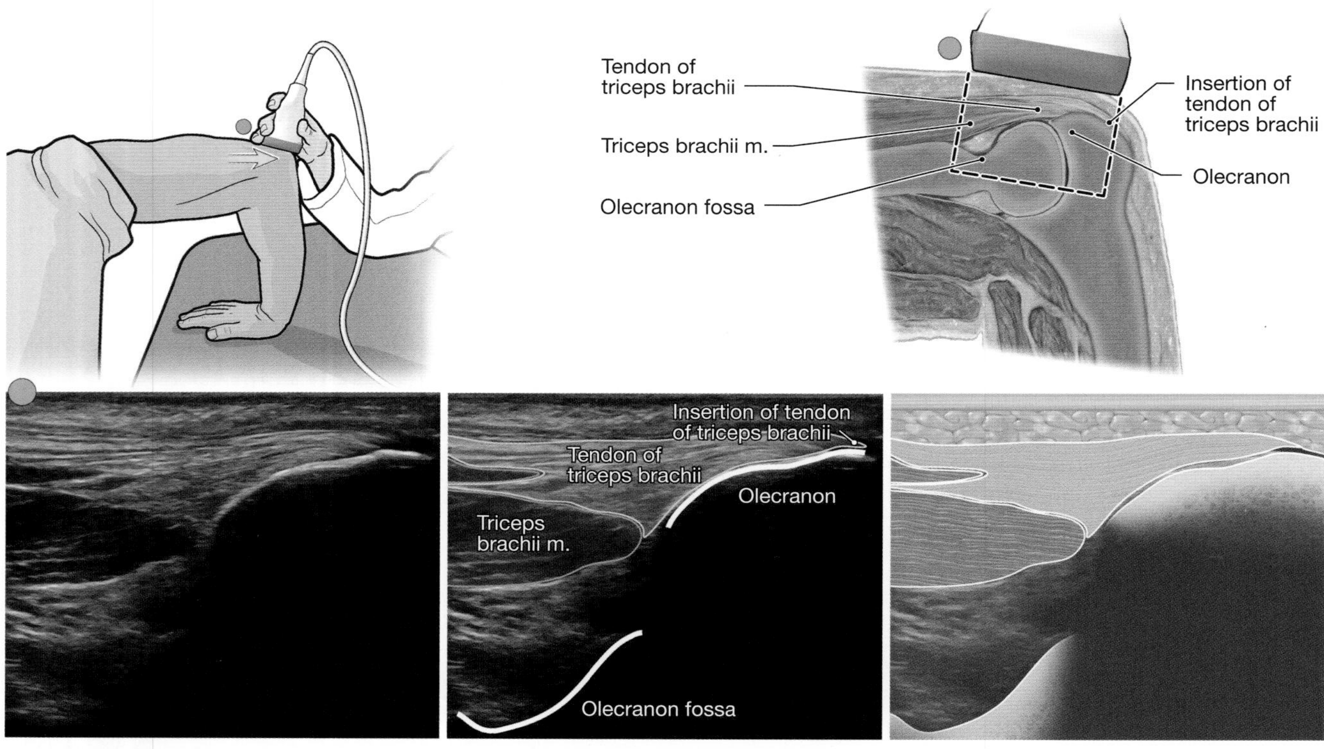

Figure 4.27 Longitudinal view of the tendon of triceps brachii inserting onto the olecranon process of the ulna.

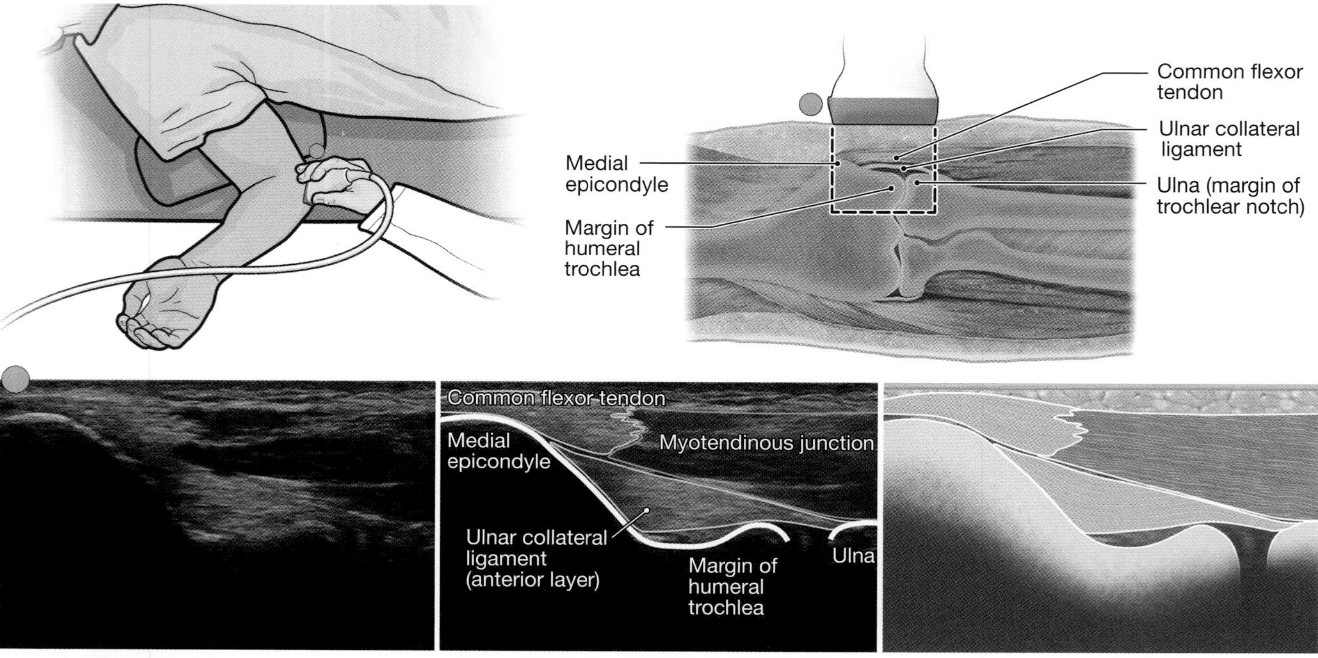

Figure 4.28 Longitudinal view of the anterior layer of the ulnar collateral ligament and overlying common flexor tendon.

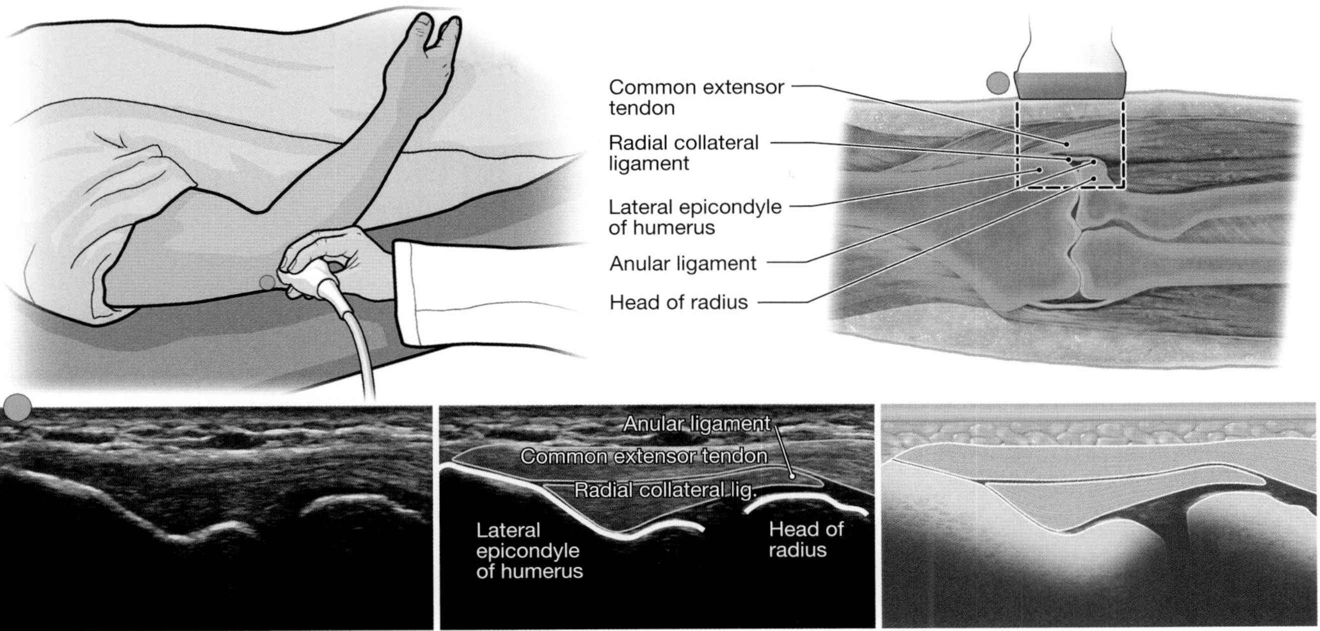

Figure 4.29 Longitudinal view of the radial collateral ligament and overlying common extensor tendon.

Forearm, Wrist, and Hand

Review of the Anatomy

Anterior Compartment Tendons and Carpal Tunnel

The muscles of the anterior compartment of the forearm include the flexors of the wrist, the superficial and deep digital flexors, flexor pollicis longus, and the two pronators of the forearm. The tendons of the flexor digitorum superficialis, flexor digitorum profundus, and flexor pollicis longus enter the hand through the carpal tunnel, along with the median nerve. The floor and sides of the tunnel are formed by the arch of the proximal and distal rows of carpal bones (and associated radiocarpal, ulnocarpal, and palmar intercarpal ligaments), and the roof is formed by the transverse carpal ligament (flexor retinaculum), which attaches medially to the pisiform and hamate bones and laterally to the tubercles of the scaphoid and trapezium. The tendon of the flexor carpi radialis crosses into the hand along the medial surface of the scaphoid just outside the carpal tunnel, between the two layers of the transverse carpal ligament.

Median Nerve

The median nerve travels through the anterior compartment of the forearm in the plane between the flexor digitorum superficialis and flexor digitorum profundus. The median nerve and its anterior interosseous branch innervate most of the muscles of the anterior forearm (except the medial half of the flexor digitorum superficialis and flexor carpi ulnaris, which are supplied by the ulnar nerve). At the wrist, the median nerve moves superficially between the tendon of the flexor carpi radialis and those of flexor digitorum superficialis and crosses into the hand through the carpal tunnel (along with the tendons of the digital flexor muscles) just under cover of the transverse carpal ligament.

Ulnar Nerve

The ulnar nerve enters the anterior compartment of the forearm between the two heads of the flexor carpi ulnaris and courses through the forearm between the flexor carpi ulnaris and flexor digitorum profundus. In the forearm, the ulnar nerve supplies motor innervation to the flexor carpi ulnaris and ulnar half of flexor digitorum profundus. The ulnar nerve, accompanied by the ulnar artery, crosses the wrist through Guyon canal, between the pisiform bone and the hook of the hamate bone. The roof of the Guyon canal is the palmar carpal ligament (a thickened region of deep forearm fascia), and the floor is the transverse carpal ligament.

Radial and Ulnar Arteries

The brachial artery divides into its terminal branches, the radial and ulnar arteries, in the cubital fossa. The radial artery, accompanied by the superficial radial nerve, crosses superficially to the pronator teres tendon, first lying just underneath the brachioradialis muscle/tendon and then lateral to the tendon of the flexor carpi radialis in the distal forearm. The ulnar artery passes deep to the pronator teres muscle and joins the ulnar nerve between the flexor carpi ulnaris and flexor digitorum profundus for the remainder of its course in the forearm and then through the Guyon canal into the hand.

Posterior Compartment Muscles, Tendons, and Extensor Retinaculum

The muscles of the posterior compartment of the forearm include the brachioradialis, supinator, extensors of the wrist and digits, abductor pollicis longus, extensors pollicis longus and brevis, and extensor indicis. The muscles of the posterior compartment are innervated by the radial nerve or its deep branch/posterior interosseous nerve. As the radial nerve emerges between the brachialis and brachioradialis, it divides into its terminal branches just anterior to the lateral epicondyle. These are the superficial branches that are sensory in nature, and the deep branch is motor. The deep branch travels deep to the extensor carpi radialis muscle, anterior to the humeroradial joint and then pierces the supinator muscle to supply the muscles of the extensor compartment of the forearm.

The tendons of the wrist and digital extensors and abductor pollicis longus, cross into the hand through six compartments formed by the extensor retinaculum related to the lateral surface of the radius, the dorsal surface of the radius, and the medial surface of the ulna. Just distal to the extensor retinaculum, the tendon of extensor pollicis longus forms the medial/posterior boundary of the anatomical snuffbox, and the tendons of extensor pollicis brevis and abductor pollicis longus form its lateral/anterior boundary. The floor of the snuffbox is formed by the scaphoid and trapezium, and its roof is formed by the skin and superficial fascia. The radial artery curves dorsally from the anterior forearm compartment through the snuffbox into the hand, and branches of the superficial radial nerve and the cephalic vein course through the superficial fascia of the snuffbox roof.

Intrinsic Muscles of the Hand

The intrinsic muscles of the hand include the palmar and dorsal interosseous muscles, four lumbrical muscles, adductor pollicis, three hypothenar muscles, and three thenar muscles: abductor pollicis brevis, flexor pollicis brevis, and opponens pollicis. The largest of the thenar muscles, opponens pollicis, originates from the tubercles of the scaphoid and trapezium and the adjacent palmar surface of the flexor retinaculum and wraps over the first metacarpal to insert along its lateral surface. The opponens lies deep to the two smaller thenar muscles. The tendon of the flexor pollicis longus leaves the carpal tunnel and passes between the adductor pollicis muscle and the thenar muscles to reach its fibrous tunnel. Emerging from the carpal tunnel, the median nerve divides into its terminal branches, the recurrent branch to the thenar muscles, small motor branches for the first and second lumbrical muscles, and common palmar digital branches for the radial 3.5 digits. Just distal to the pisiform bone, the ulnar nerve divides into its terminal branches, the superficial (palmar cutaneous) branch, and the deep (motor) branch. The ulnar nerve innervates all the intrinsic hand muscles except the thenar muscles and the first and second lumbricals, which are supplied by the median nerve, and provides common dorsal digital branches (via the dorsal cutaneous branch, which leaves the nerve proximal to the wrist) and common palmar digital branches to the ring and little fingers.

Digits and Digital Flexor Tendons

Each digit is associated with a metacarpal bone and proximal, middle, and distal phalanges (the thumb only has proximal and distal phalanges). The joints of the digits are the metacarpophalangeal (head of the metacarpal and base of the proximal phalanx), proximal interphalangeal (head of the proximal phalanx and base of the middle phalanx), and distal interphalangeal (head of the middle phalanx and base of the distal phalanx). After emerging from the carpal tunnel, the flexor tendons of the digits cross the palm and enter fibrous sheaths, which begin just proximal to the metacarpophalangeal joints, for their course along the palmar surfaces of the digits. The fibrous sheaths are made up by five annular pulleys (short fibrous canals or arches) and intervening X-shaped (cruciate) ligaments, which are attached to palmar plates (palmar ligaments) of the metacarpophalangeal joints and the palmar surfaces of the phalanges. Palmar plates (ligaments) are wedge-like fibrocartilaginous ligaments that reinforce the joint capsules of the metacarpophalangeal and interphalangeal joints.

Technique

Proximal Forearm

PROXIMAL FOREARM
SUPINATOR MUSCLE POSTERIOR INTEROSSEOUS NERVE
Transverse
FIG. 4.30

The patient should be supine (this exam can also be performed with the patient sitting up) with the elbow flexed to about 90° and the pronated forearm resting across the lower abdomen. Place the probe transverse to the posterior forearm a short distance below the lateral epicondyle of the humerus with the probe marker directed superiorly (laterally with respect to the anatomical position). Adjust the probe position until the supinator muscle can be identified wrapping around the neck of the radius. Slide the probe face proximally and distally over the supinator muscle and radial neck until the hyperechoic posterior interosseous nerve can be clearly identified in its course between the superficial and deep layers of the muscle. Center the nerve in the image and slide the probe distally until the nerve can be seen to emerge from under the distal margin of the supinator muscle onto the superficial surface of the abductor pollicis longus muscle. In this position, the nerve is deep to the extensor digitorum muscle.

PROXIMAL FOREARM
SUPINATOR MUSCLE POSTERIOR INTEROSSEOUS NERVE
Longitudinal
FIG. 4.31

The patient should be supine with the elbow flexed to about 90° and the pronated forearm resting across the lower abdomen, as described hereinbefore and illustrated in Figure 4.30. Once identified, follow the posterior interosseous nerve in a transverse orientation, and rotate the probe approximately 90° clockwise such that the probe face is aligned along the longitudinal axis of the nerve with the probe marker directed

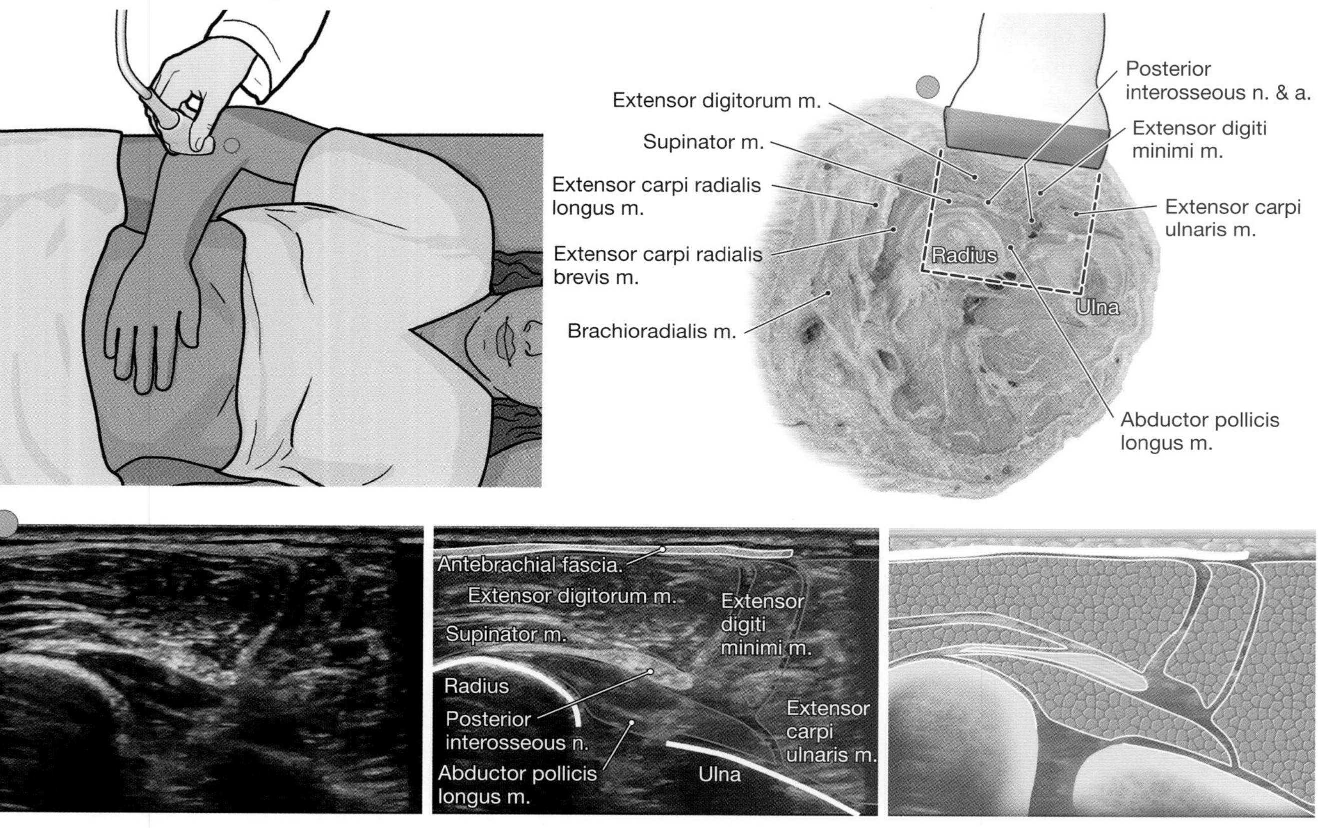

Figure 4.30 Transverse view of the posterior interosseous nerve emerging from the distal edge of the supinator muscle.

proximally/superiorly. Carefully adjust the probe position and alignment until the hyperechoic nerve can be seen as far as possible across the image from the proximal to distal end. Keeping the nerve in view, slowly slide the probe distally until the nerve can be seen to emerge from underneath the distal margin of the supinator muscle onto the superficial surface of the abductor pollicis longus.

Distal Forearm

DISTAL FOREARM
MEDIAN NERVE
Transverse
Figure 4.32

The patient should be supine with the arm slightly abducted, the forearm supinated, and the limb resting on the examination table. Place the probe transversely over the anterior surface between the middle and distal thirds of the forearm and identify the hyperechoic profiles and acoustic shadows of the radius and ulna. Adjust the probe position and tilt/fan the probe until the hyperechoic honeycomb appearance of the median nerve can be identified. The nerve is in the plane between the flexor digitorum superficialis and flexor digitorum profundus, and the flexor pollicis longus is just laterally to the nerve. Identify the myotendinous junction/tendon of the flexor carpi radialis at the superficial surface of the flexor digitorum superficialis. Just lateral to the tendon of the flexor carpi radialis identify the radial artery. The superficial radial nerve is seen immediately lateral to the radial artery. Slide the probe distally a short distance until the pronator quadratus muscle can be identified crossing between the ulna and radius.

DISTAL FOREARM
ULNAR NERVE
ULNAR ARTERY
Transverse
FIG. 4.33

Place the probe transversely over the anterior surface just beyond the middle of the forearm and once again identify the flexor digitorum superficialis and flexor digitorum profundus. Slide the probe medially until the flexor carpi ulnaris muscle appears at the medial border of the anterior compartment, medial to the digital flexor muscles. Identify the ulnar nerve and artery in the plane between the flexor carpi ulnaris and flexor digitorum profundus and just deep to the flexor digitorum superficialis.

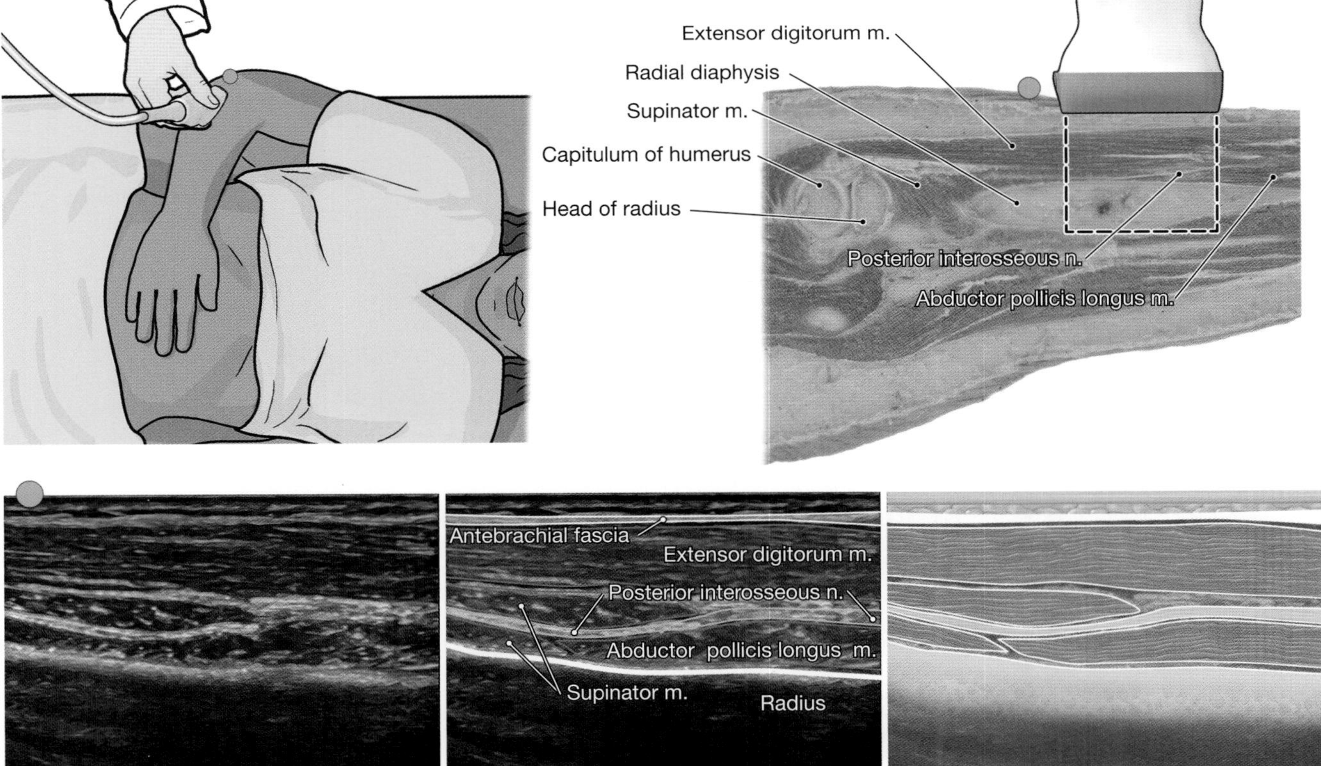

Figure 4.31 Longitudinal view of the posterior interosseous nerve coursing between layers of the supinator muscle and emerging onto the superficial surface of abductor pollicis longus muscle.

Wrist: Carpal Tunnel and Guyon Canal

CARPAL TUNNEL MEDIAN NERVE
Transverse
FIG. 4.34

The patient should be supine with the forearm supinated and the back of the wrist resting on a small pillow/bolster. Place the probe transversely over the distal wrist crease and adjust the position until the hyperechoic profiles of the scaphoid tubercle and pisiform bone can be identified at the lateral and medial borders of the carpal tunnel. By carefully tilting/fanning the probe, identify the hyperechoic reflection of the transverse carpal ligament (flexor retinaculum) and the digital flexor tendons. Owing to anisotropy, the appearance of the ligament and tendons changes dramatically by slightly tilting the probe face. The median nerve usually appears as a hypoechoic oval structure just deep to the transverse carpal ligament (flexor retinaculum). The honeycomb appearance of the nerve can usually be accentuated by careful tilting/fanning of the probe (again because of anisotropy). The tendon of flexor pollicis longus is usually located immediately deep/lateral to the median nerve, but is sometimes difficult to see because of anisotropy. Slide the probe proximally, keeping the nerve in view, and follow the nerve back out of the carpal tunnel into the distal forearm between the digital flexor muscles and the junctions of their tendons/myotendinous. Return the probe to the position between the scaphoid tubercle and pisiform bone. By recalling the effects of anisotropy on tendon appearance, identify the tendon of flexor carpi radialis in a shallow groove along the medial aspect of the scaphoid tubercle, just outside the carpal tunnel. Just lateral to the pisiform bone, identify the pulsating ulnar artery with the ulnar nerve on its medial side, as they cross over the flexor retinaculum through the Guyon canal. Note the hyperechoic fibers of the palmar carpal ligament roofing over the artery and nerve in this position.

GUYON CANAL ULNAR NERVE ULNAR ARTERY
Transverse
FIG. 4.35

Slide the probe medially, bringing the ulnar artery and nerve in the Guyon canal closer to the center of the image. By carefully tilting/fanning the probe, again identify the ulnar nerve and artery along with the roof (palmar carpal ligament) and floor (flexor

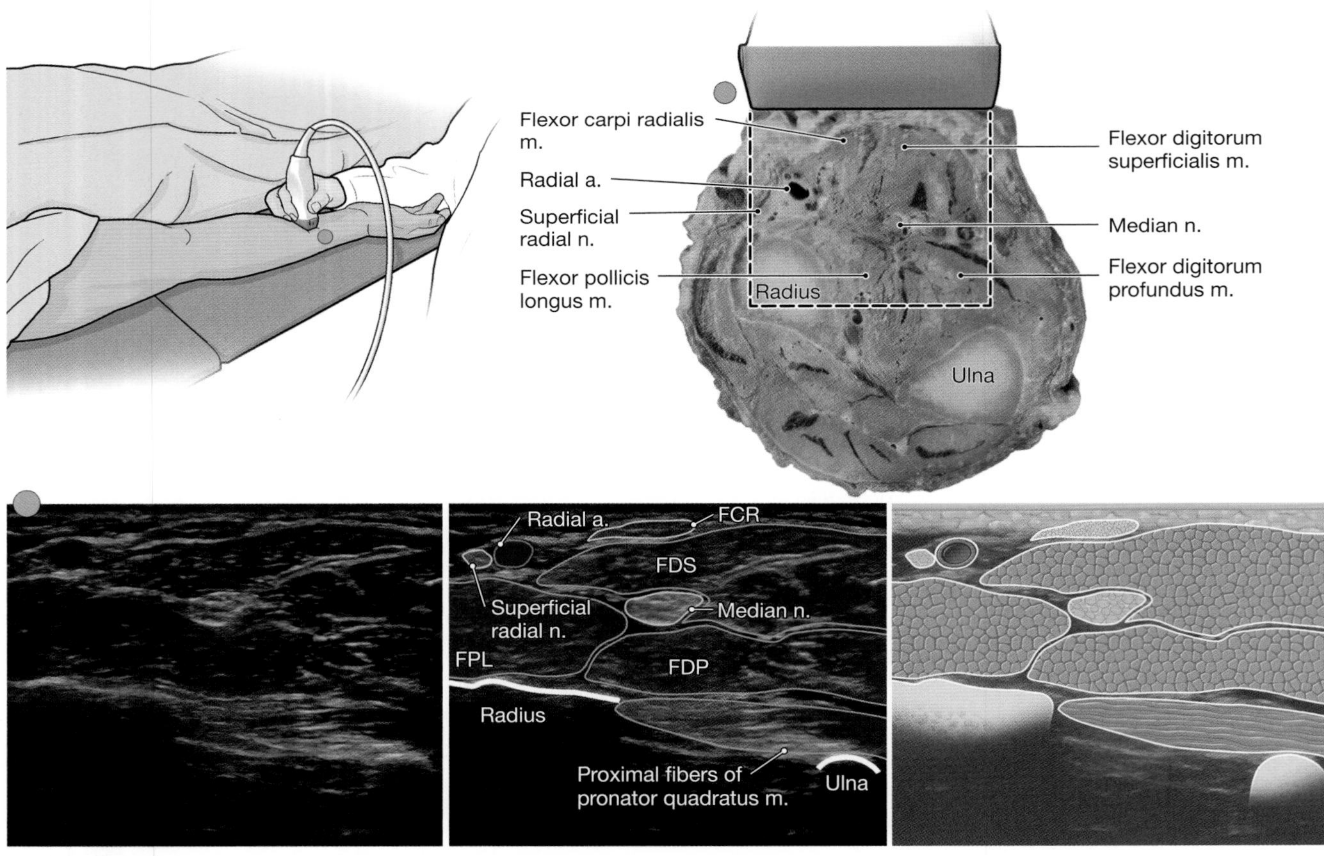

Figure 4.32 Transverse view of the median nerve in the distal forearm, in the plane between flexor digitorum superficialis (FDS) and flexor digitorum profundus (FDP). FCR, flexor carpi radialis.

retinaculum) of the canal. The nerve can often be seen dividing into its superficial and deep branches just distal to the pisiform bone.

Wrist: Extensor Retinaculum Compartments

COMPARTMENTS 3, 4, AND 5 TENDON OF EXTENSOR POLLICIS LONGUS TENDON OF EXTENSOR DIGITORUM TENDON OF EXTENSOR INDICIS TENDON OF EXTENSOR DIGITI MINIMI
Transverse
FIG. 4.36

The patient should be supine with the forearm pronated and the forearm and palm resting on the examination table. Place the probe transversely over the dorsum of the wrist with the non-marker side of the probe over the prominence of the head of the ulna. Identify the head of the ulna and the expanded distal end of the radius. Slide back and forth over this position until you can identify the small prominence on the dorsal surface of the radius, the dorsal radial tubercle. Identify the tendon of extensor pollicis longus in extensor compartment 3 at the medial surface of the dorsal radial tubercle (often in a shallow bony groove). Medial to compartment 3, identify the large compartment 4 containing the tendons of extensor digitorum and extensor indicis. Just medial to compartment 4, over the radial side of the head of the ulna, identify the tendon of extensor digiti minimi in compartment 5. By carefully tilting/fanning the probe, identify the hyperechoic extensor retinaculum and its fibrous bands separating the compartments.

COMPARTMENT 6 TENDON OF EXTENSOR CARPI ULNARIS
Transverse
FIG. 4.37

Slide the probe medially onto the ulnar side of the wrist. Adjust the probe position until it is centered over the rounded prominence of the ulnar head and the base of the ulnar styloid process. The tendon of extensor carpi ulnaris is located in compartment 6, in the groove between the ulnar head and base of the styloid process. Because of the narrow bony surface at the side of the wrist, it is not possible to maintain skin contact all the way across the probe face.

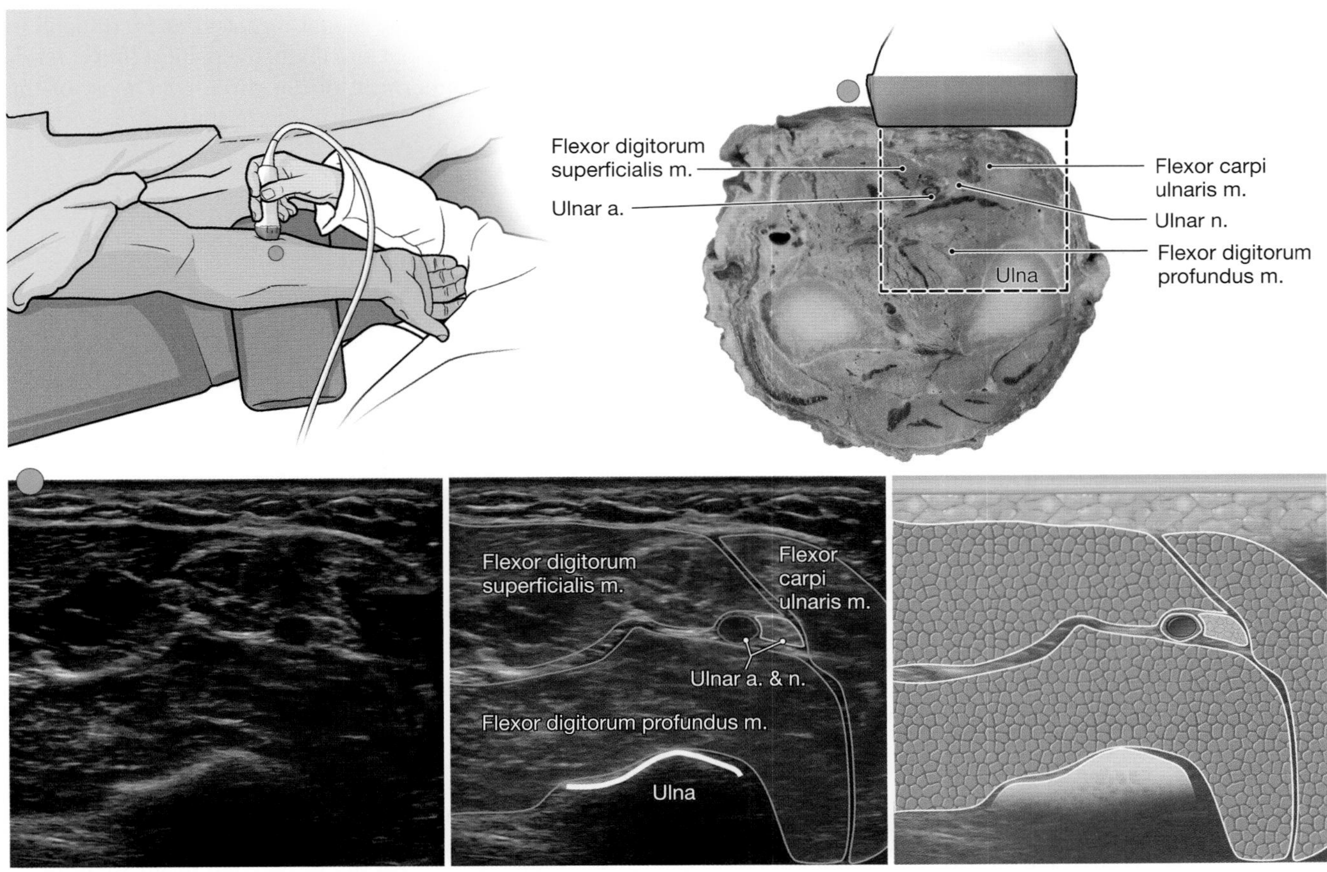

Figure 4.33 Transverse view of the ulnar artery and nerve in the plane between flexor digitorum profundus and the flexor carpi ulnaris.

COMPARTMENT 2 TENDON OF EXTENSOR CARPI RADIALIS LONGUS TENDON OF EXTENSOR CARPI RADIALIS BREVIS
Transverse
FIG. 4.38

Slide the probe back laterally across the dorsum of the wrist and again identify the dorsal radial tubercle. Continue laterally just beyond the tubercle onto the posterolateral surface of the radius (where again it is impossible to maintain skin contact across the entire probe face). In compartment 2, identify the tendons of extensor carpi radialis brevis and extensor carpi radialis longus. The tendon of extensor carpi radialis brevis lies alongside the lateral surface of the dorsal radial tubercle. Slide the probe distally and observe the tendon of extensor pollicis longus as it moves laterally across the radial carpal extensor tendons.

COMPARTMENT 1 TENDON OF EXTENSOR POLLICIS BREVIS TENDON OF ABDUCTOR POLLICIS LONGUS
Transverse
FIG. 4.39

Return the probe to the view of the radial carpal extensor tendons in compartment 2, and slide the probe further laterally/anteriorly onto the narrow lateral surface of the radius, at the base of the radial styloid process. Identify the tendons of extensor pollicis brevis and abductor pollicis longus in compartment 1. These tendons are often separated by a dense fibrous band spanning the compartment. Look for the cephalic vein and branches of the superficial radial nerve near compartment 1 in this position (which is just proximal to the anatomical snuffbox).

Hand: Thenar Eminence

THENAR MUSCLES TENDON OF FLEXOR POLLICIS LONGUS ADDUCTOR POLLICIS FIRST DORSAL INTEROSSEOUS MUSCLE
Transverse
FIG. 4.40

The patient should be supine with the forearm fully supinated and the dorsum of the hand resting on the examination table. Place the probe over the middle of the thenar eminence, transverse to the long axis of the first metacarpal bone. Adjust the probe position until the first and second metacarpal bones can be identified. The scan depth should be adjusted until the bright skin/air interface can be seen at the dorsum of the hand. The hyperechoic tendon of flexor pollicis longus is easily seen passing over the palmar surface of the adductor pollicis, between the adductor pollicis and the thenar muscles. Identify the adductor pollicis muscle, the first dorsal interosseous muscle lying posterior to it, and the thenar muscles. The thenar muscles can be difficult to identify definitively, but the abductor pollicis brevis tends to be the most superficial of the three over most of the

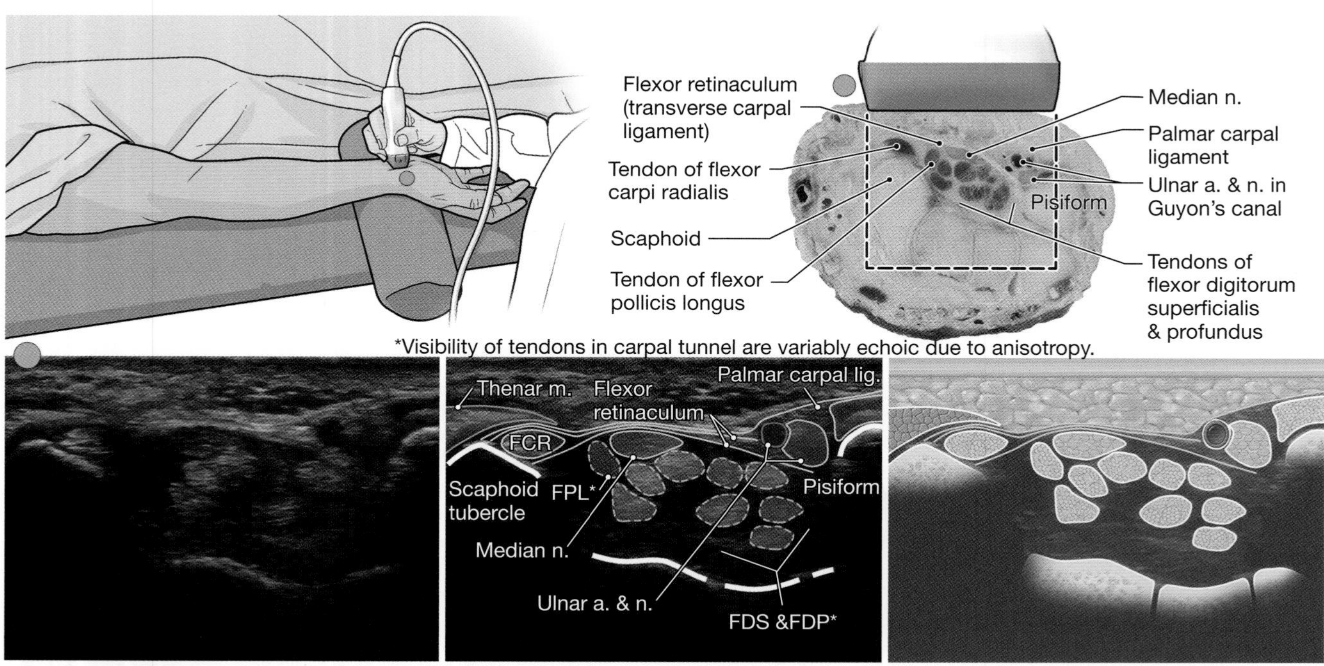

Figure 4.34 Transverse view of the median nerve in the carpal tunnel along with the tendons of flexor digitorum superficialis (FDS), flexor digitorum profundus (FDP), and flexor pollicis longus (FPL). The tendon of flexor carpi radialis (FCR) is just outside the carpal tunnel; FPL, flexor pollicis longus.

thenar eminence. By sliding the probe proximally and distally, the inserting fibers of opponens pollicis can be seen as they curve over the first metacarpal along its lateral margin. By sliding the probe distally and slightly medially, the hypoechoic oval profile of the first lumbrical muscle can be identified as it originates from the flexor digitorum profundus tendon of the index finger.

Hand: Flexor Tendons of the Digits

METACARPOPHALANGEAL JOINT FLEXOR TENDONS OF THE DIGITS
Longitudinal
FIG. 4.41

The patient should be supine with the forearm supinated, the digits adducted and extended, and the dorsum of the hand resting on the examination table. Place the probe along the longitudinal axis of a digit over the location of the metacarpophalangeal joint. Adjust the probe position until the head of the metacarpal, the metacarpophalangeal joint, and the base of the proximal phalanx are near the center of the image. Identify the flexor tendons overlying the bones and joint, and carefully adjust the probe orientation until the hyperechoic fibrillar appearance of the tendons can be seen throughout the image. Look for the area proximal to the metacarpal head where the tendons of flexor digitorum superficialis and flexor digitorum profundus converge near their entry into the fibrous digital sheath. At the metacarpal head and for some distance proximally, the tendons are separated from the surface of the metacarpal bone by the hyperechoic palmar plate (palmar metacarpal ligament) reinforcing the joint capsule. The palmar ligament (palmar plate) of the metacarpophalangeal joint is attached along the base of the proximal phalanx and tapers proximally, blending with the metacarpophalangeal joint capsule. Immediately superficial to the tendons, at the metacarpal head, attempt to identify the first annular (A1) pulley by carefully sliding/tilting/fanning the probe while centered over the

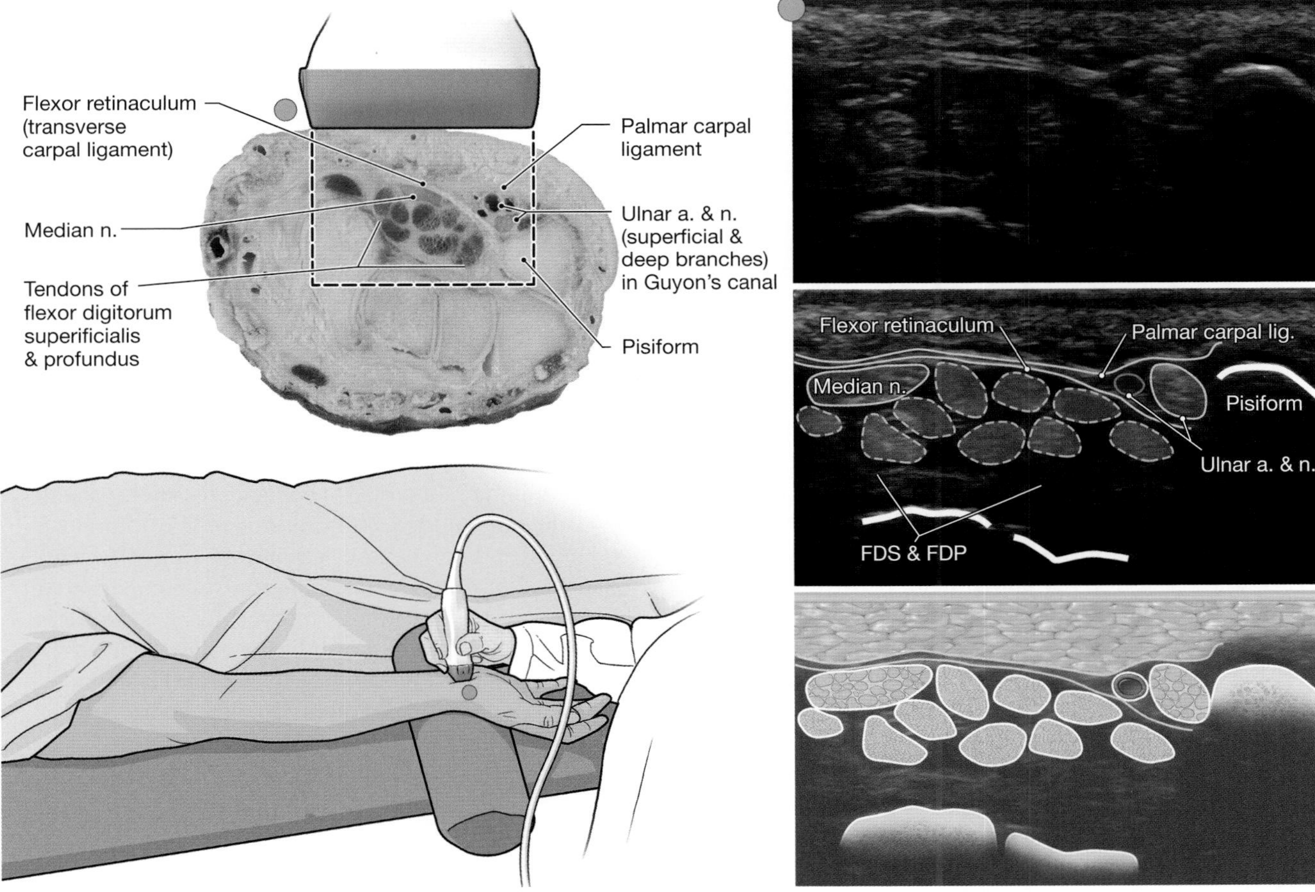

Figure 4.35 Transverse view of the ulnar artery and nerve in Guyon canal. FDP, flexor digitorum profundus; FDS, flexor digitorum superficialis.

metacarpal head. In their long axis, normal pulleys are seen as relatively thin anechoic/hypoechoic bands with thin hyperechoic margins on both sides.

METACARPOPHALANGEAL JOINT FLEXOR TENDONS OF THE DIGITS
Transverse
FIG. 4.42

By centering over the metacarpal head, rotate the probe 90° into the transverse axis. Identify the hyperechoic profile of the metacarpal head, the palmar plate, and the flexor tendons within their fibrous sheath. The first annular (A1) pulley is seen as a thin anechoic horseshoe-shaped band arching over the flexor tendons and attaching along the sides of the palmar plate. Look for the pulsations of palmar digital arteries and hyperechoic digital nerves on either side of the fibrous tendon sheath.

PROXIMAL PHALANX FLEXOR TENDONS OF THE DIGITS
Longitudinal
FIG. 4.43

Rotate the probe back into the longitudinal axis over the metacarpophalangeal joint, and while keeping the tendons and proximal phalanx in view, slide the probe a short distance distally until the central part of the palmar surface of the proximal phalanx is near the center of the image. Immediately superficial to the flexor tendons, look for the "bright to dark-bright" appearance of the second annular (A2) pulley, which is typically much easier to identify in its longitudinal axis than is the first annular pulley. The second annular pulley tends to be slightly thicker distally than it is at its proximal edge. Note that the fibrillar appearance and direction of the tendon fibers change distally as the superficialis tendon separates into bands that insert on the middle phalanx and allow the profundus tendon to continue on to the distal phalanx.

PROXIMAL PHALANX FLEXOR TENDONS OF THE DIGITS
Transverse
FIG. 4.44

By centering over the second annular (A2) pulley, rotate the probe 90° into the transverse axis of the digit. Identify the diaphysis of the proximal phalanx, the flexor tendons in their fibrous sheath, and the second annular pulley. The pulley appears as a thin anechoic horseshoe-shaped band (with occasional internal echoes) arching over the flexor tendons and attaching along the margins of the anterior surface of the proximal phalanx. Look for the proper palmar digital neurovascular bundles on either side of the fibro-osseous tendon tunnel.

CLINICAL APPLICATION

Posterior Interosseous Nerve Entrapment

Along its route, the posterior interosseous nerve is susceptible to several types of injuries such as compression as it passes beneath the arching of the tendinous proximal portion of the superficial head of the supinator muscle, clinically referred to as the arcade of Frohse; compression by tumors; iatrogenic injury during surgery to the proximal radius compression by branches of the radial recurrent artery (leash of Henry); or even as a rare complication of autoimmune diseases such as rheumatoid arthritis. The posterior interosseous nerve syndrome is a rare peripheral neuropathy that leads to upper extremity muscle weakness and can have devastating functional deficits. The diagnosis is often difficult to make but is characterized by an insidious onset, often presenting with weakness in finger and thumb extension at the metacarpophalangeal joint. It progresses with decrease in grip strength and tenderness over the lateral epicondyle over the supinator muscle.

These techniques can be used for guiding needles into position to inject local anesthetic agents along the median and ulnar nerves in the distal forearm or wrist to produce regional anesthesia for conducting surgical procedures on the hand. Ultrasound examination is also used for the evaluation of potential nerve compression injuries such as the median nerve in the carpal tunnel or the ulnar nerve in the Guyon canal.

Ultrasound examination is being increasingly used in the evaluation and treatment of a variety of muscular, tendinous, and ligamentous strains/tears or other dysfunctions. For example, the first extensor compartment is involved in De Quervain's tenosynovitis, which causes pain and dysfunction of the abductor pollicis longus and extensor pollicis brevis. Nodularity and/or thickening of the first annular pulley is often associated with "trigger finger," and the other annular pulleys (especially the second and fourth) may be torn or ruptured in rock climbing injuries.

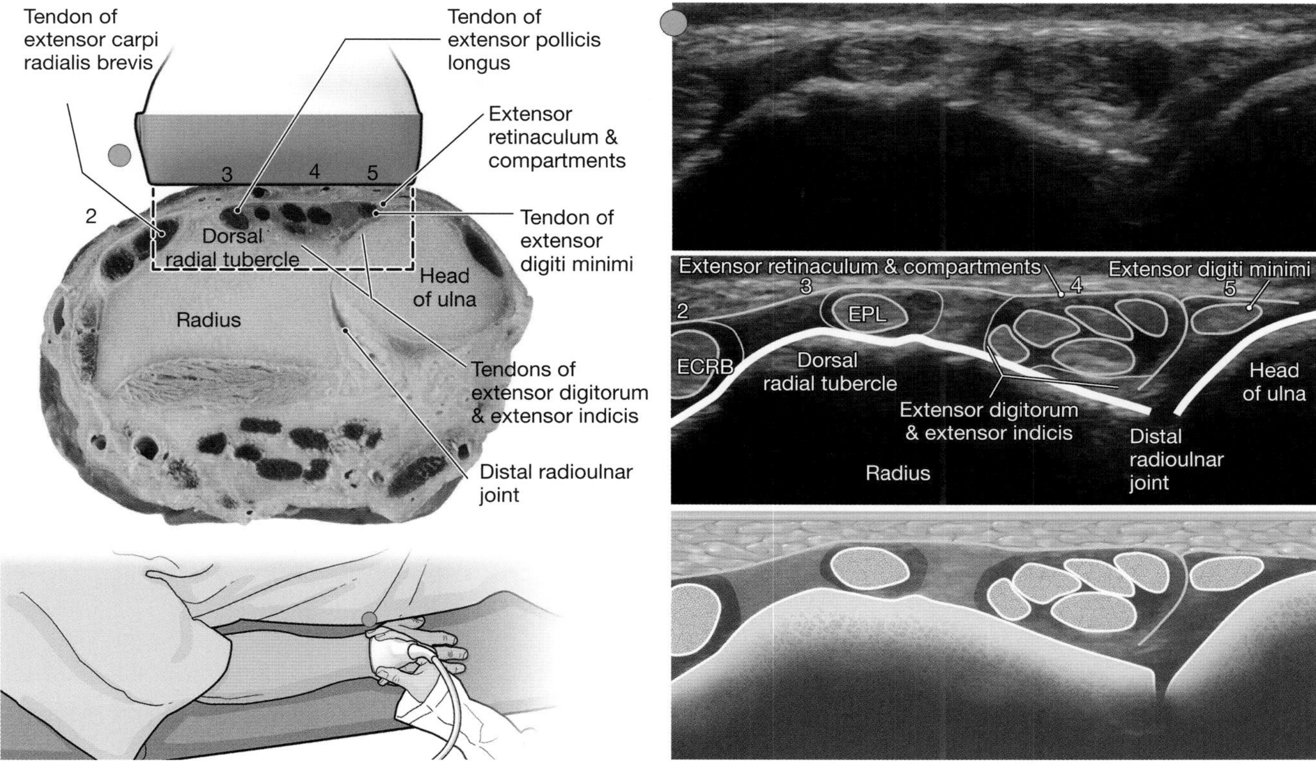

Figure 4.36 Transverse view of extensor retinaculum compartments 3, 4, and 5. Compartment 3 contains the tendon of extensor pollicis longus (EPL). Compartment 4 contains the tendons of extensor digitorum and extensor indicis. Compartment 5 contains the tendon of extensor digiti minimi.

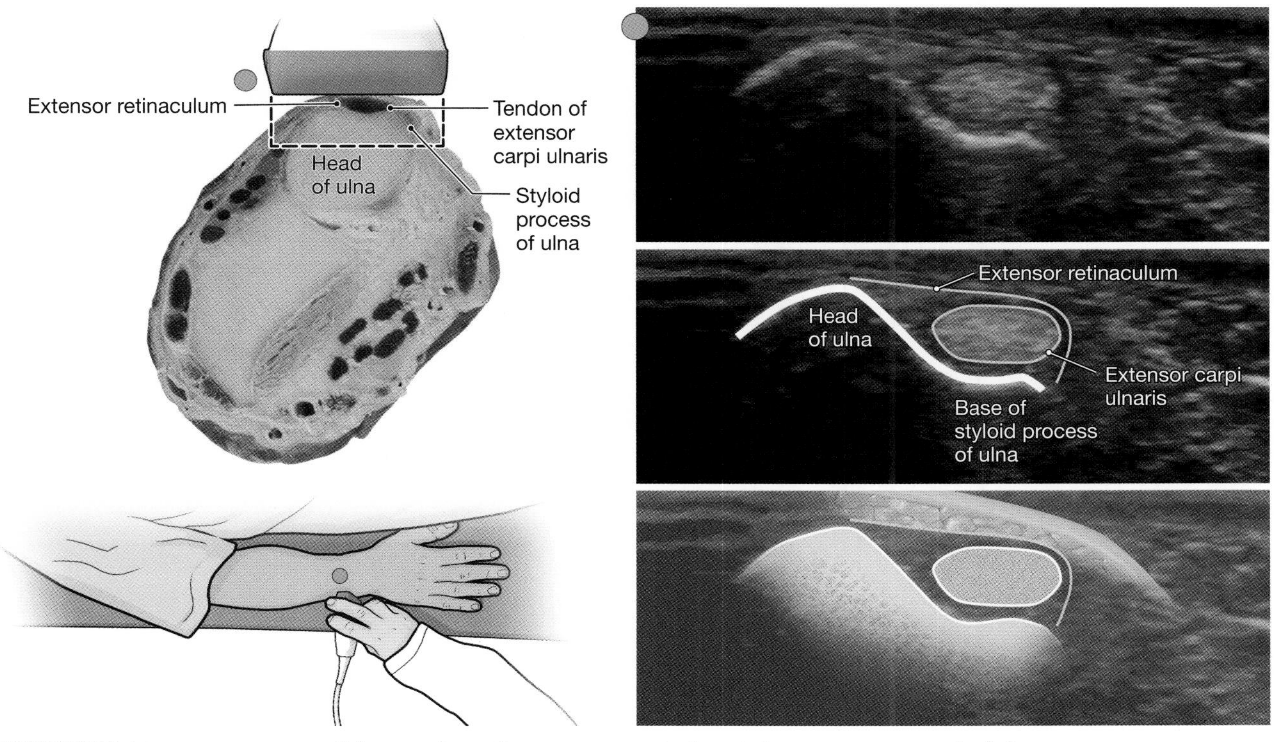

Figure 4.37 Transverse view of the tendon of extensor carpi ulnaris in compartment 6 of the extensor retinaculum.

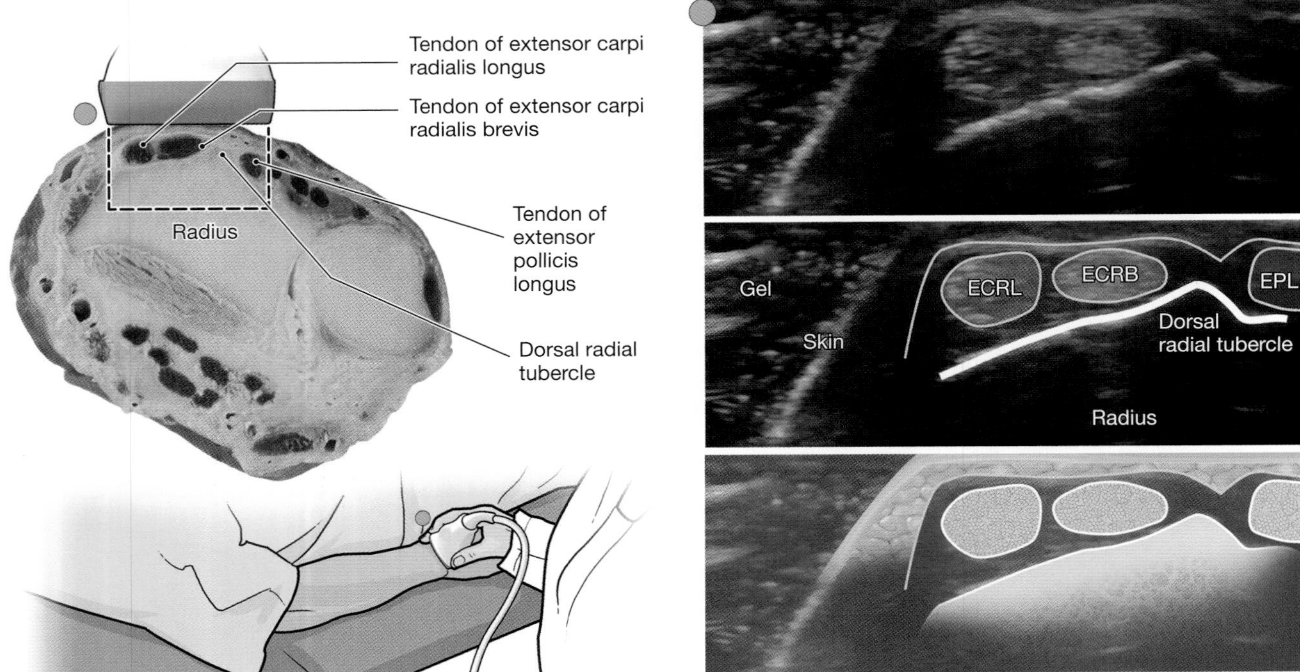

Figure 4.38 Transverse view of the tendons of extensor carpi radialis longus (ECRL) and extensor carpi radialis brevis (ECRB) in compartment 2 of the extensor retinaculum. EPL, extensor pollicis longus.

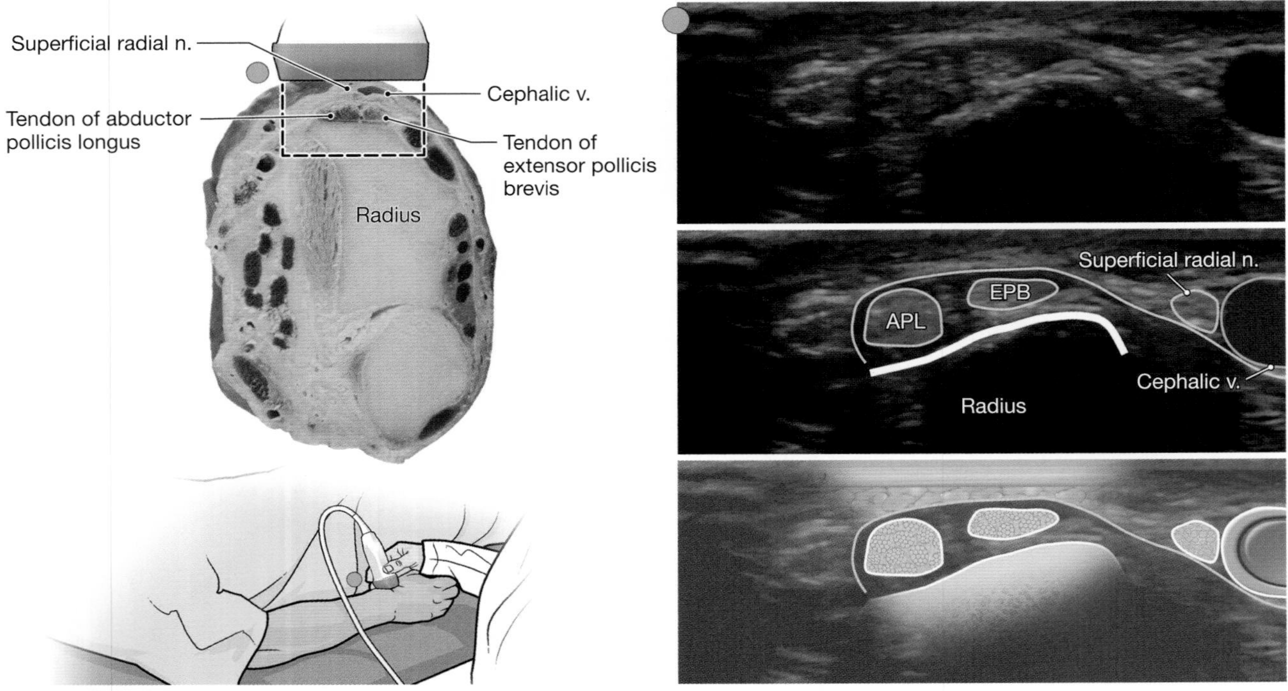

Figure 4.39 Transverse view of the tendons of extensor pollicis brevis (EPB) and abductor pollicis longus (APL) in compartment 1 of the extensor retinaculum.

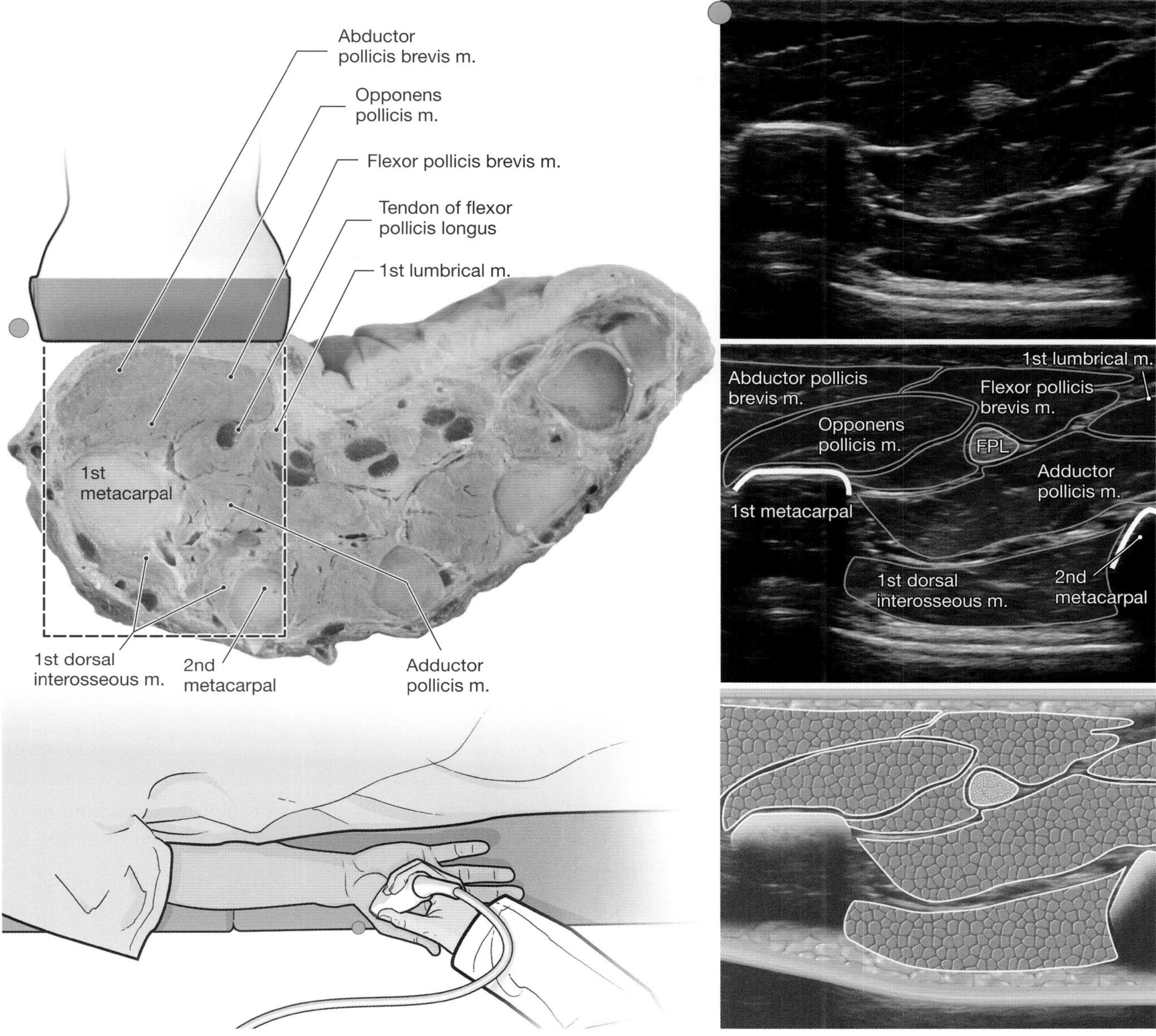

Figure 4.40 Transverse view of the thenar muscles, the tendon of flexor pollicis longus, adductor pollicis, and the first dorsal interosseous muscle.

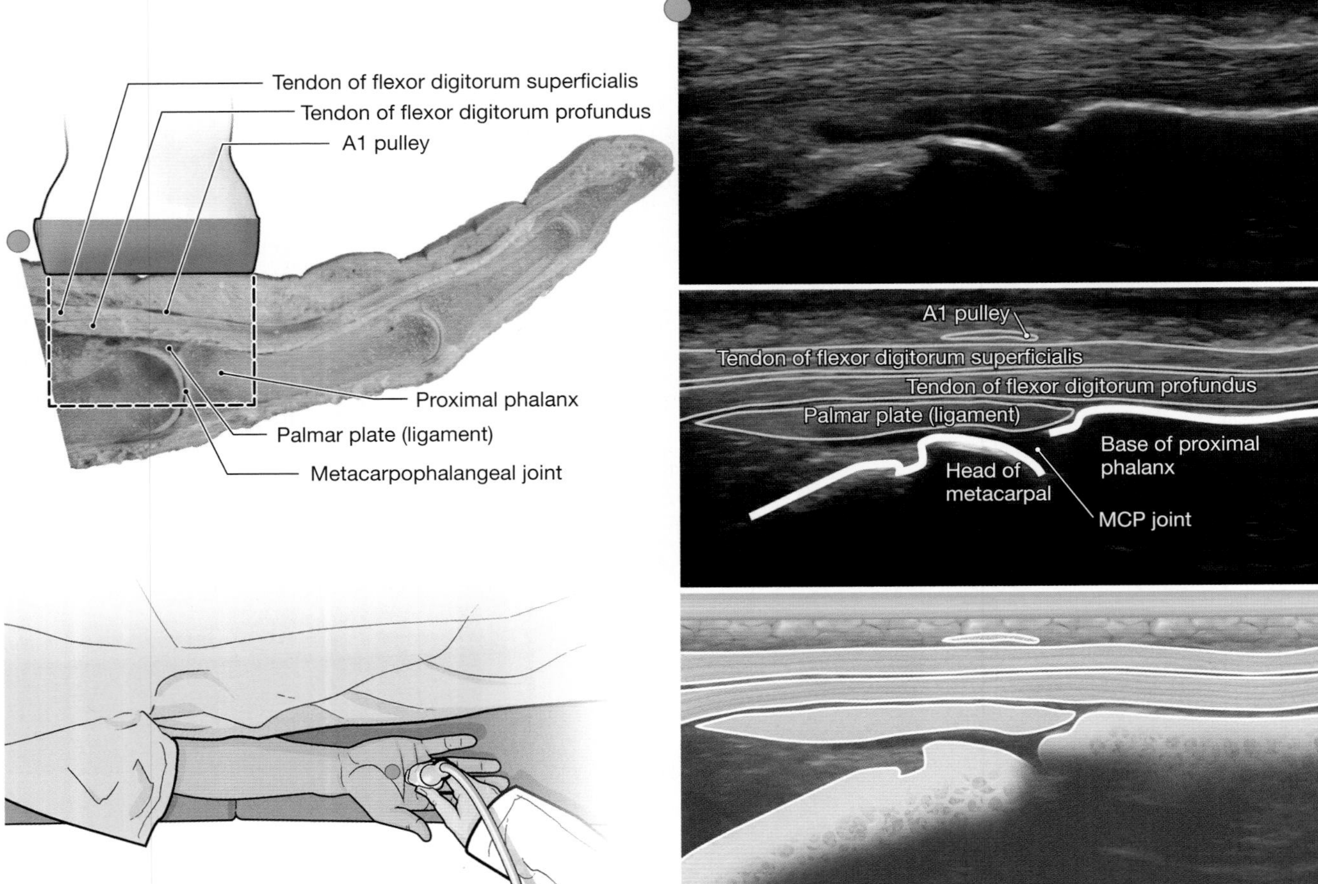

Figure 4.41 Longitudinal view of the tendons of flexor digitorum superficialis and flexor digitorum profundus at the metacarpophalangeal (MCP) joint, along with the palmar ligament of the joint and the first annular (A1) pulley of the fibrous tendon sheath.

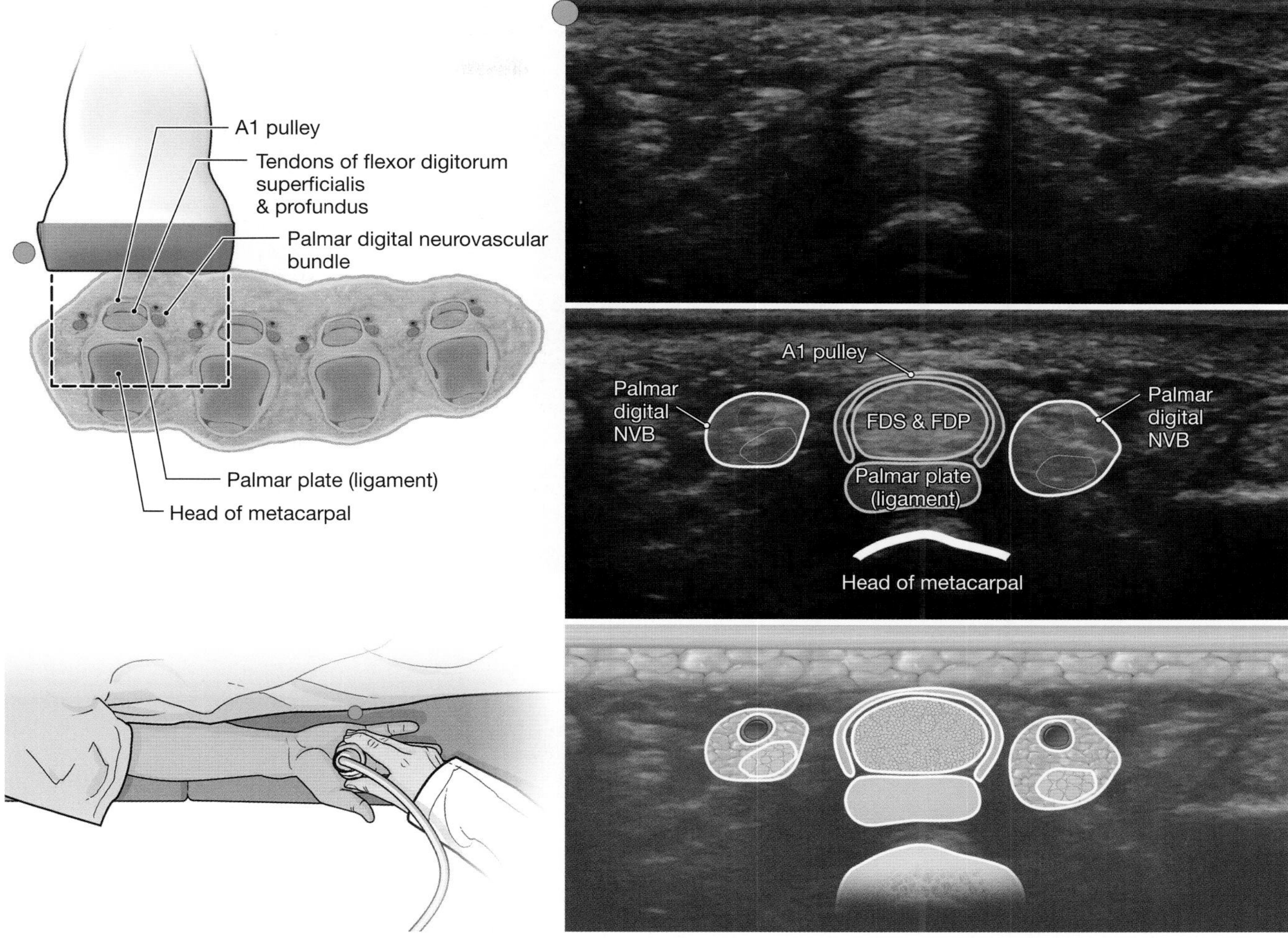

Figure 4.42 Transverse view of the tendons of flexor digitorum superficialis (FDS) and flexor digitorum profundus (FDP) over the head of the metacarpal bone, along with the palmar ligament of the metacarpophalangeal joint and the first annular (A1) pulley of the fibrous tendon sheath. NVB, neurovascular bundle.

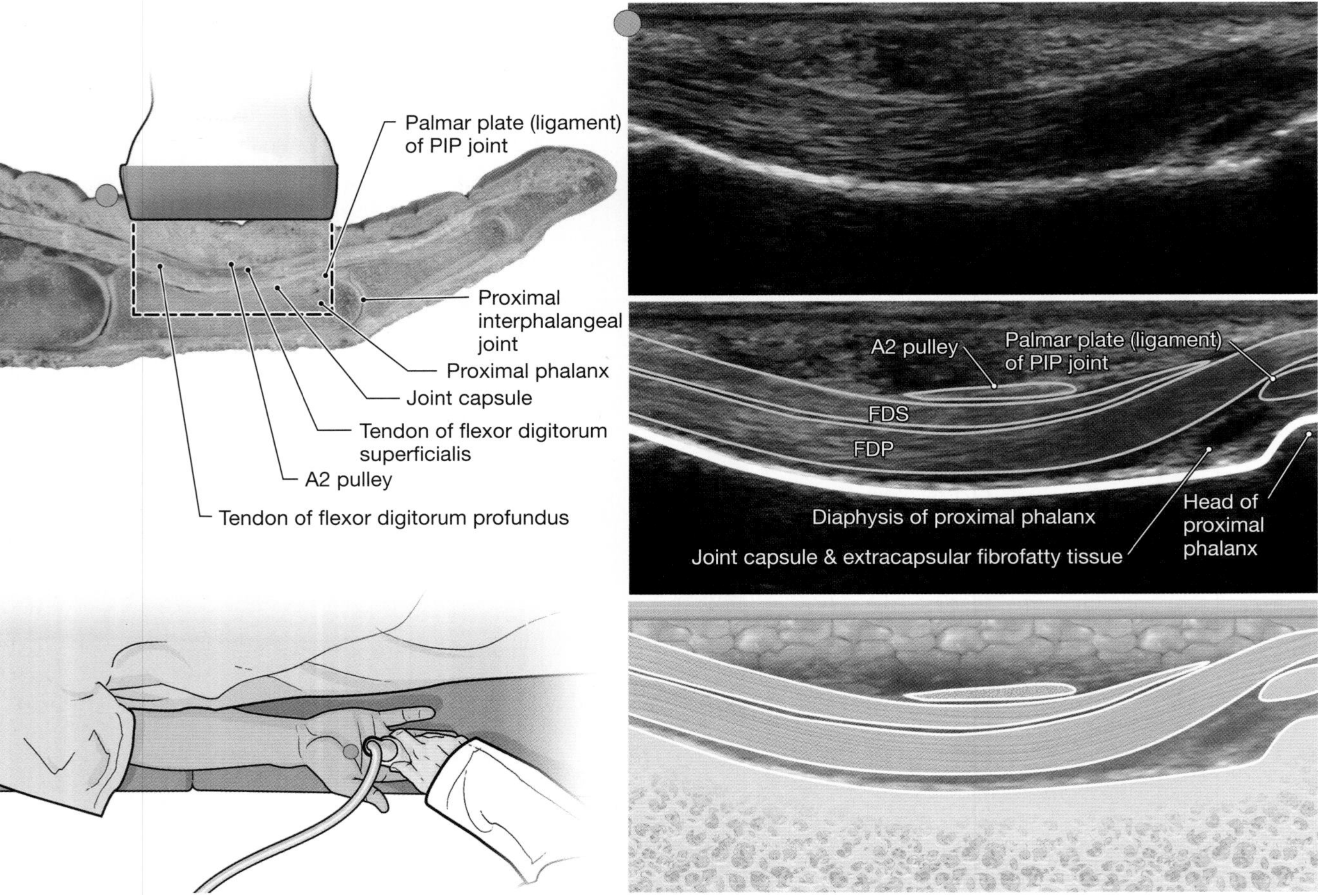

Figure 4.43 Longitudinal view of the tendons of flexor digitorum superficialis (FDS) and flexor digitorum profundus (FDP over the diaphysis of the proximal phalanx, along with second annular (A2) pulley of the fibrous tendon sheath. PIP, proximal interphalangeal.

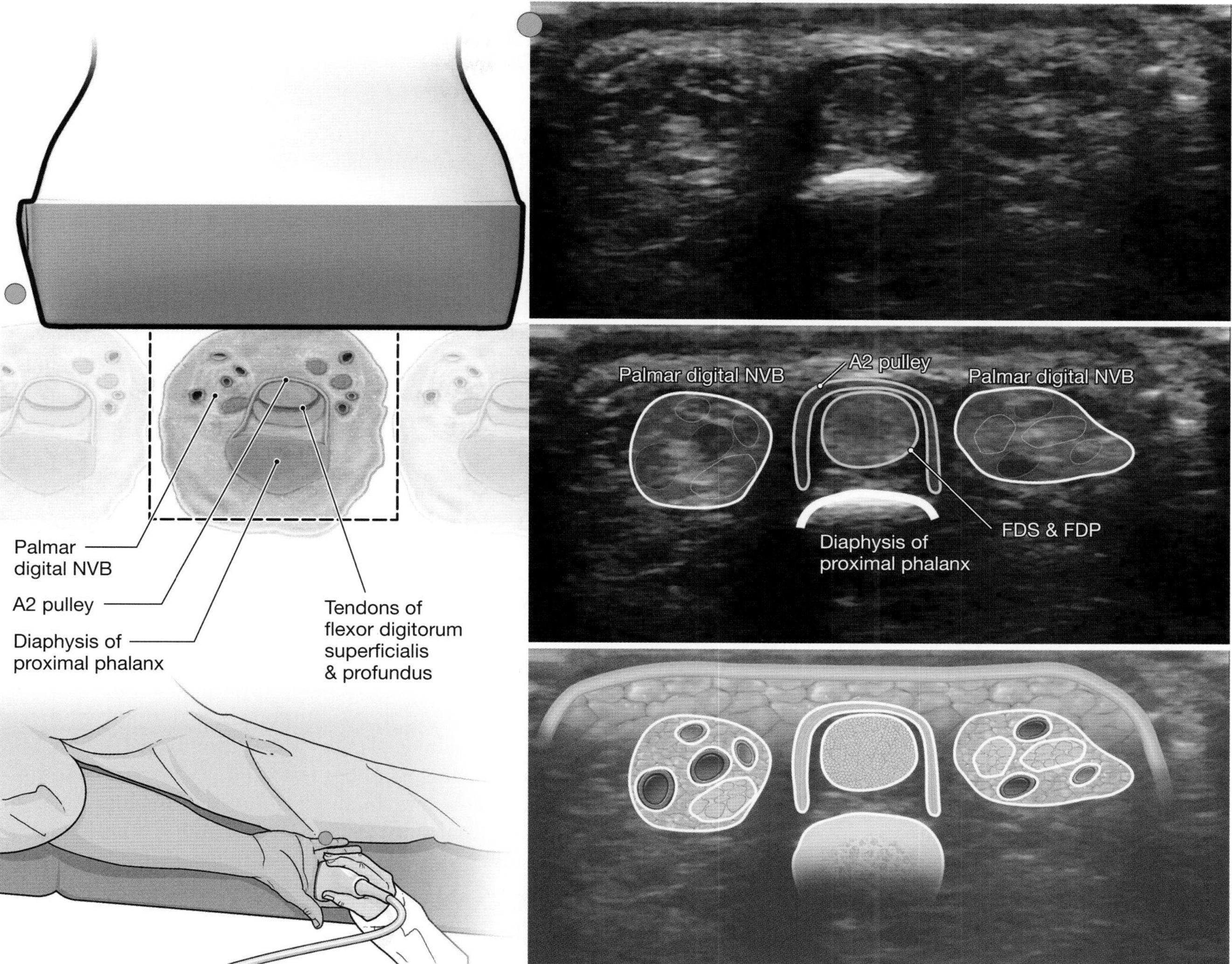

Figure 4.44 Transverse view of the tendons of flexor digitorum superficialis (FDS) and flexor digitorum profundus (FDP) over the diaphysis of the proximal phalanx, along with second annular (A2) pulley of the fibrous tendon sheath. NVB, neurovascular bundle.

4 Upper Limb

Multiple Choice Questions

1. A 27-year-old cricket bowler is undergoing an ultrasound-guided interscalene brachial plexus block before surgical repair of the radial collateral ligament of his elbow. This patient will most likely require additional regional anesthesia at another site. Which of the following structures must be encroached if the surgical field needs to be expanded?

A. Annular ligament
B. Lateral epicondyle of the humerus
C. Origin of brachioradialis muscle
D. Supinator muscle
E. Ulnar collateral ligament

2. Following a motor vehicle collision that resulted in a comminuted fracture of the right clavicle, a 25-year-old man has developed extensive weakness/paralysis in his right upper limb. Physical examination shows weakness of both abduction and adduction of the arm, extension of the elbow, and extension of the wrist and digits. There is decreased sensation over the shoulder, posterior and lateral aspects of the arm, posterior aspect of the forearm, and dorsum of the hand laterally. In which of the following components of the brachial plexus will an ultrasound examination of the axilla most likely show posttraumatic changes?

A. Upper trunk
B. Lower trunk
C. Lateral cord
D. Posterior cord
E. Medial cord

3. A 20-year-old college tennis player comes to the physician because of a 6-month history of progressive shoulder pain, especially while serving. Physical examination shows that flexion of the shoulder to 90° accompanied by internal rotation results in severe pain under her acromion process. Which of the following tendons will an ultrasound examination of her shoulder most likely show an injury?

A. Biceps brachii, long head
B. Infraspinatus
C. Subscapularis
D. Supraspinatus
E. Teres minor

4. A 60-year-old woman comes to the physician because of a deep aching pain in the anterior part of her shoulder for the past several weeks. Physical examination shows tenderness to palpation over her anterior shoulder, and the pain is reproduced by supination of the forearm against resistance and by flexion of the shoulder against resistance with the forearm extended and supinated. In which of the following tendons is an ultrasound examination of the shoulder most likely to show inflammatory changes?

A. Biceps brachii, long head
B. Infraspinatus
C. Subscapularis
D. Supraspinatus
E. Teres minor

5. A 78-year-old woman with end-stage renal disease and a left brachial artery/basilic vein arteriovenous fistula is admitted to the hospital because of a 2-month history of pain in her upper limb. Physical examination shows numbness and tingling in her palm, palmar aspect of the thumb, and index and middle fingers of her left hand. An ultrasound examination shows an aneurysm of the brachial artery in the distal third of the arm. Which of the following muscles is most likely to exhibit weakness?

A. Adductor pollicis
B. Brachialis
C. Extensor carpi ulnaris
D. Flexor carpi ulnaris
E. Pronator teres

6. An 82-year-old woman is admitted to the emergency department because of severe pain in her right upper limb after falling forward onto her hands and knees, while rising from a chair. An x-ray of her arm shows an oblique fracture at the mid-shaft of her right humerus. Immediately after closed reduction of the fracture, she developed numbness and tingling in the limb. Which of the following nerves would most likely show injury in an ultrasound examination?

A. Deep radial nerve
B. Posterior cutaneous nerve of the forearm
C. Posterior interosseous nerve
D. Radial nerve
E. Superficial radial nerve

7. Following a bar fight, a 26-year-old man is brought to the emergency department with multiple defensive stab wounds along the anterior surface of the left forearm and medial surface of the elbow and arm. An ultrasound examination shows a hematoma a few centimeters below the elbow between the flexor digitorum superficialis and flexor digitorum profundus muscles. Which of the following nerves is most likely to be affected by a hematoma in this location?

   A. Deep radial nerve
   B. Medial cutaneous nerve of the forearm
   C. Median nerve
   D. Superficial radial nerve
   E. Ulnar nerve

8. A 45-year-old man comes to the physician because of a 5-week history of numbness and tingling in the ring and little fingers of his right hand. He is now concerned that he seems to be losing strength in the hand. Physical examination shows altered sensation in the palmar aspect of the ring and little fingers on the right, along with weakness of adduction of all the digits of his right hand. Strength for flexion at the proximal and distal interphalangeal joints of all fingers is normal and equal bilaterally. An ultrasound examination shows a compression of the ulnar nerve. In which of the following locations is the compression most likely taking place?

   A. Cubital tunnel
   B. Supinator muscle
   C. Between the heads of pronator teres muscle
   D. Guyon canal
   E. Carpal tunnel

9. A 23-year-old woman comes to the physician because of a 1-month history of numbness and tingling over the lateral side of the wrist, thumb, and dorsum of her hand. A month ago, she underwent a fixator pin placement for a complicated fracture of the distal radius. Physical examination shows no loss of motor function in the wrist or hand. An ultrasound examination shows a nerve entrapment. Which of the following nerves is most likely entrapped?

   A. Anterior interosseous nerve
   B. Dorsal cutaneous branch of the ulnar nerve
   C. Posterior cutaneous nerve of the forearm
   D. Posterior interosseous nerve
   E. Superficial radial nerve

10. A 22-year-old woman comes to the physician because of a progressive weakening of her grip that has rendered her unable to hold her racquet during tennis practice. She has no history of trauma, infection, or autoimmune disorder. Physical examination shows atrophy of the thenar eminence, inability to oppose the thumb, and difficulty flexing the middle interphalangeal joint of the digits. Which of the following diagnoses would an ultrasound examination confirm?

   A. Hypertrophy of the supinator
   B. Pronator syndrome
   C. Medial supracondylar fracture
   D. Tennis elbow
   E. Golfer's elbow

5

Lower Limb

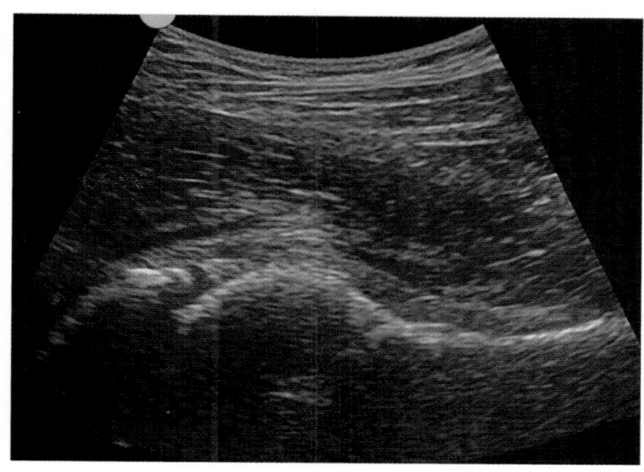

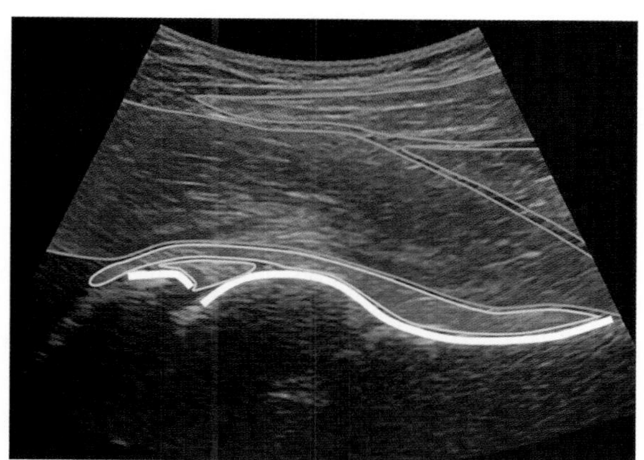

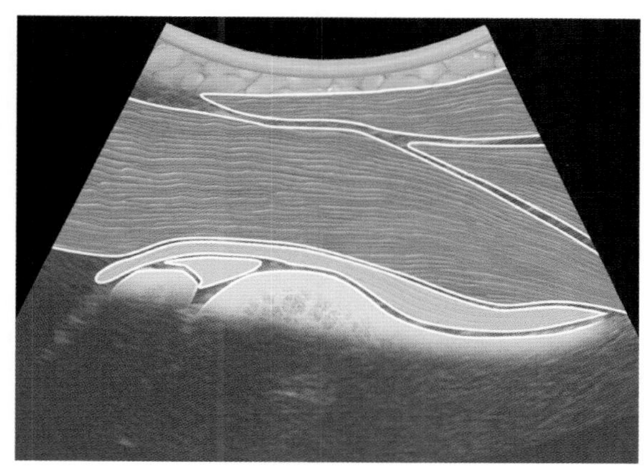

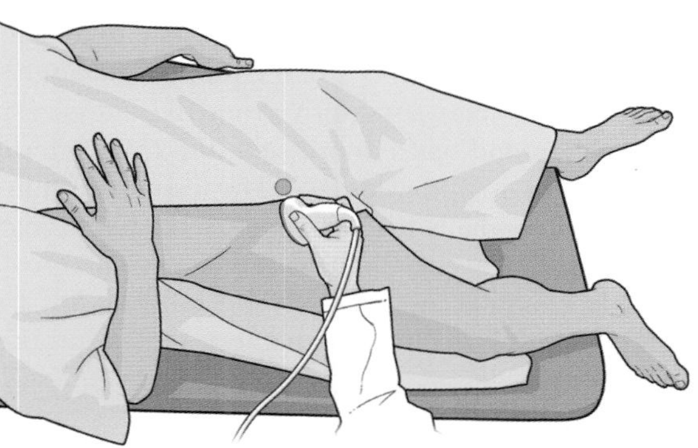

Proximal Thigh and Inguinal Region

Review of the Anatomy

Bones

The bones of the proximal thigh and groin are those of the pelvis and femur.

Pelvic Bones

The pelvic bones (os coxae) are formed by the fusion of the ilium, ischium, and pubis. The expanded upper part of the ilium, the wing (ala), has an anterior surface that forms part of the posterior abdominal wall and a posterior surface that is part of the gluteal region. The iliac crest is superior to the ala and extends from the anterior superior iliac spine (ASIS) anteriorly to the posterior superior iliac spine posteriorly. The anterior inferior iliac spine projects from the anterior edge of the ilium a few centimeters inferior and medial to the ASIS just above the lateral aspect of the socket of the hip joint, the acetabulum. The acetabulum is located laterally on the pelvic bone where the three bones come together, just inferior to the approximate midpoint of the inguinal ligament.

Femur

The head of the femur articulates with the acetabulum of the pelvic bone to form the hip joint. The head of the femur is attached to the body of the femur by the neck of the femur, which projects inferolaterally (and slightly anteriorly) from the head of the femur to the proximal part of the body of the femur, at an angle between 120° and 135° in the frontal plane. The greater and lesser trochanters and intertrochanteric areas are adjacent to the junction between the neck and body of the femur. The large greater trochanter projects superiorly from the lateral aspect of this junction and has a depression, the trochanteric fossa, along its posteromedial surface. The lesser trochanter projects posteromedially from the body of the femur just below the junction between the neck and body. The greater and lesser trochanters are connected posteriorly by a prominent bony ridge, the intertrochanteric crest. Anteriorly, the trochanters are connected by a small bony ridge, the intertrochanteric line.

Hip Joint Capsule

The fibrous capsule of the hip joint attaches along the acetabural neck adjacent to the intertrochanteric fossa. A synovial membrane attaches along the margins of the articular surfaces of the acetabulum and femoral head and descends along the neck of the femur before reflecting to line the interior of the fibrous membrane. The fibrous membrane is reinforced by three thickenings: the iliofemoral, pubofemoral, and ischiofemoral ligaments. The iliofemoral ligament is attached to the margin of the acetabulum proximally and the intertrochanteric line distally, reinforcing the joint capsule anteriorly. Although the hip joint is inherently much more stable than the glenohumeral joint, the bony rim of the acetabulum is additionally elevated by a fibrocartilaginous acetabular labrum.

Muscles

The muscles of the thigh are divided into three compartments by the fascia lata and its intermuscular septae. In addition, iliacus and psoas major enter the thigh from the posterior abdominal wall and insert through a common tendon (iliopsoas) onto the lesser trochanter of the femur. The anterior compartment muscles include sartorius and quadriceps femoris. The medial compartment muscles are pectineus, adductor brevis, adductor longus, adductor magnus, gracilis, and obturator externus. The posterior compartment muscles are the hamstrings: biceps femoris, semitendinosus, and semimembranosus.

With respect to muscular anatomy, this section focuses on a small subset of muscles in the proximal-most part of the thigh related to the ASIS, femoral triangle, and hip joint, plus a brief overview of the medial compartment muscles in the proximal thigh. The anterior and posterior compartments are discussed in additional detail in subsequent sections.

Iliacus and Psoas Major

Iliacus originates from the anterior abdominal surface (iliac fossa) of the pelvic bone. The psoas major muscle originates from transverse processes and adjacent bodies of the lumbar vertebrae. The two muscles enter the thigh inferior to the inguinal ligament and form the lateral half of the floor of the femoral triangle, passing over the hip joint and medial aspect of the neck of the femur to insert through a common tendon (iliopsoas tendon) onto the lesser trochanter of the femur.

Sartorius

Sartorius originates from the medial aspect of the ASIS, crosses the thigh from lateral to medial and inserts along with gracilis and semitendinosus on the medial aspect of the proximal tibia.

Tensor Fasciae Latae

The tensor fasciae latae muscle originates along a line that begins at the lateral aspect of the ASIS and extends a few centimeters posteriorly along the iliac crest as far as the tubercle of the crest, and inserts via the iliotibial tract, a thickened band of the fascia lata, onto the proximal tibia.

Gluteus Medius and Minimus

The gluteus medius and minimus muscles originate from the gluteal surface of the iliac ala nearly as far anteriorly as the ASIS and so come partially into view in ultrasound (US) images of proximal thigh muscles near the ASIS.

Rectus Femoris

The rectus femoris muscle originates mainly from the anterior inferior iliac spine (a few centimeters inferomedial to the ASIS) and inserts along with the vastus muscles via the quadriceps femoris tendon. Near its origin, the rectus femoris muscle is just deep to sartorius and tensor fasciae latae as these muscles diverge medially and laterally, respectively, from the ASIS.

Medial Compartment Muscles

Pectineus muscle originates from the pectineal line of the superior pubic ramus, just above the inguinal ligament, enters the thigh deep to the inguinal ligament, forming the medial half of the floor of the femoral triangle, and inserts on the body of the femur immediately below the lesser trochanter. The adductor longus, adductor brevis, and adductor magnus muscles originate from the pelvic bone medial to pectineus (part of the adductor magnus' origin is posterior to pectineus). Adductor longus is the most superficial of these three medial compartment muscles. Adductor brevis is just deep to adductor longus, and adductor magnus, in turn, is deep to adductor brevis (and its lateral-most fibers are deep to pectineus). Adductor longus originates from the superior part of the body of the pubic bone and inserts onto the middle third of the body of the femur (linea aspera) posteriorly. Adductor brevis originates from the lower part of the pubic body and adjacent ischiopubic ramus and inserts onto the proximal third of the femoral shaft (linea aspera) posteriorly. Adductor magnus originates from the ischiopubic ramus and adjacent ischial tuberosity, and inserts in two parts: a hamstring part and an adductor part. The hamstring part inserts onto the adductor tubercle of the medial femoral condyle and the adductor part inserts onto the body of the femur immediately lateral to the lines of insertion of both the adductors brevis and longus.

Nerves and Vessels

The peripheral nerves that innervate the lower limb originate from the lumbar (L1-L4) and lumbosacral plexuses (L4-S4). The main blood supply of the lower limb is provided by the femoral artery, the continuation of the external iliac artery distal to beyond the plane of the inguinal ligament. The nerves and vessels pass between the pelvis or posterior abdominal wall and the lower limb through several openings, mainly via the subinguinal space anteriorly and the greater sciatic foramen posteriorly.

Femoral Nerve

The femoral nerve, a branch of the lumbar plexus, leaves the posterior abdominal wall in a groove between iliacus and psoas major below the inguinal ligament to enter the femoral triangle. The femoral nerve innervates the iliacus, pectineus (usually), sartorius, and quadriceps femoris and the cutaneous supply to areas of the anterior thigh, medial leg, and medial aspect of the foot.

Femoral Vessels

The femoral artery, the continuation of the external iliac artery as it passes under the inguinal ligament, lies just medial to the femoral nerve in the femoral triangle. The femoral vein lies just medial to the artery. Typically, in the proximal part of the femoral triangle, the femoral artery gives rise to the deep femoral artery and then continues to the apex of the triangle, wherein it enters the adductor (subsartorial) canal accompanied by the femoral vein and two branches of the femoral nerve, the nerve to vastus medialis and the saphenous nerve.

Lateral Femoral Cutaneous Nerve

The lateral femoral cutaneous nerve, a branch of the lumbar plexus, passes from the posterior abdominal wall to the lower limb, below the inguinal ligament, and medial to the ASIS along the superficial surface of the sartorius muscle at its origin. The nerve initially occupies a space within the fascia lata between the sartorius and tensor fasciae latae muscles and then pierces the fascia lata a few centimeters below the ASIS to supply a cutaneous area along the lateral aspect of the thigh.

Femoral Triangle

The subinguinal space is the area between the inguinal ligament (spanning between the ASIS and the pubic tubercle) and the pelvic bone, which opens from the posterior abdominal wall into a triangular depression in the proximal thigh, the femoral triangle. The inguinal ligament forms the base of the triangle, and the medial margin of sartorius muscle and the lateral margin of the adductor longus muscle form its lateral and medial borders, respectively. The floor of the triangle is made up of iliacus and psoas muscles (joining to form iliopsoas) laterally and by pectineus muscle medially. The main contents of the triangle are, from lateral to medial, the femoral nerve and branches, the femoral artery and branches, the femoral vein and tributaries, and deep inguinal lymph nodes and lymphatic channels (within the femoral canal).

Technique

Anterior Superior Iliac Spine

ANTERIOR SUPERIOR ILIAC SPINE
Transverse
FIG. 5.1

The patient should be supine and appropriately draped to allow for palpation of landmarks and for placing and manipulating the probe while maintaining patient privacy and comfort.

Locate the ASIS and adjacent iliac crest by palpation. Place the face of the probe transversely over the ASIS such that the marker side of the probe is on the ASIS with the remainder of the probe face on the skin of the anterior abdominal wall medial to ASIS. Identify the smooth hyperechoic arc of the ASIS and its dense acoustic shadow. The iliacus muscle is readily identifiable on the anterior abdominal surface of the iliac bone. Medial to the ASIS, identify the three muscle layers of the anterior abdominal wall: external abdominal oblique aponeurosis, internal abdominal oblique, and transversus abdominis. Locate the peritoneum at the deep surface of transversus abdominis. Observe for respiratory movements and peristalsis of abdominal contents deep to the peritoneum. The origins of sartorius and tensor fasciae latae are difficult to identify at the ASIS, but both muscles can be readily identified by scanning a short distance (1-2 cm) inferior to the ASIS. Scan up and down along sartorius (medially and inferiorly

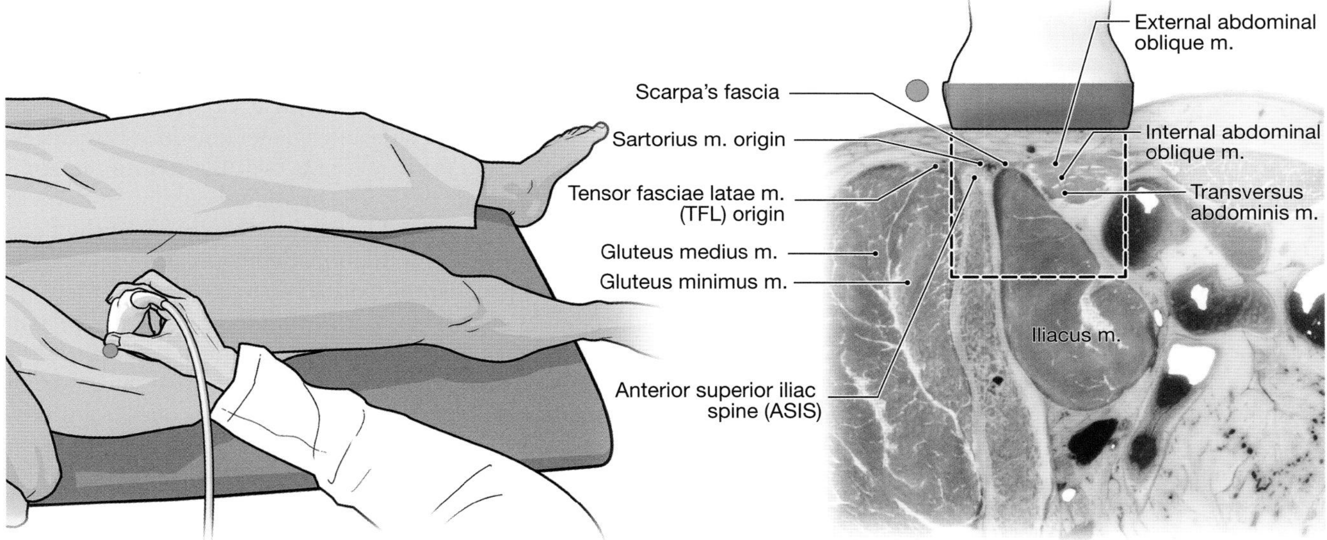

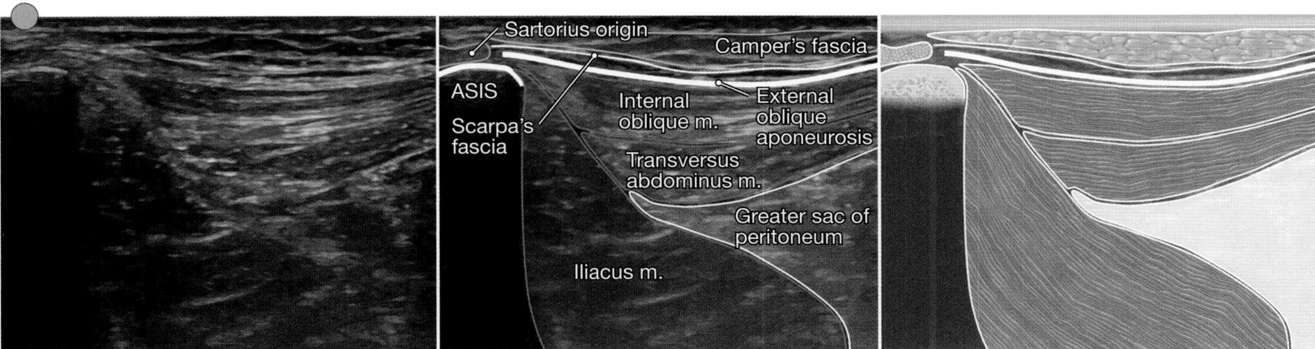

Figure 5.1 Transverse view of anterior superior iliac spine (ASIS) and related muscles including gluteus medius and minimus and abdominal wall muscles, and the origins of sartorius and tensor fasciae latae (TFL).

from the ASIS) for several centimeters. The muscle profile appears just below the ASIS, and the muscle enlarges rapidly to its familiar "strap" shape (flattened oval profile). Place the probe back over the ASIS and scan up and down over tensor fasciae latae (laterally/posteriorly and inferiorly from the ASIS) for several centimeters. Like the sartorius, the tensor fasciae latae quickly enlarges and its oval muscle tissue profile becomes obvious a very short distance below the ASIS.

Sartorius, Tensor Fasciae Latae, and Rectus Femoris

SARTORIUS TENSOR FASCIAE LATAE RECTUS FEMORIS
Transverse
FIG. 5.2

Starting with the same patient position and draping, place the probe over the ASIS and slowly slide the probe inferiorly until both tensor fasciae latae and sartorius can be identified within the image. Keeping both tensor fasciae latae and sartorius in the image, continue slowly scanning inferiorly until the rectus femoris muscle begins to appear immediately deep to these two muscles. After identifying the rectus femoris, slide the probe face back superiorly to the point where the rectus femoris muscle disappears, and attempt to identify the hyperechoic profile and the acoustic shadow of anterior inferior iliac spine. Return the probe distally to the point where tensor fasciae latae, sartorius, and rectus femoris can be clearly identified within the same image. In the medial aspect of the image, deep to sartorius and the medial aspect of rectus femoris, identify the iliopsoas muscle. The hyperechoic reflection of the femoral head and proximal part of the femoral neck (viewed obliquely) covered by fibrous hip joint capsule and iliofemoral ligament can be seen just deep to iliopsoas in this position. The anterior-most extent of the gluteus medius can be identified deep to tensor fasciae latae.

Lateral Femoral Cutaneous Nerve

LATERAL FEMORAL CUTANEOUS NERVE
Transverse
FIG. 5.3

Beginning with the probe in the last position above, scan slowly a short distance inferiorly until, as tensor fasciae latae moves posteriorly/laterally and sartorius moves medially, rectus femoris comes to occupy a more superficial position between these two muscles. Observe that the lateral femoral cutaneous nerve has pierced the deep surface of the fascia lata to occupy a small fatty compartment within the fascia lata between the tensor fasciae latae and the sartorius and just superficial to the rectus femoris. Attempt to follow the nerve until it pierces the superficial surface of the fascia lata into a cutaneous position.

Hip Joint, Iliopsoas, and Iliofemoral Ligament

HIP JOINT
Longitudinal
FIG. 5.4

The patient should be supine and appropriately draped, with the limb to be examined rotated externally. Using a curved array abdominal probe, place the probe face just below the center of the inguinal fold, oriented obliquely (roughly perpendicular to the inguinal fold) from superomedial to inferolateral. Adjust the probe position and tilt until the hyperechoic profile of the femoral head and neck can be identified. Adjust the probe position and tilt until the hyperechoic profile of the acetabular rim can be seen along with the femoral head and neck. Identify the acetabular labrum projecting a short distance over the femoral head from the rim of the acetabulum. Just superficial to the acetabular rim, labrum, femoral head, and femoral neck, identify the joint capsule and iliofemoral ligament, which typically appear hypoechoic with multiple linear hyperechoic bands. The capsule and ligament begin at the acetabular margin superiorly and pass over the labrum, femoral head, and femoral neck. The capsule should be uniform in thickness (4-6 mm) and parallel to the profile of the head and neck of the femur. Identify the iliopsoas muscle superficial to the joint capsule with its characteristic hyperechoic deep tendinous part in contact with the capsule (there is an intervening iliopsoas bursa, which cannot be seen unless it is inflamed) as it passes over the hip joint and femoral neck to insert at the lesser trochanter (just out of view posteromedially in Figure 5.4). Sartorius muscle is the most superficial muscle in this view, and in the distal part of the image, a portion of rectus femoris can often be identified between sartorius and iliopsoas.

Femoral Triangle

FEMORAL TRIANGLE FEMORAL VESSELS AND NERVE
Transverse
FIG. 5.5

The patient should be supine and appropriately draped, with the limb to be examined rotated externally. Place the probe (high-frequency linear) just below the inguinal fold and oriented obliquely about halfway between parallel to the inguinal ligament and a true horizontal plane. Adjust the probe position until the pulsating femoral artery is visible near the center of the image. Identify the iliopsoas in the floor of the triangle laterally and the

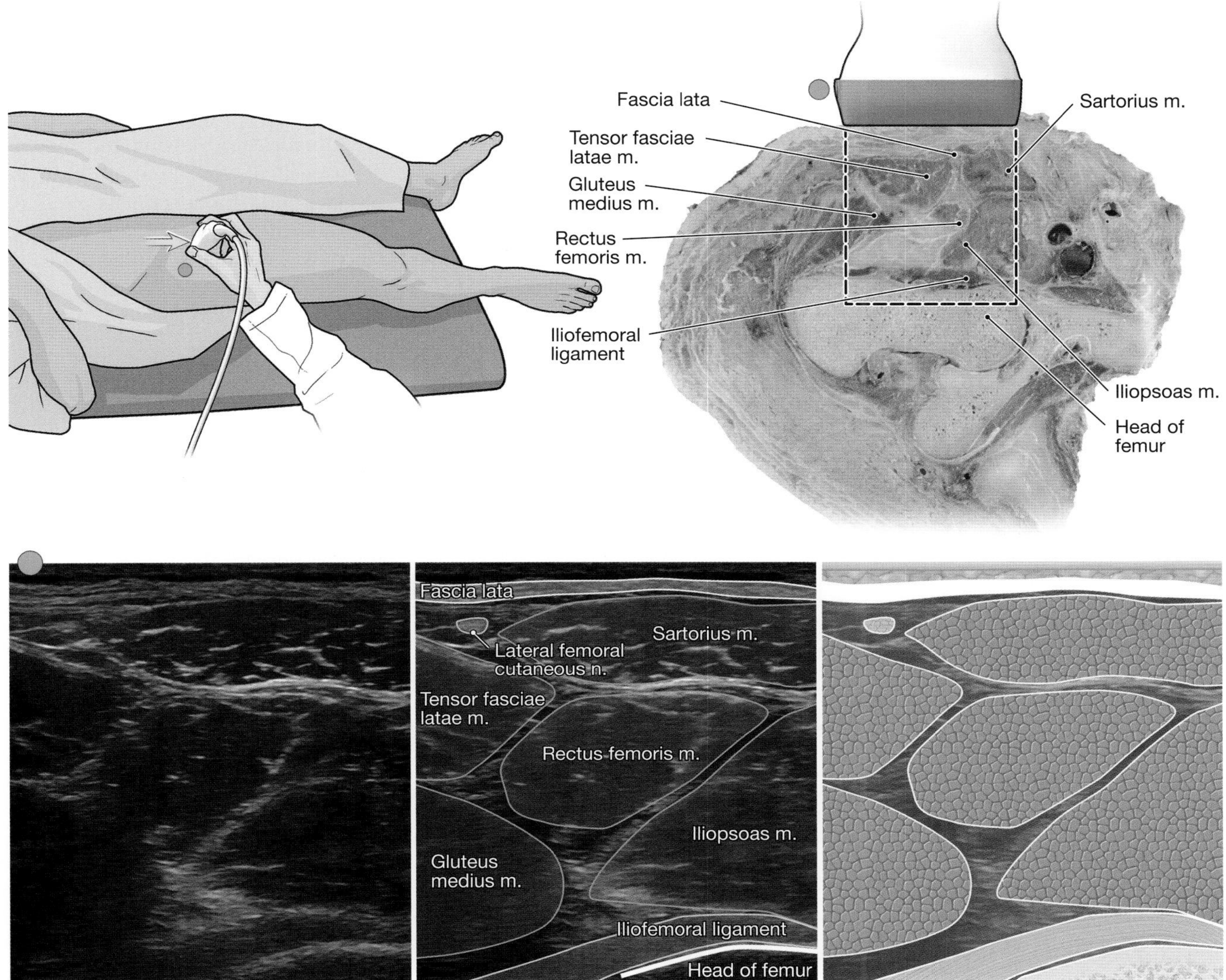

Figure 5.2 Transverse view of sartorius, tensor fasciae latae, rectus femoris, and iliopsoas a short distance below anterior inferior iliac spine, crossing anterior to the femoral head.

pectineus in the floor of the triangle medially. Identify the femoral vein medial to the femoral artery, and observe the effects of varying probe face pressures on the vein. Identify the femoral nerve on the lateral side of the artery, by adjusting the probe position, pressure, and tilting it to optimize the "honeycomb" echotexture of the nerve, which commonly has a triangular profile in this view. Scan inferiorly a short distance along the femoral artery to observe its deep femoral branch. Using as little probe pressure as possible, slide the probe superiorly along the femoral vein and attempt to identify the point where the great saphenous vein enters the femoral vein through a defect in the fascia lata, the saphenous opening. Observe the motion of the venous valves in the femoral vein and its tributaries.

Deep Inguinal Lymph Node

DEEP INGUINAL LYMPH NODE
Transverse
FIG. 5.6

With the probe over the femoral triangle as described hereinbefore, slide the probe a short distance medially until the femoral artery is at the lateral extent of the image and the pectineus muscle is well seen. Look for one or more deep inguinal lymph nodes between the fascia lata and pectineus muscle near the medial aspect of the femoral vein (in this image the probe pressure is nearly completely compressing the vein). The typical US appearance of a lymph node is a hypoechoic oval or bean-shaped structure with a linear hyperechoic band/zone in the center. The capsule of the lymph node may be seen as a very thin echogenic line. Although the precise histology/cytoarchitecture of lymph nodes cannot be identified with US, generally the hypoechoic area represents the node cortex and paracortex, and the hyperechoic band represents fat tracking along nodal blood vessels and efferent lymphatic vessel through the hilum and into the medullary zone of the node.

Pectineus and Adductor Muscles in the Proximal Thigh

PECTINEUS AND ADDUCTOR MUSCLES
Transverse
FIG. 5.7

Starting from the probe position and orientation described hereinbefore for viewing the medial aspect of the femoral triangle including the pectineus muscle, slide the probe medially keeping the pectineus muscle in view. Continue scanning medially until the medial edge of the pectineus is just in view at the lateral aspect of the image and the three adductor muscles

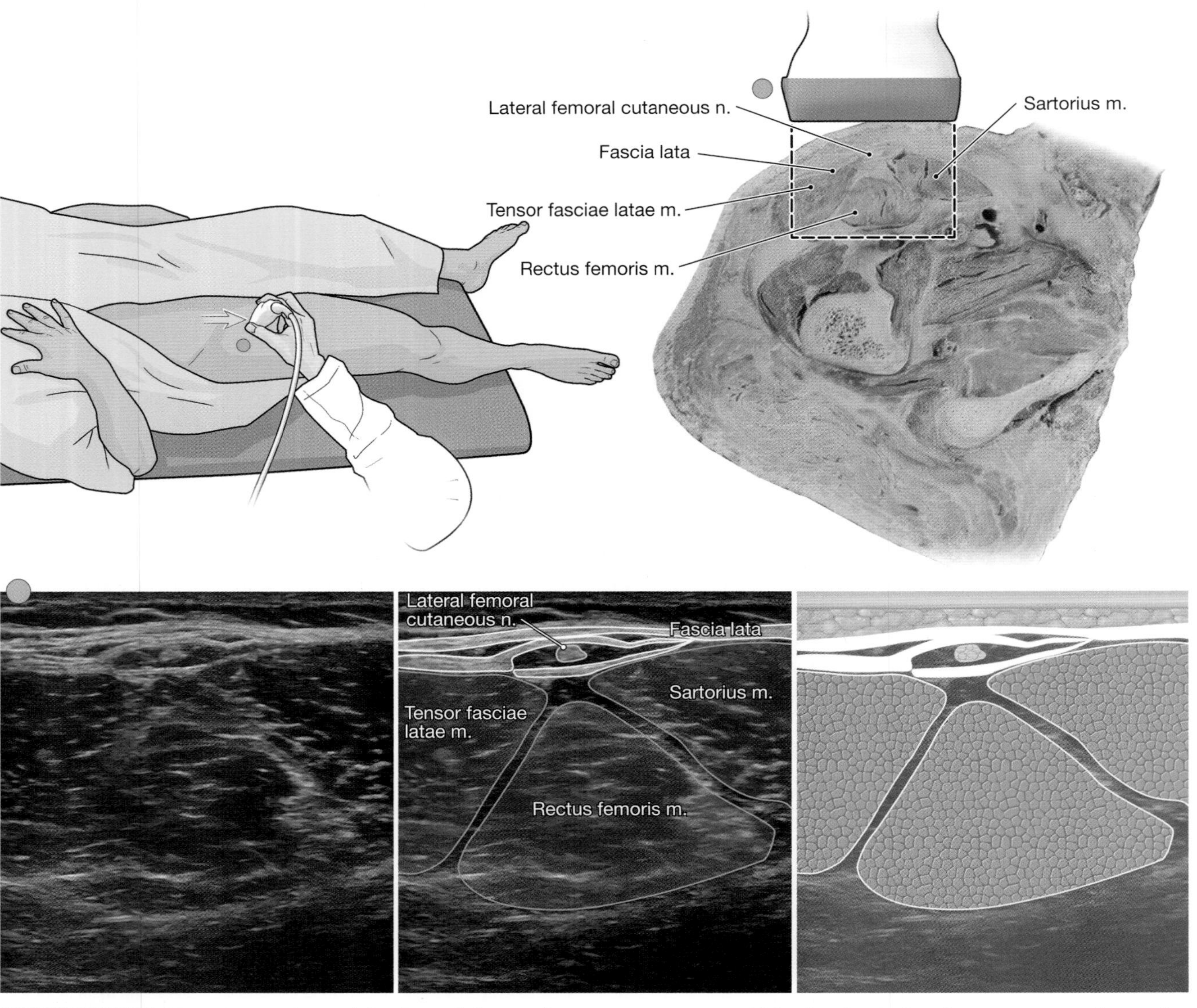

Figure 5.3 Transverse view of the lateral femoral cutaneous nerve within the fascia lata between sartorius and tensor fasciae latae.

can be seen medial to the pectineus. The most superficial of the three is the adductor longus. Immediately deep to adductor longus is adductor brevis. Deep to the adductor brevis is adductor magnus. Note that the lateral-most part of adductor magnus is also deep to the pectineus. Scan inferiorly and superiorly along the adductor brevis muscle and attempt to identify branches of the obturator nerve at the deep and superficial surfaces of the muscle.

CLINICAL APPLICATION

US examination is commonly used in the evaluation of the painful hip resulting from musculoskeletal injuries or degenerative disorders, such as iliopsoas tendinosis/tendonitis, partial or complete tendon tears, iliopsoas bursitis, tears or cysts of the acetabular labrum, and effusions resulting from inflammatory conditions affecting the hip joint. US can also be used for guiding needles for hip joint aspiration or injection of anti-inflammatory drugs and local anesthetic agents. These techniques can be used for guiding needles for access and catheter placement in the femoral vein or artery. US examination, including Doppler US, is commonly used for the detection of deep vein thrombi in lower limb veins, including the femoral vein and its tributaries. Doppler US is also used for the measurement of flow velocity profiles in the femoral artery in suspected peripheral artery disease. US-guided femoral nerve blocks are used in surgeries involving the anterior thigh and for postoperative pain control in anterior thigh and knee surgery. Femoral nerve block combined with sciatic nerve block can be used in a wide variety of lower limb surgeries. Lateral femoral cutaneous nerve blocks are used in the evaluation and management of lateral thigh pain syndromes resulting from compression or entrapment of the nerve (meralgia paresthetica). Incidental pathologies such as femoral or inguinal hernias may also be detected during US examinations in the proximal thigh.

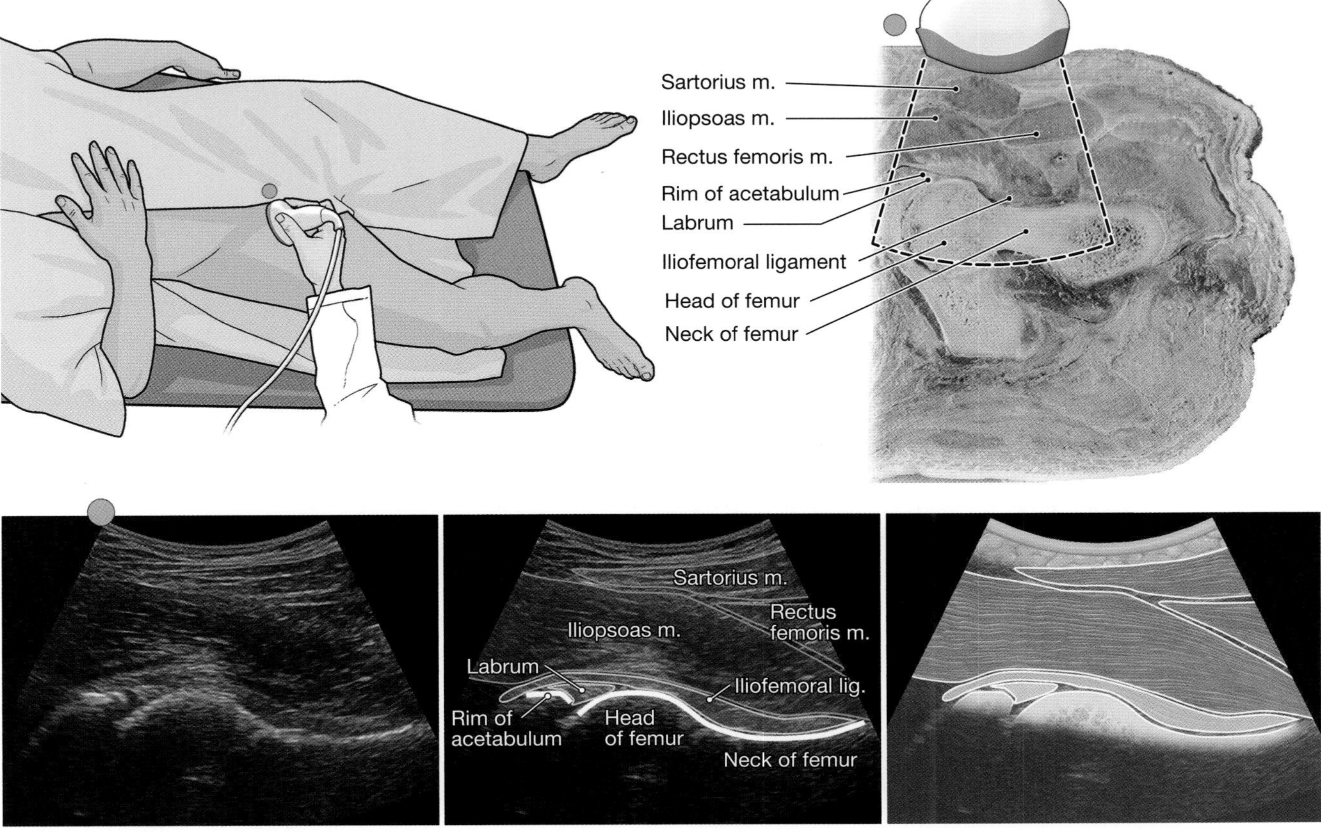

Figure 5.4 Longitudinal view of the hip joint including the rim of the acetabulum, acetabular labrum, femoral head and neck, iliofemoral ligament, and iliopsoas muscle/tendon.

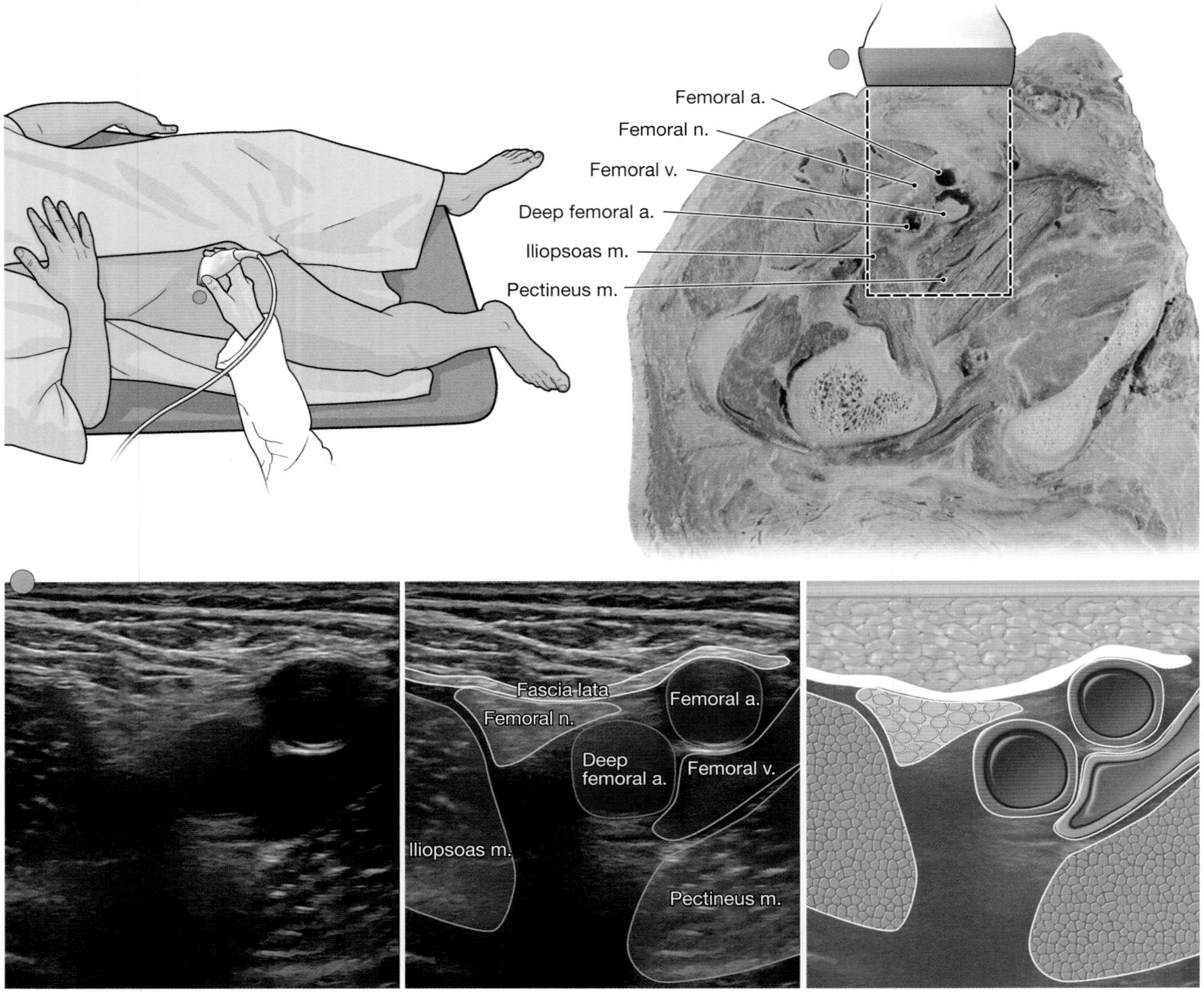

Figure 5.5 Transverse view of the femoral nerve, femoral artery, and femoral vein in the femoral triangle.

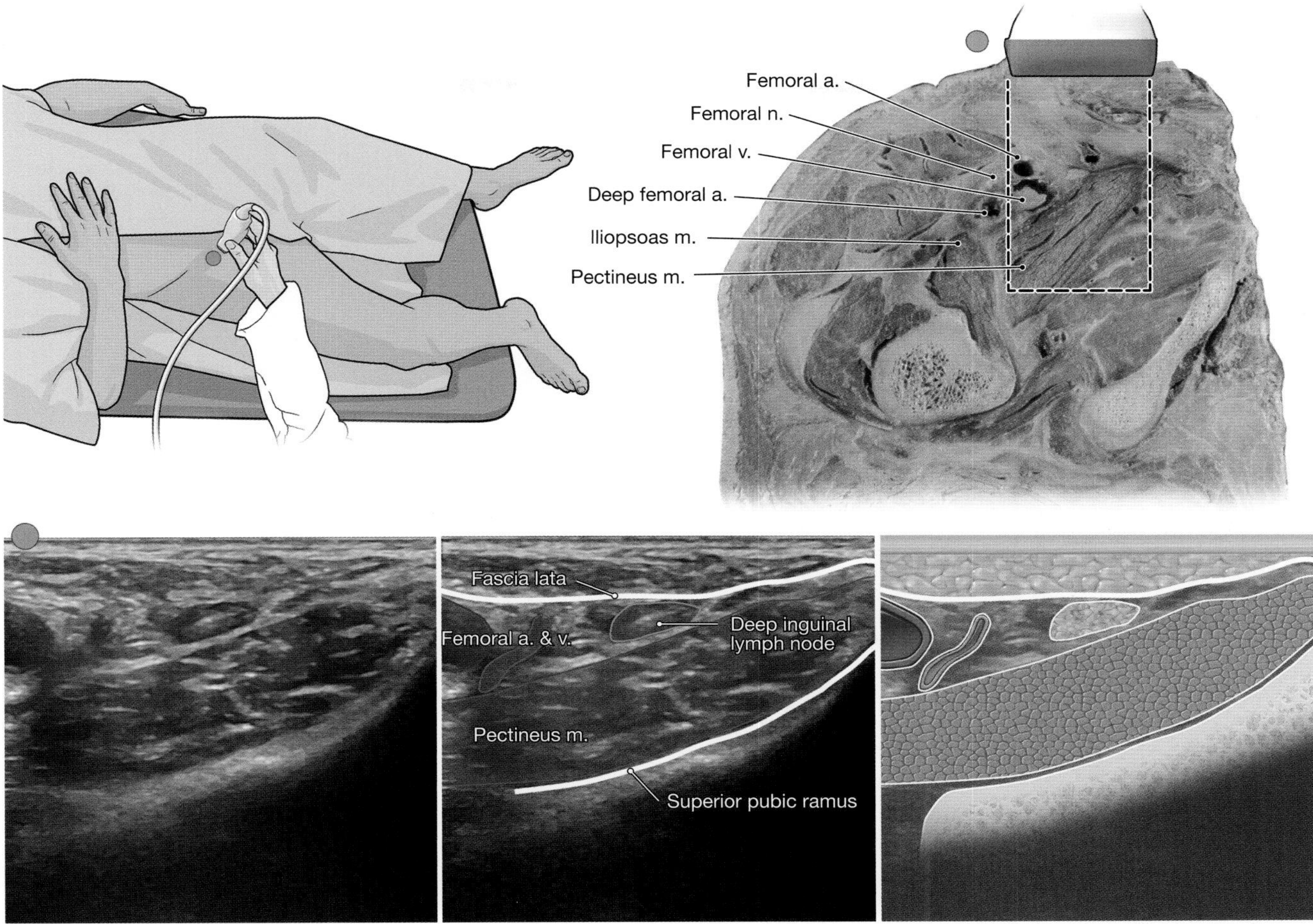

Figure 5.6 Transverse view of a deep inguinal lymph node in the medial aspect of the femoral triangle.

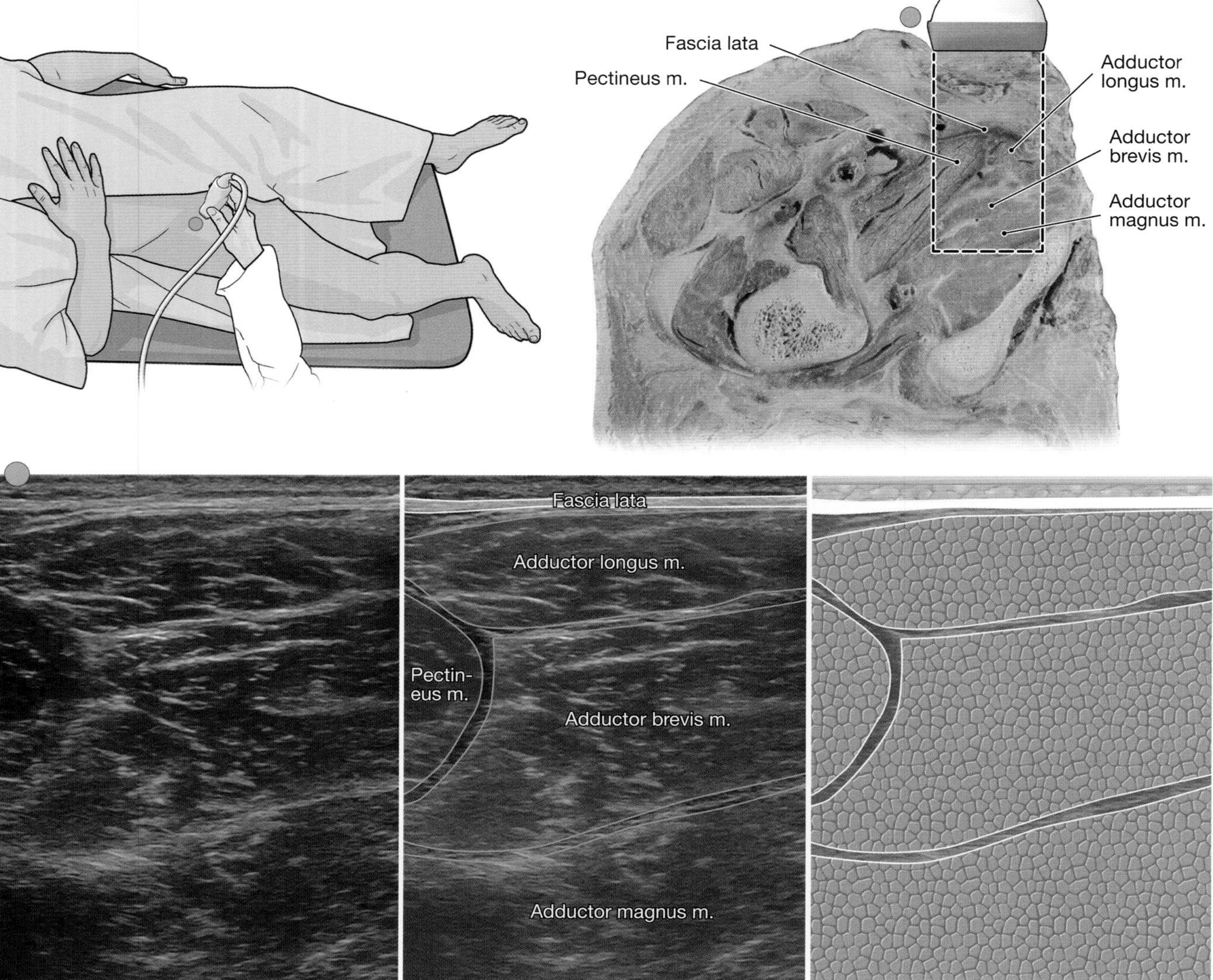

Figure 5.7 Transverse view of pectineus, adductor longus, adductor brevis, and adductor magnus just medial to the femoral triangle.

Gluteal Region

Review of the Anatomy

Bones

The bones of the gluteal region are the pelvic bones, sacrum, coccyx, and greater trochanter, intertrochanteric crest, and gluteal tuberosity of the proximal femur.

Greater and Lesser Sciatic Foramina

Two ligaments, the sacrospinous and sacrotuberous, stabilize the sacrum relative to the pelvic bone and form parts of the borders of two openings, the greater and lesser sciatic foramina. The greater sciatic foramen is superior to the sacrospinous ligament and ischial spine, and the lesser sciatic foramen is inferior to the sacrospinous ligament and ischial spine. The bony margins of the two foramina are formed by the greater sciatic and lesser sciatic notches of the posterior margin of the pelvic bone. The gluteal region communicates with the pelvis through the greater sciatic foramen and with the perineum through the lesser sciatic foramen.

Muscles and Fascia

Fascia Lata and Iliotibial Tract

The fascia lata is the deep fascia of the gluteal region and thigh. The fascia lata covers only the superficial surface of the gluteus medius, but splits into two layers to cover both the deep and superficial surfaces of gluteus maximus and tensor fasciae latae. It has a thickened band laterally, the iliotibial tract, which begins proximally as fibrous extensions from the superficial and deep surfaces of gluteus maximus and from the superficial and deep surfaces of tensor fasciae latae, which join together in the anterior part of the gluteal region. The iliotibial tract continues distally along the lateral aspect of the thigh and then crosses the knee joint to attach at the anterolateral surface of the tibia.

Gluteal Maximus, Medius, and Minimus

The posterior (gluteal) surface of the ala of the ilium serves as a site of origin for gluteus maximus, medius, and minimus.

Gluteus maximus is a large rhomboid-shaped muscle that originates from the posterior surface of the ilium posterior to the posterior gluteal line, the posterior surface of the sacrum, and the posterior surface of the sacrotuberous ligament and inserts into the posterior edge of the iliotibial tract and the gluteal tuberosity of the proximal femur. Gluteus maximus is the largest and most superficial muscle of the gluteal region. Gluteus medius originates from the gluteal surface of the ilium between the posterior and anterior gluteal lines and inserts onto the lateral surface of the greater trochanter of the femur. Lying deep to gluteus medius, gluteus minimus originates from the surface of the ilium between the anterior and inferior gluteal lines and inserts onto the anterior surface of the greater trochanter.

Tensor Fasciae Latae

The tensor fasciae latae originates from the iliac crest along a line between the ASIS and the tubercle of the crest and uses the iliotibial tract to gain attachment to the tibia. In this position, the tensor fasciae latae is superficial to gluteus medius and minimus.

Deep Group of Muscles

Several lateral rotators of the femur, comprising the deep group of gluteal region muscles, originate from the pelvic bone and pass through the gluteal region to insert on the proximal femur. Piriformis originates from the pelvic surface of the sacrum, enters the gluteal region through the greater sciatic foramen, and inserts onto the medial surface of the apex of the greater trochanter of the femur. The obturator internus originates from the deep surface of the margin of the obturator foramen and obturator membrane, turns approximately 90° over the lesser sciatic notch, and its tendon passes laterally through the floor of the gluteal region between gemellus superior and inferior muscles to insert onto the trochanteric fossa of the greater trochanter. The gemellus superior and inferior originate from the posterior surfaces of the ischial spine and tuberosity, respectively, and insert onto the intervening tendon of obturator internus and the trochanteric fossa. Quadratus femoris, the most inferior of the lateral rotators of the hip, originates from the lateral surface of the ischium adjacent to the ischial tuberosity and inserts onto the intertrochanteric crest of the femur.

Hamstring Origin

The hamstring muscles of the posterior compartment of the thigh originate from a large common tendon attached along the posterior/posterolateral surface of the ischial tuberosity.

Nerves and Arteries

Sciatic Nerve

The sciatic nerve, a major source of innervation in the lower limb, is the largest branch of the lumbosacral plexus with nerve fibers from L4 to S3. The nerve leaves the pelvis through the greater sciatic foramen inferior to piriformis and descends through the gluteal region immediately deep to the gluteus maximus and coursing over the gemellus superior, the tendon of obturator internus, the inferior gemellus, and finally, the quadratus femoris. At the inferior extent of the gluteal region, the nerve is located between the gluteus maximus and the quadratus femoris, where it lies in a shallow groove between the intertrochanteric crest laterally and the ischial tuberosity medially, adjacent to the common hamstring tendon of origin. At the inferior border of quadratus femoris, the sciatic nerve enters the thigh wherein it continues to descend deep to the long head of biceps femoris muscle in the posterior compartment of the thigh. In the distal thigh, the sciatic nerve divides into its terminal branches, the tibial and common fibular nerves.

Other Branches of the Lumbosacral Plexus

Other branches of the lumbosacral plexus that enter the gluteal region through the greater sciatic foramen include the superior gluteal nerve (gluteus medius, gluteus minimus, and tensor fasciae latae), inferior gluteal nerve (gluteus maximus), pudendal nerve (perineum), posterior femoral cutaneous nerve (cutaneous supply in the posterior thigh), the nerve to obturator internus (obturator internus and gemellus superior), and the nerve to quadratus femoris (gemellus inferior and quadratus femoris).

Superior and Inferior Gluteal Arteries

The superior and inferior gluteal arteries, branches off the internal iliac artery in the pelvis, enter the gluteal region through the greater sciatic foramen, respectively, above and below the piriformis muscle. These arteries supply muscles and other structures of the gluteal region and hip joint and provide anastomotic branches for collateral circulation with the femoral artery.

The superior gluteal artery, accompanied by the superior gluteal nerve, courses anteriorly between gluteus medius and gluteus minimus.

Technique

Anterior Gluteal Region

TENSOR FASCIA LATA GLUTEUS MEDIUS AND MINIMUS
Longitudinal
FIG. 5.8

For examination of the anterior gluteal region on the right, the patient should be in left lateral decubitus position and appropriately draped to allow for palpation of landmarks and probe positioning. Orient the probe in the long axis of the thigh halfway between the ASIS and the tubercle of the iliac crest, a few centimeters inferior to the crest. The probe face should be directed slightly posteriorly (as opposed to true coronal orientation). Identify the tensor fasciae latae muscle and the layers of fascia lata on its superficial and deep surfaces. Identify the gluteus medius muscle deep to the tensor fasciae latae. Deep to the gluteus medius, and with a slightly different fiber orientation and connective tissue density, identify the gluteus minimus muscle.

GLUTEUS MEDIUS GLUTEUS MINIMUS GLUTEAL SURFACE OF ILIUM
Longitudinal
FIG. 5.9

From the aforementioned position, slide the probe posteriorly, maintaining the same orientation, to just beyond the lateral/posterior border of tensor fasciae latae. Adjust the probe position slightly superiorly until, from superficial to deep, the fascia lata, gluteus medius muscle, gluteus minimus muscle, and the posterior (gluteal) surface of the iliac ala can be clearly seen and identified.

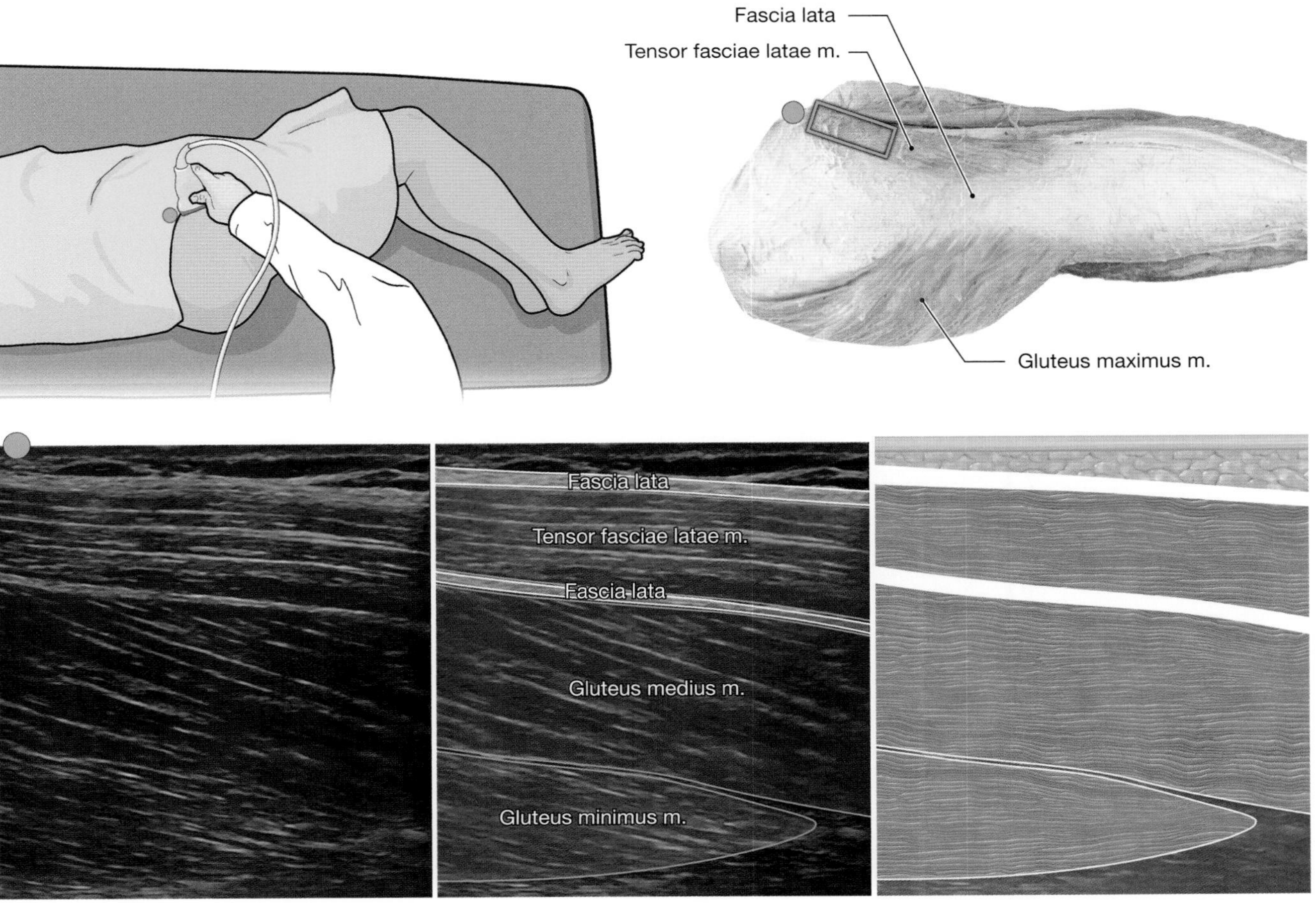

Figure 5.8 Longitudinal view of tensor fasciae latae, gluteus medius, and gluteus minimus at the anterior-most extent of the gluteal region.

Greater Trochanter: Tendons of the Gluteus Medius and Minimus

ILIOTIBIAL TRACT
TENDONS OF GLUTEUS MEDIUS AND MINIMUS
Transverse
FIG. 5.10

The patient should be in the lateral decubitus position and appropriately draped to allow for palpation of landmarks and probe positioning. Locate the greater trochanter by palpation and place the probe transversely near its superior aspect. Identify the hyperechoic reflection and the acoustic shadow of the greater trochanter and adjust the probe position as needed to obtain an image that includes the following bony features: a relatively flat lateral surface parallel to the skin (lateral surface), which ends anteriorly with a steep drop onto a surface directed anteriorly/anterolaterally (anterior surface) and which curves posteriorly onto a surface directed posterolaterally. This area of the greater trochanter is often clinically referred to as the trochanteric apex. The gluteus medius inserts onto the lateral surface, and its tendon can be seen in transverse view along the lateral surface of the trochanter. The gluteus minimus inserts onto the anterior surface, and its tendon can be seen in this position, although it is commonly hypoechoic due to **anisotropy**. The gluteus maximus crosses along the posterior surface of the greater trochanter (not a true tendinous

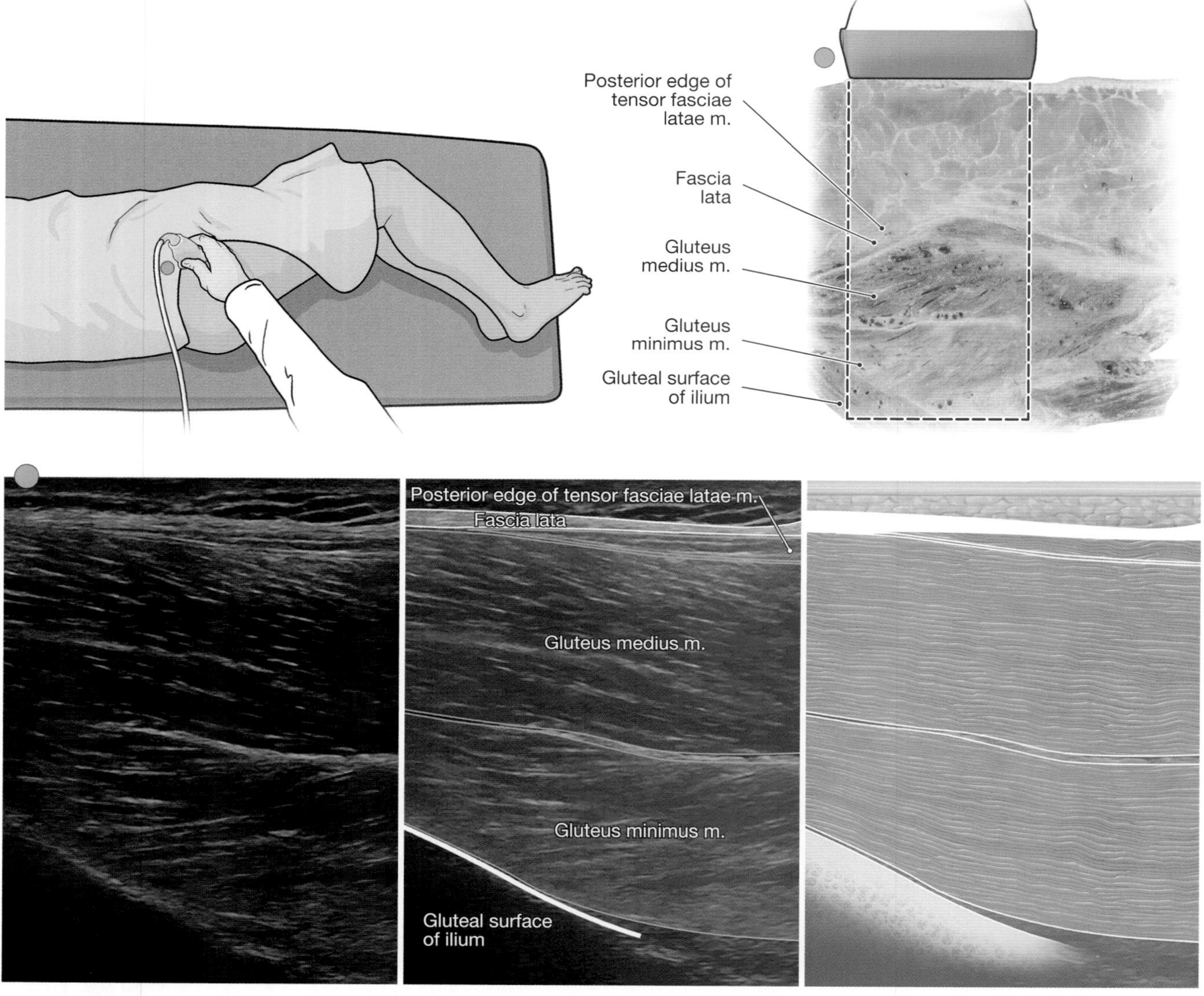

Figure 5.9 Longitudinal view of gluteus medius, gluteus minimus, and the posterior (gluteal) surface of the ala of the ilium, just posterior to the lateral/posterior border of tensor fasciae latae.

attachment surface), separated from the bone surface by the trochanteric bursa (only visible when inflamed), and inserts into the posterior edge of the iliotibial tract of the fascia lata.

TENDON OF GLUTEUS MEDIUS
Longitudinal
FIG. 5.11

Beginning from the transverse view of the greater trochanter above, center the lateral facet in the image and carefully rotate the probe 90° (probe marker directed superiorly) into a longitudinal orientation over the lateral surface. Adjust the probe position as needed (usually a short distance superiorly) until the insertion of the gluteus medius tendon can be identified. Fanning and "heel-toe" tilting of the probe face are helpful to visualize the fibrillar architecture of the tendon, which may be obscured because of anisotropy. Identify the iliotibial tract overlying the tendon. Fibers of the gluteus maximus muscle can also be seen inserting into the iliotibial tract from the inferior aspect of the image.

Sciatic Nerve in the Gluteal Region

SCIATIC NERVE
GLUTEUS MAXIMUS
QUADRATUS FEMORIS
Transverse
FIG. 5.12

The patient should be prone and appropriately draped to allow for palpation of landmarks and probe manipulation. By palpation, identify the posterior edge of the greater trochanter/intertrochanteric crest laterally and the ischial tuberosity medially. Place a curved array abdominal probe, oriented transversely, between these two landmarks (probe marker directed laterally) and adjust the probe position until the hyperechoic profile of the intertrochanteric crest can be identified along the lateral edge of

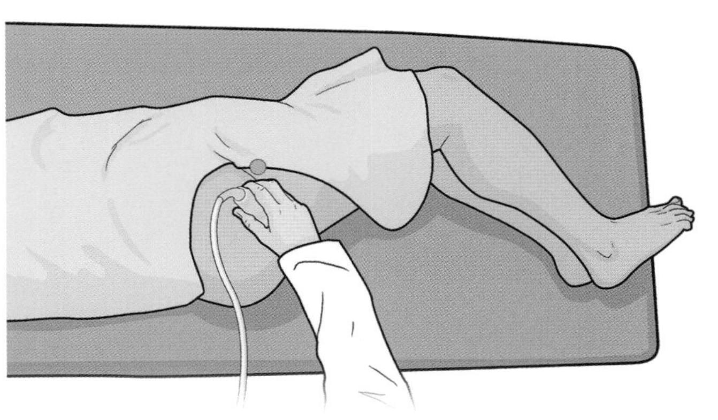

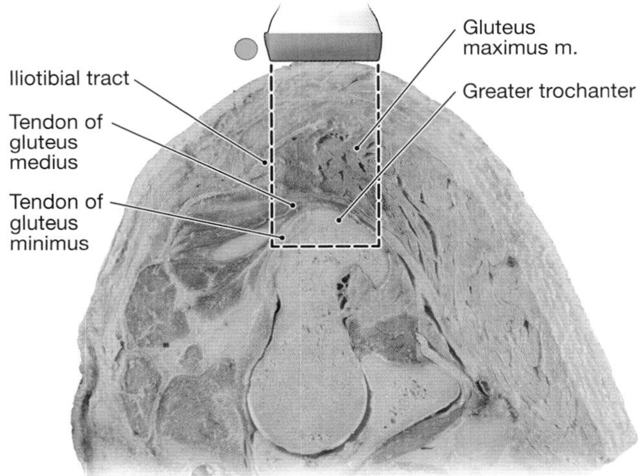

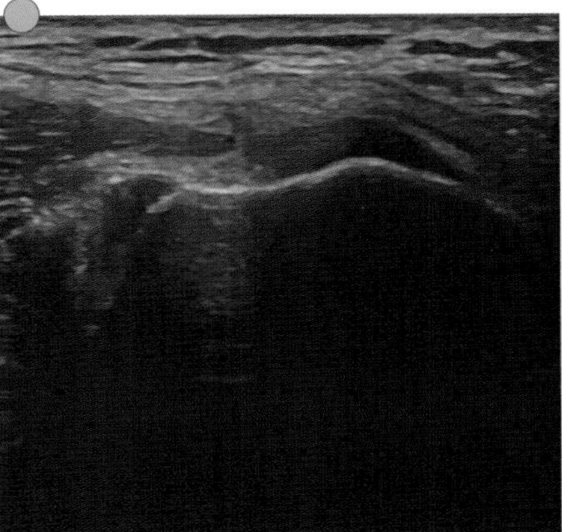

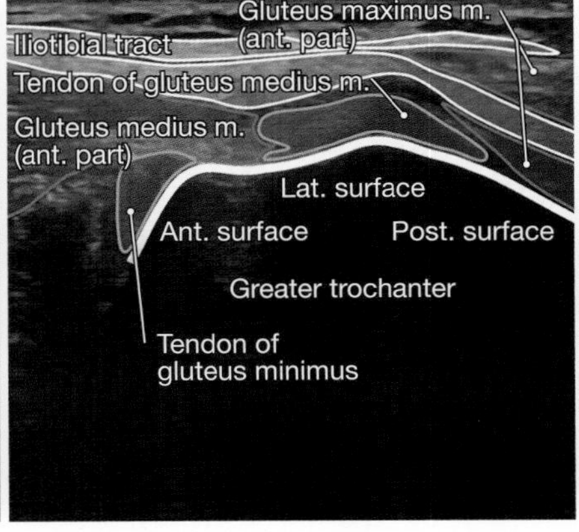

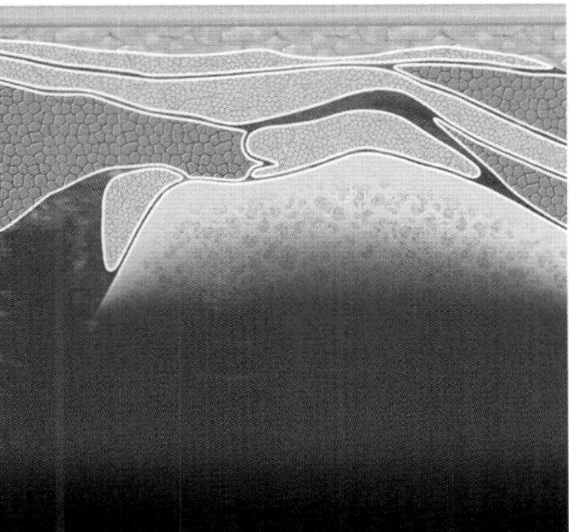

Figure 5.10 Transverse view of the tendons of gluteus minimus and gluteus medius at the anterior and lateral surfaces of the greater trochanter. Muscle fibers of gluteus maximus are seen attaching at the posterior edge of the iliotibial tract.

the image and the hyperechoic ischial tuberosity with the overlying hypoechoic/anechoic (due to anisotropy) common hamstring tendon can be seen at the medial aspect of the image. Identify the quadratus femoris muscle spanning between the lateral surface of the ischium adjacent to the tuberosity and the intertrochanteric crest. Adjacent to the ischial tuberosity and common hamstring tendon, between the quadratus femoris and the gluteus maximus muscles, identify the ovoid or triangular profile of the sciatic nerve with its typical hyperechoic honeycomb appearance (fanning and tilting the probe face as needed to minimize anisotropy).

CLINICAL APPLICATION

US examination is being increasingly used in the evaluation of lateral hip pain resulting from musculoskeletal injuries or overuse disorders, such as the gluteus medius or gluteus minimus tendinosis/tendonitis, partial/complete tendon tears, or associated trochanteric bursopathy/bursitis. US is also used for guiding needles for peritendinous or intrabursal injection of local anesthetics and/or anti-inflammatory steroids. Lateral "snapping" hip syndrome results from the iliotibial tract or the anterior border of gluteus maximus sliding back and forth across the greater trochanter, and this sudden movement can be detected in real-time images as the examiner passively flexes and externally rotates the hip.

US-guided sciatic nerve blocks are used in surgeries involving the knee, posterior leg, Achilles (calcaneal) tendon, ankle, and foot and for postoperative control of posterior knee pain. Sciatic nerve block combined with femoral nerve block is used in a wide variety of lower limb surgeries.

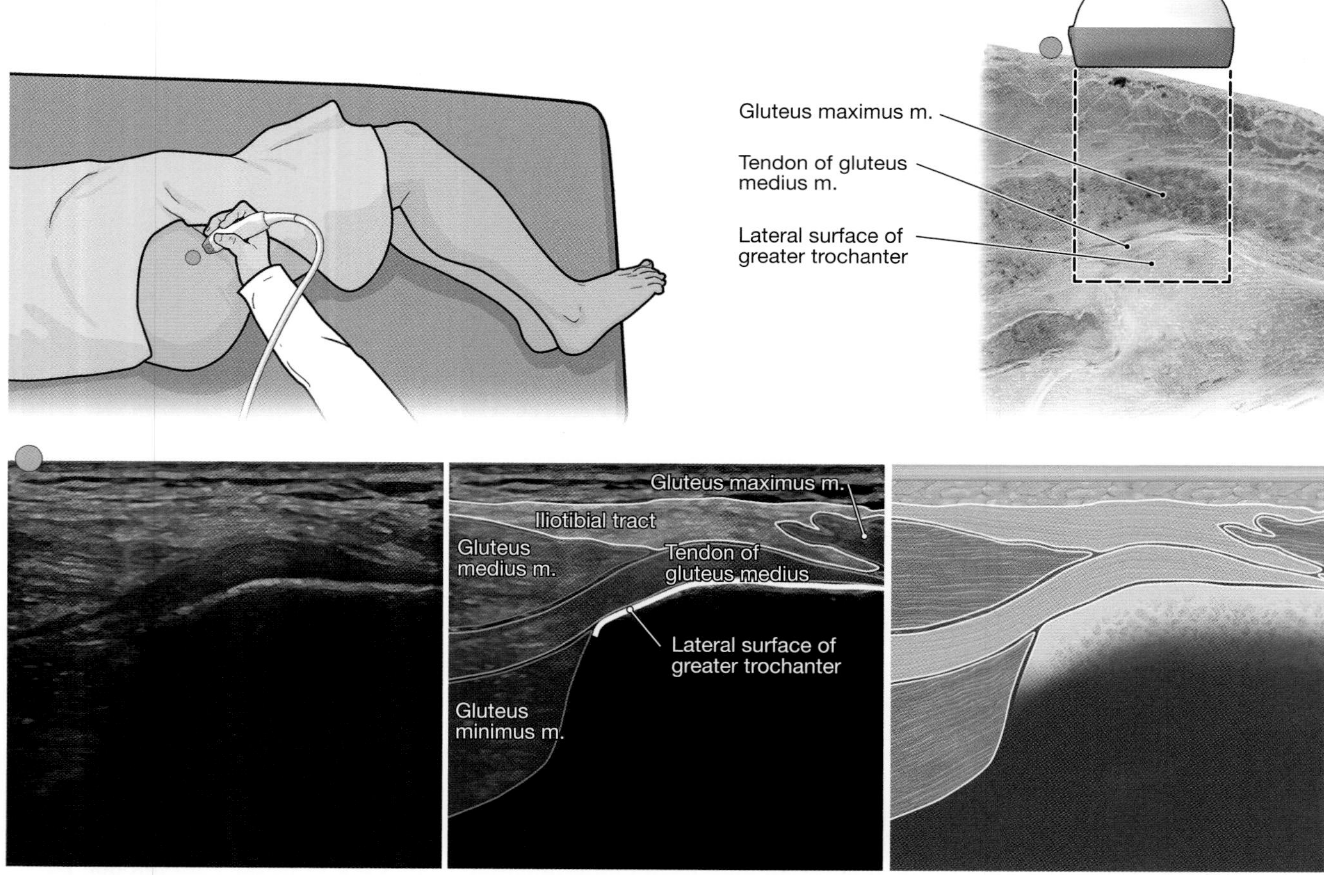

Figure 5.11 Longitudinal view of the tendon of gluteus medius inserting onto the lateral surface of the greater trochanter of the femur.

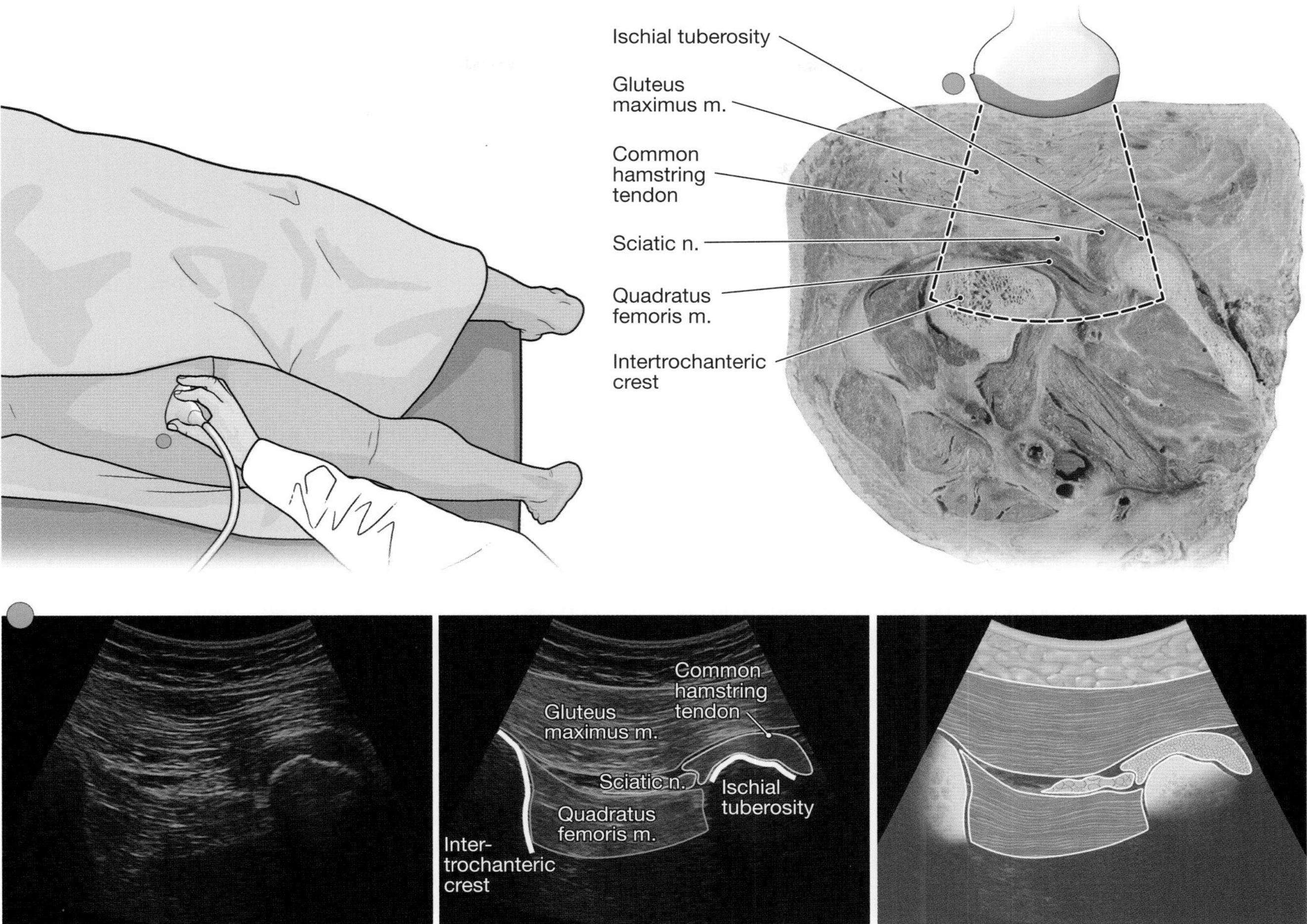

Figure 5.12 Transverse view of the sciatic nerve in the gluteal region, between gluteus maximus and quadratus femoris, and adjacent to the common hamstring tendon of origin at the ischial tuberosity.

Thigh

Review of the Anatomy

Bones

The femur is the bone of the thigh. From the junction of the femoral neck with the trochanteric region, the body of the femur descends obliquely from lateral to medial and ends at the medial and lateral condyles, which articulate with corresponding articular surfaces of the medial and lateral condyles of the tibial plateau. The proximal half of the body of the femur is triangular in profile, with smooth borders between the anterior surface and its posteromedial and posterolateral surfaces, and with a coarse ridge, the linea aspera, at its posterior border. The distal half of the body widens as it approaches the condyles, and the linea aspera divides into medial and lateral supracondylar lines, forming an additional posterior surface as the femur approaches the popliteal fossa.

Muscles and Fascia

Compartments

The muscles of the thigh are divided into three compartments by the fascia lata and its intermuscular septae. The anterior compartment muscles include the quadriceps femoris and sartorius. The posterior compartment muscles are the hamstrings: biceps femoris, semitendinosus, and semimembranosus. The medial compartment muscles were briefly reviewed in an ealier section.

Anterior Compartment

The quadriceps femoris muscle consist of rectus femoris, vastus lateralis, vastus intermedius, and vastus medialis.

- The *rectus femoris* muscle is the most superficial of the quadriceps group and the only quadriceps femoris muscle that crosses both the hip and knee joints. It originates via a straight tendon from the anterior inferior iliac spine and a second reflected tendon from the ilium just superior to the acetabulum and inserts along with the vastus muscles via the quadriceps femoris tendon onto the patella.
- The *vastus lateralis* originates from the distal inferior surface of the greater trochanter of the femur, the superolateral part of the intertrochanteric line, and from a line along the lateral lip of the linea aspera.
- The *vastus intermedius* originates from a wide area along the posterolateral and anterior surfaces, and medial border of the body of the femur, separating the vastus lateralis from most of the posterolateral surface of the femur.
- The *vastus medialis* originates along a line beginning at the inferomedial aspect of the intertrochanteric line, continues along the medial lip of the linea aspera and adjacent posteromedial surface of the body of the femur, and ends in the distal femur, a short distance along the medial supracondylar line. The vastus muscles, along with the rectus femoris, insert onto the patella via the quadriceps femoris tendon.

Sartorius originates from the medial aspect of the ASIS and crosses the thigh from lateral to medial. In the first part of its course, sartorius forms the lateral border of the femoral triangle. Beyond the apex of the triangle, sartorius forms the roof or anterior wall of the adductor canal throughout the middle third of the thigh. Sartorius inserts on the medial surface of the proximal tibia along with gracilis and semitendinosus. The anterior compartment muscles are innervated by the femoral nerve.

The *fascia lata* is the deep fascia of the gluteal region and thigh. The fascia lata has a thickened band laterally, the *iliotibial tract*, which begins proximally in the anterior part of the gluteal region and continues distally along the vastus lateralis muscle, crosses the knee joint, and attaches to the anterolateral surface of the lateral tibial condyle.

Posterior Compartment

The three hamstring muscles of the posterior compartment are biceps femoris, semitendinosus, and semimembranosus.

- The long head of the *biceps femoris* originates from a common tendon with the semitendinosus attached to the medial half of the ischial tuberosity and inserts via a common tendon with the short head at the head of the fibula. The short head originates along a line beginning about the midfemur at the lateral lip of the linea aspera and ending at the proximal part of the lateral supracondylar line. The biceps femoris is the most lateral of the posterior compartment muscles and has an oblique medial to the lateral course through the thigh.

- The *semitendinosus* originates from a conjoined tendon with the biceps femoris attached to the medial half of the ischial tuberosity. The muscle belly, which lies just medial to the biceps femoris in the upper half of the thigh, tapers about the midthigh to a long thin tendon that inserts onto the anteromedial surface of the proximal tibia along with the sartorius and gracilis.
- The *semimembranosus* originates from the lateral half of the ischial tuberosity via a tendon that expands into a broad flattened aponeurosis with a prominent ovoid lateral free margin lying deep to the semitendinosus muscle belly. Muscle fibers arise from the surface of the aponeurosis and enlarge to form the belly of the semimembranosus, which lies medial and deep to the semitendinosus muscle and tendon through the posterior compartment of the thigh. The muscle tapers to a thick tendon just above the knee joint, which passes over the knee joint capsule at the medial femoral condyle and inserts onto a horizontal groove in the posteromedial aspect of the medial tibial condyle.

The posterior compartment muscles are innervated by the sciatic nerve.

Nerves and Vessels

Femoral Artery and Adductor Canal

The femoral artery is the major blood supply of the lower limb, and its course and relationships through the femoral triangle and adductor canal in the thigh are anatomically important. The femoral artery is the continuation of the external iliac artery as it passes under the inguinal ligament, where it comes to lie just medial to the femoral nerve in the femoral triangle. The femoral vein lies just medial to the artery. Typically, in the proximal part of the triangle, the femoral artery gives rise to the deep femoral artery and then continues to the apex of the triangle, where it enters the adductor canal.

The adductor canal begins at the apex of the femoral triangle and ends in the distal thigh at the adductor hiatus, the gap between the hamstring part of the adductor magnus and the adductor part of the muscle, which opens into the popliteal fossa. The canal is roughly triangular in profile with a lateral wall formed by vastus medialis, a posteromedial wall formed by the adductor longus, and an anterior wall formed by the sartorius.

The femoral artery descends in the canal accompanied by the femoral vein and two branches of the femoral nerve, the nerve to the vastus medialis and the saphenous nerve. The femoral vessels leave the canal through the adductor hiatus, and become the popliteal vessels. The saphenous nerve continues through the thigh along the deep surface of the sartorius, emerges between the sartorius and the tendon of gracilis just above the knee joint, and then pierces the deep fascia to provide cutaneous supply to the medial surface of the leg from the knee joint to the medial aspect of the foot.

The deep branch of the femoral artery descends in the thigh across the pectineus, then passes posterior (deep) to the adductor longus, where it first lies between the adductor longus and adductor brevis, and then beyond the distal edge of the adductor brevis, it lies between the adductor longus and adductor magnus. In the femoral triangle, the deep femoral artery has medial and lateral femoral circumflex branches, and has three perforating branches beyond the triangle, which provide arterial supply to the structures of the posterior compartment.

Sciatic Nerve

The sciatic nerve continues into the thigh from the gluteal region as it passes beyond the inferior margin of quadratus femoris and comes to lie immediately anterior (deep) to the biceps femoris. The nerve lies along the anteromedial surface of the long head of the biceps femoris through most of the thigh and typically divides just proximal to the popliteal fossa into its terminal branches, the tibial nerve and the common fibular nerve. In the posterior compartment, the sciatic nerve innervates the long head of the biceps, semitendinosus, and semimembranosus via its tibial division, whereas the short head of the biceps femoris receives its motor supply from the common fibular division of the nerve. The tibial nerve continues through the central part of the popliteal fossa and into the posterior compartment of the leg. The common fibular nerve diverges laterally along the medial edge of the biceps femoris muscle and tendon, then crosses subcutaneously along the fibular neck into the lateral compartment of the leg.

Technique

Adductor Canal

FEMORAL ARTERY AND VEIN SAPHENOUS NERVE
Transverse
FIG. 5.13

The patient should be supine with the thigh laterally rotated, appropriately draped for US examination from just below the ASIS through the proximal third of the thigh anteromedially. Place the probe in a transverse orientation just below and medial to the ASIS. Identify the sartorius and center the muscle in the image. Slide the probe distally along the oblique (lateral to medial) course of the sartorius for a short distance and observe as the muscle crosses superficially over the femoral vessels beyond the apex of the femoral triangle. Continue sliding the probe distally for another 2

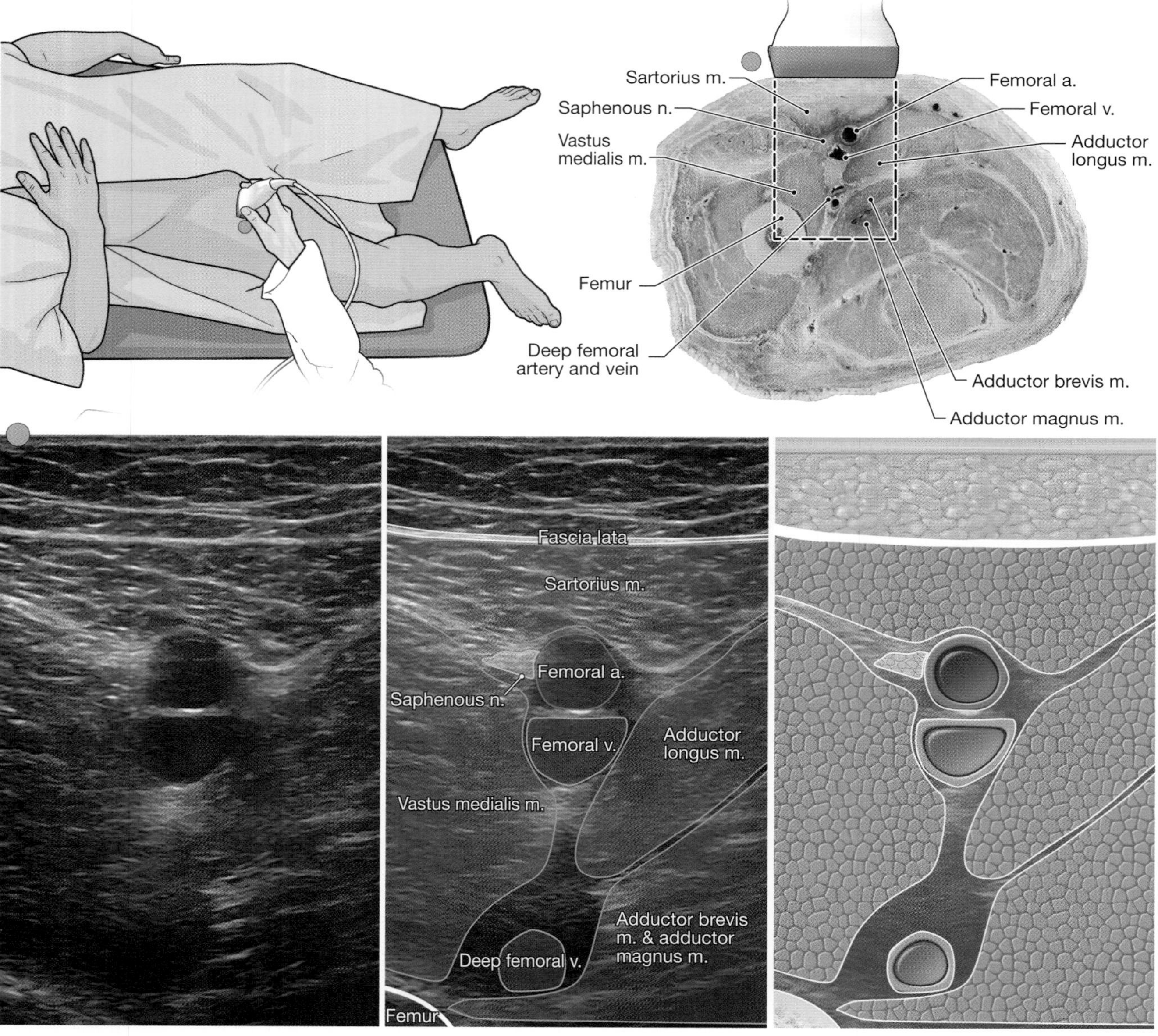

Figure 5.13 Transverse view of the femoral artery, femoral vein, and saphenous nerve in the adductor canal.

to 4 cm until the femoral vessels can be seen to occupy a triangular cleft between the sartorius anteriorly, vastus medialis laterally, and adductor longus posteromedially. Note the pulsations of the more superficial femoral artery and the effects of changing the probe pressure on the femoral vein, which lies just deep to the artery. Fan and tilt the probe face (to minimize anisotropy) to identify the saphenous nerve, which usually lies immediately lateral to the artery along the deep surface of the sartorius in the upper part of the canal. The deep femoral vessels may be visible in the deepest part of the image, where they are separated from the canal by the adductor longus muscle.

Quadriceps Femoris

RECTUS FEMORIS
VASTUS MUSCLES
Transverse
FIG. 5.14

The patient should be supine with minimal lateral rotation of the thigh. Slight flexion at the knee, supported by a small bolster behind the knee, may help to relax the quadriceps muscles for US examination. Place the probe in a transverse orientation over the anterior surface of the midthigh and adjust the probe position as necessary to center the rectus femoris muscle, the most superficial of the quadriceps group, in the image. Identify the vastus intermedius immediately deep to the central part of the rectus femoris and note its relationship to the anterior and posterolateral surfaces of the femur. Medial to the vastus intermedius, identify the vastus medialis and note its position from deep to the medial aspect of the rectus femoris to the medial border and posteromedial surface of the femur. Identify the vastus lateralis between the lateral aspect of the rectus femoris and the anterior surface of the vastus intermedius. Most of the vastus lateralis is beyond the field of view, separated from the femur by the broad attachment of vastus intermedius to the anterior surface, lateral border, and posterolateral surface of the femur. Slide the probe distally along the rectus femoris muscle and note that the rectus femoris becomes tendinous more proximally than the vastus muscles.

Iliotibial Tract

ILIOTIBIAL TRACT
TENSOR FASCIAE LATAE VASTUS LATERALIS
Longitudinal
FIG. 5.15

The patient should be supine and appropriately draped, with minimal external rotation of the thigh and the knee slightly flexed (a small bolster behind the knee may be helpful). Begin by placing the probe in a transverse orientation below the lateral aspect of the ASIS. Identify the muscle belly of the tensor fasciae latae and center the muscle in the image. Slide the probe distally a short distance while keeping the muscle centered in the image and observe that the course of the tensor fasciae latae is slightly anterior to posterior. Carefully rotate the probe into a longitudinal orientation parallel to the muscle belly. Continue sliding the probe distally along the path of the muscle until the distal tapered end of the muscle can be seen clearly, as it inserts into the iliotibial tract. Observe that the iliotibial tract receives fibers from layers of fascia lata on both the superficial and deep surfaces of tensor fasciae latae muscle at this point. Identify vastus lateralis, deep to the fascia lata covering the deep surface of the tensor fasciae latae and then more distally, deep to the iliotibial tract. Deep to the vastus lateralis identify the vastus intermedius, which is in contact with the surface of the body of the femur.

ILIOTIBIAL TRACT
VASTUS LATERALIS
VASTUS INTERMEDIUS
Transverse
FIG. 5.16

The patient should be in the lateral decubitus position with the knee slightly flexed. A small bolster should be positioned between the patient's knees. Place the probe in a transverse orientation over the lateral surface of the anterior compartment at about the junction of the middle and distal thirds of the thigh. Note the multilaminar appearance (hyperechoic, hypoechoic, and hyperechoic) of the iliotibial tract covering the lateral surface of the vastus lateralis. The vastus intermedius can be clearly identified covering the posterolateral surface of the femur. Slide the probe a short distance posteriorly and attempt to identify the slightly rounded (teardrop) appearance of the posterior edge of the iliotibial tract as it blends with the fascia lata posteriorly.

Posterior Compartment: Hamstring Muscles and Sciatic Nerve

HAMSTRING MUSCLES
SCIATIC NERVE
Transverse
FIGS. 5.17-5.20

The patient should be prone and appropriately draped to allow for palpation of landmarks and probe positioning. A small bolster placed under the distal leg/ankle may be helpful in relaxing the posterior compartment muscles. Locate the ischial tuberosity by palpation. Place the probe transversely over the tuberosity, and identify the hypoechoic hamstring tendon of origin over the hyperechoic profile of the bone (as shown in the gluteal region). Slide the probe distally a short distance until the muscle fibers of the long head of the biceps femoris and the semitendinosus begin to appear, joined by a curving tendinous band. At this point, the long head of the biceps femoris should be just underneath the inferior border of the gluteus maximus muscle. Identify the sciatic nerve at the deep (anterior) surface of the biceps muscle. Slide the probe medially and identify the semitendinosus muscle covered by the fascia lata posteriorly. Identify the hyperechoic

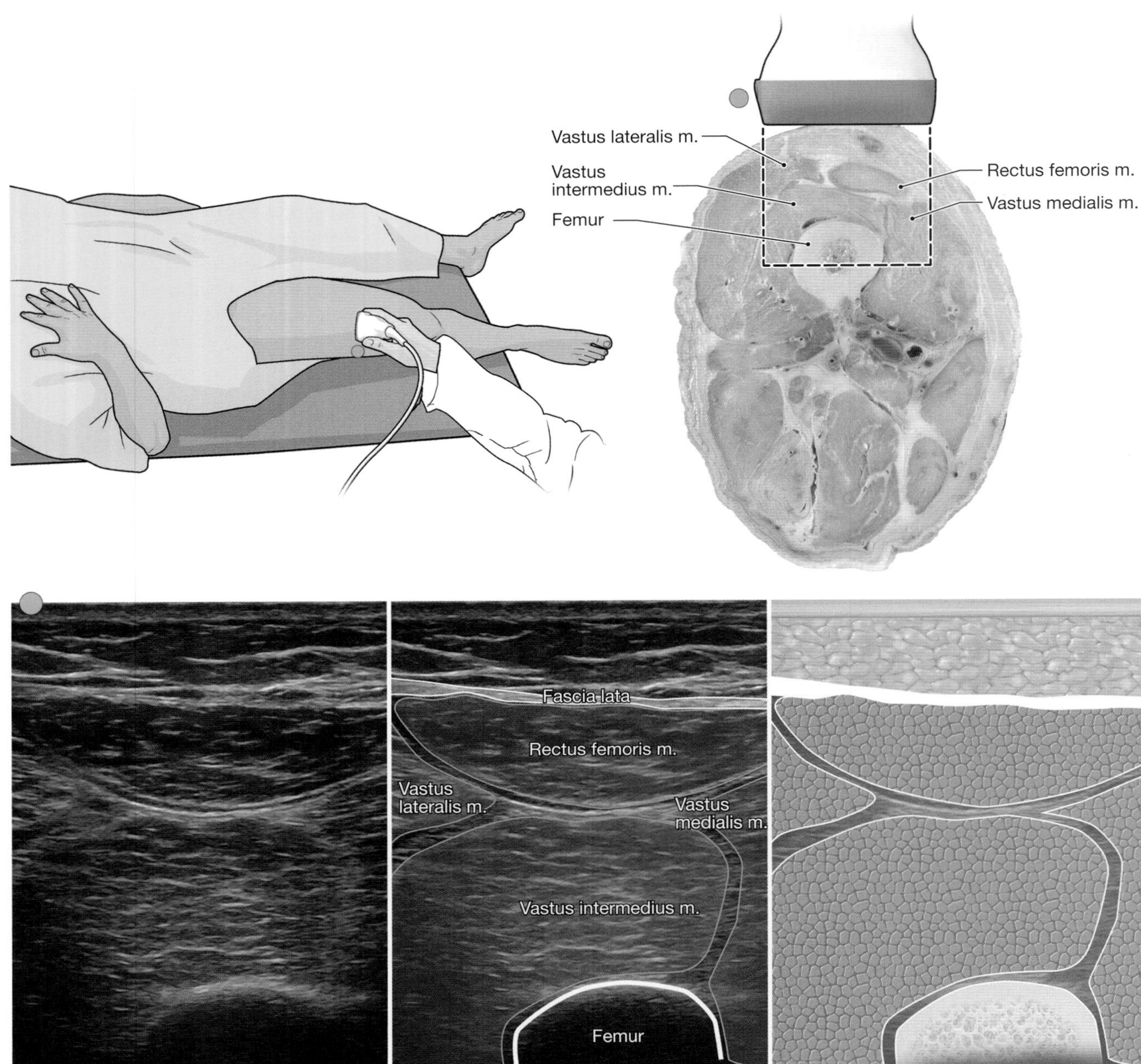

Figure 5.14 Rectus femoris, vastus intermedius, vastus medialis, and vastus lateralis at the midthigh.

aponeurotic tendon of the semimembranosus at the deep surface of the semitendinosus. Note the prominent teardrop expansion at its lateral edge tapering to a broad flat tendon, which continues medial to the deep surface of the semitendinosus, where muscle fibers of the semimembranosus begin to form at the posterior surface of the tendon. The adductor magnus muscle can be seen deep to the sciatic nerve and hamstring muscles in this position. For this sequence, an extended field of view (EFOV) US image is shown to demonstrate all these relationships in a single image, followed by three separate standard (non-EFOV) US images, moving from lateral to medial, to demonstrate the same structures and their relationships.

BICEPS FEMORIS
SCIATIC NERVE
Transverse
FIG. 5.21

Slide the probe laterally to center of the long head of the biceps femoris in the image. Next, slide the probe distally along the oblique (medial to lateral) course of the muscle. About the midthigh, muscle fibers of the short head of biceps begin to appear at the deep (anterolateral) surface of the long head.

Continue following the biceps femoris distally and observe as the muscle belly of the short head enlarges and the belly of the long head begins to taper as it approaches the common biceps insertion tendon a short distance above the popliteal fossa. The hyperechoic sciatic nerve can be seen along the deep (anteromedial) surface of the long head of the biceps.

SEMIMEMBRANOSUS MUSCLE SEMITENDINOSUS TENDON
Transverse
FIG. 5.22

Return the probe to the transverse view of the hamstring muscles near their origin. Slide the probe medially to center the semitendinosus and semimembranosus muscles in the image. Next, slide the probe distally along the two muscles. Observe that as muscle fibers emerge from the posterior surface of the semimembranosus aponeurotic tendon, the muscle enlarges rapidly and comes to occupy a position directly deep to the semitendinosus. Continuing distally, the semitendinosus muscle begins tapering to a relatively thin tendon at about the midthigh. Continue scanning distally along the semitendinosus tendon and semimembranosus muscle belly to about the junction of the middle and distal thirds of the thigh, a short distance above the popliteal fossa. Identify the fascia lata, semitendinosus tendon, and semimembranosus muscle belly.

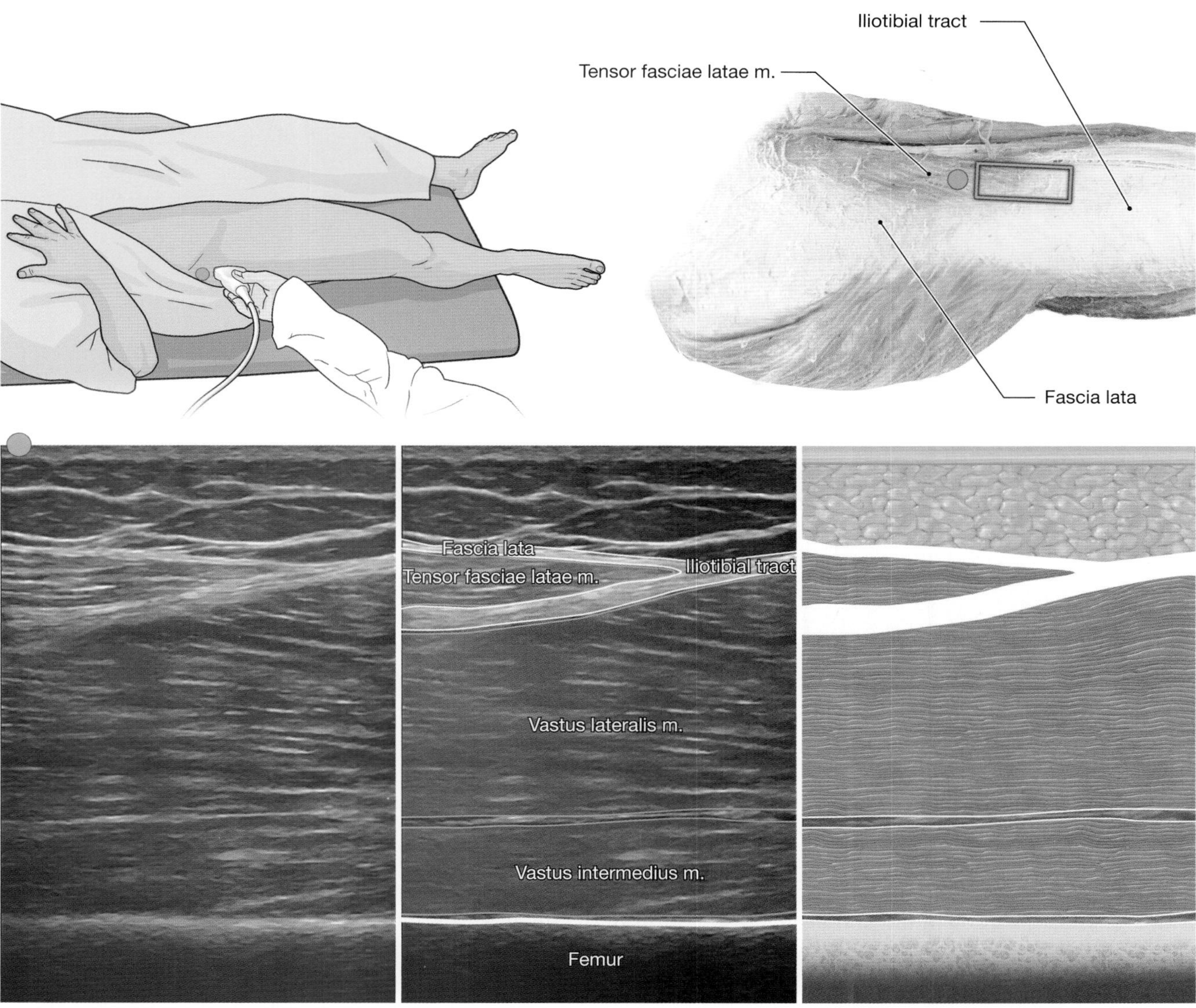

Figure 5.15 Longitudinal view of the distal end of tensor fasciae latae and the iliotibial tract along the lateral aspect of vastus lateralis muscle in the proximal third of the thigh. Vastus intermedius is seen between the deep surface of vastus lateralis and the body of the femur.

CLINICAL APPLICATION

US examination is used for musculoskeletal injuries or disorders such as hamstring origin tendinosis/tendonitis, partial and complete tendon tears/avulsions, and/or muscle tears.

US examination, including Doppler US, is commonly used for the detection of deep vein thrombi in lower limb veins, including the femoral vein and its tributaries. Doppler US is also used for the measurement of flow velocity profiles in the femoral artery in suspected peripheral artery disease.

US guidance is used for saphenous nerve blocks in the adductor canal. Saphenous nerve blocks are used for surgeries involving the medial leg, ankle, and foot or, more commonly, in combination with the sciatic nerve block for surgeries below the knee (the saphenous nerve is the only nerve with sensory distribution below the knee that is not derived from the sciatic nerve).

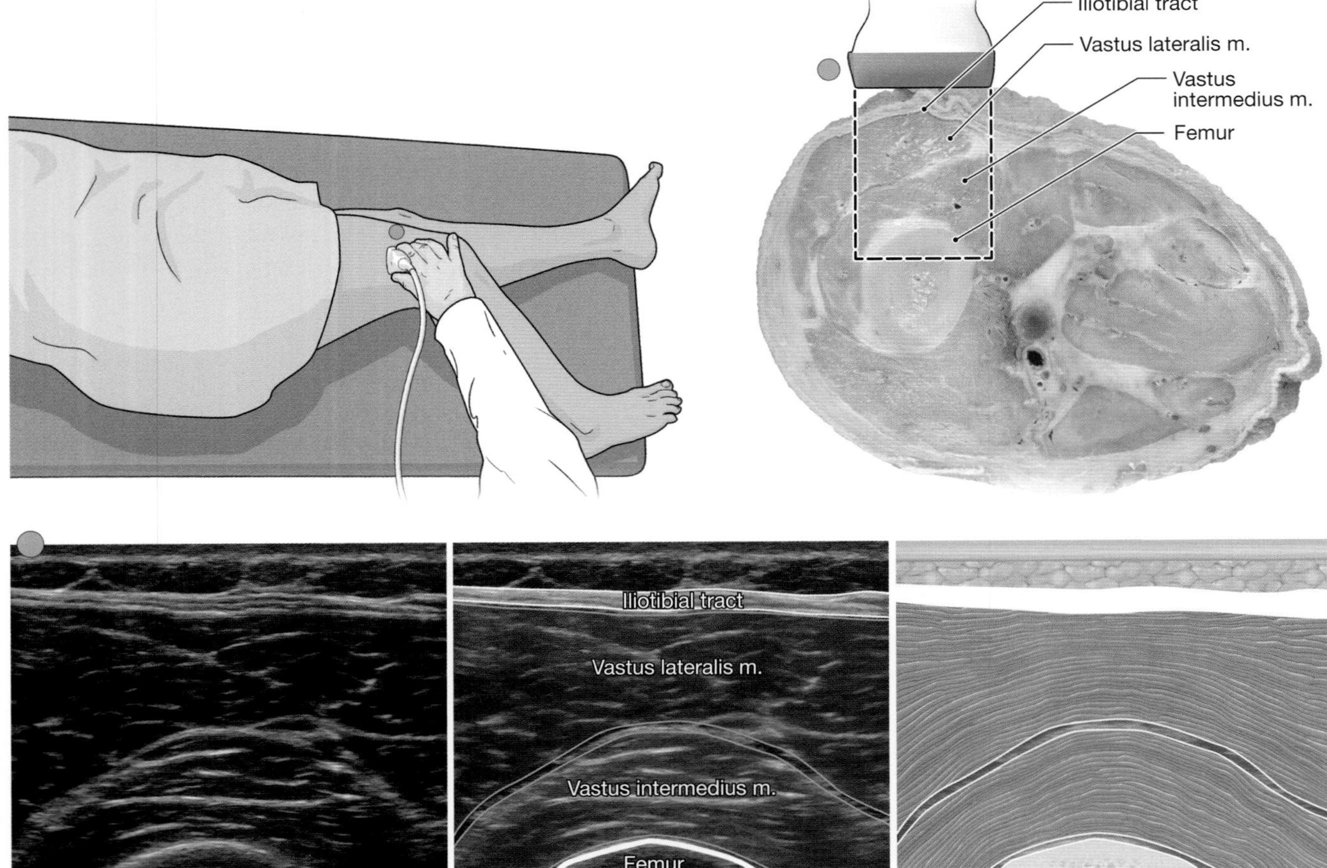

Figure 5.16 Transverse view of the iliotibial tract along the lateral surface of vastus lateralis muscle at the junction of the middle and distal thirds of the thigh. Vastus intermedius is seen between the deep surface of vastus lateralis and the body of the femur.

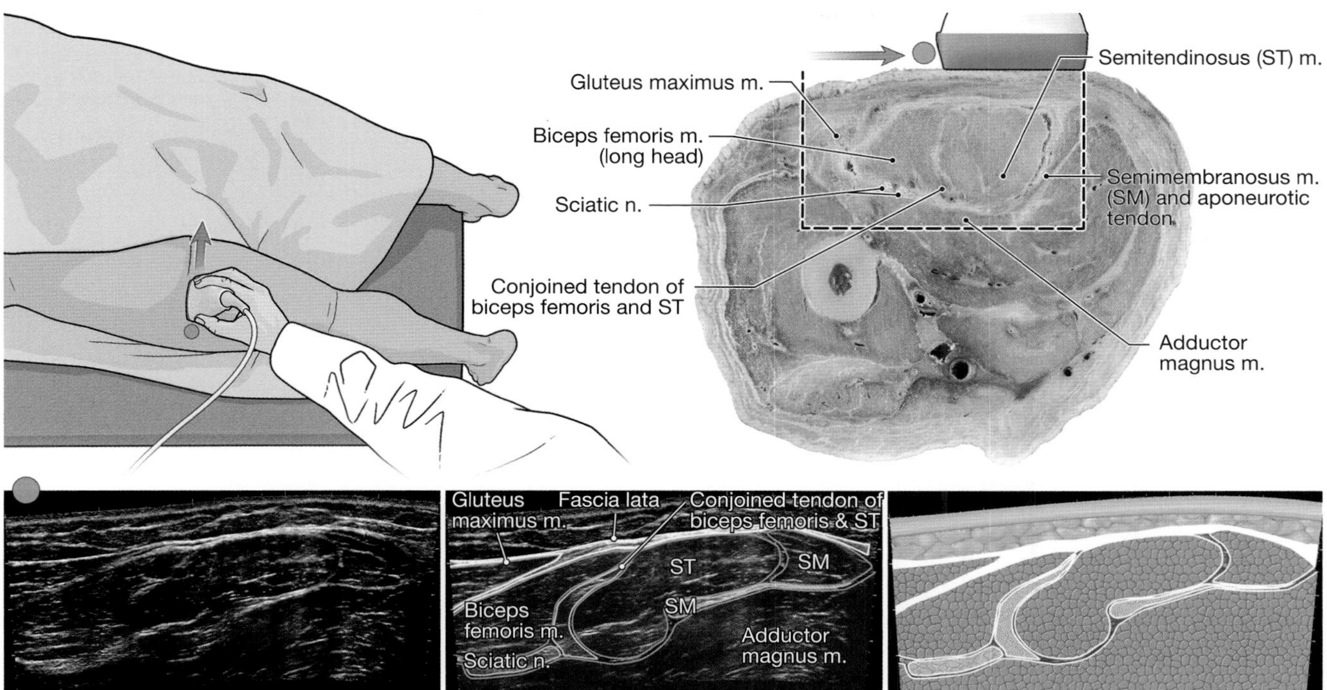

Figure 5.17 Transverse extended field of view (EFOV) of the hamstring muscles (long head of biceps femoris, semitendinosus, and semimembranosus) in the proximal-most part of the posterior thigh. The sciatic nerve can be seen in contact with the deep surface of biceps femoris (long head).

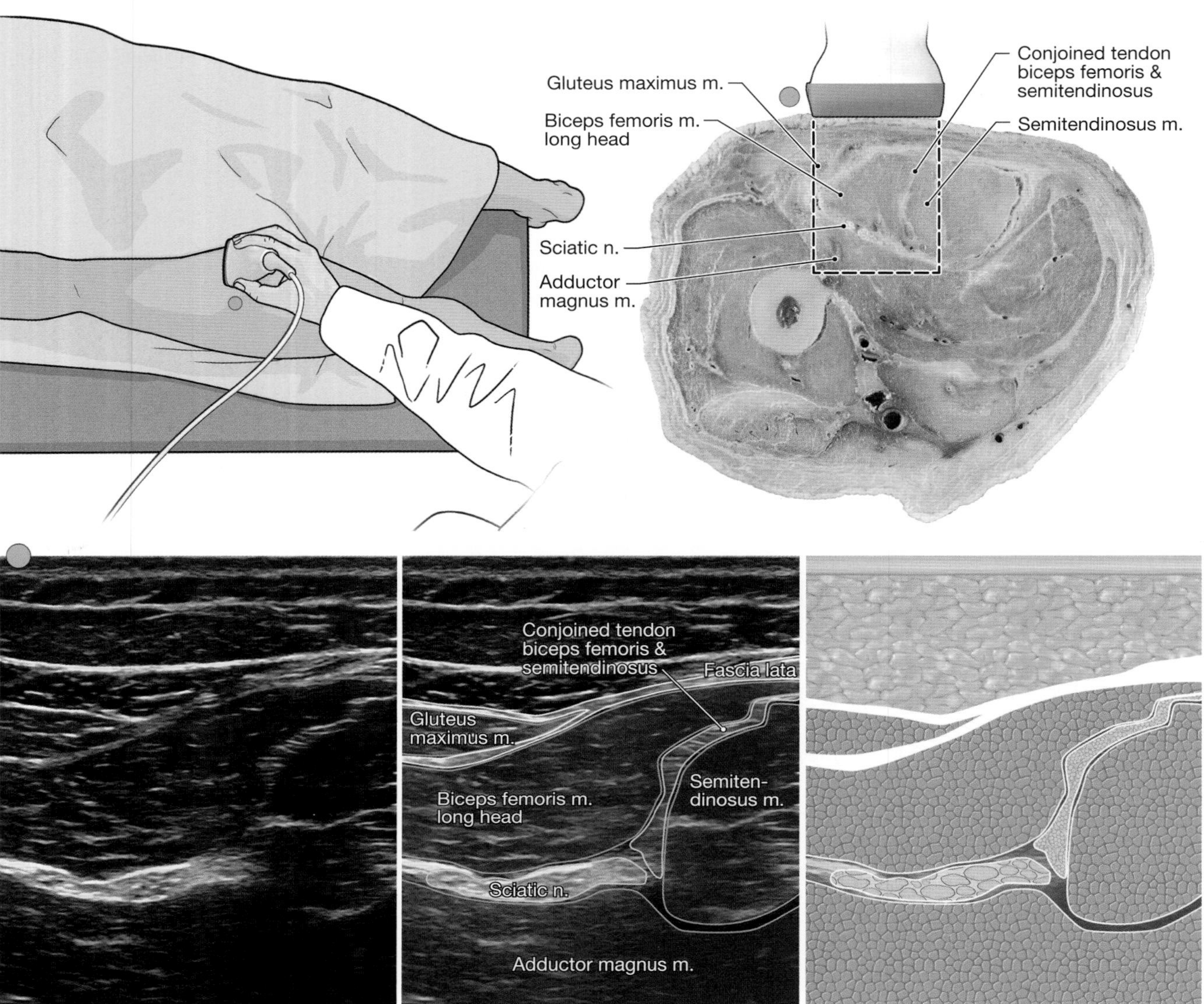

Figure 5.18 Transverse view of the long head of biceps femoris and semitendinosus muscles joined by a curving tendinous band, in the proximal-most part of the thigh. The sciatic nerve is seen deep to the biceps femoris long head, which is partially overlapped by inferior fibers of gluteus maximus. Compare with Figure 5.17.

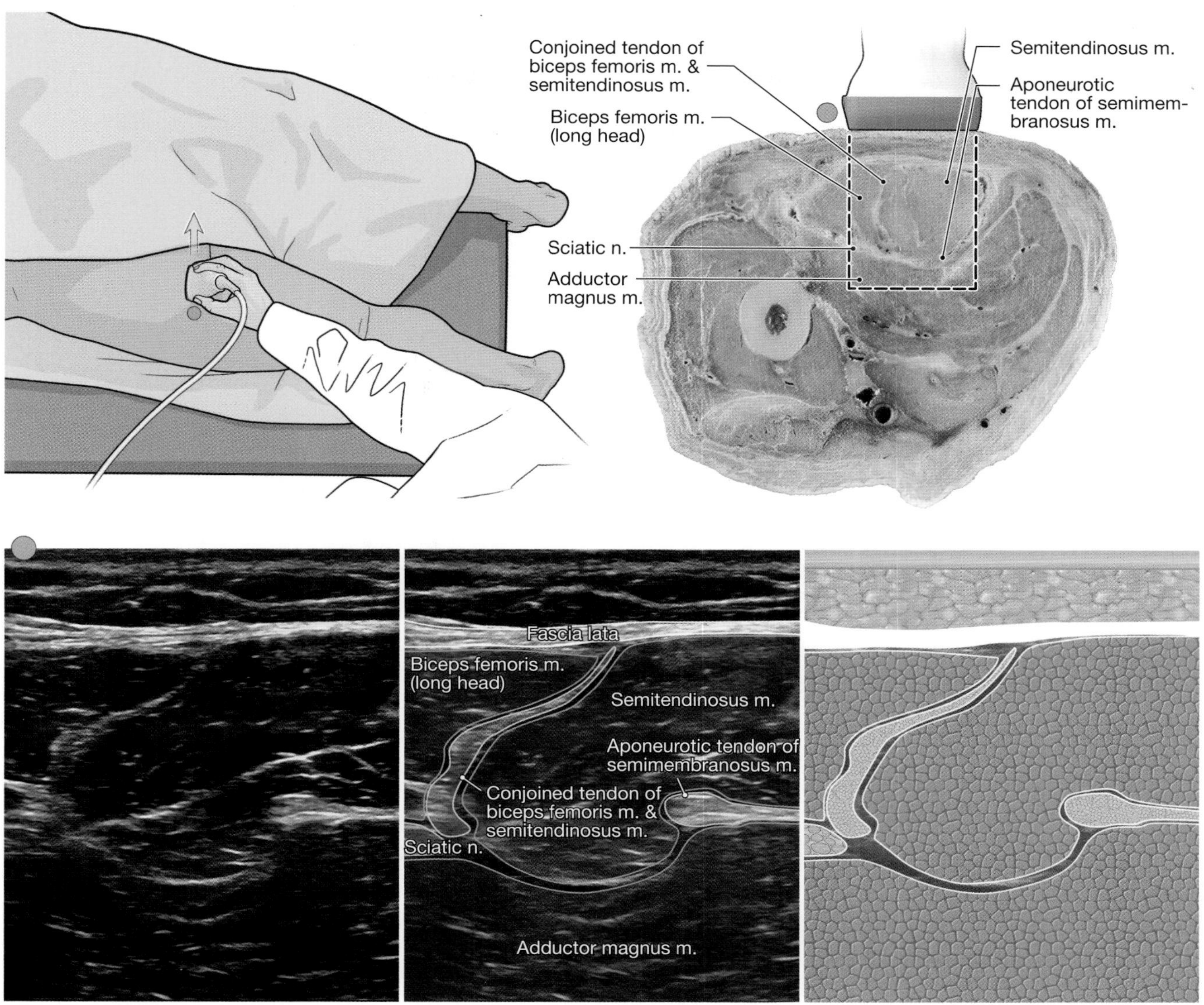

Figure 5.19 Transverse view of the long head of biceps femoris and semitendinosus muscles, along with the lateral ovoid edge of the aponeurotic tendon of semimembranosus, in the proximal thigh. Compare with Figure 5.17.

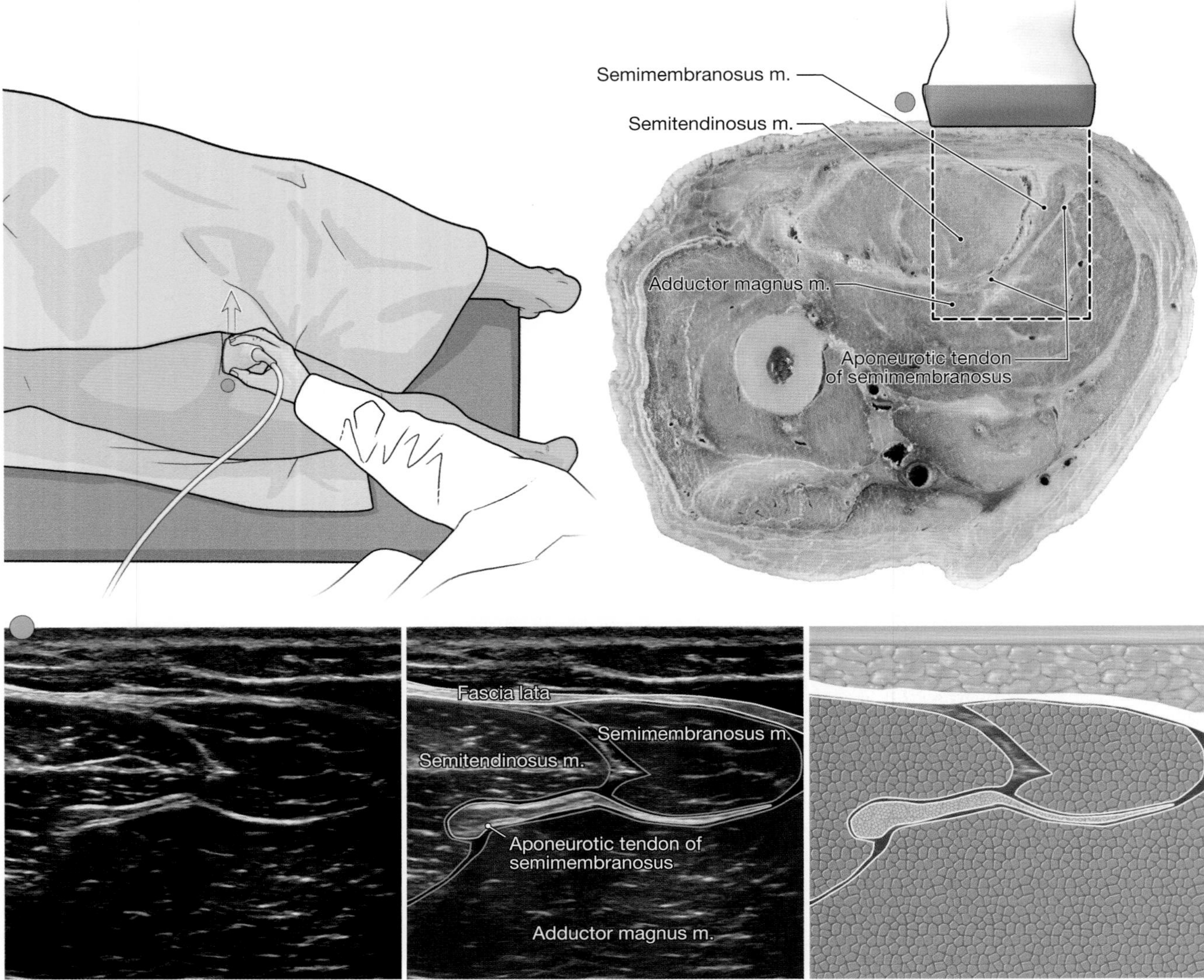

Figure 5.20 Transverse view of semitendinosus muscle and the aponeurotic tendon of semimembranosus with muscle fibers forming along its posterior surface, in the proximal thigh. Compare with Figure 5.17.

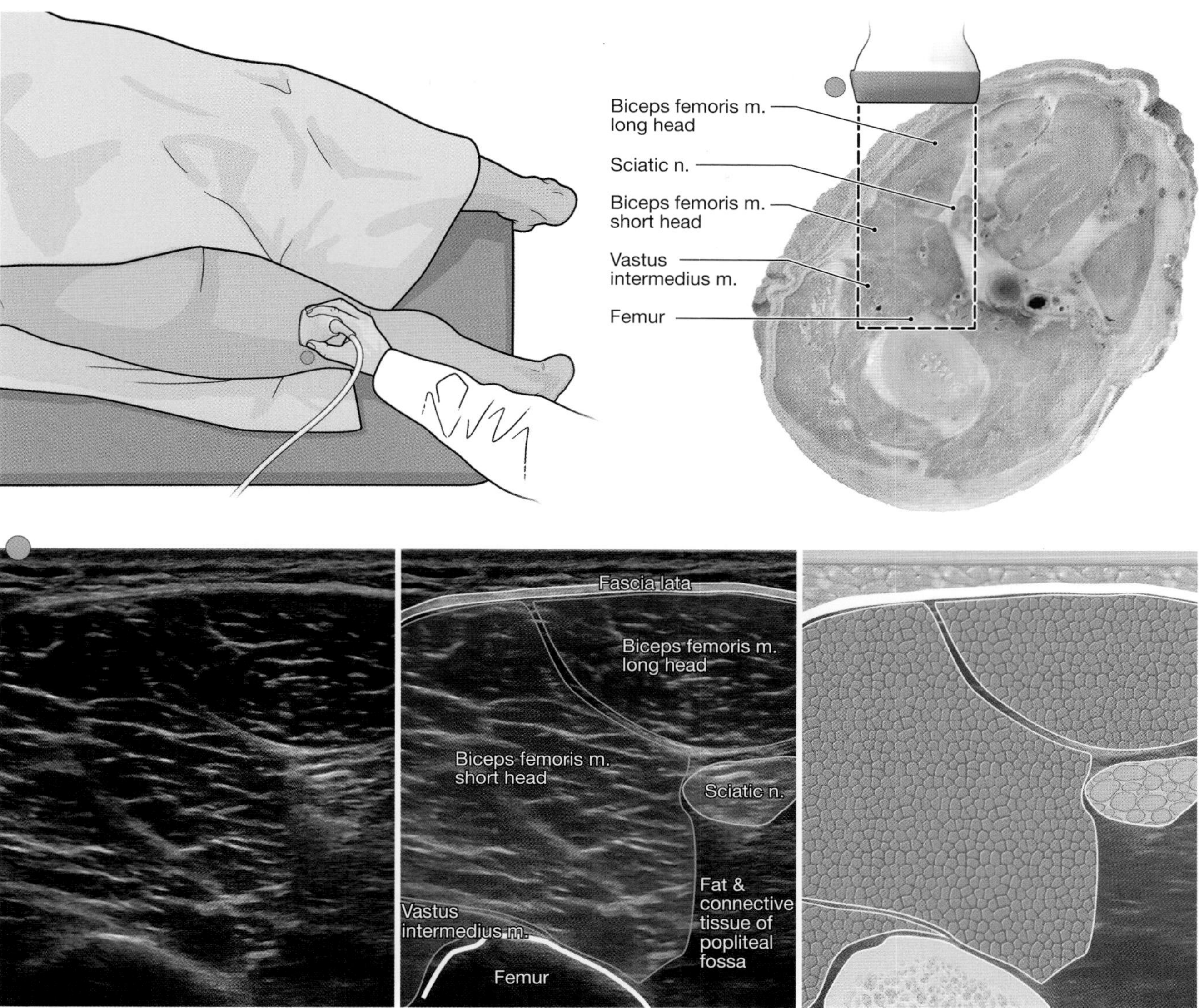

Figure 5.21 Transverse view of the long and short heads of biceps femoris, along with the sciatic nerve, in the distal third of the thigh.

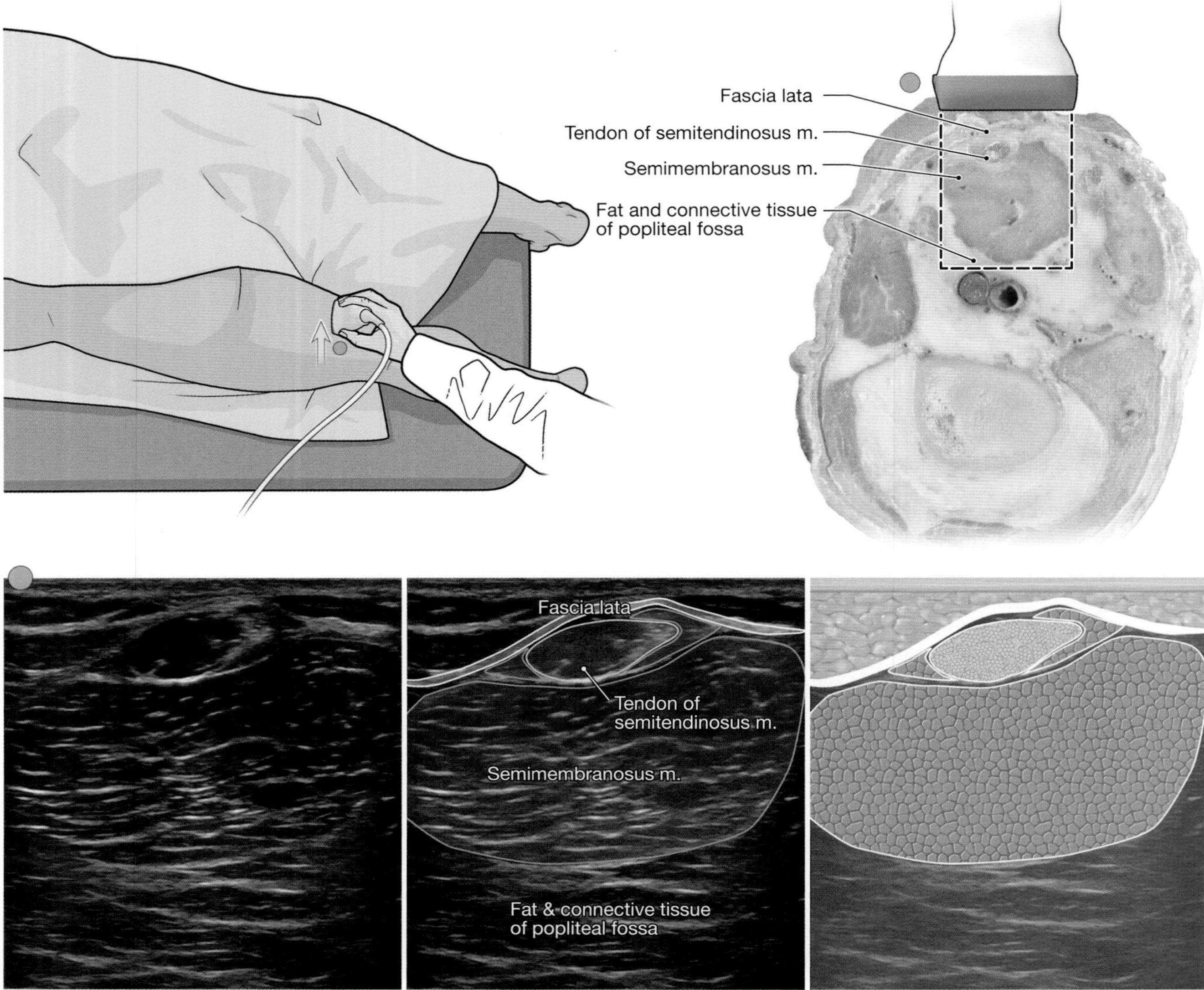

Figure 5.22 Transverse view of the tendon of semitendinosus at the surface of semimembranosus muscle in the distal third of the thigh.

Knee

Review of the Anatomy

Knee Joint

The knee joint is a large complex synovial joint with articulations between the femoral condyles and the corresponding surfaces of the tibial condyles and between the posterior surface of the patella and the femoral trochlea.

Bones, Articular Surfaces, and Menisci

Distally, the body of the femur widens as it approaches the medial and lateral condyles, and an additional femoral surface forms under the floor of the popliteal fossa. The femoral condyles, separated posteriorly and inferiorly by the intercondylar fossa, are joined anteriorly to form the femoral trochlea, the femoral articular surface for the **patella**. The trochlea, like the condyles, is covered by articular cartilage. The trochlea has sloping lateral and medial surfaces that form a groove along its central region and that are congruent with the medial and lateral articular facets (and intervening ridge) of the posterior surface of the patella. The condyles are rounded posteriorly and slightly flattened inferiorly, where they meet the articular facets of the medial and lateral condyles of the tibial plateau.

Between the tibial condyles is the intercondylar region of the tibial plateau, which has facets for the attachment of the anterior and posterior horns of the medial and lateral **menisci** and for the anterior and posterior cruciate ligaments. The fibrocartilaginous menisci are semilunar in shape and wedgelike in profile with thicker outer edges and thinner inner margins. They are described as having anterior and posterior horns connected by a middle portion, the body. The menisci cover large areas of the articular surfaces of the tibial condyles, intervening between the femoral and tibial condyles. The inferior surface of the lateral condyle of the tibia has an articular facet for the head of the fibula.

Below the condyles, the tibia tapers to its triangular body, with anteromedial, anterolateral, and posterior surfaces. At the proximal body anteriorly, there is an ovoid anterior prominence that tapers distally, the tibial tuberosity, which serves as the site of attachment of the patellar ligament.

Joint Capsule

The synovial membrane of the knee joint attaches above to the margins of the articular surfaces of the femoral condyles, below to the margins of the articular surfaces of the tibial condyles (and outer edges of the menisci), and anteriorly along the margins of the articular facets of the patella. It has a large superior recess, the suprapatellar bursa, which extends superiorly from between the patellar and trochlear articular surfaces to between the triangular suprapatellar fat pat and posterior surface of the quadriceps femoris tendon anteriorly and the prefemoral fat pad covering the anterior surface of the femur posteriorly.

The fibrous capsule of the knee has similar attachments as the synovial membrane with the prominent exception of its anterior femoral attachment. Anteriorly, the fibrous capsule attaches to the femoral body several centimeters above the articular margin of the trochlea, accommodating the suprapatellar bursa of the synovial membrane. The fibrous membrane is incompletely lined by the synovial membrane, separated from the synovial membrane in several sites by fat pads, including the suprapatellar fat pad at the superior pole of the patella and the infrapatellar fat pad (of Hoffa), which intervenes between the two membranes anteriorly, behind the patellar ligament. The fibrous capsule is reinforced by fibrous extensions from the vastus medialis and lateralis, the quadriceps femoris tendon, the semimembranosus tendon, the tibial collateral ligament, and the iliotibial tract.

Ligaments

Tibial Collateral Ligament

The tibial collateral ligament of the knee also known as the medial collateral ligament of the knee, is a long (8-10 cm) flattened band attached superiorly to the medial epicondyle of the femur. The ligament passes across the medial surface of the knee joint and attaches distally to the anteromedial surface of the body of the tibia 4 to 5 cm below the tibiofemoral joint line. The ligament is described as having superficial and deep parts. The superficial part (tibiofemoral ligament), often referred to as the vertical component of the tibial collateral ligament, is the main structural component of the ligament. It is fused with the overlying deep fascia. The deep part is fused with the underlying fibrous capsule of the knee joint, which also attaches along the outer margin of the body of medial meniscus, resulting in the attachment of the tibial collateral ligament to the body of the medial meniscus. There are short extensions superiorly and inferiorly from the deep layer, the meniscofemoral and meniscotibial ligaments. Just below the tibial condyle, the ligament crosses over the medial inferior genicular vessels. Near its inferior end, the ligament is partly overlapped by the attachments of the tendons of the sartorius, gracilis, and semitendinosus (pes anserinus). The tibial collateral ligament resists the valgus stress at the knee joint.

Fibular Collateral Ligament

The fibular collateral ligament of the knee, also known as the lateral collateral ligament of the knee, is a narrow, rounded cord that attaches superiorly to the lateral epicondyle of the femur just above the groove for the popliteus tendon, crosses the lateral aspect of the knee joint directed slightly posteriorly and attaches below to the lateral surface of the fibular head, along with the biceps femoris tendon. The fibular collateral ligament is separated from the fibrous capsule of the knee joint by a bursa (ie, is not attached to the capsule or lateral meniscus). The fibular collateral ligament resists varus stress at the knee joint.

Tendons

Multiple muscles cross and act on the knee joint including the quadriceps femoris anteriorly and the hamstrings and gastrocnemius muscles posteriorly. The iliotibial tract also crosses the knee joint at its lateral aspect.

Quadriceps Femoris

The quadriceps femoris tendon is a thick strong tendon formed by contributions from the rectus femoris and the vastus muscles. The tendon is commonly described as trilaminar with a superficial layer formed by the rectus femoris, an intermediate layer formed by the vastus lateralis and medialis, and a deep layer formed by vastus intermedius. The quadriceps femoris tendon attaches to the superior surface of the patella, which is in turn attached to the tibial tuberosity via the patellar ligament.

Iliotibial Tract

The iliotibial tract courses distally along the vastus lateralis muscle, crosses the tibiofemoral joint laterally, and attaches to the tubercle of the iliotibial tract (Gerdy's tubercle) at the anterolateral surface of the lateral tibial condyle. Near its tibial attachment, the posterior edge of the iliotibial tract lies a short distance anterior to the fibular collateral ligament.

Hamstring Tendons

Biceps Femoris

From the posterior compartment of the thigh, the long and short heads of the biceps femoris converge distally to insert onto the lateral surface of the fibular head via a round cord-like common tendon. The tendon is readily palpable at the posterolateral aspect of the knee for several centimeters proximal to the head of the fibula.

Semimembranosus

Just above the knee joint, the semimembranosus muscle tapers to a thick tendon that passes medially over the knee joint capsule at the medial femoral condyle alongside the medial head of gastrocnemius and inserts mainly onto a groove in the posteromedial aspect of the medial tibial condyle and partly into the fibrous joint capsule of the knee via fibrous expansions.

Semitendinosus

The semitendinosus muscle tapers to a long thin tendon just beyond the midthigh. The semitendinosus tendon continues distally along the superficial surface of the semimembranosus and crosses the knee joint posteromedially accompanying the tendons of the gracilis and sartorius to insert on the anteromedial surface of the body of the tibia near the inferior end of the tibial collateral ligament.

Posterior Compartment of the Leg

The posterior compartment of the leg has superficial and deep muscle groups. Because of its relationship to the knee joint, an overview of the superficial muscle group (plus popliteus muscle and tendon) is provided here. The superficial muscles of the posterior leg include the medial and lateral heads of gastrocnemius, soleus, and plantaris.

Gastrocnemius

The two heads of the gastrocnemius along with soleus form the triceps surae muscle, which inserts onto calcaneus via the thick strong calcaneal (Achilles) tendon. The medial head of the gastrocnemius originates from the posterior surface of the femur just above the medial condyle. The thick tendinous medial edge of the muscle lies alongside the tendon of semimembranosus just outside the joint capsule over the medial condyle. The lateral head of the gastrocnemius originates from the posterior surface of the femur just above the lateral condyle. The small plantaris muscle originates from the lateral supracondylar line just above the origin of the lateral head of the gastrocnemius. The two heads of the gastrocnemius converge at the inferior extent of the popliteal fossa forming the belly (gaster) of the calf contour and then taper to a broad flattened tendinous band about the midleg.

Soleus

Soleus muscle, deep to the gastrocnemius, originates from the posterior surfaces of the fibula and tibia and an intervening tendinous arch. In the distal leg the tendon of soleus fuses with the overlying tendon of gastrocnemius to form the calcaneal tendon. Part of the small muscle belly of the plantaris and its long thin tendon pass between the gastrocnemius and soleus to insert along the medial aspect of the calcaneal tendon.

Popliteus

In the deep group of muscles, which includes popliteus, tibialis posterior, flexor digitorum longus, and flexor hallucis longus, popliteus is particularly relevant to a discussion of the knee. The popliteus tendon attaches to the anterior part of the groove for popliteus on the lateral surface of the lateral femoral epicondyle, just below the proximal attachment of the fibular collateral ligament. Within the groove, the tendon is inside the fibrous capsule of the knee, surrounded by a small recess of the synovial space (popliteal recess). The tendon crosses the knee joint across the posterolateral aspect of the lateral meniscus and emerges from the fibrous capsule at its inferior attachment. The tendon then expands into the fan-shaped belly of popliteus, which attaches to the posterior surface of the body of the tibia above the soleal line.

Popliteal Fossa and Contents

Popliteal Fossa

The popliteal fossa is a diamond-shaped space posterior to the knee joint, formed by the muscles of the posterior compartments of the thigh and leg, through which major neurovascular structures cross between the thigh and the leg. The upper borders of the fossa are formed by the biceps femoris laterally and semimembranosus and semitendinosus medially. The lower borders are formed by the medial and lateral heads of the gastrocnemius muscle. The floor of the fossa is formed by the capsule of the knee joint and posterior surface of the femur, and the roof is formed by the skin, superficial fascia, and popliteus muscle.

Popliteal Vessels

The femoral artery becomes the popliteal artery as it leaves the subsartorial canal and enters the popliteal fossa through the adductor hiatus of the adductor magnus. The popliteal vein lies superficial to the artery in the fossa and becomes the femoral vein when it leaves the fossa through the adductor hiatus to enter the subsartorial canal.

Sciatic Nerve

The sciatic nerve approaches the popliteal fossa along the deep surface of the biceps femoris. Typically, the sciatic nerve divides into its terminal branches, the tibial and common fibular nerves, just proximal to the popliteal fossa. The tibial nerve travels through the central part of the fossa, immediately superficial to the popliteal vein, whereas the common fibular nerve diverges laterally along the medial margin of the biceps femoris and its tendon.

Tibial Nerve

The tibial nerve and popliteal vessels pass between the medial and lateral heads of the gastrocnemius and under the tendinous arch of the soleus to enter the posterior compartment of the leg at the inferior extent of the popliteal fossa, passing superficial to the popliteus muscle and deep to triceps surae. The popliteal artery has genicular branches in its course through the fossa and divides into its terminal branches, the anterior and posterior tibial arteries, shortly after entering the posterior compartment of the leg.

Common Fibular Nerve

The common fibular nerve follows the biceps tendon to the posterolateral aspect of the fibular head. The nerve then crosses the neck of the fibula subcutaneously and divides into its terminal divisions, the deep and superficial fibular nerves, which enter the anterior and lateral compartments of the leg, respectively.

Technique

Suprapatellar Knee

QUADRICEPS FEMORIS TENDON SUPERIOR POLE OF THE PATELLA
Longitudinal
FIG. 5.23

The patient should be supine with minimal thigh rotation, and the knee should be flexed over a small bolster placed behind the knee. Place the probe in a longitudinal orientation over the distal end of the quadriceps femoris tendon in the midline of the thigh just above the patella. Identify the hyperechoic fibrillar appearance of the quadriceps femoris tendon and slide the probe distally until the attachment of the tendon to the superior pole of the patella can be seen. The patella can be readily identified by its hyperechoic bony surface and dense acoustic shadow. At the superior pole of the patella, immediately deep to the quadriceps femoris tendon, identify the generally hyperechoic triangular profile of the suprapatellar fat pad. Along the anterior surface of the femur, identify the hyperechoic prefemoral fat pad. While concentrating on the space between the two fat pads, slide the probe face medially and laterally until the anechoic/hypoechoic synovial fluid within the suprapatellar bursa can be clearly identified.

FEMORAL TROCHLEA QUADRICEPS FEMORIS TENDON
Transverse
FIG. 5.24

Ask the patient to flex the knee as much comfortably as possible, placing the sole of the foot on the examination table. Place the probe transversely over the anterior surface of the knee, just proximal to the patella. Identify the sloping medial and lateral bony surfaces of the femoral trochlea covered by an anechoic layer of hyaline cartilage. The lateral surface of the trochlea tends to be longer and steeper than the medial surface. Identify the large hyperechoic quadriceps femoris tendon superficial to the articular cartilage. Fanning/tilting the probe face alters the echogenicity of the tendon from anechoic to hyperechoic (because of anisotropy). At the

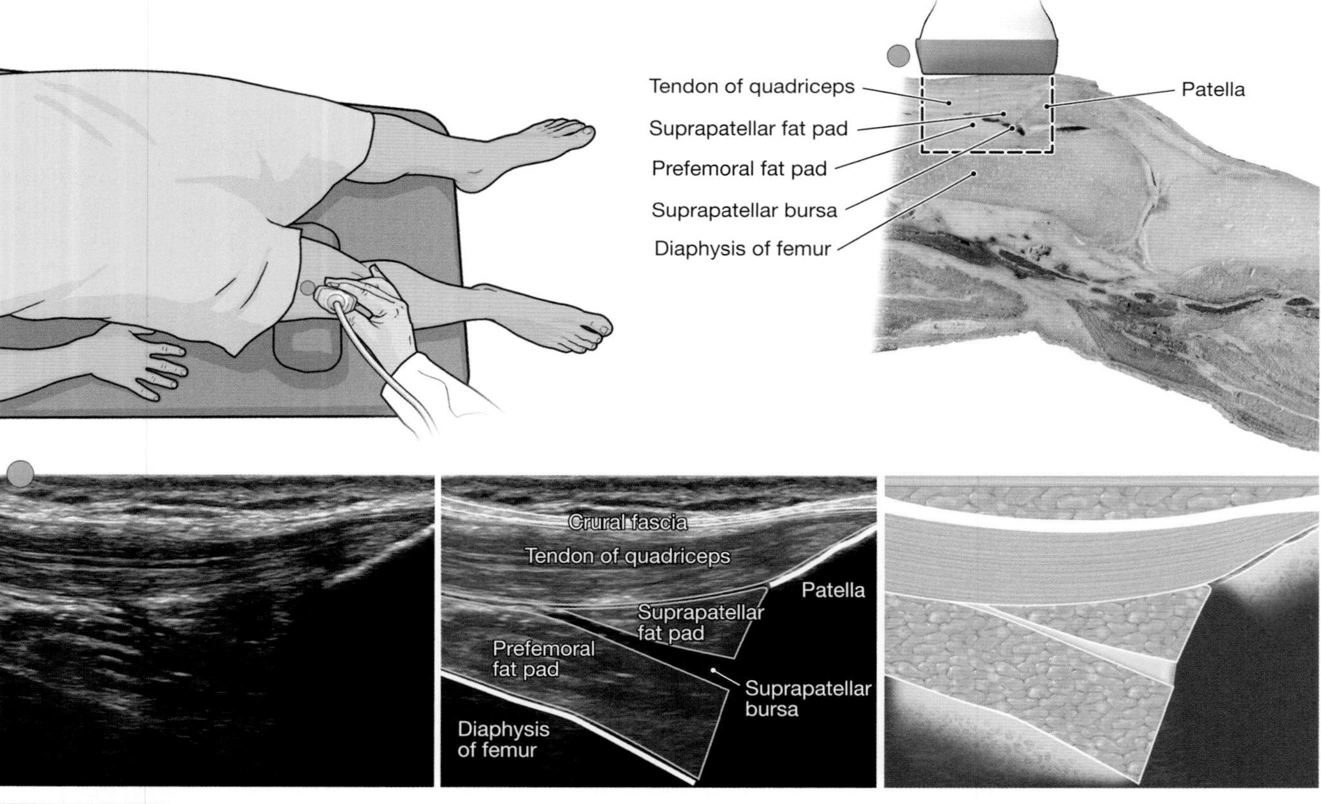

Figure 5.23 Longitudinal view of the quadriceps femoris tendon, superior pole of the patella, suprapatellar fat pad, suprapatellar bursa, and prefemoral fat pad.

medial side of the tendon, look for the distal muscle tissue of the vastus medialis joining the tendon.

Infrapatellar Knee

INFERIOR POLE OF PATELLA PATELLAR LIGAMENT
Longitudinal
FIG. 5.25

The patient should be supine with the knee flexed over a small bolster placed under the knee, with minimal thigh rotation. Place the probe longitudinally over the patellar ligament at the inferior pole of the patella. Adjust the probe position until the inferior pole of the patella and the attaching fibers of the patellar ligament are clearly seen at the superior aspect of the image. Identify the hyperechoic fibrillar appearance of the ligament spanning across the image (the tibia and distal attachment of the tendon are just beyond the inferior extent of the image). Deep to the patellar tendon and fibrous joint capsule is the large infrapatellar fat pad (of Hoffa) with its hypoechoic fat mixed with hyperechoic strands of connective tissue fibers. Distal to the acoustic shadow of the patella, in the deep central part of the image, the hyperechoic bony profile of the femoral trochlea covered by anechoic hyaline cartilage can be seen.

PATELLAR LIGAMENT TIBIAL TUBEROSITY
Longitudinal
FIG. 5.26

Next, slide the probe distally along the patellar ligament until the hyperechoic anterior surface of the tibia leading inferiorly to the rounded prominence of the tibial tuberosity with attached fibers of the ligament can be clearly seen and identified. The deep infrapatellar bursa is located between the posterior surface of the tendon and the tibia just proximal to the tuberosity. The bursa is often difficult to identify when it is not inflamed. Deep to the patellar ligament and fibrous joint capsule, the inferior extent of the infrapatellar fat pad is readily identifiable.

Collateral Ligaments and Iliotibial Tract

MEDIAL COLLATERAL LIGAMENT
Longitudinal
FIG. 5.27

The patient should be supine, with the thigh externally rotated and the knee flexed over a small bolster. Place the probe longitudinally over the medial knee, centered across the tibiofemoral joint line. Adjust the probe position and tilt until the hyperechoic profile of the medial femoral condyle proximally and the medial tibial condyle distally can be seen and identified. In the joint space between the femur

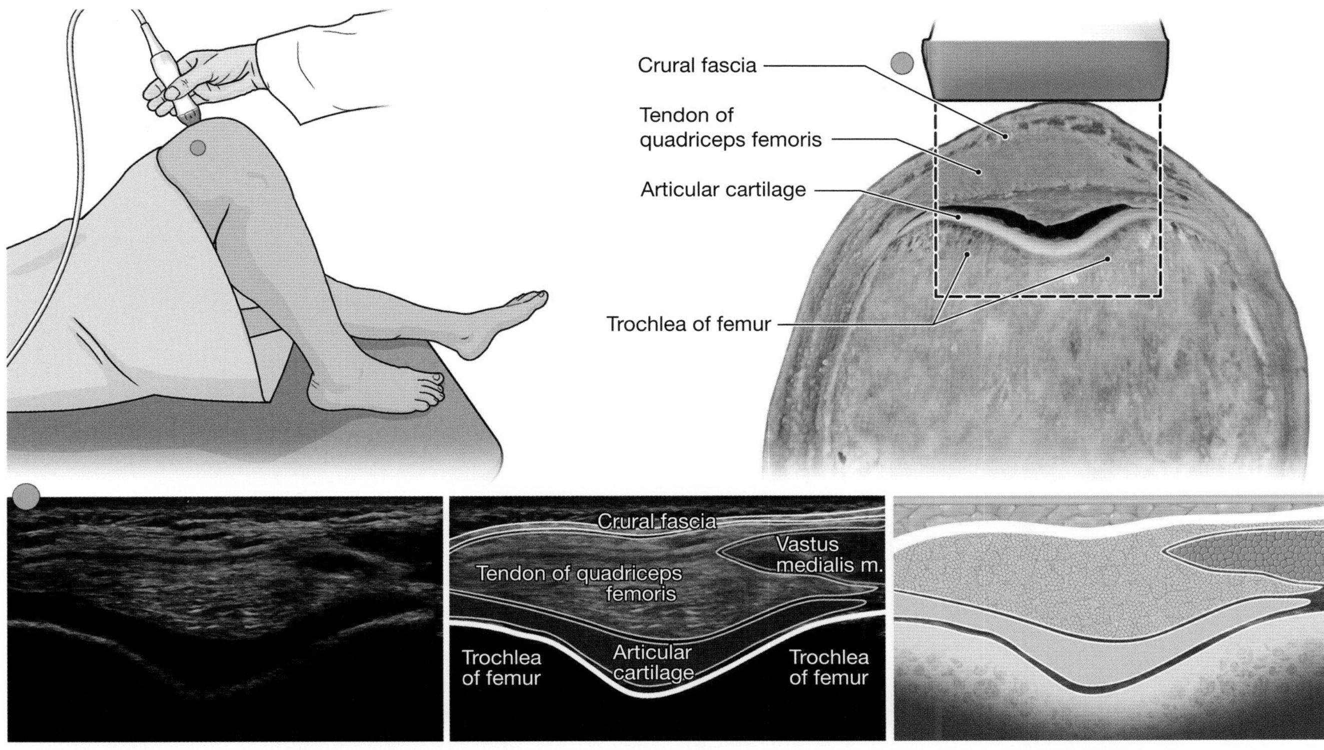

Figure 5.24 Transverse view of the articular surface of the femoral trochlea, the quadriceps femoris tendon, and distal muscle fibers of vastus medialis.

and tibia, identify the wedge-shaped slightly hyperechoic profile of the body of the medial meniscus (tilting and fanning the probe face as needed to minimize anisotropy). In contact with the superficial surface of the meniscus, locate the hyperechoic deep layer of the medial (tibial) collateral ligament and its superior and inferior extensions, the meniscofemoral and meniscotibial ligaments. Superficial to the deep layer, identify the slightly less echogenic fibrillar pattern of the superficial layer of the ligament spanning across the entire image. The attachments of the superficial layer are beyond the superior and inferior edges of the image. A small bursa can sometimes be seen between the superficial and deep layers of the ligament. The superficial layer is covered by, and fused with, the hyperechoic deep fascia. Sliding the probe distally while concentrating on the superficial layer of the medial (tibial) collateral ligament, attempt to follow the ligament to its attachment at the anteromedial surface of the tibia several centimeters below the joint line.

ILIOTIBIAL TRACT ATTACHMENT
Longitudinal
FIG. 5.28

The patient should be in the lateral decubitus position with a pillow or a small bolster between the knees. The hip and knee joints should be slightly flexed. By palpation, locate the biceps femoris tendon posteriorly just proximal to the fibular head. Slide fingers anteriorly from the tendon across a soft depression leading to a firm edge, the posterior edge of the iliotibial tract. Place the probe longitudinally just anterior and parallel to the edge of the iliotibial tract. Identify the characteristic laminar appearance (hyperechoic superficial surface, hypoechoic central part, hyperechoic deep surface) of the distal iliotibial tract. Continue sliding distally toward the anterolateral surface of the lateral tibial condyle until the rounded prominence of the tubercle of iliotibial tract (Gerdy's) tubercle can be seen. Observe that the central hypoechoic part of the iliotibial tract expands over the surface of the tubercle where it attaches. In the proximal part of the image, deep to the iliotibial tract, the tibiofemoral joint, the body/anterior horn of the lateral meniscus and inferior lateral genicular vessels can be seen.

LATERAL COLLATERAL LIGAMENT TENDON OF POPLITEUS
Longitudinal
FIG. 5.29

By palpation, locate the head of the fibula, the tendon of biceps femoris, and the posterior edge of the iliotibial tract. Place the probe longitudinally over the

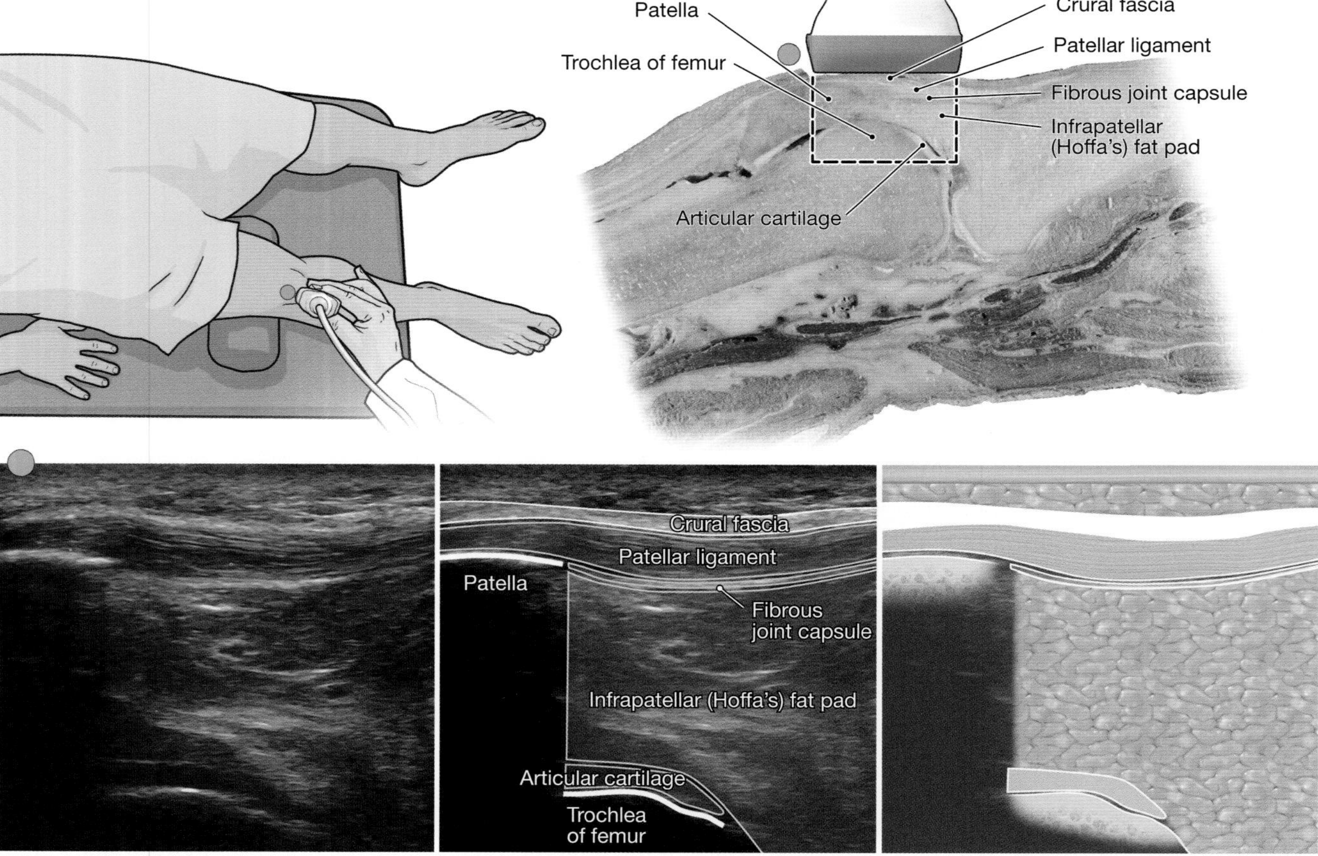

Figure 5.25 Longitudinal view of the inferior pole of the patella, patellar ligament, infrapatellar fat pad (of Hoffa), and femoral trochlea.

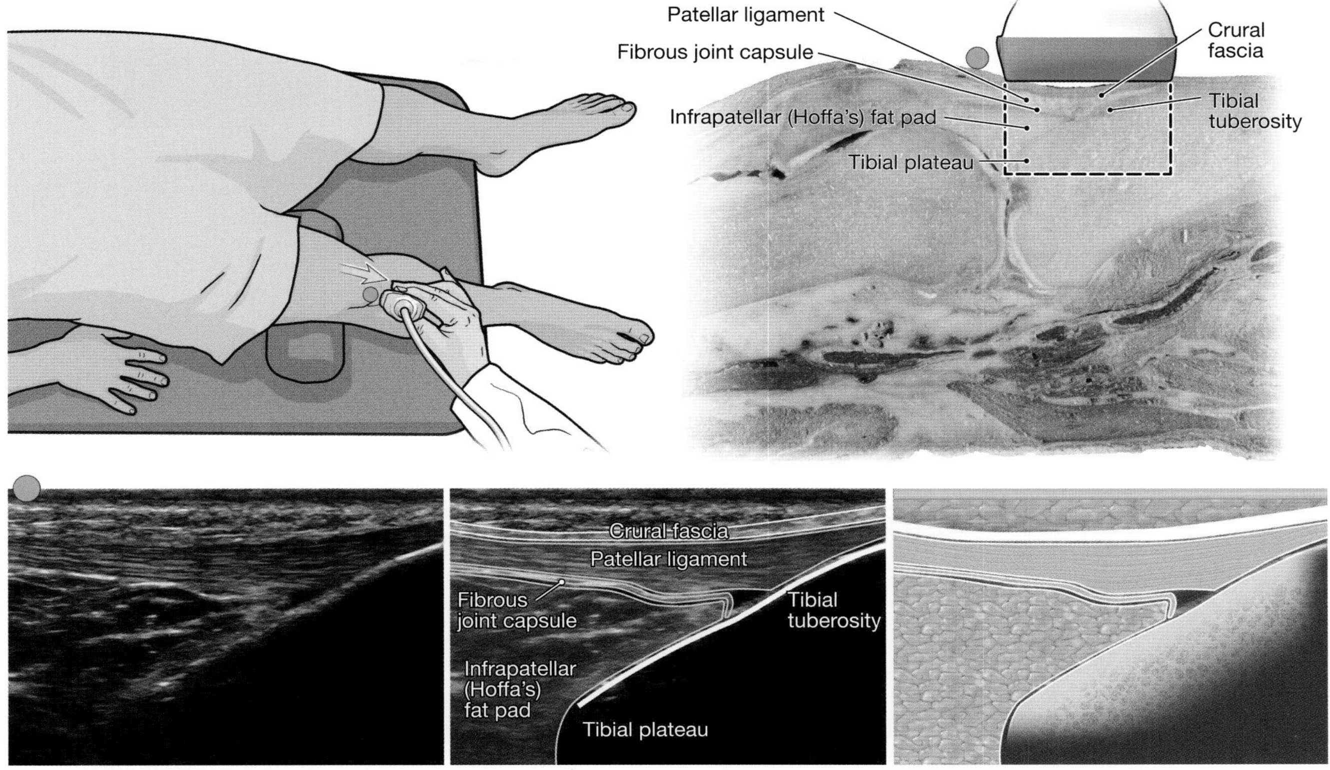

Figure 5.26 Longitudinal view of the patellar ligament and its insertion at the tibial tuberosity.

lateral surface of the lateral femoral condyle just posterior to the edge of the iliotibial tract with the probe marker directed superiorly and the heel of the probe face directed toward the head of the fibula. While maintaining the same orientation, adjust the probe position until the groove for popliteus along the lateral surface of the lateral femoral condyle can be clearly identified. This bony landmark is critical for locating the proximal attachment of the small cordlike lateral (fibular) collateral ligament. While fanning and tilting the probe face in this position, locate the hyperechoic popliteus tendon within the groove. Immediately superior to the groove, the hyperechoic fibers of the lateral (fibular) collateral ligament can be seen attaching to the surface of the lateral epicondyle and then narrowing into the cordlike central part of the ligament over the groove for popliteus. The ligament is separated from the popliteus tendon by the fibrous joint capsule. Attempt to follow the ligament distally to the fibular head. Take care not to misidentify the iliotibial tract (just anterior to the ligament) or the biceps femoris tendon (just posterior to the ligament) as the lateral collateral ligament. At the lateral surface of the head of the fibula, the lateral collateral ligament fibers merge with fibers of the biceps femoris tendon.

Popliteal Fossa

TIBIAL NERVE
COMMON FIBULAR NERVE POPLITEAL VESSELS
Transverse
FIG. 5.30

The patient should be prone with a small bolster placed under the distal leg to slightly flex the knee, for relaxing the posterior muscles around the knee joint. Place the probe transversely over the biceps femoris muscle superior to the popliteal fossa. Identify the hyperechoic honeycomb appearance of the sciatic nerve deep to the muscle, along its anteromedial surface. Adjust the probe position to center the nerve in the image. While concentrating on the nerve, slide the probe distally toward the popliteal fossa until the nerve can be seen to divide into a smaller lateral branch, the common fibular nerve, and a larger medial branch, the tibial nerve. Typically, this division occurs just proximal to the popliteal fossa. While continuing to slide a short distance distally, observe that the tibial nerve descends more or less vertically into the fossa, whereas the common fibular nerve moves laterally to a position along the medial edge of the biceps femoris muscle. While keeping the tibial nerve near the center of the image, apply as little pressure as possible to the probe face to avoid compression/effacement of the popliteal vein, which lies immediately deep to the tibial nerve. Passively flexing the knee to 90° may also

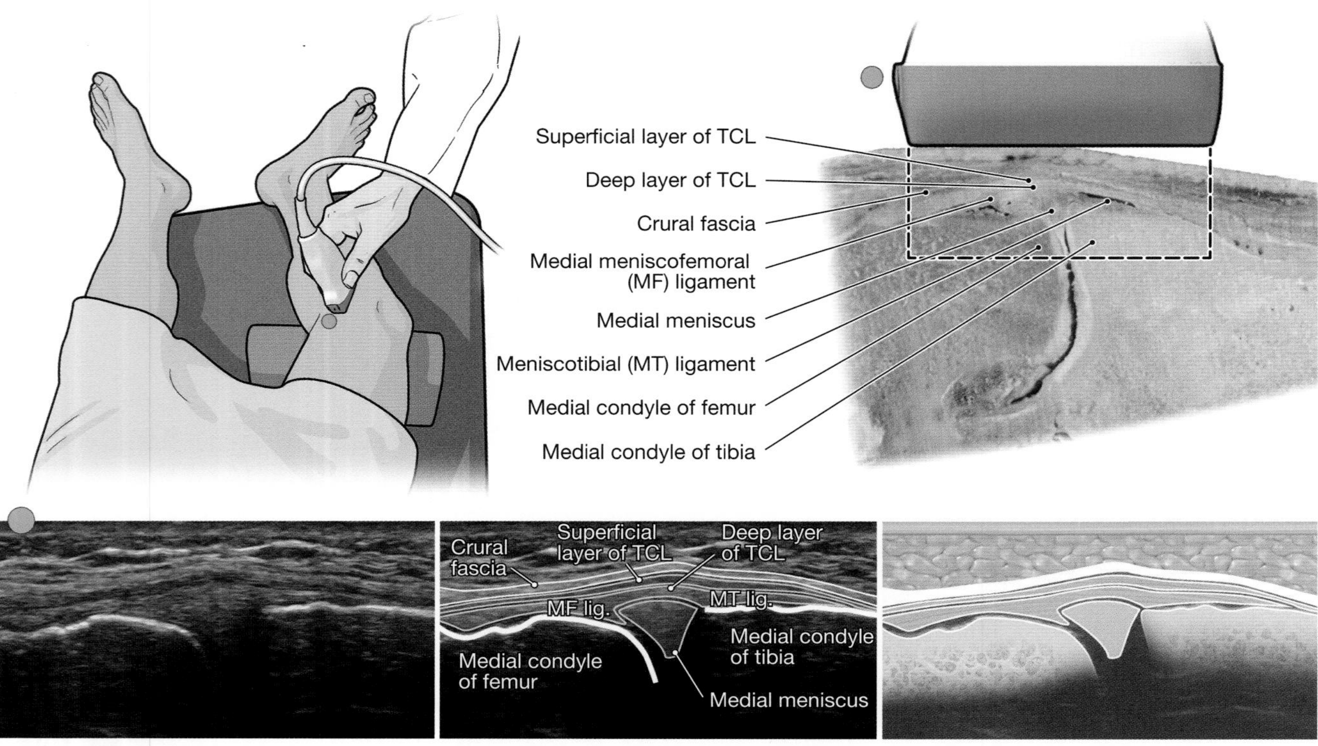

Figure 5.27 Longitudinal view of the tibial collateral ligament of the knee and the body of the medial meniscus.

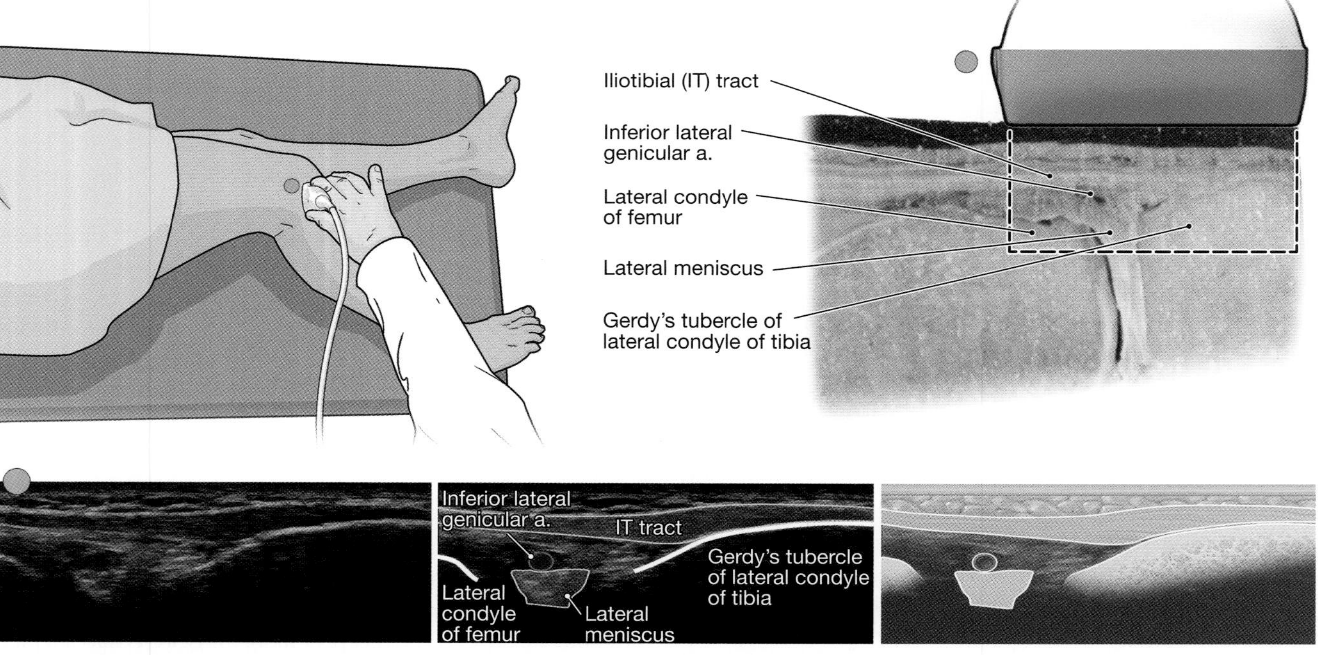

Figure 5.28 Longitudinal view of the iliotibial tract crossing the knee joint to its attachment at the anterolateral surface of the lateral tibial condyle (Gerdy tubercle).

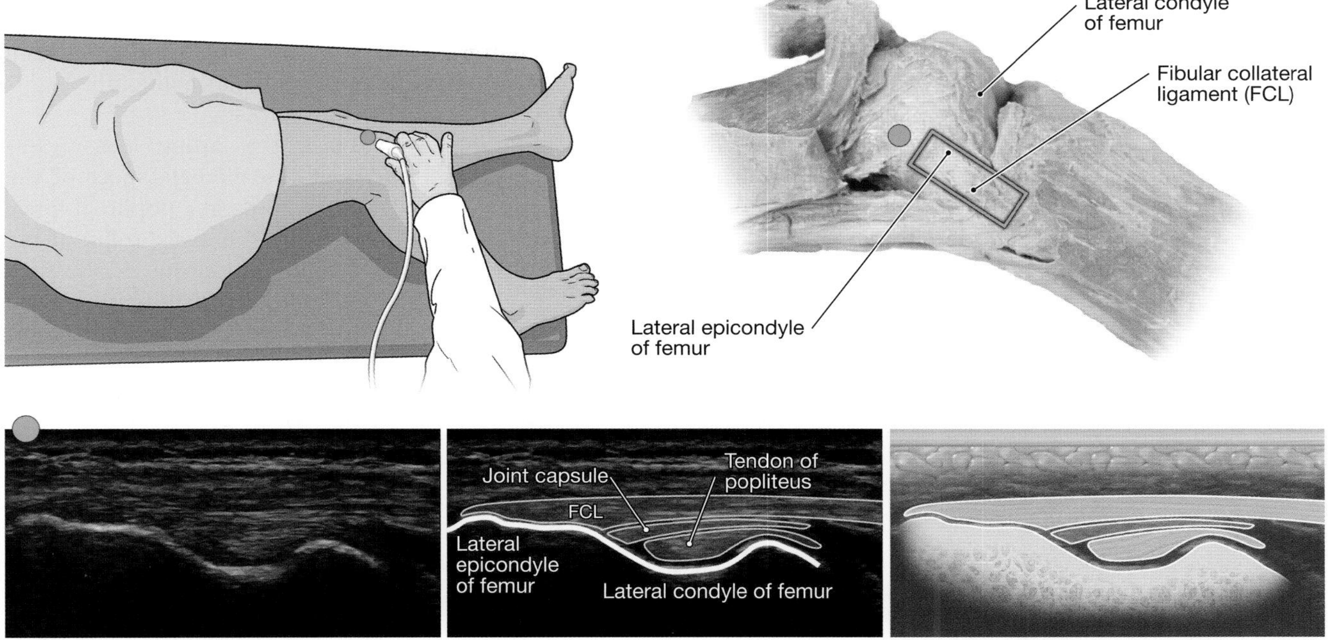

Figure 5.29 Longitudinal view of the femoral attachment of the fibular collateral ligament and the tendon of popliteus.

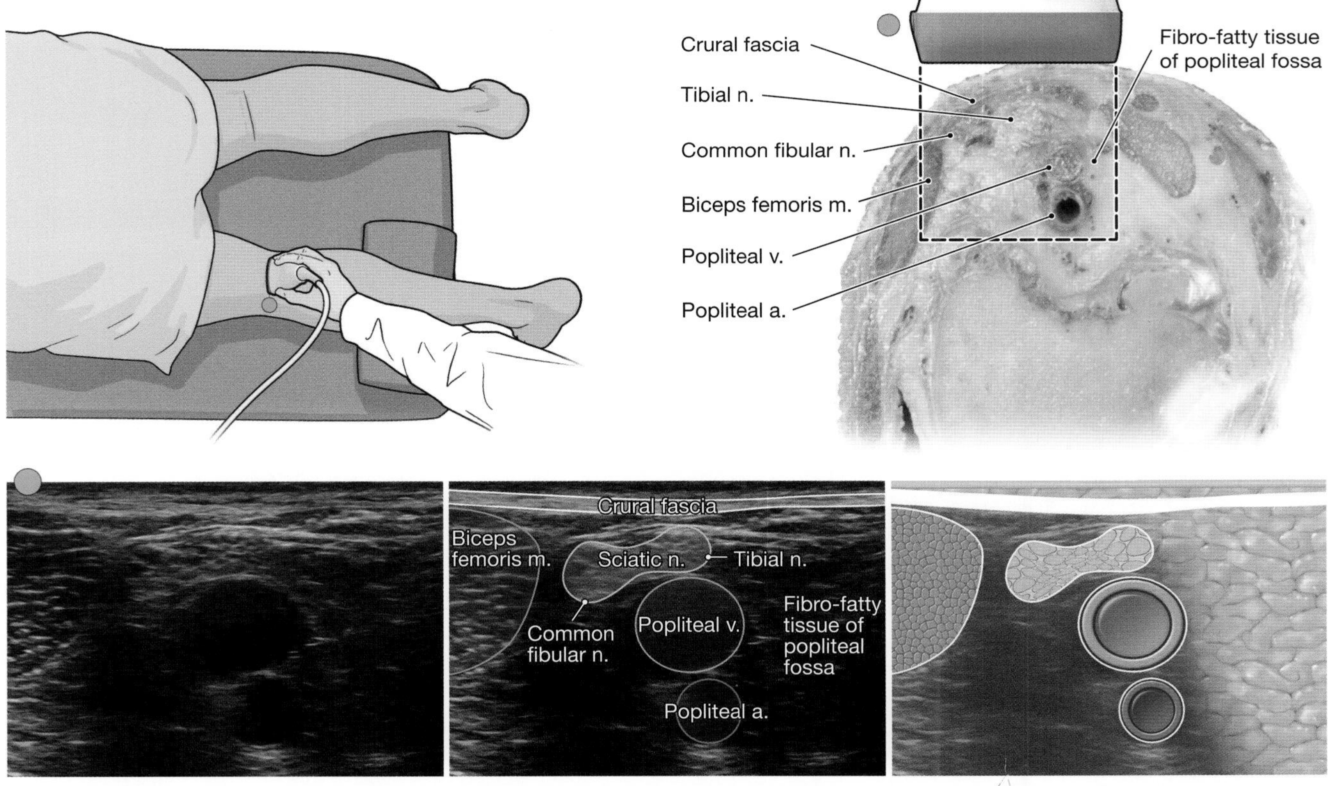

Figure 5.30 Transverse view of the sciatic nerve dividing into the tibial and common fibular nerves, popliteal vein, and popliteal artery in the superior part of the popliteal fossa.

help fill the vein by increasing venous return from the foot and leg. Gently squeezing the calf muscles also briefly fills the vein. Deep to the vein, look for pulsations of the popliteal artery.

POPLITEAL ARTERY
POPLITEUS MUSCLE
Longitudinal
FIG. 5.31

Center the popliteal artery in the image and carefully rotate the probe into a longitudinal orientation over the artery. Slide the probe distally along the artery through and just beyond the popliteal fossa. Locate the hyperechoic bony profile of the tibial plateau sloping down to the posterior surface of the proximal body of the tibia, which is covered by the popliteus muscle belly. The popliteal artery can be seen coursing over the popliteus muscle and deep to the lateral head of the gastrocnemius and then soleus as it enters the posterior compartment of the leg.

MEDIAL HEAD OF THE GASTROCNEMIUS
SEMIMEMBRANOSUS TENDON MEDIAL FEMORAL CONDYLE
Transverse
FIG. 5.32

Place the probe transversely over the medial aspect of the thigh above the popliteal fossa. Identify the oval profile of the semimembranosus muscle with the tendon of semitendinosus at its posterior surface and center

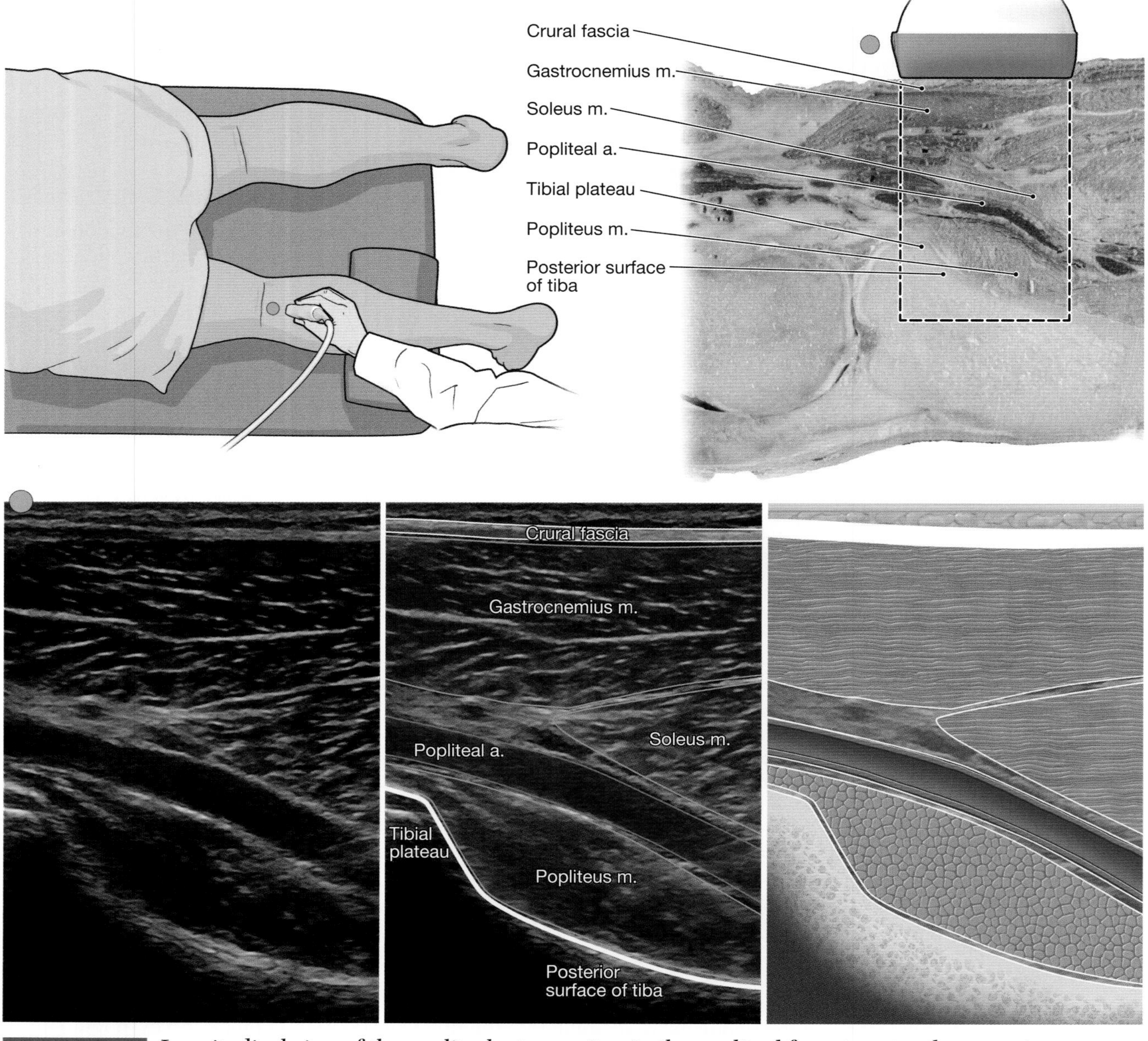

Figure 5.31 Longitudinal view of the popliteal artery as it exits the popliteal fossa to enter the posterior compartment of the leg.

them in the image. Slide the probe distally along the muscle and tendon until the semimembranosus can be seen to taper to a broad thick tendon. While continuing distally a short distance, observe that the semimembranosus tendon crosses behind the medial condyle in contact with the fibrous joint capsule. Immediately lateral to the tendon in this position, identify the hypoechoic medial tendinous edge and muscle tissue of the medial gastrocnemius. The semimembranosus tendon is separated from the tendinous edge of the medial gastrocnemius by a (normally) thin bursa communicating with the knee joint. The tendon of semitendinosus can be seen superficial to the semimembranosus tendon. At the medial aspect of the image (adjust probe position as needed), the small gracilis tendon can be found at the posterolateral edge of the sartorius. The sartorius is still muscular at this point, but quickly tapers to a thin tendon distally.

CLINICAL APPLICATION

US examination is used in the evaluation of several potential causes of a painful knee, mainly related to the external structures of the knee joint. These techniques are useful for evaluating disorders including tendonitis/tendinosis and partial or complete muscle/tendon tears (quadriceps femoris, patellar ligament, semitendinosus, semimembranosus, gracilis, and biceps femoris), bursitis/bursopathy (prepatellar bursa, deep infrapatellar bursa, semimembranosus-gastrocnemius bursa, and Baker's cyst), and ligamentous injuries (tibial collateral ligament, fibular collateral ligament, and iliotibial tract). US is useful for evaluating and detecting even very small knee joint effusions and for needle guidance into the suprapatellar bursa (this bursa is continuous with the knee joint proper, so is not a true bursa) of the knee joint to aspirate fluid and/or to inject anti-inflammatory steroids and local anesthetic agents.

Popliteal (Baker's) cyst is one of the most common conditions of the knee joint characterized by the formation of a fluid-filled sac (cyst) that usually protrudes at the popliteal fossa causing stiffness, discomfort, and pain. The development of the cyst is usually linked to the underlying knee joint problems such as osteoarthritis, rheumatoid arthritis, meniscal tear, or cruciate ligament tear. These conditions cause excess synovial fluid production in the knee joint that accumulates at the popliteal bursa leading to the cyst formation. In most cases, Nonsteroidal anti-inflammatory drugs and rest improve the clinical picture.

Evaluation of the hyaline cartilage of the femoral trochlea can be used for detecting cartilage thinning, marginal erosions, and/or increased echogenicity as a marker for the extent of cartilage loss/changes in the knee as a result of osteoarthritis or other inflammatory arthropathies. Because of the acoustic shadowing behind bony surfaces, US has more limited usefulness for the evaluation of the cruciate ligaments and the menisci, although tears involving the meniscal bodies and meniscal cysts are often visible.

US examination, including Doppler US, is commonly used for the detection of deep vein thrombi in the lower limb veins, including the popliteal vein and its tributaries. Doppler US is also used for the measurement of flow velocity profiles in the popliteal artery in suspected peripheral artery disease and for the detection and measurement of popliteal artery aneurysms.

US-guided sciatic nerve blocks are used in surgeries involving the knee, posterior leg, Achilles (calcaneal) tendon, ankle, and foot and for postoperative control of posterior knee pain.

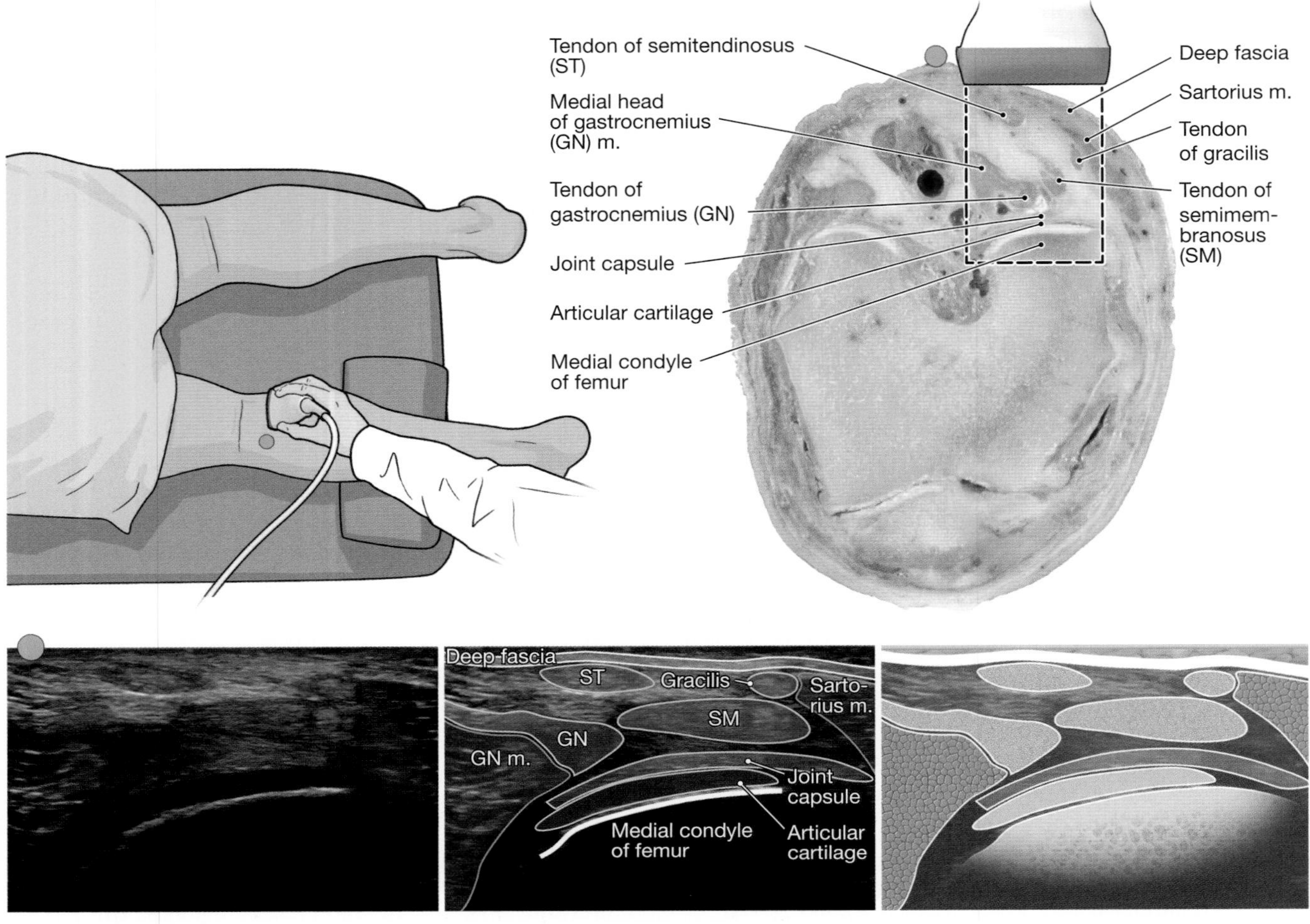

Figure 5.32 Transverse view of the tendon of semimembranosus adjacent to the medial tendinous edge of the medial head of gastrocnemius, posterior to the medial femoral condyle. B, Transverse view as in Figure 5.32 demonstrating the neck and proximal part of a popliteal (Baker) cyst. The neck of a true popliteal cyst always emerges from between the tendinous edge of the medial head of gastrocnemius and the semimembranosus tendon, as demonstrated in this image.

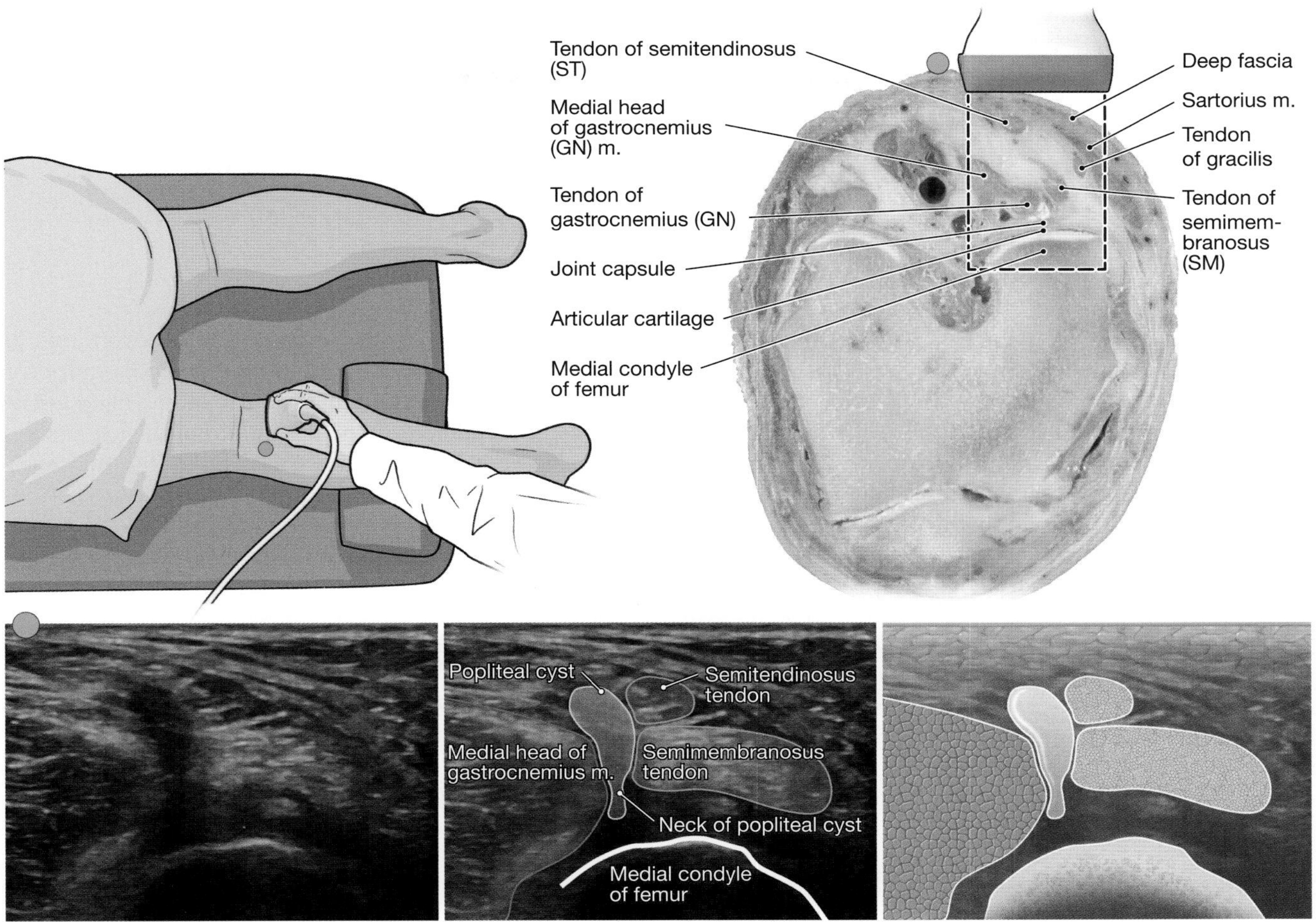

Tendon of semitendinosus (ST)
Medial head of gastrocnemius (GN) m.
Tendon of gastrocnemius (GN)
Joint capsule
Articular cartilage
Medial condyle of femur
Deep fascia
Sartorius m.
Tendon of gracilis
Tendon of semimem-branosus (SM)
Popliteal cyst
Semitendinosus tendon
Medial head of gastrocnemius m.
Semimembranosus tendon
Neck of popliteal cyst
Medial condyle of femur

Figure 5.32 *(Continued)*

Leg

Review of the Anatomy

Bones

The bones of the leg are the tibia and fibula.

Tibia

The tibia, which forms the distal part of the knee joint and most of the proximal part of the ankle joint, is the large weight-bearing bone of the leg. The body of the tibia is triangular in profile, with the posterior, anterolateral, and anteromedial surfaces delineated by anterior, medial, and interosseous (lateral) borders. The anteromedial surface is subcutaneous throughout its length. The expanded distal end of the tibia forms the superior and medial (medial malleolus) surfaces of the bony arch of the ankle joint, articulating with the upper surface (trochlea) of the talus.

Fibula

The non-weight-bearing fibula is a much smaller bone. At its proximal end, the head of the fibula articulates with a facet on the inferior surface of the lateral tibial condyle. The neck of the fibula is continuous with the body, which is triangular in profile with the posterior, lateral, and medial surfaces delineated by anterior, lateral, and medial borders. Along the medial surface is an additional border, the interosseous crest, representing the line of attachment of the tibiofibular interosseous membrane, which spans between the fibula and the interosseous border of the tibia. The fibula expands distally to the lateral malleolus, which forms the lateral surface of the ankle joint.

Muscles

The deep (crural) fascia and its intermuscular septae, along with the tibiofibular interosseous membrane, divide the leg into three muscular compartments: anterior, posterior, and lateral.

Anterior Compartment

The anterior compartment muscles, innervated by the deep fibular nerve, are tibialis anterior, extensor digitorum longus, fibularis tertius, and extensor hallucis longus.

Tibialis Anterior

Tibialis anterior originates from the upper two-thirds of the lateral surface of the body of the fibula, the adjacent interosseous membrane, and the surrounding deep fascia. It becomes tendinous in the distal third of the leg, crosses the ankle joint deep to the extensor retinacula, and turns under the medial side of the foot to insert at the base of the first metatarsal and adjacent plantar surface of medial cuneiform. The tibialis anterior extends (dorsiflexes) and inverts the foot.

Extensor Digitorum Longus

Extensor digitorum longus originates from the lateral tibial condyle, the medial surface of the fibular shaft and adjacent upper part of the interosseous membrane, the anterior intermuscular septum, and the surrounding deep fascia. Its tendon forms in the distal leg and crosses the ankle joint deep to the extensor retinacula. On the dorsum of the foot, the tendon divides into four slips that insert into the extensor expansions of the lateral toes. The extensor digitorum longus dorsiflexes the foot and extends at the joints of the lateral toes.

Fibularis Tertius

Fibularis tertius originates from the medial surface of the fibula just below the extensor digitorum longus, and the two muscles are usually joined. On the dorsum of the foot, the tendon of fibularis tertius separates from the digital extensor tendon and inserts over the dorsal surface of the base of the fifth metatarsal distal to the insertion of the fibularis brevis. This small muscle assists in dorsiflexion and eversion of the foot. This muscle is often absent.

Extensor Hallucis Longus

Extensor hallucis longus originates from the middle third of the medial surface of the fibula and adjacent interosseous membrane, between the origins of tibialis anterior medially and extensor digitorum longus laterally. At its origin, the extensor hallucis longus is covered by these two muscles, emerging between the two in the distal leg to cross the ankle joint between their tendons.

Lateral Compartment

The two lateral compartment muscles, fibularis longus and brevis, are innervated by the superficial fibular nerve. They evert the foot and assist in plantar flexion at the ankle joint. The fibularis longus additionally assists, along with tibialis anterior and posterior, in dynamic support of the transverse arch of the foot.

Fibularis Longus

Fibularis longus, which is superficial to fibularis brevis, originates from the lateral surface of the head of the fibula, the upper half of the lateral surface of the body of the fibula, the anterior and posterior intermuscular septae that bound the compartment, and from the surrounding deep fascia. The fibularis longus becomes tendinous about the midleg, and the long tendon descends along the superficial surface of the fibularis brevis muscle. In the distal third of the leg, the fibularis longus tendon descends along the posterior surface of the fibula and lateral malleolus where it is immediately posterolateral to the tendon of fibularis brevis as both tendons cross the ankle joint.

Fibularis Brevis

Fibularis brevis originates from the distal two-thirds of the lateral surface of the body of the fibula, the anterior and posterior intermuscular septae, and from the surrounding deep fascia. The muscle becomes tendinous as it descends along the posterior surface of the distal fibula and lateral malleolus, as it crosses the ankle joint with the tendon of fibularis longus.

Posterior Compartment

The posterior compartment muscles, innervated by the tibial nerve, are arranged in superficial and deep layers.

Superficial Layer

The muscles of the superficial group include the medial and lateral heads of gastrocnemius, soleus, and plantaris, all three of which insert via the calcaneal tendon onto the posterior surface of the calcaneus to plantarflex of the foot. The two heads of the gastrocnemius plus the small plantaris muscle cross the knee joint from their origins and therefore flex the leg.

Gastrocnemius

The medial head of the gastrocnemius originates from the posterior surface of the femur just above the medial condyle, and the lateral head originates from the posterior surface of the femur just above the lateral condyle. The plantaris muscle originates from the lateral supracondylar line just above the lateral head of the gastrocnemius. The two heads of the gastrocnemius converge at the inferior extent of the popliteal fossa and then taper to a broad flattened tendinous band (gastrocnemius aponeurosis) at about the midleg.

Soleus

Soleus muscle, deep to the gastrocnemius, originates from the posterior surface of the head, neck, and proximal third of the fibula, from the soleal line of the posterior surface of the tibia, and from an intervening tendinous arch. The tendon of soleus fuses with the overlying tendon of gastrocnemius to complete the formation of the calcaneal tendon in the distal third of the leg.

Plantaris

The long thin plantaris tendon courses between the gastrocnemius and soleus to insert along the posteromedial aspect of the calcaneal tendon.

Deep Layer

The muscles of the deep group include the popliteus, tibialis posterior, flexor digitorum longus, and flexor hallucis longus. The popliteus muscle is a short muscle related to the knee joint and was discussed hereinbefore along with the structures of the knee. The tendons tibialis posterior, flexor digitorum longus, and flexor hallucis longus cross the medial side of the ankle joint through the tarsal tunnel to enter the plantar aspect of the foot. The detailed anatomy of the tarsal tunnel and its contents have been discussed along with structures of the ankle.

Tibialis posterior originates from the upper half of the interosseous membrane and adjacent surfaces of the tibia and fibula, between the origins of the flexor hallucis longus laterally and flexor digitorum longus medially. The flexor hallucis longus originates from the middle half of the posterior surface of the body of the fibula and adjacent interosseous membrane. The flexor digitorum longus originates from the middle third of the posterior surface and lateral border of the tibia. All three tendons cross the ankle joint into the plantar aspect of the foot through the tarsal tunnel on the medial side of the ankle.

Kager Fat Pad

Kager fat pad is located in the distal leg and posterior to the ankle joint. The fat pad has a triangular shape, with the base formed by the superior cortical surface of the calcaneus, the anterior border formed by the flexor hallucis longus muscle and tendon, and the posterior border formed by the anterior surface of the calcaneal tendon. The apex of the triangle extends superiorly between the distal fibers of soleus and the muscles of the deep group.

Vessels and Nerves

The major neurovascular structures of the leg enter the leg from the thigh by passing through the popliteal fossa.

Popliteal Vessels

The femoral artery becomes the popliteal artery as it leaves the adductor canal of the thigh and enters the popliteal fossa through the adductor hiatus. The accompanying popliteal vein becomes the femoral vein when it leaves the fossa through the adductor hiatus to enter the adductor canal. The popliteal artery, along with the vein and tibial nerve, descends through the popliteal fossa and enters the posterior compartment of the leg by passing deep to the gastrocnemius and the tendinous arch of soleus. The artery ends just beyond the tendinous arch of soleus by dividing into its terminal branches, the anterior and posterior tibial arteries.

Anterior Tibial Artery

The anterior tibial artery leaves the posterior compartment to enter the anterior compartment by passing over the superior edge of the tibiofibular interosseous membrane. The anterior tibial artery continues through the anterior compartment and ends by changing its name to the dorsalis pedis artery after crossing the ankle joint onto the dorsum of the foot.

Posterior Tibial Artery

The posterior tibial artery has an important lateral branch near its origin, the fibular artery, which descends in the lateral aspect of the posterior compartment giving out perforating branches to supply the tissues of the lateral compartment, through which no artery runs. The posterior tibial artery continues through the posterior compartment along with the tibial nerve between the superficial and deep muscle layers and then leaves the leg through the tarsal tunnel to enter the foot.

Sciatic Nerve

The sciatic nerve approaches the popliteal fossa from the deep surface of the biceps femoris and divides into its terminal branches, the tibial and common fibular nerves, just proximal to the popliteal fossa.

Tibial Nerve

The tibial nerve travels through the central part of the fossa between the medial and lateral heads of the gastrocnemius muscle and enters the posterior compartment of the leg by passing under the tendinous arch of the soleus muscle, accompanied by the popliteal vessels. The tibial nerve descends through the posterior compartment of the leg between the superficial and deep layers of the muscles, and provides motor innervation to the muscles of the posterior compartment of the leg. Along with the posterior tibial vessels, the tibial nerve leaves the leg to enter the foot through the tarsal tunnel.

Sural Nerve

The medial sural cutaneous nerve branches from the tibial nerve in the popliteal fossa and, along with a communicating branch from the lateral sural cutaneous nerve (from the common fibular nerve), forms the sural nerve. The sural nerve joins the small saphenous vein in the shallow groove between the medial and lateral heads of the gastrocnemius and pierces the crural fascia at about the midleg to provide cutaneous innervation to the distal half of the posterolateral leg and lateral side of the foot.

Common Fibular Nerve

In the proximal part of the popliteal fossa, the common fibular branch of the sciatic diverges laterally along the medial margin of the biceps femoris and its tendon, following the tendon to the posterolateral aspect of the fibular head. The nerve then crosses the fibular neck subcutaneously and enters the lateral compartment between the attachments of the fibularis longus muscle and divides into its terminal divisions, the deep and superficial fibular nerves.

Superficial Fibular Nerve

The superficial fibular nerve descends in the lateral compartment (supplying motor innervation to the compartment) deep to the fibularis longus and then emerges between the fibularis brevis and extensor digitorum longus in the distal third of the leg where it pierces the deep fascia to provide cutaneous innervation to the anterolateral surface of the leg distally and to most of the dorsum of the foot.

Deep Fibular Nerve

The deep fibular nerve pierces the anterior intermuscular septum to enter the anterior compartment wherein it accompanies the anterior tibial vessels. The deep fibular nerve supplies the muscles of the anterior compartment, crosses the ankle joint onto the dorsum of the foot accompanying the dorsalis pedis artery, supplies motor branches to the extensor digitorum brevis and extensor hallucis brevis, and then pierces the deep fascia between the first and second metatarsal bones to supply cutaneous innervation to the web space between the great and second toes.

Technique

Anterior Compartment

ANTERIOR COMPARTMENT PROXIMAL
Transverse
FIG. 5.33

The patient should be supine with the knee flexed to 90° and the sole of the foot should rest on the examination table. By palpation, identify the tibial tuberosity and anterior border of the tibia. Place the probe transversely over the proximal part of the anterior compartment just below the inferior extent of the tibial tuberosity. Identify the hyperechoic anterolateral surface of the tibia and its dense acoustic shadow. Adjust the probe position until the fibula is in view at the lateral extent of the image. Locate the hyperechoic tibiofibular interosseous membrane spanning between the medial surface of the fibula and the anterolateral surface of the tibia in the deep part of the image. Tibialis anterior is the large muscle seen along the tibia and medial half of the interosseous membrane. Identify the extensor digitorum longus muscle between the tibialis anterior and the hyperechoic anterior intermuscular septum, which spans between the medial surface of the fibula and the deep surface of the crural fascia. The fibularis longus muscle is partly in view lateral to the anterior intermuscular septum, in the lateral compartment. Toggle (tilt and fan) the probe face to locate the anterior tibial artery and deep fibular nerve in contact with the interosseous membrane deep to the extensor digitorum longus. Part of the tibialis posterior muscle can be seen along the posterior surface of the interosseous membrane.

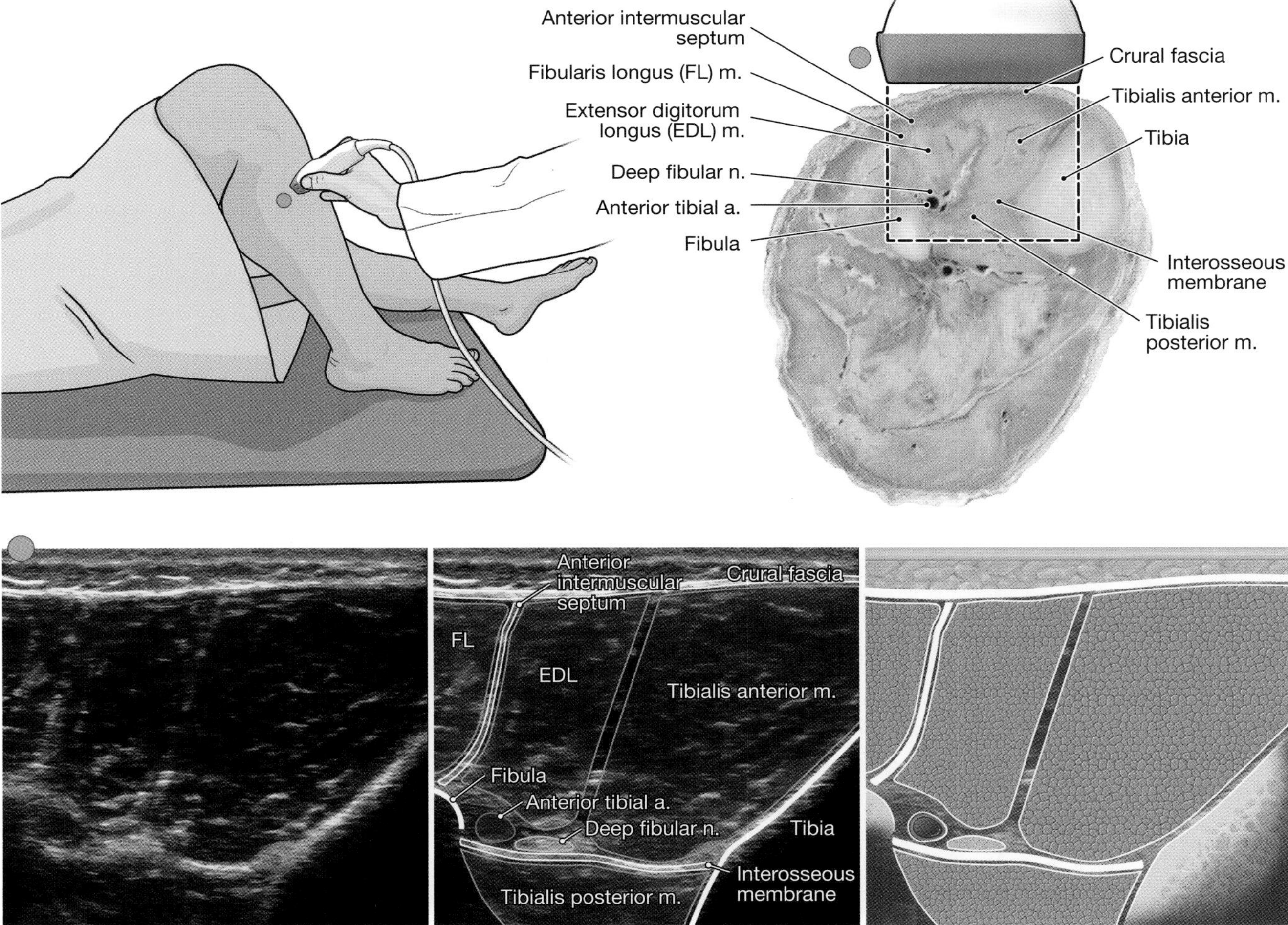

Figure 5.33 Transverse view of the proximal third of the anterior compartment of the leg.

ANTERIOR COMPARTMENT MIDLEG
Transverse
FIG. 5.34

Starting from the previous probe position, slide the probe distally along the anterior compartment to the midleg (or just beyond midleg) keeping the tibialis anterior, extensor digitorum longus, tibia, fibula, and tibiofibular interosseous membrane in view. While sliding the probe distally, passively flex and extend the big toe and watch for flashes of corresponding motion in the deep part of the compartment along the medial surface of the fibula and adjacent interosseous membrane, to identify the extensor hallucis longus muscle and to delineate its borders. Note the characteristic hyperechoic central tendon of the tibialis anterior muscle in the midleg. The fibularis brevis muscle is partly in view lateral to the flexor digitorum longus and along the lateral surface of the fibula. The anterior intermuscular septum separating the fibularis brevis from the extensor digitorum longus may be difficult to see because of anisotropy. Toggle (tilt and fan) the probe face to locate the anterior tibial artery and deep fibular nerve in the deep part of the image between the extensor hallucis longus, the tibialis anterior, and the tibiofibular interosseous membrane.

Lateral Compartment

LATERAL COMPARTMENT NECK OF THE FIBULA
Transverse
FIG. 5.35

The patient should be in a lateral decubitus position with a small pillow/bolster between the knees and the knee flexed to 90°. Locate the head and neck of the fibula by palpation and place the probe transversely (marker directed anteriorly) over the lateral aspect of the leg at the junction of the fibular head and neck. Identify the hyperechoic surface of the fibula and its acoustic shadow. Slide the probe superiorly and inferiorly a short distance and observe the change in profile from the larger ovoid head to the narrow neck. Adjust the probe position and toggle/tilt the probe face to identify the hyperechoic

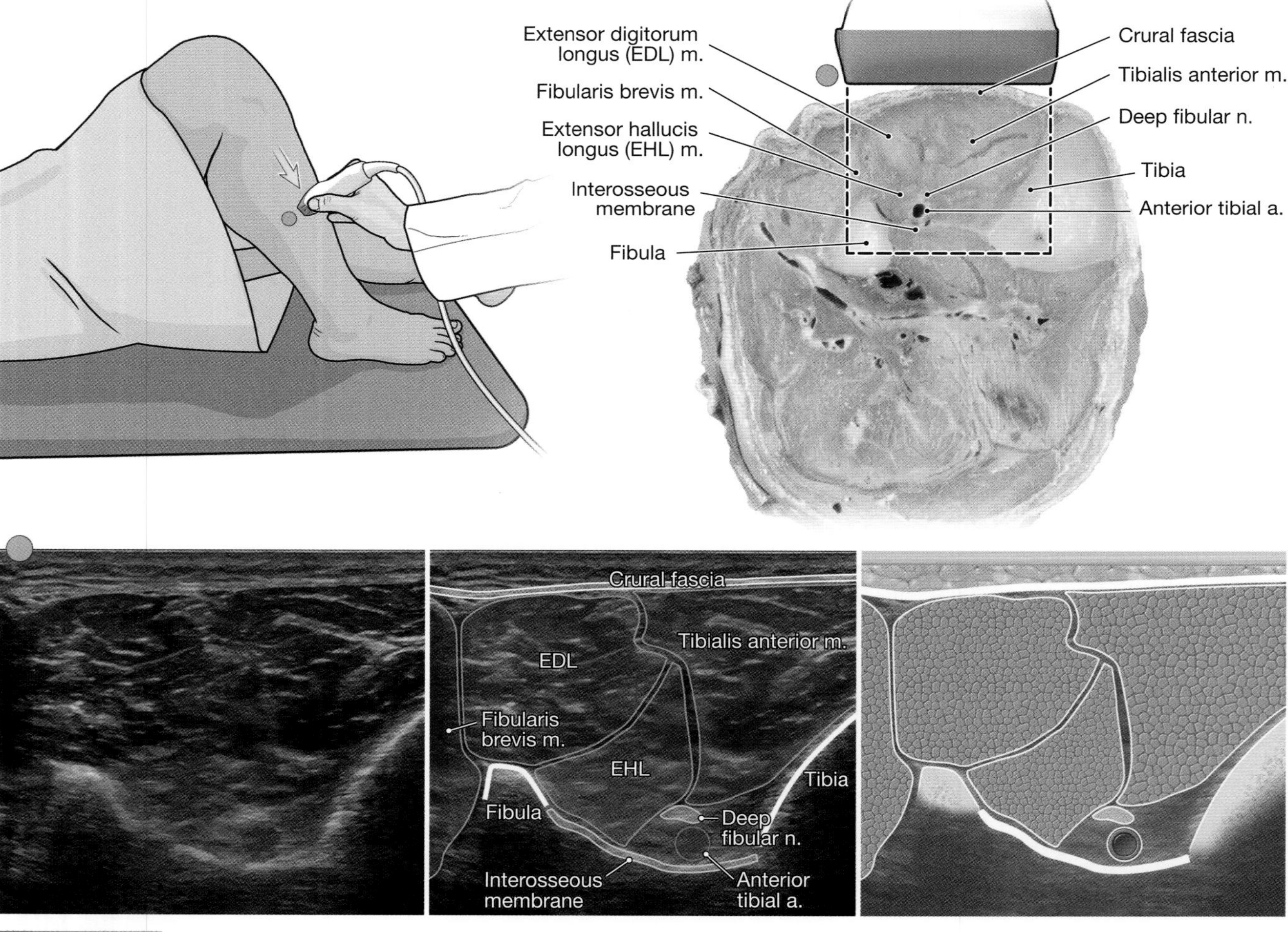

Figure 5.34 Transverse view of the anterior compartment at the midleg.

common fibular nerve as it courses obliquely across the neck of the fibula deep to the fibularis longus muscle. Identify the fibularis longus muscle with its rounded anterior and posterior edges. The hyperechoic anterior intermuscular septum is seen along the deep surface of the anterior part of the fibularis longus, extending from the fibula to the deep (crural) fascia, separating the lateral and anterior compartments of the leg. The posterior intermuscular septum is seen along the deep surface of the posterior part of the fibularis longus, extending from the fibula to the crural fascia, separating the lateral and posterior compartments.

LATERAL COMPARTMENT MIDLEG
Transverse
FIG. 5.36

Starting from the previous probe position, slide the probe distally along the lateral compartment to about the midleg, keeping the fibularis longus muscle centered in the image. The fibularis longus begins to narrow in its lateral-medial dimension, and its connective tissue density increases as the fibularis brevis muscle appears and enlarges along the lateral surface of the fibula, between the fibula and fibularis longus. Again, identify the anterior intermuscular septum separating the lateral and anterior compartments and the posterior intermuscular septum separating the lateral and posterior compartments.

LATERAL COMPARTMENT DISTAL THIRD OF THE LEG
Transverse
FIG. 5.37

Beginning from the previous probe position, slide the probe distally along the lateral compartment to the junction between the proximal and distal thirds of the leg, keeping the fibularis longus and brevis centered in the image. Approaching the distal third of the leg, the fibularis longus narrows to a tendinous band along the superficial surface of the fibularis brevis. More distally, the tendinous band becomes an oval tendon posterior to the tendon of the fibularis brevis. The anterior part of the fibularis brevis muscle narrows to form an oval tendon at the posterior surface of the distal fibula, whereas the posterior muscular part persists as far as the posterior surface of the lateral malleolus. Identify the anterior intermuscular septum separating the lateral and anterior compartments and the posterior intermuscular septum separating the lateral and posterior compartments.

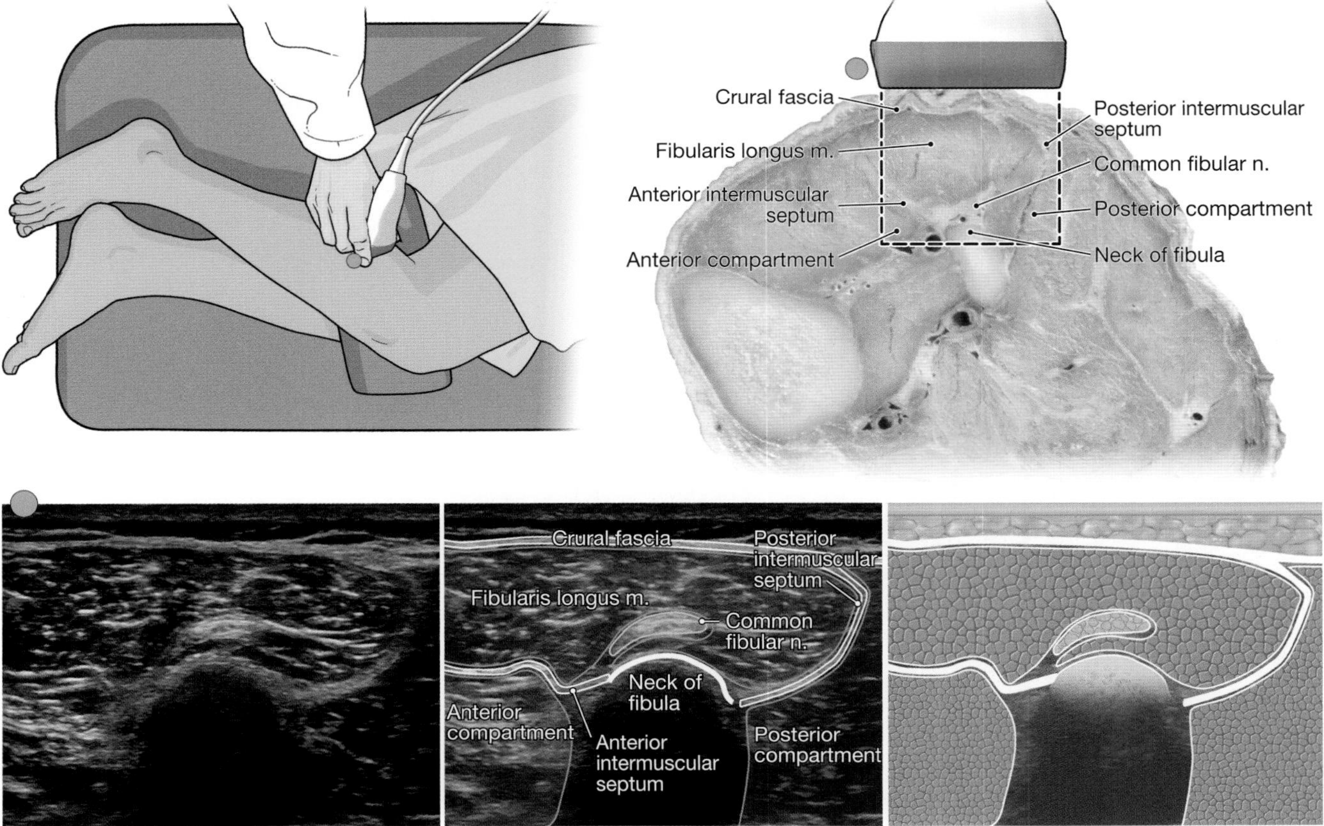

Figure 5.35 Transverse view of the lateral compartment of the leg at the level of the neck of the fibula.

Posterior Compartment

POSTERIOR COMPARTMENT MIDLEG
Transverse
FIG. 5.38

The patient should be prone with the ankles and feet over the end of the examination table. Place the probe transversely over the center of the posterior aspect of the leg at the inferior extent of the calf belly, at or just below the midleg (probe marker directed laterally). Adjust the probe position as needed to identify the inferior extent of the medial and lateral heads of the gastrocnemius and their intervening aponeurotic tendon overlying the soleus muscle and its tendinous superficial surface. Applying minimal pressure to the probe face, slide the probe superiorly and inferiorly while toggling/tilting the probe to identify the small saphenous vein and the accompanying sural nerve within a compartment of the crural fascia superficial to the aponeurotic tendon between the heads of the gastrocnemius. Adjust the probe position and tilt as needed to identify the rounded oblong contour of the soleus muscle. Deep to the medial aspect of soleus, between the soleus and the deep muscles of the posterior compartment, identify the tibial nerve and posterior tibial vessels.

POSTERIOR COMPARTMENT MIDLEG
Longitudinal
FIG. 5.39

Starting from the previous probe position, slide the probe medially bringing the lower part of the medial head of the gastrocnemius into the center of the image. Rotate the probe by 90° (marker side directed superiorly) into the longitudinal axis of the leg and adjust the probe position to bring the tapering distal end of the medial head of the gastrocnemius into view. Deep to the gastrocnemius, identify the soleus muscle and note the tendinous layer along its superficial surface. At the distal end of the gastrocnemius, the gastrocnemius aponeurotic tendon joins the soleus tendon forming the

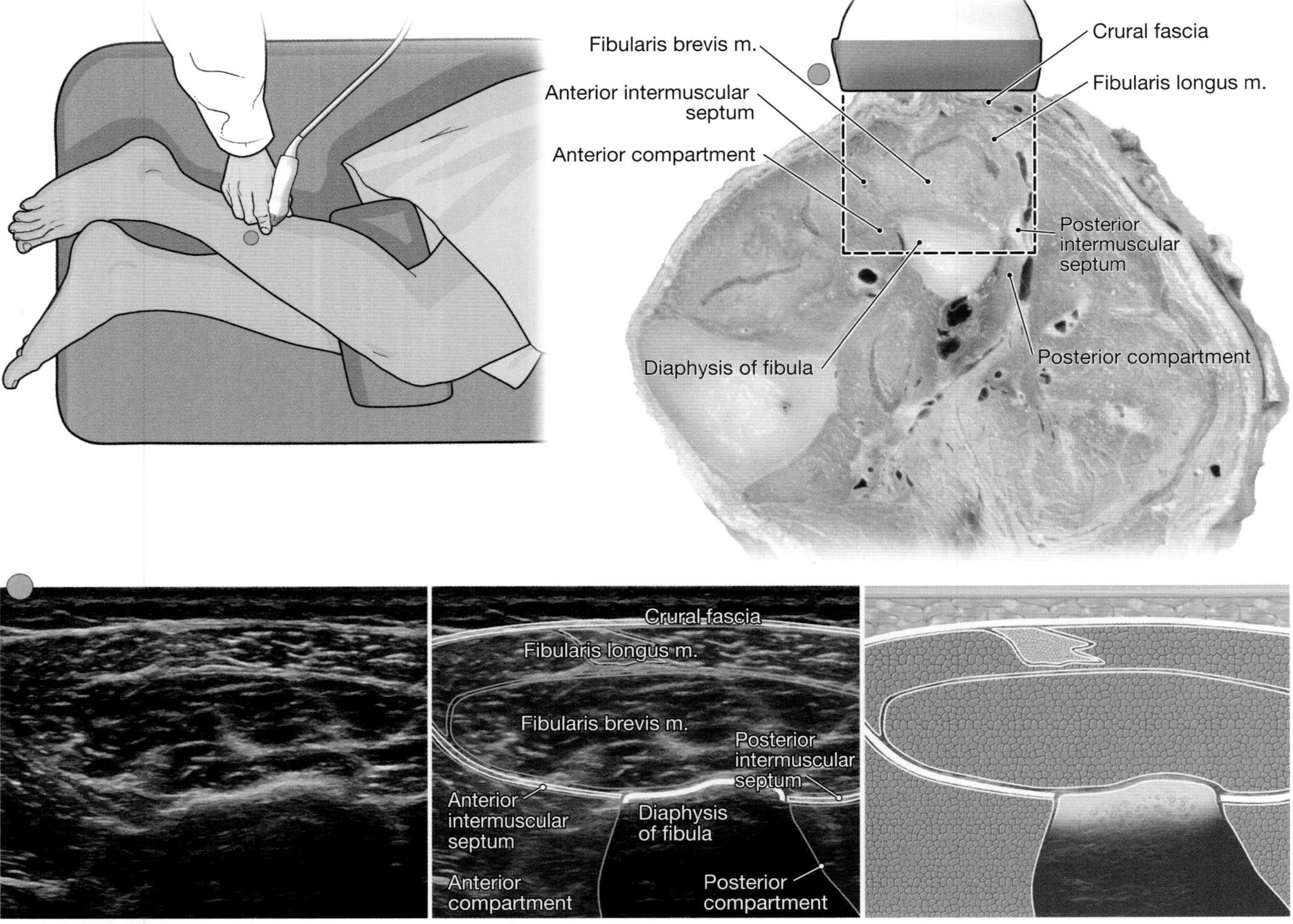

Figure 5.36 Transverse view of the lateral compartment muscles at the midleg.

calcaneal tendon. Sliding distally in the same plane, the calcaneal tendon progressively thickens as tendon fibers from soleus are added to it. Deep to the soleus, identify the deep muscle layer of the posterior compartment. From medial to lateral, the deep muscles are the flexor digitorum longus, tibialis posterior, and flexor hallucis longus. Tilt the probe face as needed to identify the hyperechoic posterior surface of the tibia and its acoustic shadow.

POSTERIOR COMPARTMENT CALCANEAL TENDON DISTAL LEG
Longitudinal
FIG. 5.40

By palpation, locate the calcaneal tendon in the distal leg. Place the probe over the tendon in its longitudinal axis 4 to 6 cm above the heel (marker directed superiorly). Note the hyperechoic fibrillar appearance of the thick calcaneal tendon. Adjust the probe position superiorly/inferiorly along the tendon until the tapering inferior end of the soleus can be clearly seen. Look for the numerous parallel hyperechoic lines of the connective tissue (perimysium) within the soleus to help distinguish the distal end of the soleus from Kager fat pad beyond (the hyperechoic connective tissue lines in the fat pad are much less-organized). The triangular profile of Kager fat pad is seen deep to the calcaneal tendon with its apex projecting between the distal end of the soleus and the deep group of muscles. The flexor hallucis longus is the main muscle of the deep group seen in this position. Look for the hyperechoic posterior surface of the tibia, which curves posteriorly into a rounded hump at its distal end, clinically referred to as the posterior malleolus.

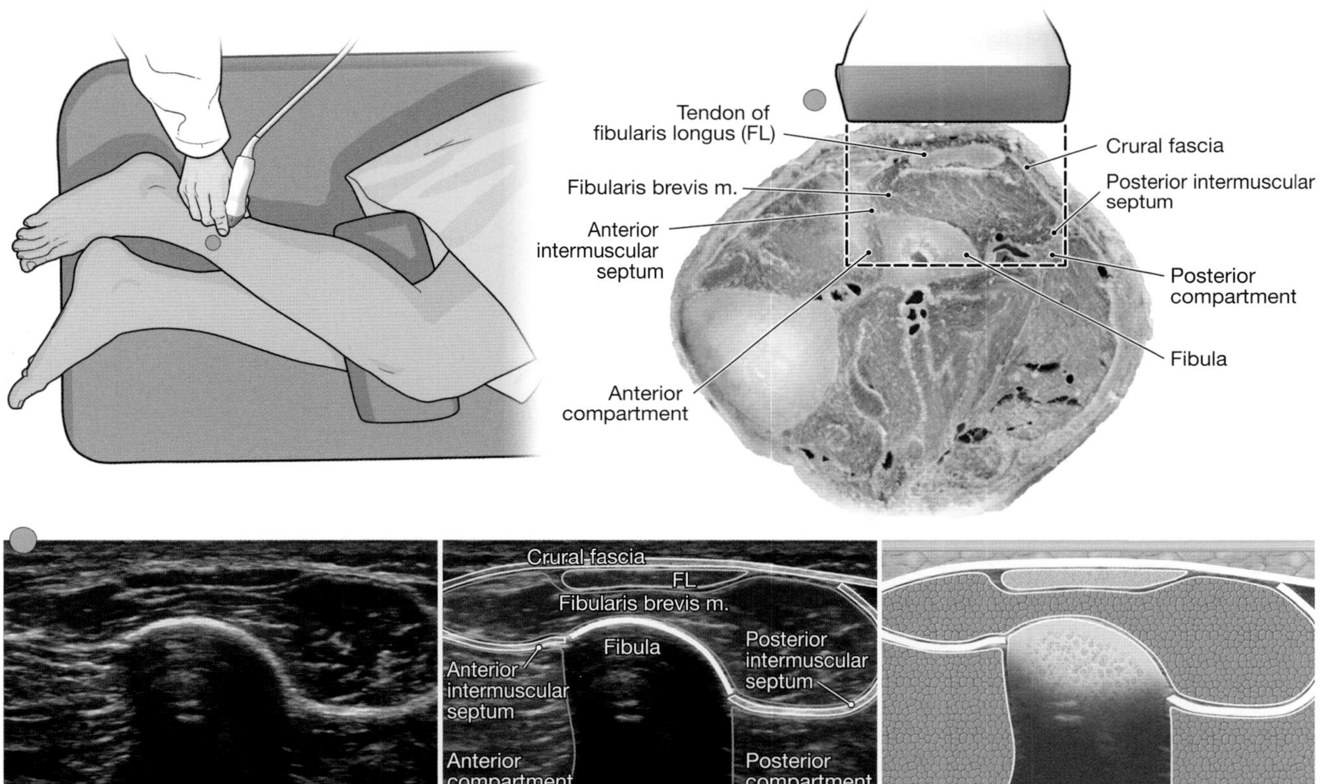

Figure 5.37 Transverse view of the lateral compartment in the distal third of the leg.

CLINICAL APPLICATION

US examination is useful for the evaluation of muscle and tendon injuries, including tendinosis/tendonitis and partial or complete tears of the gastrocnemius and/or soleus muscles and their aponeurotic tendons, the calcaneal tendon, and the ankle extensor (dorsiflexor) tendons (tibialis anterior, extensor digitorum longus, and extensor hallucis longus). Most injuries of the fibularis tendons occur at the ankle joint.

US measurement of anterior compartment thickness before and after a period of exertion is being increasingly used in the diagnosis of chronic exertional compartment syndrome.

US examination and measurement may be used in the evaluation of entrapment/compression of the common fibular nerve in its course along the fibular head and neck, the superficial fibular nerve as it pierces the deep fascia in the distal leg, the deep fibular nerve in its course through the anterior compartment (by osteophytes, space-occupying lesions, or scar tissue), the sural nerve where it pierces deep fascia in the distal leg, and the tibial nerve where it passes under the tendinous arch of the soleus muscle origin into the posterior leg compartment.

US-guided nerve blocks are used in a variety of surgeries involving the distal leg, ankle, and foot, including blocks of the tibial nerve, common fibular nerve, superficial fibular nerve, deep fibular nerve, saphenous nerve, and sural nerve. US examination is used for evaluating the posterior tibial and fibular veins when deep vein thrombosis is suspected. The anterior tibial veins are much less commonly involved in deep vein thrombosis and so are not routinely scanned. In the evaluation of peripheral artery disease, arteries that are included in Doppler US studies of the leg include the popliteal, posterior tibial, fibular, and anterior tibial.

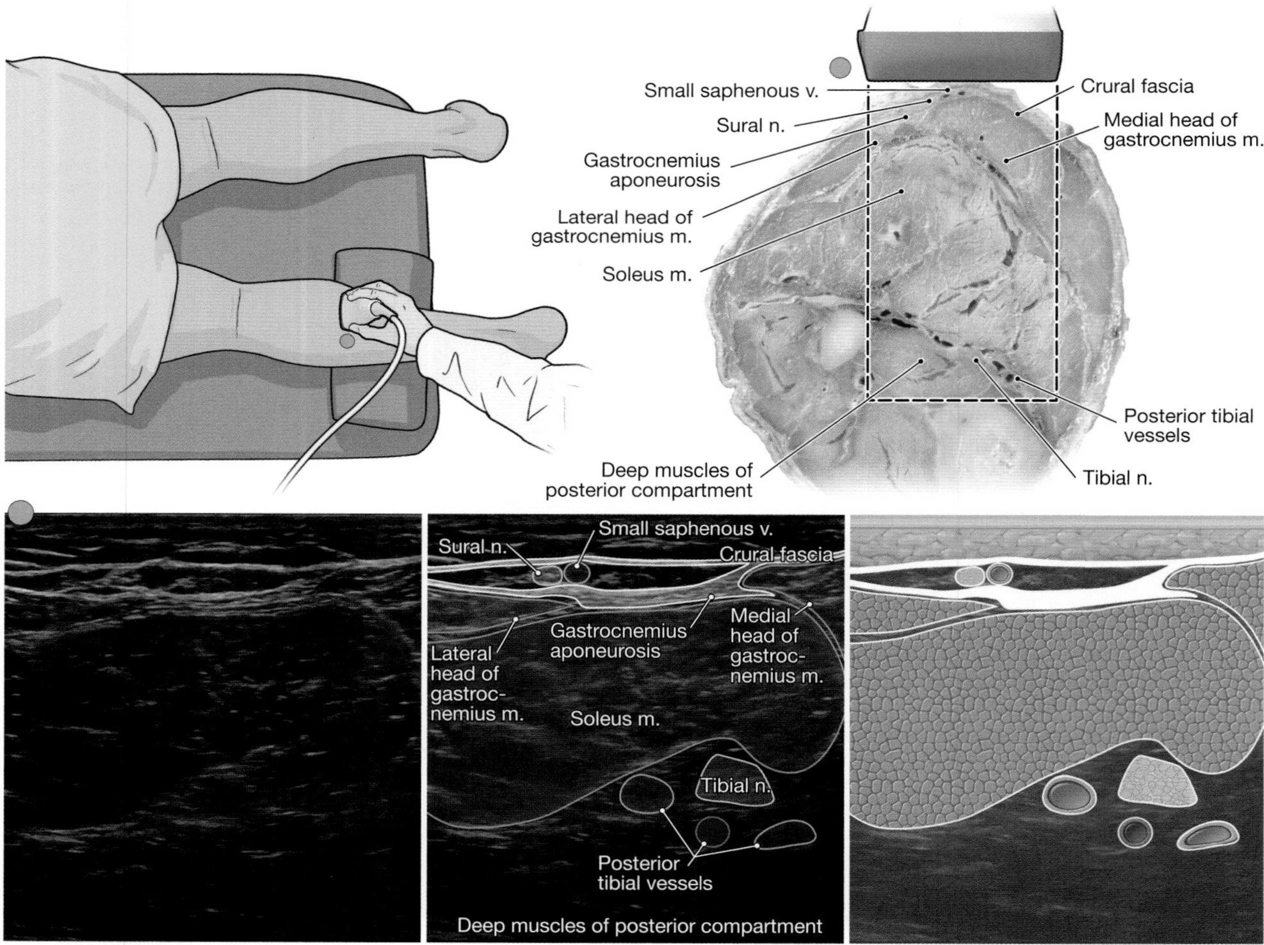

Figure 5.38 Transverse view of the posterior compartment at midleg, including the small saphenous vein and sural nerve.

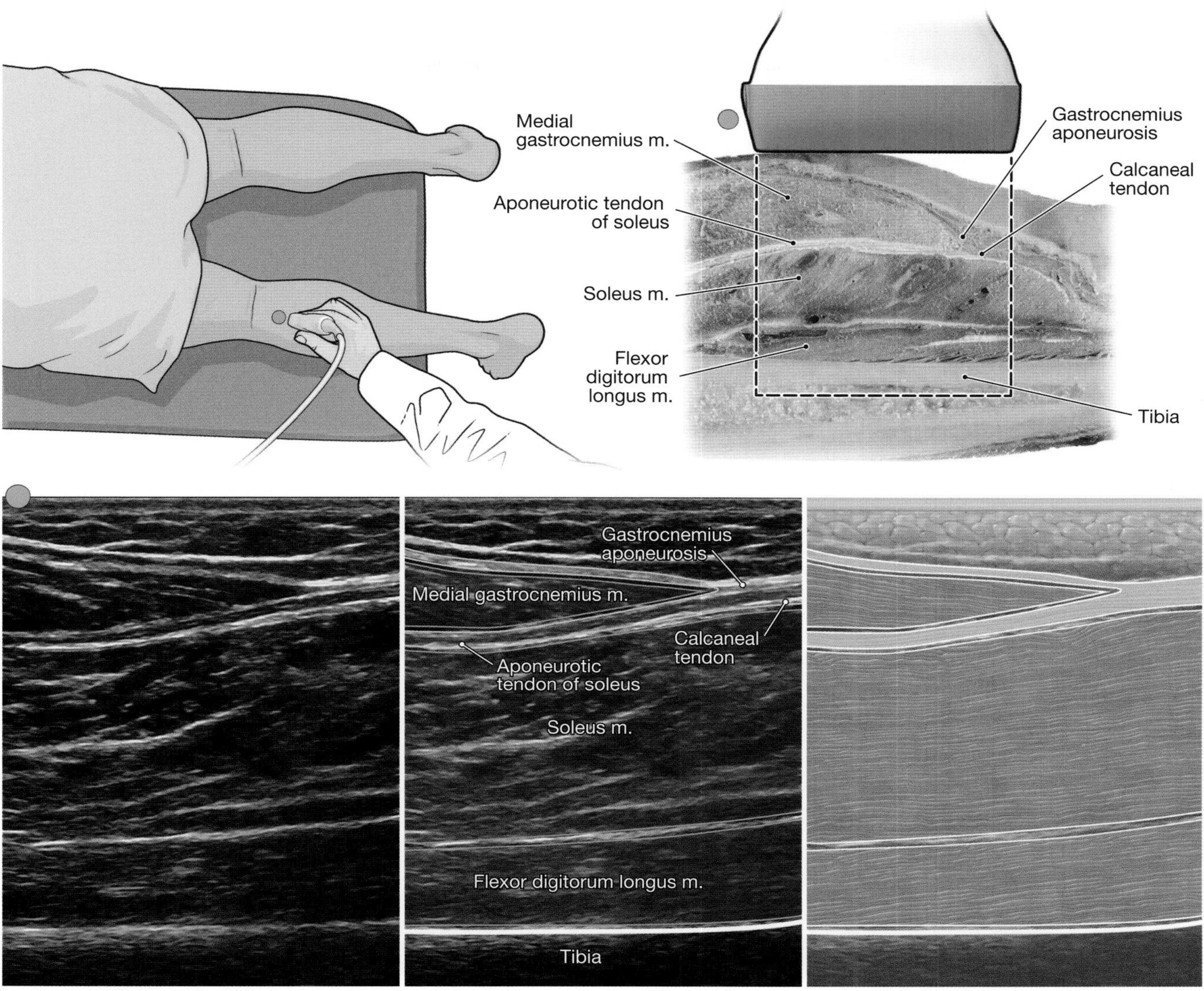

Figure 5.39 Longitudinal (parasagittal) view of the medial aspect of the posterior compartment at the midleg.

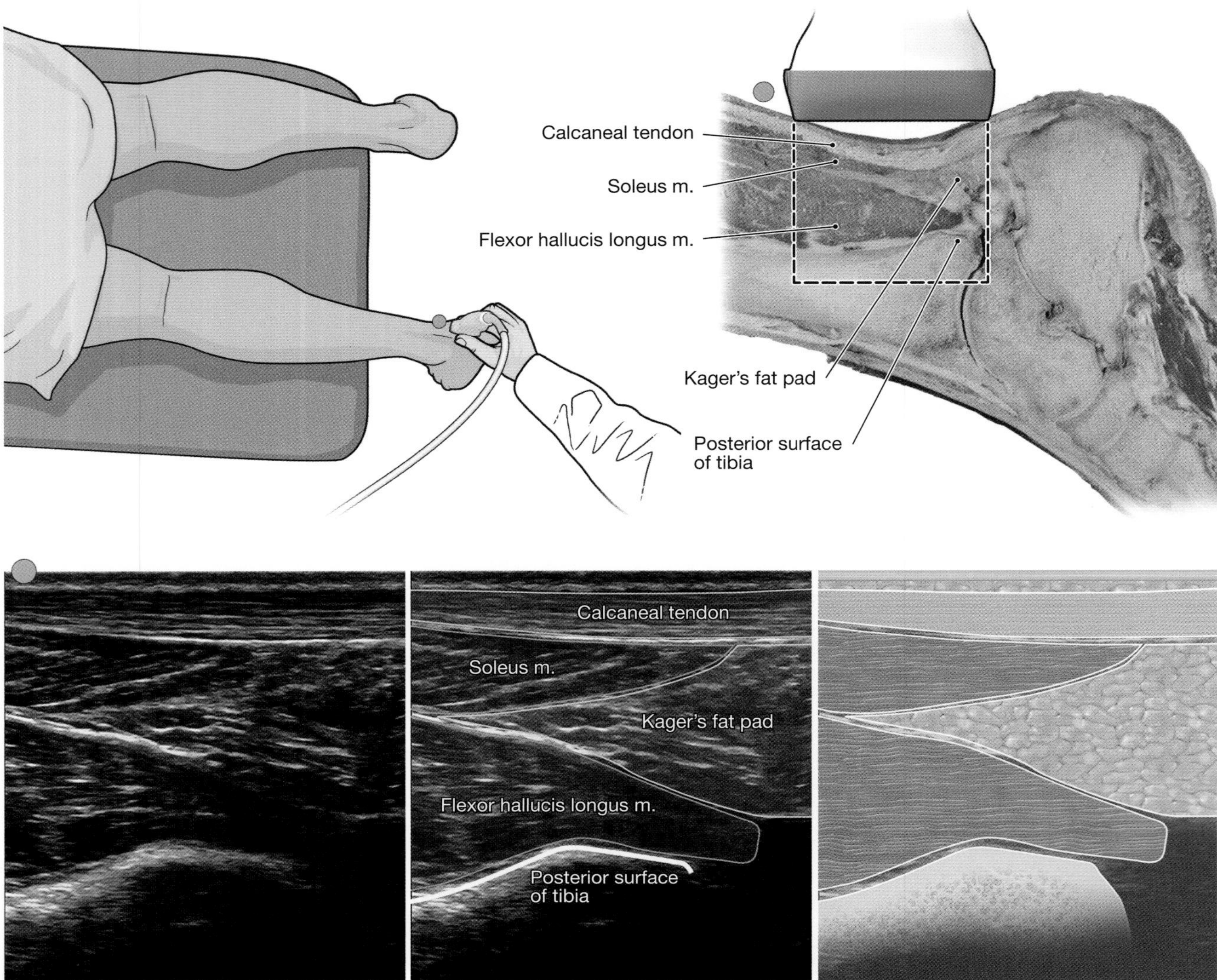

Figure 5.40 Longitudinal view of the posterior compartment in the distal leg, including the calcaneal tendon, the distal end of soleus, and Kager fat pad.

Ankle and Foot

Review of the Anatomy

Bones

The bones of the foot include seven tarsal bones, five metatarsals, and three phalanges for each toe except the big toe, which has only two phalanges.

Tarsal Bones

Talus

The main part of the talus is referred to as the body. The trochlea of the talus, which articulates with the tibia and fibula to form the ankle joint, projects superiorly from the body. A small lateral process projects laterally from the body over the lateral surface of the calcaneus. The posterior process of the talus projects posteriorly from the body and has two rounded projections, the medial and lateral tubercles, with a groove between them for the tendon of flexor hallucis longus. A short neck projects anteriorly from the body to the rounded head at the anterior surface of the talus, which articulates with the navicular bone. The talus sits on top of and is supported by the calcaneus.

Calcaneus

The calcaneus is the largest of the tarsal bones. The superior surface of the calcaneus has three articular facets for the talus forming the subtalar joint. Part of the calcaneus projects behind the ankle joint to form the heel. The posterior surface is semicircular with a facet for insertion of the calcaneal tendon posteriorly and expands below to the calcaneal tuberosity at the plantar surface of the heel. At its anterior aspect, the calcaneal tuberosity has two projections separated by a shallow groove, the medial and lateral processes. The plantar aponeurosis attaches to the larger medial process and the intervening groove.

A thick bony shelf, the sustentaculum tali, projects medially from the upper anterior part of the calcaneus. Its superior surface supports and articulates with the talus at the junction of the head and neck, and there is a groove for the tendon of the flexor hallucis longus along its undersurface.

The tendons of fibularis longus and brevis course across the lateral surface of the calcaneus and are separated by a small projection, the fibular trochlea, as they pass through separate compartments of the inferior fibular retinaculum.

The anterior surface of the calcaneus articulates with the cuboid bone.

Other Tarsal Bones

The navicular bone articulates posteriorly with the head of the talus and anteriorly with the medial, intermediate, and lateral cuneiform bones, which articulate anteriorly with the bases of the metatarsal bones I, II, and III, respectively. The cuboid bone articulates posteriorly with calcaneus, medially with the medial cuneiform bone, and anteriorly with the bases of metatarsals IV and V. There is a groove along the plantar surface of the cuboid bone for the tendon of fibularis longus.

Metatarsals

The metatarsal bones, numbered I through V from medial to lateral, have bases proximally and heads distally, joined by their bodies. The metatarsal heads articulate with the medial, intermediate, and lateral cuneiform bones (I, II, and III, respectively), and with the cuboid bone (IV and V), as well as with one another. There is a prominent posterolateral projection, the tubercle, from the base of the metatarsal V, which serves as a site of attachment for the tendon of fibularis brevis. The heads of the metatarsals articulate with the proximal phalanges of the toes.

Ankle Joint

The ankle joint is formed between the distal ends of the leg bones, the tibia and fibula, and the talus. The expanded distal end of the tibia forms the superior and medial (medial malleolus) surfaces of the bony arch of the ankle joint, often clinically referred to as the ankle *mortise*. The lateral malleolus of the fibula forms the lateral surface of the ankle joint arch or mortise. The cylindrical trochlea of the talus projects superiorly from the body of the talus into the arch formed by the tibia and fibula. A synovial membrane attached along the margins of the articular surfaces of the tibia, fibula, and trochlea of the talus lines the joint. The synovial membrane is in turn covered by a fibrous capsule with similar bony attachments. The ankle joint is stabilized by medial and lateral collateral ligament complexes, which also reinforce the joint capsule medially and laterally. The capsule is lax anteriorly and posteriorly (the anterior and posterior recesses) where it is not reinforced by ligaments.

A number of tendons cross the ankle joint to reach their attachments in the foot. The tendons of tibialis posterior, flexor digitorum longus, and flexor hallucis longus cross the ankle joint posteromedially through the tarsal tunnel. The calcaneal tendon crosses the joint posteriorly. The tendons of fibularis longus and brevis cross the ankle joint posterolaterally along the posterior surface of the lateral malleolus. The tendons of tibialis anterior, extensor hallucis longus, and extensor digitorum longus cross the joint anteriorly.

Ligaments

Tibiofibular Ligaments

The tibia and fibula are joined by the tibiofibular interosseous membrane. Reinforcing the interosseous membrane just above the ankle joint, the distal tibia and fibula are joined by anterior and posterior tibiofibular ligaments.

Fibular Collateral Ligament Complex

The anterior talofibular, posterior talofibular, and calcaneofibular ligaments are the 3 components of the fibular collateral ligament of the ankle. The lateral ligaments of the ankle are not as strong as the medial (tibial) ligaments. The anterior talofibular ligament, the weakest and most commonly injured of the lateral ligaments, spans between the anterior edge of the lateral malleolus and the dorsal aspect of the neck of the talus. The posterior talofibular ligament spans between the posterior nonarticular part of the medial surface of the lateral malleolus and the lateral tubercle of the posterior process of the talus. The calcaneofibular ligament attaches between the tip of the lateral malleolus and a small tubercle on the posterolateral surface of the calcaneus just behind the ankle joint. The tendons of fibularis brevis and longus cross over the ligament as they turn anteriorly from the posterior surface of the lateral malleolus.

Tibial Collateral Ligament Complex (Deltoid Ligament)

Collectively referred to as the **deltoid ligament**, the medial ligament complex of the ankle has four named parts: the anterior tibiotalar ligament, the tibionavicular ligament, the tibiocalcaneal ligament, and the posterior tibiotalar ligament. The components of the deltoid ligament are larger and stronger than the lateral ankle ligaments.

The tibionavicular ligament attaches between the anterior inferior surface of the medial malleolus to the medial surface of the navicular bone and the superior/medial margin of the plantar calcaneonavicular (spring) ligament just behind the navicular. The anterior tibiotalar ligament, deep to the tibionavicular ligament, attaches between the anterior inferior edge of the medial malleolus and the medial surface of the talus from the head to the body. The tibiocalcaneal ligament, nearly vertical, spans between the inferior edge of the medial malleolus and the sustentaculum tali of the calcaneus. The posterior tibiotalar ligament attaches between the posterior inferior edge of the medial malleolus and the medial surface of the talus from the medial tubercle of the posterior process to the body. Most of the superficial surface of the deltoid ligament is crossed by the tendons of tibialis posterior and flexor digitorum longus in their course through and just beyond the tarsal tunnel.

Tendons, Nerves, and Arteries Crossing the Ankle

Anterior Compartment of the Leg

The anterior compartment muscles, innervated by the deep fibular nerve, are tibialis anterior, extensor hallucis longus, extensor digitorum longus, and fibularis tertius. Their tendons cross the anterior aspect of the ankle joint deep to superior and inferior extensor retinacula onto the dorsum of the foot. The deep fibular nerve and anterior tibial vessels descend through the anterior compartment to cross the ankle joint anteriorly along with the tendons of the anterior compartment muscles.

Anterior Compartment Tendons

Tibialis anterior becomes tendinous in the distal third of the leg, crosses the ankle joint as the most medial of the anterior compartment tendons, and turns under the medial side of the foot to insert at the base of the first metatarsal and adjacent plantar surface of the medial cuneiform bone.

The extensor hallucis longus is covered at its origin by tibialis anterior medially and by the extensor digitorum longus laterally. Its tendon emerges between the two in the distal third of the leg to cross the ankle joint between their tendons, continuing across the dorsum of the foot to insert onto the dorsal surface of the base of the distal phalanx of the great toe.

The tendon of extensor digitorum longus forms in the distal leg and crosses the ankle joint lateral to the tendon of extensor hallucis longus. On the dorsum of the foot, the tendon divides into four slips that insert into the extensor expansions of the lateral toes.

Dorsalis Pedis Artery

The dorsalis pedis artery (usually the continuation of the anterior tibial artery beyond the ankle joint) crosses the ankle just lateral to the tendon of extensor hallucis longus and continues alongside the tendon onto the dorsum of the foot, where it has dorsal metatarsal branches and a deep plantar branch, which anastomoses with the deep plantar arterial arch.

Deep Fibular Nerve

The deep fibular nerve is lateral to the anterior tibial artery as it crosses the ankle onto the dorsum of the foot. Just after crossing the ankle, it gives out a motor branch to the extensor digitorum brevis and continues distally, becoming cutaneous in the web space between the great and second toes.

Lateral Compartment of the Leg

The two lateral compartment muscles, fibularis longus and brevis, are innervated by the superficial fibular nerve. Their tendons cross the ankle joint along the posterior surface of the lateral malleolus.

Lateral Compartment Tendons

The fibularis longus becomes tendinous about the midleg and descends along the superficial surface of fibularis brevis and more distally along the posterior surface of the distal fibula and lateral malleolus, where it is immediately lateral to the tendon of fibularis brevis. The fibularis brevis becomes tendinous as it descends along the posterior surface of the distal fibula and lateral malleolus.

At the posterior edge of the tip of the lateral malleolus, both tendons cross under the small superior fibular retinaculum and then over the calcaneofibular ligament as they begin to turn anteriorly across the lateral surface of the calcaneus. A short distance anteriorly, they cross through separate compartments of the small inferior fibular retinaculum where they are separated by the fibular trochlea of calcaneus. The tendon of fibularis brevis lies above the trochlea and the tendon of fibularis longus lies below it.

Beyond the fibular trochlea, the tendon of fibularis brevis continues anteriorly along the lateral surface of the calcaneus and the lateral surface of the cuboid bone to insert at the tubercle of the base of the fifth metacarpal.

The tendon of fibularis longus continues anteriorly across the lateral surface of the calcaneus, curving deeply at the anterior aspect of the calcaneus to approach the cuboid bone where it enters a groove along its plantar surface. The tendon turns medially in the groove and courses obliquely across the plantar foot to attach at the base of the first metatarsal and adjacent medial cuneiform bone. A sesamoid bone may be present adjacent to the base of the fifth metatarsal, where the tendon turns into the groove in the cuboid bone.

Superficial Fibular Nerve

The superficial fibular nerve descends in the lateral compartment, which it supplies, deep to the fibularis longus and then emerges between the fibularis brevis and extensor digitorum longus in the distal third of the leg. It pierces the deep fascia a variable distance above the lateral malleolus and divides into its terminal branches, the medial and intermediate dorsal cutaneous nerves. The medial dorsal cutaneous branch supplies the medial aspect of the dorsum of the foot and proximal part of the great toe. The intermediate dorsal cutaneous nerve supplies most of the remainder of the dorsum of the foot and proximal parts of the second through fifth toes.

Posterior Compartment of the Leg

The posterior compartment muscles, innervated by the tibial nerve, are arranged in the superficial and deep layers.

Superficial Layer

The muscles of the superficial group include the medial and lateral heads of gastrocnemius, soleus, and the small plantaris muscle. The two heads of gastrocnemius converge at the inferior extent of the popliteal fossa and taper to a broad flattened tendinous band (gastrocnemius aponeurosis) about the midleg. Tendinous fibers begin to appear along the central posterior part of the soleus muscle in the midcalf. The tendon of soleus fuses with the overlying tendon of gastrocnemius to complete the formation of the calcaneal tendon in the distal third of the leg.

The calcaneal tendon continues distally, superficial to Kager fat pad, to insert onto the midportion of the posterior surface of the calcaneus.

Kager Fat Pad and Subtendinous Calcaneal (Retrocalcaneal) Bursa

Kager fat pad is located in the distal leg and posterior to the ankle joint. The fat pad is triangular shaped, with the base formed by the superior cortical surface of the calcaneus, the anterior border formed by the flexor hallucis longus muscle and tendon, and the posterior border formed by the anterior (deep) surface of the calcaneal tendon. The apex of the triangle extends superiorly between the distal fibers of soleus and the muscles of the deep group. The subtendinous calcaneal (retrocalcaneal) bursa, which intervenes between the upper posterior surface of calcaneus and the calcaneal tendon, is located at the posterior inferior corner of the triangle. The bursa may not be seen unless it is inflamed.

Deep Layer

The muscles of the deep group include the popliteus, tibialis posterior, flexor digitorum longus, and flexor hallucis longus. The popliteus is a short muscle related to the knee joint discussed earlier along with structures of the knee. The tendons tibialis posterior, flexor digitorum longus, and flexor hallucis longus cross the medial side of the ankle joint through the tarsal tunnel to enter the plantar aspect of the foot.

Tarsal Tunnel

The tarsal tunnel is a fibro-osseous tunnel consisting of a shallow depression along the posterior surface of the medial malleolus, the medial surface of the posterior process and body of the talus, and the medial surface of calcaneus, spanned by the flexor retinaculum. The flexor retinaculum is a band of fibrous connective tissue attached anteriorly along the inferior margin of the medial malleolus and posteriorly to the medial surface of the calcaneus. Fibrous septae from the deep surface of the retinaculum form separate compartments within the tarsal tunnel for the tendons of the deep posterior compartment muscles and for the neurovascular bundle consisting of the posterior tibial vessels and the tibial nerve.

In the distal leg, the tendon of flexor digitorum longus crosses the tendon of tibialis posterior superficially from anterior to posterior, so that in the tarsal tunnel, the tibialis posterior tendon lies along the posterior surface of the medial malleolus immediately anterior to the flexor digitorum longus tendon. The tendon of the flexor hallucis longus enters the tarsal tunnel in a groove between the medial and lateral tubercles of the posterior process of the talus and thus separated from the tendons of tibialis posterior and flexor digitorum longus. Beyond the groove in the posterior process of the talus, the flexor hallucis longus tendon enters a groove along the inferior surface of the sustentaculum tali of calcaneus. The neurovascular bundle is located in the space between the tendon of flexor digitorum longus anteriorly and the tendon of flexor hallucis longus posteriorly. The vessels, the posterior tibial artery and two or three accompanying veins are just behind the tendon of flexor digitorum longus with the tibial nerve just posterior to the vessels. Within the tunnel, the neurovascular bundle is slightly anterior and superficial (medial) to the tendon of flexor hallucis longus.

Tendons and Insertions

All three tendons turn anteriorly in the tunnel, exiting the tunnel deep to the abductor hallucis muscle and curving under the medial aspect of the foot to reach their attachments. The tendon of tibialis posterior fans out to attach to the plantar surfaces of the navicular bone and adjacent cuneiform bones along the medial aspect of the foot. The tendon of flexor hallucis longus continues distally, inserting at the plantar surface of the base of the distal phalanx of the great toe. The tendon of flexor digitorum longus crosses under (inferior or superficial to) the flexor hallucis longus tendon and divides into four slips that insert onto the plantar surfaces of the bases of the distal phalanges of the lateral toes.

Posterior Tibial Artery

In the distal part of the tarsal tunnel, or just after exiting the tunnel, the posterior tibial artery and its accompanying veins divide into three branches: medial calcaneal, lateral plantar, and medial plantar. The lateral plantar artery crosses to the lateral side of the foot deep to the flexor digitorum brevis, a superficial intrinsic muscle of the foot, and then curves medially to form the deep plantar arterial arch. The medial plantar artery continues distally along the medial aspect of the foot.

Tibial Nerve

The tibial nerve has a similar course and branching pattern as the posterior tibial artery. A medial calcaneal branch accompanies the similarly named artery onto the plantar surface of the posterior part of the calcaneus, and lateral medial and plantar nerves accompany the similarly named arteries. The large lateral plantar nerve provides cutaneous supply to most of the plantar aspect of the foot and lateral 3½ toes and motor supply to most of the intrinsic muscles of the foot. The smaller medial plantar nerve provides cutaneous innervation to the medial aspect of the plantar foot and medial 1½ toes and motor innervation to 4 intrinsic muscles of the foot not supplied by the lateral plantar nerve.

Plantar Aponeurosis

The plantar aponeurosis is a distinct thickened band of deep fascia that attaches posteriorly to the periosteum of the medial process of the calcaneal tubercle and extends anteriorly along the central part of the sole of the foot, over the superficial surface of the flexor digitorum brevis muscle. At about midfoot, the aponeurosis begins to expand medially and laterally, dividing into separate bands for each of the toes, which attach to the metatarsophalangeal joint capsules and associated ligaments.

Technique

Anterior Aspect of the Ankle Joint

Anterior Compartment Tendons

ANTERIOR COMPARTMENT TENDONS ANKLE JOINT
Transverse
FIG. 5.41

The patient should be supine with the knee flexed to 90° and the sole of the foot resting on the examination table. Place the probe transversely over the distal part of the anterior compartment a few centimeters above the medial and lateral malleoli. In the distal leg, the muscles of the anterior compartment become progressively smaller as their tendinous components enlarge and become more evident. Tilt/toggle the probe face to identify the hyperechoic tendons (and the remaining muscle tissue) of tibialis anterior, extensor hallucis longus, and extensor digitorum longus.

Slide the probe distally, keeping the tendons in view, to a position between the medial and lateral malleoli. Look for the shallow concave hyperechoic surface of the trochlea of the talus covered by an anechoic layer of hyaline cartilage, occupying most or the entire deep part of the image. The joint capsule and synovial lining of the anterior recess of the ankle joint can be seen superficial to the trochlea of the talus. Superficial to the joint capsule, identify the tibialis anterior tendon at the medial aspect of the image, toggling the probe face as needed to minimize anisotropy. A short distance lateral to the tibialis anterior tendon, identify the tendon/myotendinous junction of the extensor hallucis longus. Lateral to the extensor hallucis longus, identify the tendon/myotendinous junction of the extensor digitorum longus. Deep to the lateral edge of the extensor hallucis longus (toggling the probe face as needed), identify the deep fibular nerve and the anterior tibial artery.

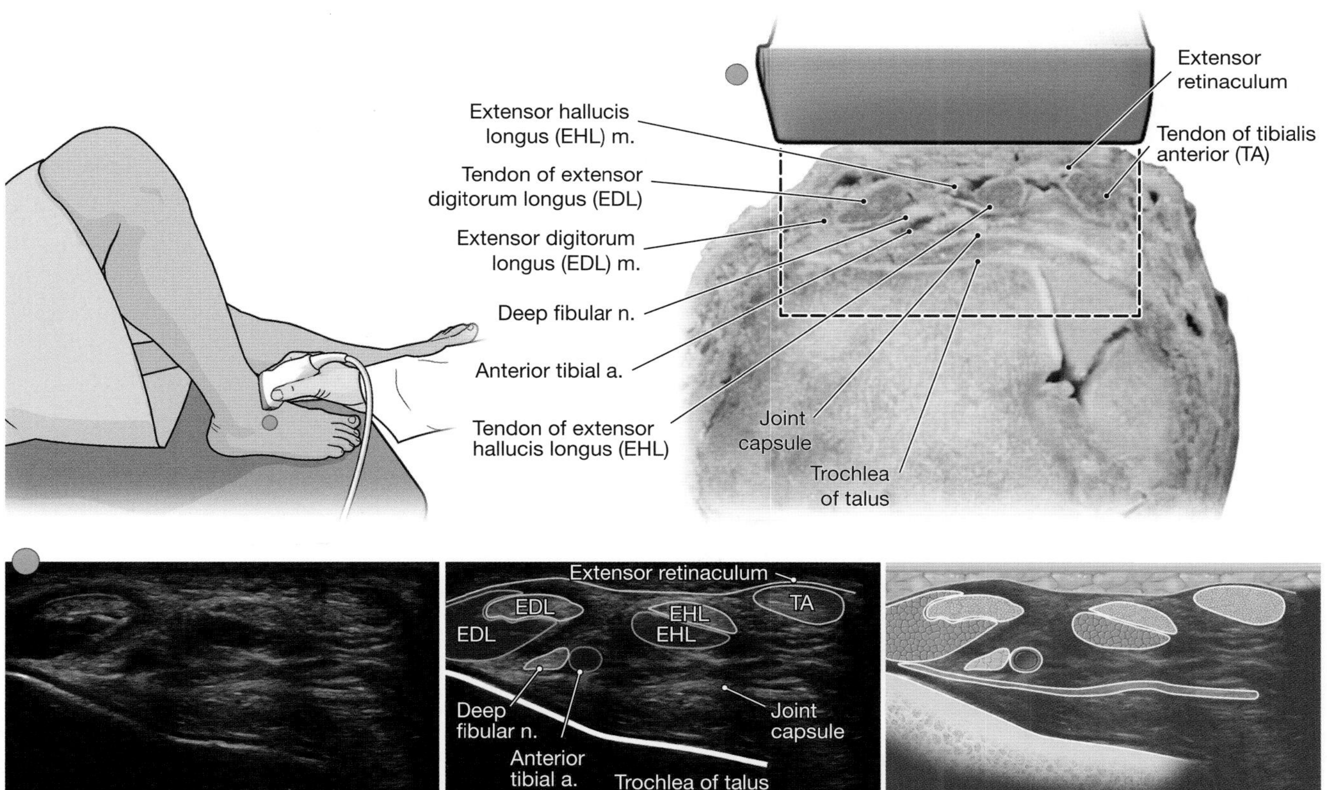

Figure 5.41 Transverse view of the anterior compartment tendons crossing the ankle joint, along with the deep fibular nerve and anterior tibial artery.

Anterior Tibiofibular Ligament

ANTERIOR TIBIOFIBULAR LIGAMENT
Longitudinal
FIG. 5.42

The patient should be supine with the knee flexed to 90° and the sole of the foot should rest on the examination table. Place the probe transversely over the anterolateral aspect of the leg, with the marker side of the probe over the anterior edge of the lateral malleolus about 1 cm above the tip of the malleolus. Identify the hyperechoic surface and the acoustic shadow of the lateral malleolus. Keeping the marker side of the probe anchored in position, rotate the heel (nonmarker side) of the probe superiorly so that it comes to lie about 2 cm higher on the leg than the marker side. This brings the probe face approximately parallel to the longitudinal axis of the anterior tibiofibular ligament. Look for the bony profile of the distal tibia and the distal tibiofibular joint to be visible. Adjust the probe position and tilt to identify the fibrillar appearance of the anterior tibiofibular ligament as it spans the tibiofibular joint between the anterior surfaces of the lateral malleolus and lateral aspect of the distal tibia. Internal rotation of the foot places tension on the ligament.

Anterior Talofibular Ligament

ANTERIOR TALOFIBULAR LIGAMENT
Longitudinal
FIG. 5.43

The patient should be supine with the knee flexed to 90° and the sole of the foot resting on the examination table. Alternatively, the patient can be positioned in lateral decubitus with the knee slightly flexed and a small bolster placed under the medial side of the ankle to allow the examiner to passively plantarflex and invert the foot, placing tension on the ligament. Starting with the probe in the position described earlier to image the anterior tibiofibular ligament, slide the probe slightly inferiorly so that the marker side of the probe is over the anterior surface of the tip of the lateral malleolus and rotate the heel of the probe downward approximately 90° across the anterior aspect of the ankle joint (the anterior tibiofibular and anterior talofibular ligaments are nearly at right angles to one another). During the rotation, the probe sweeps across the articular surface of the trochlea of the talus and onto the neck of the talus. Adjust the probe position and tilt until you can identify the hyperechoic fibrillar appearance of the anterior talofibular ligament spanning between the anterior edge of the tip of the lateral malleolus and the neck of the talus.

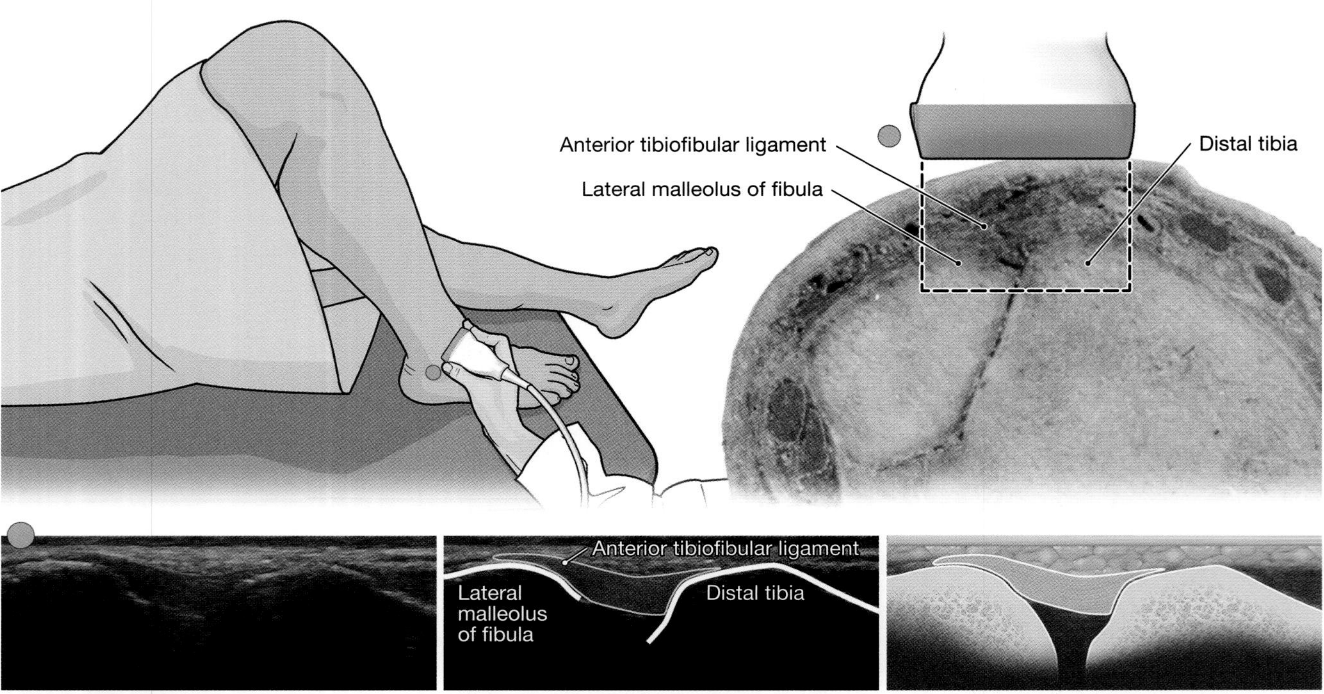

Figure 5.42 Longitudinal view of the anterior tibiofibular ligament.

Lateral Aspect of the Ankle Joint

Tendons of Fibularis Longus and Brevis

FIBULARIS LONGUS TENDON FIBULARIS BREVIS TENDON LATERAL MALLEOLUS
Transverse
FIG. 5.44

The patient should be in lateral decubitus position with a small pillow or bolster between the slightly flexed knees. Place the probe face transverse to the long axis of the leg with the marker side of the probe at the posterolateral aspect of the superior part of the lateral malleolus. Adjust the probe position and tilt/fan the probe face, minimizing anisotropy, to identify the tendon of fibularis longus. Immediately posteromedial to the fibularis longus tendon, the tendon of fibularis brevis is incompletely formed at this level and more difficult to identify definitively. A small ovoid component of the fibularis brevis muscle is seen along the posterior aspect of the forming tendon. Keeping the lateral malleolus and fibularis tendons in view, slide the probe posteriorly as needed, while minimizing the probe face pressure, to locate the small saphenous vein in the superficial fascia a short distance behind the lateral malleolus.

Calcaneofibular Ligament

CALCANEOFIBULAR LIGAMENT
Longitudinal
FIG. 5.45

With the patient in the lateral decubitus position as described earlier, dorsiflex the foot to place tension on the calcaneofibular ligament and to bring it into alignment with the long axis of the fibula. Place the marker side of the probe at the tip of the lateral malleolus with the heel of the probe positioned slightly posteriorly, bringing the probe face into alignment with the longitudinal axis of the calcaneofibular ligament. Adjust the probe position and tilt to identify the tendons of fibularis longus and brevis, and immediately deep to the tendons, the hyperechoic fibrillar calcaneofibular ligament spanning from the medial surface of the lateral malleolus (hidden in its acoustic shadow) to the lateral surface of the posterior part of the calcaneus a short distance below the tip of the malleolus.

Fibularis Brevis Tendon

FIBULARIS BREVIS TENDON INSERTION
Longitudinal
FIG. 5.46

The patient should be in the lateral decubitus position with a small pillow or bolster between the slightly flexed knees. Locate

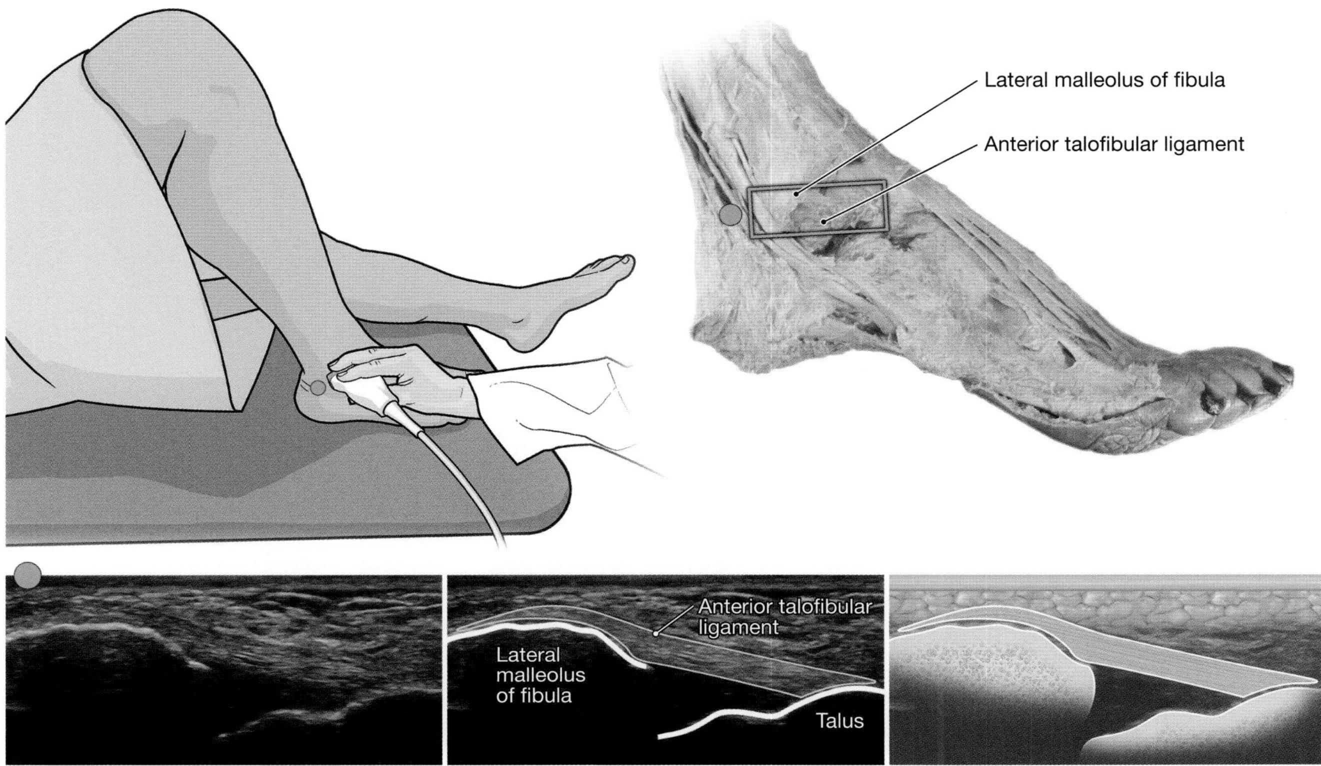

Figure 5.43 Longitudinal view of the anterior talofibular ligament.

the tubercle of the base of the fifth metatarsal by palpation. Ask the patient to evert the foot. The tendon of fibularis brevis is usually visible from just below and anterior to the tip of the lateral malleolus to its insertion at the tubercle of the fifth metatarsal base. With the muscles around the ankle relaxed again, position the probe along the longitudinal axis of the tendon with the marker side directed toward the anterior aspect of the tip of the lateral malleolus and the heel over the posterior aspect of the tubercle of the fifth metatarsal base. Identify the rounded hyperechoic surface and the acoustic shadow of the tubercle. Adjust the probe position until the hyperechoic fibrillar appearance of the fibularis brevis tendon can be seen along with its insertion onto the tubercle. Proximal to its insertion, the tendon passes over the anterior part of the lateral surface of the calcaneus and the lateral surface of the cuboid bone.

Fibularis Longus Tendon

FIBULARIS LONGUS TENDON CALCANEUS
Longitudinal
FIG. 5.47

With the patient in lateral decubitus position as described earlier, position the probe along a line interconnecting the tip of the lateral malleolus and a point about 1 cm posterior to the tubercle of the base of the fifth metatarsal. Adjust the probe position until the hyperechoic fibrillar appearance of the fibularis longus tendon can be identified. Identify the lateral surface of calcaneus deep to the tendon. As needed, slide the probe distally along the tendon until it can be seen curving toward the plantar surface of the foot along the anterior part of the calcaneus approaching the cuboid bone (the fibrillar appearance of the tendon disappears because of anisotropy).

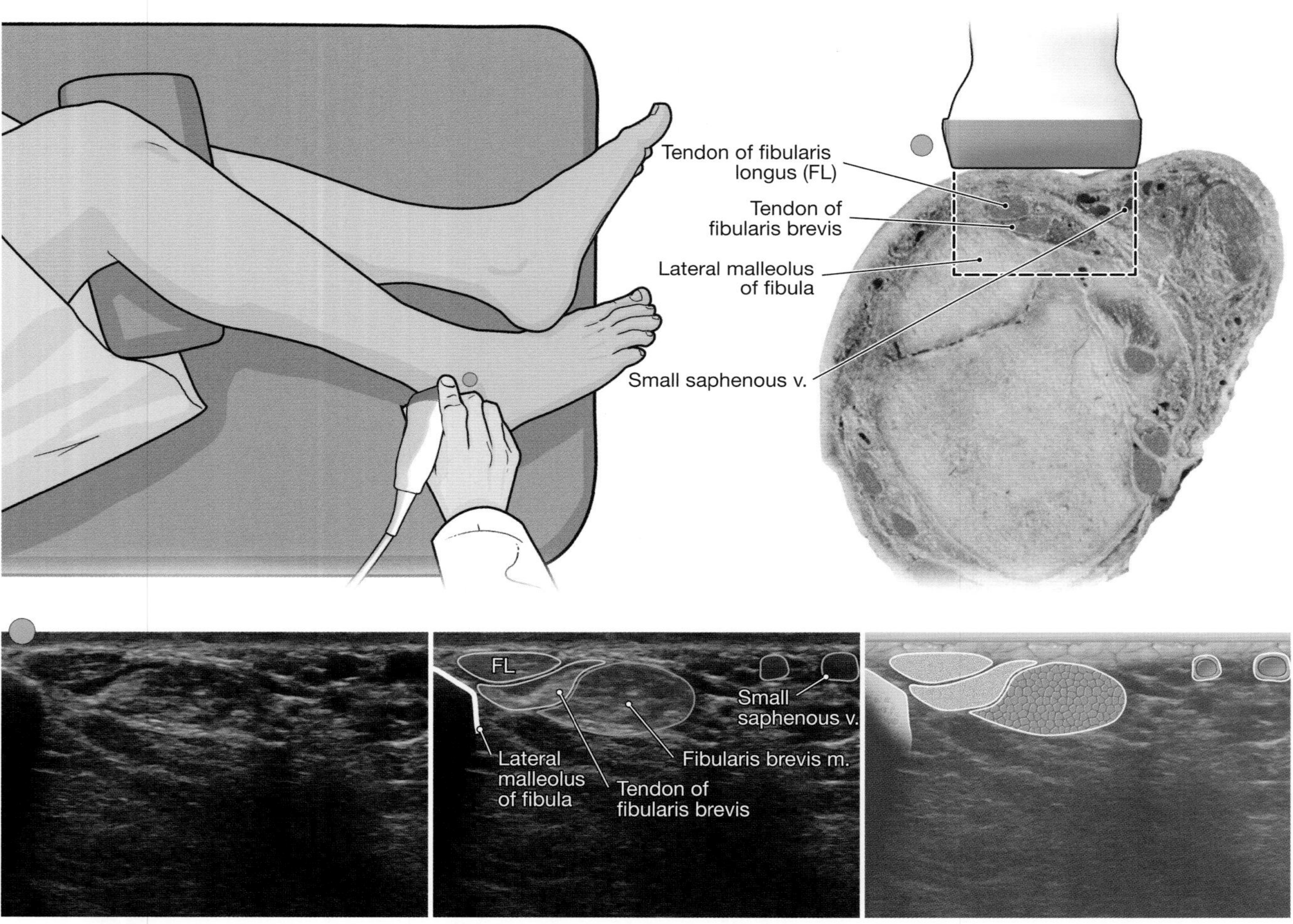

Figure 5.44 Transverse view of the tendon of fibularis longus and the tendon/myotendinous junction of fibularis brevis at the posterior aspect of the distal fibula/lateral malleolus.

Medial Aspect of the Ankle Joint

Tarsal Tunnel and Contents

TARSAL TUNNEL
MEDIAL MALLEOLUS
Transverse
FIG. 5.48

The patient should be supine with the knee slightly flexed and the thigh externally rotated ("frog-leg" position). A small pillow or bolster should be placed under the lateral aspect of the ankle to allow for eversion of the foot, to minimize the concavity of the tarsal tunnel. Place the marker side of the probe along the inferior edge of the medial malleolus with the probe face angled toward the heel. Adjust the probe position and tilt to identify the tendon of tibialis posterior along the medial malleolus. Immediately posterior (and slightly deep/medial) to the tibialis posterior tendon, identify the tendon of flexor digitorum longus (adjusting the probe position slightly and fanning/tilting the probe face as needed to minimize anisotropy). Keeping the tendons of tibialis posterior and flexor digitorum longus in view, adjust the probe position and tilt until the tendon of flexor hallucis longus can be identified in a groove along the posterior process of the talus. Owing to anisotropy, the flexor hallucis longus tendon can be somewhat difficult to identify. Locating the rounded profile of the medial tubercle of the posterior process of the talus is often helpful in identifying the position of the flexor hallucis longus tendon. Immediately deep to the hyperechoic flexor retinaculum, the posterior tibial vessels and tibial nerve are seen posterior to the tendon of flexor digitorum longus.

Tibiocalcaneal Ligament

TIBIOCALCANEAL LIGAMENT
Longitudinal
FIG. 5.49

Starting from the tarsal tunnel view described earlier, rotate the heel (nonmarker side) of the probe anteriorly while keeping the tendon of flexor hallucis longus in view. The marker end of the probe should move slightly anteriorly while rotating the nonmarker end. Slowly rotate the probe until the tendon disappears under a prominent shelf of bone, the sustentaculum tali of calcaneus. Another bony prominence, the medial surface of the body of the

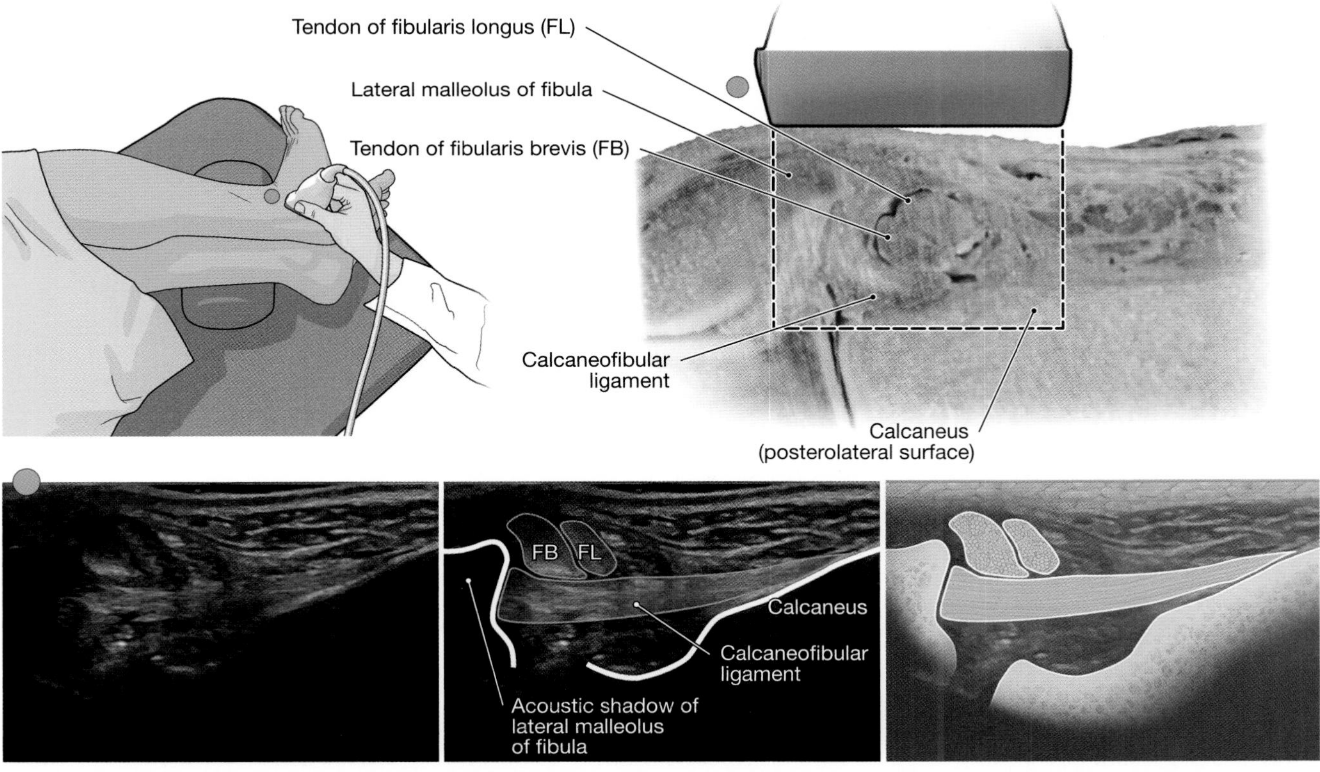

Figure 5.45 Longitudinal view of the calcaneofibular ligament. The tendons of fibularis longus and brevis cross over the ligament as they turn under the tip of the lateral malleolus.

talus, should come into view between the medial malleolus and the sustentaculum tali. These two medial bony prominences have a somewhat similar appearance, but observing the course of the tendon of flexor hallucis longus helps to identify the sustentaculum tali definitively. At this point, the probe should have a nearly vertical alignment along the long axis of the limb, with the nonmarker end of the probe directed slightly posteriorly. Identify the medial malleolus, the medial surface of the body of the talus, and the sustentaculum tali of the calcaneus. Adjust the probe position and tilt/fan the face to identify the tendon of tibialis posterior. The tendon profile is elongated in this position, as the tendon is oblique to the probe orientation. Owing to anisotropy, the tendon may appear hypoechoic. Attempt to identify the tendon of flexor digitorum longus (also oblique to the probe orientation) inferior to the tibialis posterior tendon and superficial to the medial edge of the sustentaculum tali. The tendons are seen in this position in the distal (anterior) end of the tarsal tunnel, where they are located between the flexor retinaculum superficially and the tibiocalcaneal ligament on their deep surfaces. Carefully adjust the probe position and tilt as needed, and passively evert the foot to place tension on the tibiocalcaneal ligament, so that its fibrillar appearance can be seen. The ligament spans between the medial surface and inferior margin of the medial malleolus to the superior surface of the sustentaculum tali.

Posterior Aspect of the Ankle Joint

CALCANEAL TENDON INSERTION
Longitudinal
FIG. 5.50

The patient should be prone with the ankles and feet over the end of the examination table. By palpation, locate the calcaneal tendon in the distal leg. Place the probe over the tendon in its longitudinal axis just above the heel (marker directed superiorly). Note the hyperechoic fibrillar appearance of the thick calcaneal tendon. With the probe face centered along the longitudinal axis of the calcaneal tendon, slide the probe distally until the tapered distal end of the tendon can be seen at its insertion onto the posterior surface of the calcaneus. Identify the hyperechoic posterior surface of the calcaneus and its

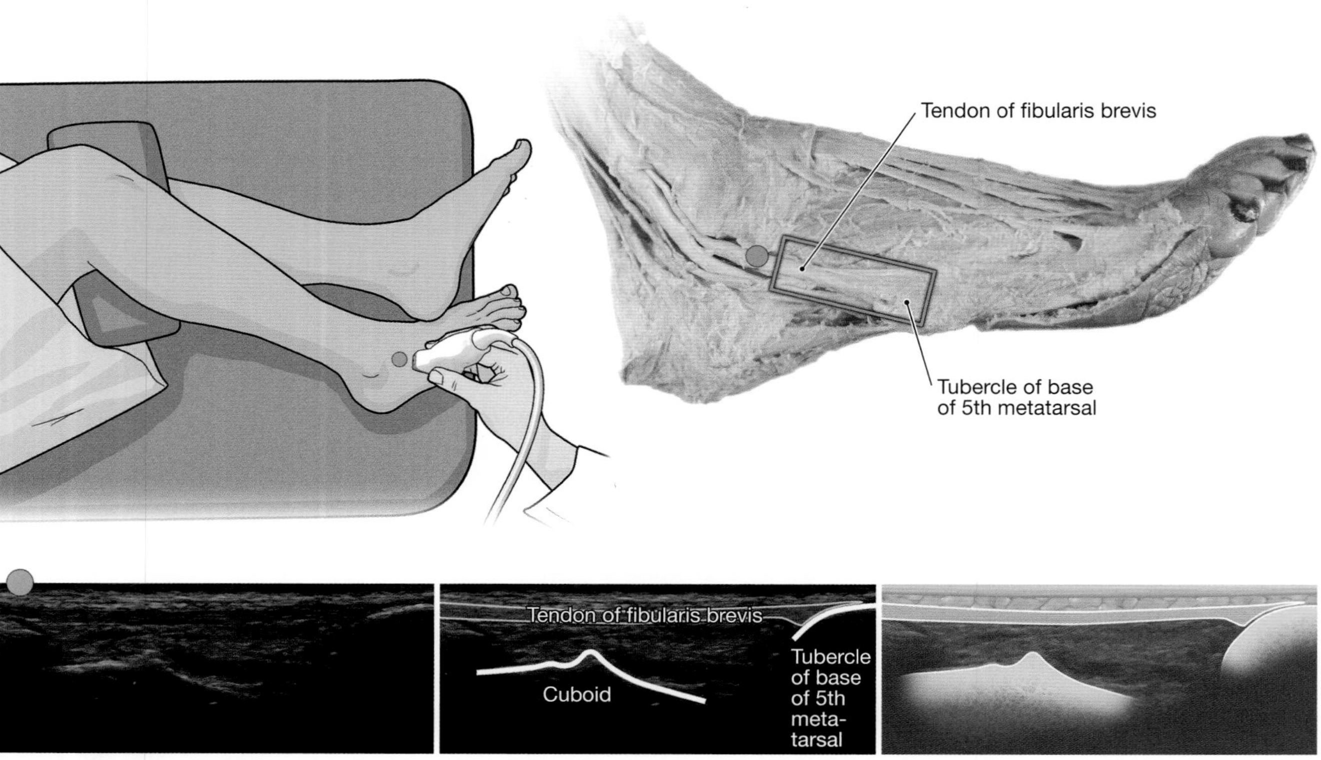

Figure 5.46 Longitudinal view of the tendon of fibularis brevis crossing over the cuboid bone to its insertion at the tubercle of the base of the fifth metatarsal.

dense acoustic shadow. Deep to the calcaneal tendon along the posterior superior margin of the calcaneus, the base of the triangular profile of Kager fat pad can be seen. The retrocalcaneal bursa is located between the calcaneal tendon and the upper posterior surface of the calcaneus, but may not be well-seen unless it is inflamed.

Plantar Aponeurosis

PLANTAR APONEUROSIS
Longitudinal
FIG. 5.51

The patient should be prone with the ankles and feet over the end of the examination table. Place the probe over the plantar surface of the heel, oriented along the long axis of the foot, with the marker side directed posteriorly. Identify the hyperechoic surface and the dense acoustic shadow of the calcaneal tuberosity. Slide the probe face medially and laterally to identify the medial process of the tuberosity. Tilt/fan the probe face until the fibrillar appearance of the thick (3-5 mm) plantar aponeurosis can be identified as it attaches to the periosteum over the medial process and then extends anteriorly along the superficial surface of the flexor digitorum brevis muscle. Because of the density of the overlying tissues, the image gain may need to be increased to image the aponeurosis and muscle adequately.

CLINICAL APPLICATION

US examination is useful for the evaluation of muscle and tendon injuries, including tendinosis/tendonitis and partial or complete tendon tears. Examples of ankle tendon injuries that are routinely examined using US include the calcaneal tendon and the fibularis longus and brevis tendons. Injuries of the ankle extensor tendons and deep posterior compartment tendons are less common, but they do occur and may be underdiagnosed.

Calcaneal tendon rupture tends to occur in older men during recreational activities, of, eg, "week-end warriors." The tendons of fibularis longus and/or brevis may subluxate owing to tearing of the superior fibular retinaculum in association with inversion ankle sprain injuries. This leads to snapping lateral ankle pain and may progress to tendinosis/tendonitis or fraying and partial or complete rupture of a fibularis tendon, most commonly fibularis brevis at the posterior surface of the lateral malleolus.

The medial and lateral ligaments of the ankle joint are stretched and partially or completely torn in inversion/eversion ankle sprains. The anterior talofibular ligament is the most commonly involved lateral ligament in inversion ankle injuries, followed by the calcaneofibular ligament. The medial (deltoid) ankle ligaments may be torn in association with injuries involving foot eversion or inversion with external rotation, but because of the strength of the medial (deltoid) ligaments, avulsion fractures of the medial malleolus are more common. Sometimes injury to the anterior tibiofibular ligament is referred to as high ankle sprain, and the ligament can be torn in association with a variety of ankle sprain injuries (and ankle fractures), especially those that involve forceful external rotation of the inverted or everted foot.

US examination is used in the diagnosis of Morton neuroma, an enlargement (perineural fibroma) of a common digital plantar nerve, usually in the space between the third and fourth metatarsal heads, leading to entrapment and pain or numbness. US examination and measurement may be used in the evaluation of entrapment or compression of the tibial nerve in its course through the tarsal tunnel.

US guidance can be used in ankle blocks (tibial nerve, sural nerve, saphenous nerve, superficial fibular nerve, and deep fibular nerve) for surgical procedures in the foot.

In the evaluation of peripheral artery disease, arteries that are included in Doppler US studies of the ankle and foot include the dorsalis pedis and posterior tibial arteries.

Plantar fasciitis is a painful condition related to overuse and repetitive stress of the plantar aponeurosis, resulting in tearing and disruption of the normal collagen fiber organization. US is useful for detecting localized changes in organization and thickness of the plantar aponeurosis, for detecting calcified areas, and in some cases, for guiding steroid injections.

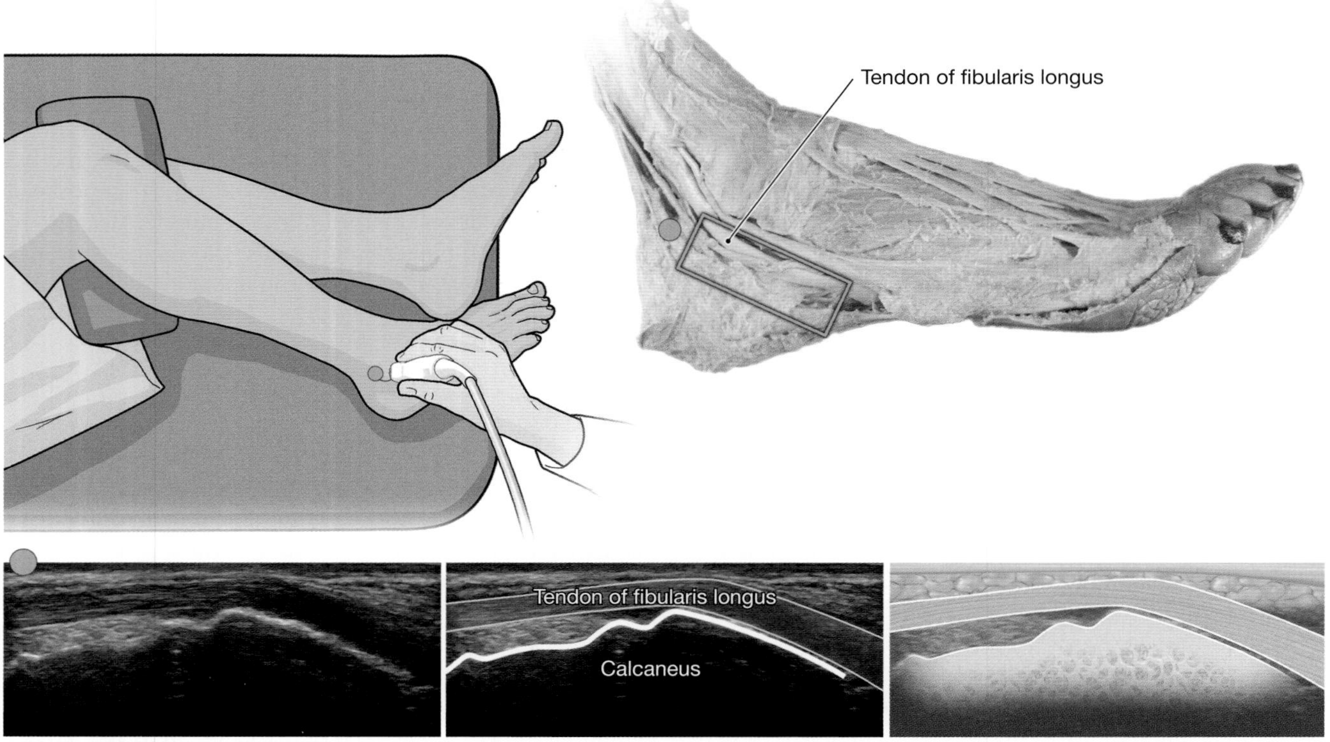

Figure 5.47 Longitudinal view of the tendon of fibularis longus crossing the lateral surface of calcaneus.

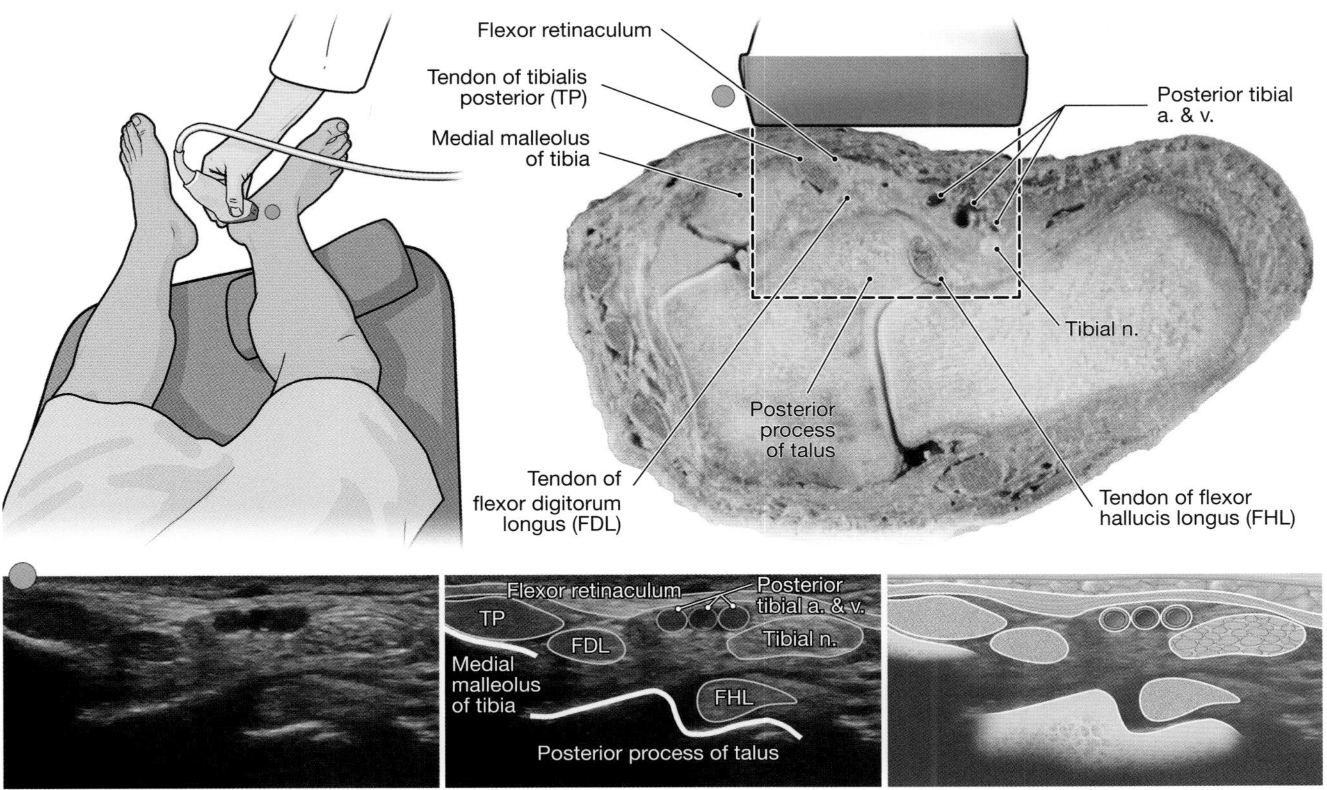

Figure 5.48 Transverse view of the contents of the tarsal tunnel.

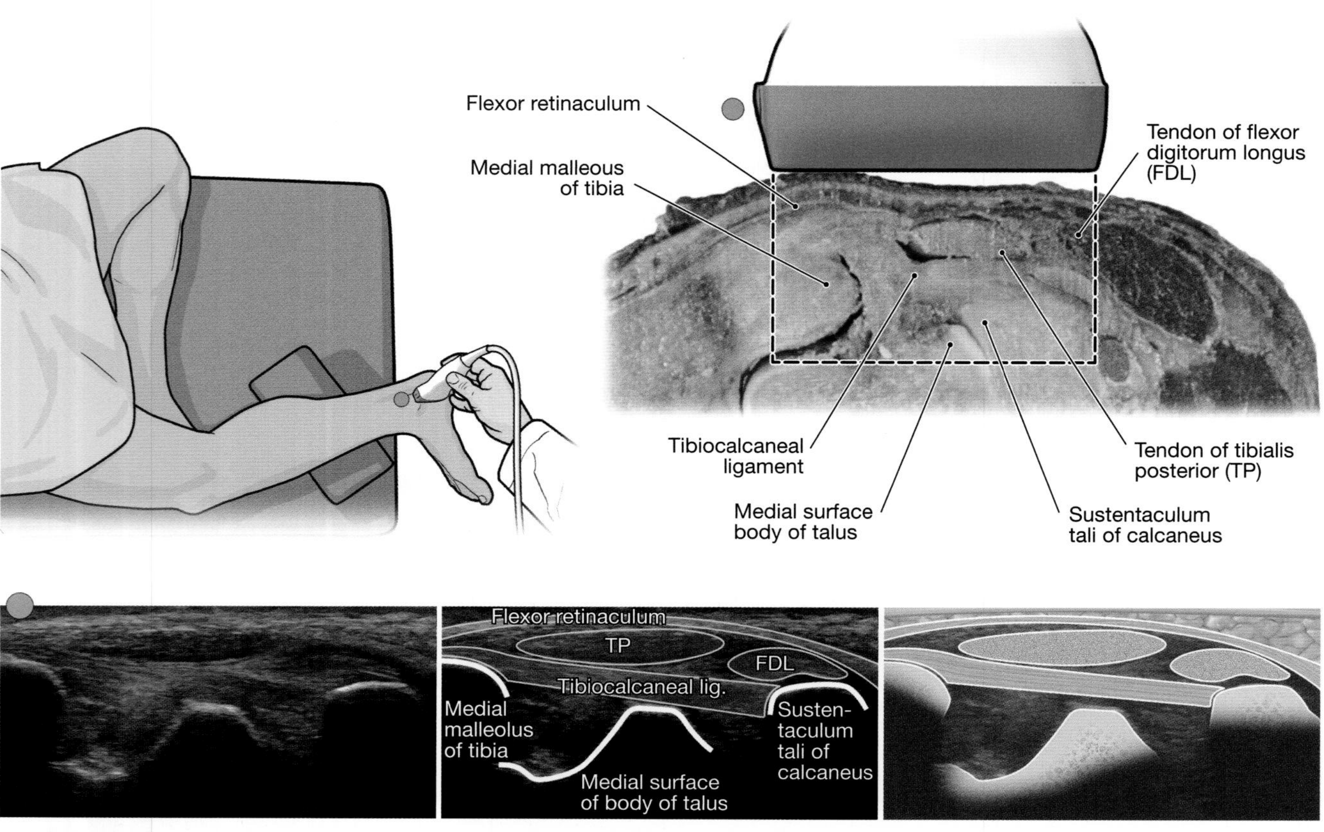

Figure 5.49 Longitudinal view of the tibiocalcaneal ligament (of the deltoid ligament complex) in the floor of the tarsal tunnel.

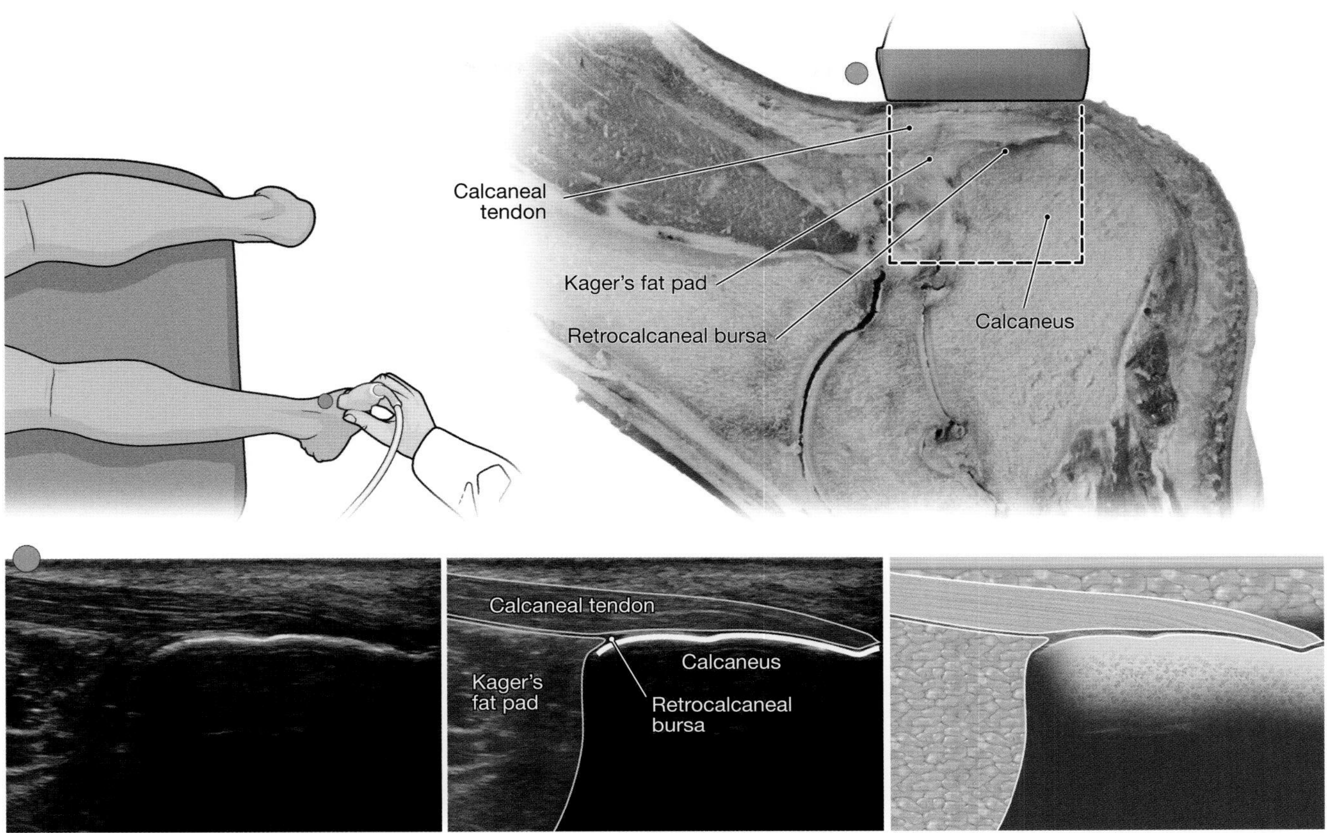

Figure 5.50 Longitudinal view of the calcaneal tendon at its insertion onto the posterior surface of the calcaneus.

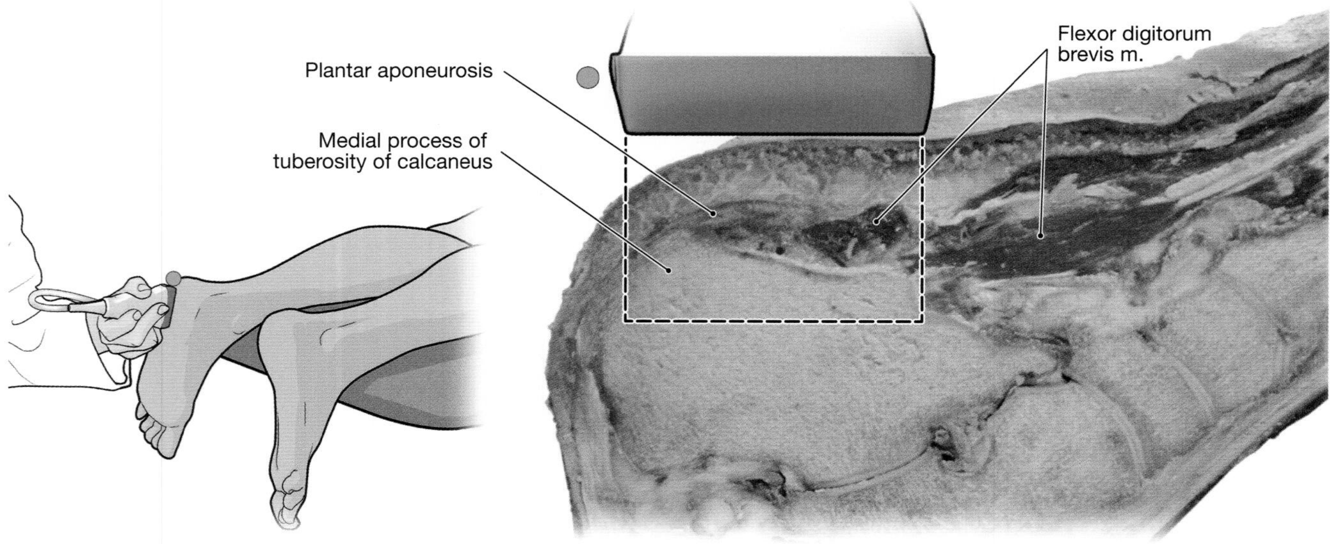

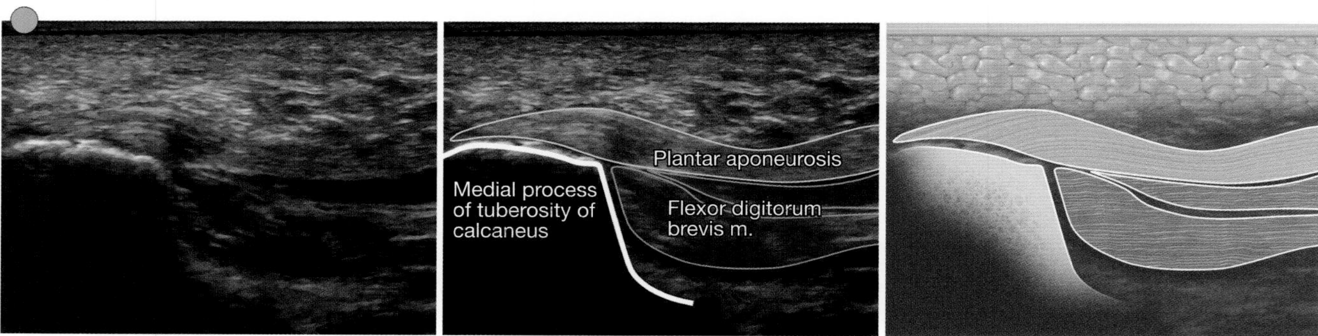

Figure 5.51 Longitudinal view of the plantar aponeurosis arising from the medial process of the calcaneal tuberosity.

Multiple Choice Questions

1. A 75-year-old woman comes to the physician because of a 6-month history of cold and pale right foot. Physical examination shows a cyanotic painful cold foot. An ultrasound Doppler examination shows a thrombotic occlusion of her popliteal artery and minimal flow at the posterior tibial artery. At which of the following locations will physical examination most likely show absence of the pulse?

   A. Lateral to the abductor hallucis
   B. Posteroinferior to the medial femoral condyle
   C. Midway between the lateral malleolus and the calcaneus
   D. Midway between the medial malleolus and the calcaneus
   E. Between the two heads of the gastrocnemius

2. An 80-year-old woman comes to the physician because of a 6-month history of progressive difficulty walking. An ultrasound Doppler examination shows occlusion of her femoral artery at the proximal part of the adductor canal and well-established collateral circulation. Which of the following arteries will most likely be responsible for the collateral circulation?

   A. Descending branch of the lateral circumflex femoral
   B. Descending genicular
   C. Medial circumflex femoral
   D. First perforating branch of deep femoral
   E. Obturator artery

3. An 85-year-old man comes to the physician because of a 6-month history of progressive difficulty walking. He was diagnosed with osteoarthritis 25 years ago. Physical examination shows pain and tightness posteriorly to his right knee. An ultrasound examination shows a large cyst in the popliteal fossa compressing the adjacent nerve descending the fossa vertically. Which of the following movement will most likely be impaired during physical examination?

   A. Dorsiflexion of the foot
   B. Flexion of the thigh
   C. Extension of the digits
   D. Extension of the leg
   E. Plantar flexion of the foot

4. A 32-year-old man is brought to the emergency department after he fell and injured his ankle during a basketball game. Physical examination shows a severe sprain of his ankle. The man is still in pain despite treatment with non-steroidal anti-inflammatory medications. Under ultrasound guidance which of the following nerves can be anesthetized to stop the pain sensation to the ankle joint?

   A. Deep fibular
   B. Femoral
   C. Obturator
   D. Posterior femoral cutaneous
   E. Sural

5. A 32-year-old woman is brought to the emergency department by her parents because of pain in her right foot. An x-ray of the foot shows a fracture of the first and second toes. Under ultrasound guidance she receives a local anesthetic injection to permit easy manipulation of the fractured toes and correction. Which of the following nerves is most likely blocked under ultrasound guidance?

   A. Saphenous
   B. Cutaneous branch of deep fibular
   C. Cutaneous branch of superficial fibular
   D. Sural
   E. Common fibular

6. A 32-year-old man is admitted to the hospital for a detoxification program. He has been an intravenous drug abuser injecting himself with heroin for the past 10 years. Physical examination reveals residual scar tissue over most of his veins. The only veins without any residual scar are the femoral veins at the femoral triangle. Which of the following relationships are the most reliable to identify these veins during ultrasound examination?

   A. The femoral vein lies medial to the femoral artery
   B. The femoral vein lies within the femoral canal
   C. The femoral vein lies lateral to the femoral artery
   D. The femoral vein lies directly medial to the femoral nerve
   E. The femoral vein lies medial to the femoral canal

6

Thorax: Chest Wall and Pleura; Breast

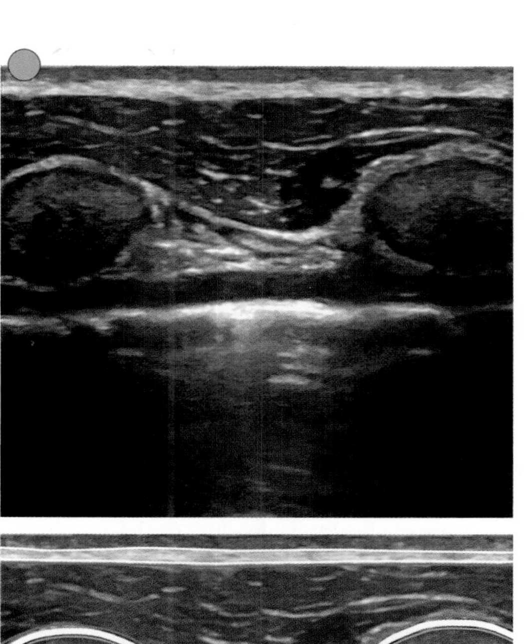

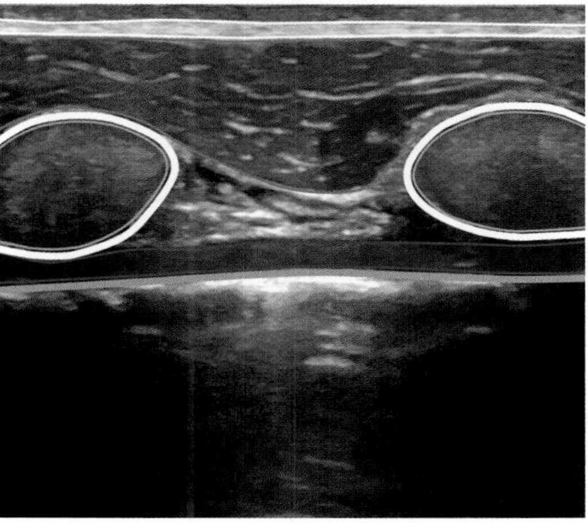

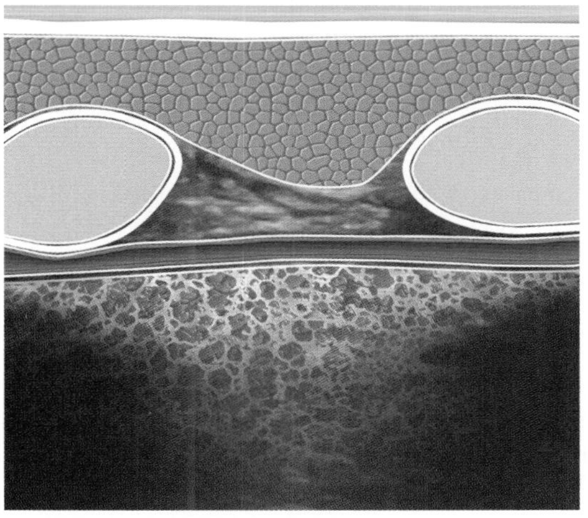

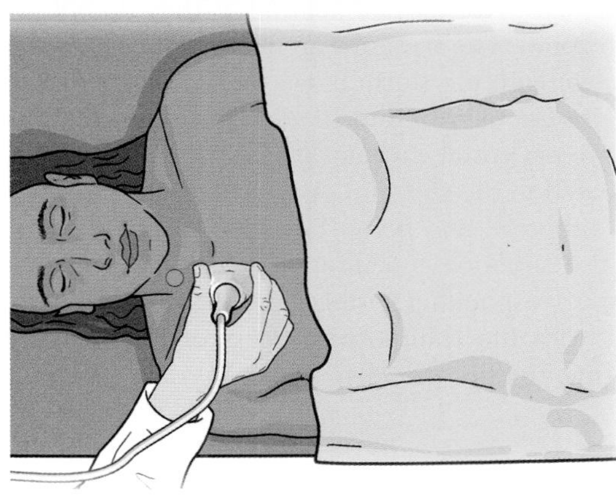

Chest Wall and Pleura

Review of the Anatomy

The thorax is the part of the body that occupies the space between the neck and abdomen. The bony cage of the thorax is conical in shape, has a narrow apex superiorly (the superior thoracic aperture, leading to the root of the neck) and a wide base inferiorly (the inferior thoracic aperture guarded by the diaphragm). The true thoracic wall includes the thoracic cage and the intercostal muscles and the musculature of the anterolateral wall. The same structures covering its posterior aspect are considered as part of the back.

Bones of the Thoracic Wall

The bones of the thoracic wall include the sternum and the ribs. The sternum is a flat bone composed of three parts: the manubrium, body, and xiphoid process.

The manubrium superiorly has the jugular notch and, on each of its lateral sides, the clavicular notch for articulating with the clavicle. The manubrium also articulates with the first rib, the second rib, and the body of the sternum. The junction between the manubrium and the body of the sternum is also known as the sternal angle (of Louis) and is the site of the manubriosternal joint. This landmark marks the following:

- second rib articulates with the sternum
- bifurcation of the trachea
- where the aortic arch begins and ends
- the inferior border of the superior mediastinum
- the T4/T5 vertebral level

The body of the sternum articulates with the second to seventh costal cartilages at the sternocostal joints and the xiphoid process at the xiphisternal joint.

There are 12 pairs of ribs classified as either true or false with the last two termed *floating* as they do not attach to the sternum. The true ribs are the ribs 1 to 7 that directly articulate with the sternum via their costal cartilages. The false ribs are the ribs 8 to 10 and are connected to the seventh rib via costal cartilages. The ribs 11 and 12 are not connected to the sternum. A typical rib consists of a head, neck, tubercle, and body. The head of the rib articulates with the superior and inferior costal facets (demifacets) of the corresponding vertebral bodies. The tubercle articulates with the transverse process of the corresponding vertebrae (except the ribs 11 and 12). The body of the rib contains a costal groove along its inferior edge in which the intercostal vein, artery, and nerve are accommodated.

Intercostal Muscles

There are three intercostal muscles: the external intercostals, internal intercostals, and the innermost intercostals. The external intercostal muscle is located superficially, and its fiber orientation runs medially and downward in a direction in line with the external abdominal oblique muscle of the anterior abdominal wall. At the level of the sternum, the external intercostal muscle is replaced by the anterior intercostal membrane. Deep to the external intercostal muscle is the internal intercostal muscle. This muscle runs in a direction opposite the external intercostals downward and laterally, in line with the internal abdominal oblique muscle. The innermost intercostal muscle is the deepest of the intercostal muscles, running in the same direction as the internal intercostal muscles.

Intercostal Arteries, Veins, and Nerves

The intercostal arteries travel between the ribs. Each intercostal space is typically supplied by a posterior intercostal artery and a pair of anterior intercostal arteries. The anterior intercostal arteries are branches of the internal thoracic arteries. Each internal thoracic artery arises from the inferior surface of the first part of the subclavian artery and descends in the thorax alongside the sternum within the endothoracic fat/fascia posterior to costal cartilages/intercostal space contents and anterior to the parietal pleura. At or just below the 6th intercostal space, the internal thoracic arteries end by dividing into their terminal branches, the musculophrenic and superior epigastric arteries. The posterior intercostal arteries are branches of the descending thoracic aorta. In addition, the first and second intercostal spaces are usually supplied by the supreme or highest intercostal artery, which is a branch of the costocervical trunk, a branch of the subclavian artery.

The intercostal veins run alongside the intercostal arteries and nerves. Similar to the arteries, there are posterior intercostal veins that drain into the azygos/hemiazygos venous system. The anterior intercostal veins are tributaries of the internal thoracic veins. The posterior intercostal veins of the first intercostal space drain into the right and left brachiocephalic veins. The posterior intercostal veins of the second and third intercostal spaces come together and form the superior intercostal vein. The right superior intercostal vein drains into the azygos vein, and the left superior intercostal vein drains into the left brachiocephalic vein.

There are 12 pairs of thoracic spinal nerves that supply the thoracic wall. These nerves exit the intervertebral foramina and immediately divide into anterior and posterior primary rami. The anterior primary rami of T1-T11 nerves run in the intercostal spaces and are thus termed intercostal nerves. The anterior primary ramus of T12 nerve runs inferior to the 12th rib and is called the subcostal nerve. The posterior primary ramus of thoracic intercostal spinal nerves run posteriorly, lateral to the articular processes of the vertebrae, and supply the joints, deep muscles of the back muscles, and their corresponding dermatomes.

The intercostal nerves give off lateral cutaneous branches in the midaxillary line and then terminate as anterior cutaneous nerves. The intercostal nerves innervate the intercostal muscles and corresponding dermatomes. In general, the intercostal veins, arteries, and nerves run between the internal and innermost intercostal muscles in the costal grooves.

Pleura

The pleura is a thin serous membrane that envelopes each lung and consists of parietal and visceral layers. The parietal pleura is subdivided into:

- costal pleura adherent to the ribs
- cervical pleura extending above the first rib into the root of the neck
- mediastinal pleura facing the mediastinum
- diaphragmatic pleura adherent to the superior surface of the diaphragm

The parietal pleura is attached to the internal surface of the thoracic wall by the endothoracic fascia. In the neck, the cervical pleura is reinforced by a condensed part of the endothoracic fascia also known as Sibson fascia (suprapleural membrane). The visceral layer invests the lungs. The costal pleura is innervated by the intercostal nerves. The mediastinal and diaphragmatic pleurae are innervated by the phrenic nerves. Thus, the parietal pleura is sensitive to pain, in contrast to the visceral pleura, which is insensitive to pain but receives vasomotor innervation for stretch and respiratory reflexes via the vagus nerve.

The internal thoracic, superior phrenic, posterior intercostal, and supreme (the highest) intercostal arteries supply the parietal pleura, whereas the visceral pleura is supplied by the bronchial arteries.

Between the parietal and visceral pleurae is a potential space, the pleural space. The pleura is composed of mesothelial cells that produce small amounts of serous fluid, which facilitate the movements of the lungs. During normal respiration, the lungs are not fully expanded and, as a result, the parietal pleura is not in contact with the visceral pleura. The areas in which the parietal pleura is not in direct contact with the lung parenchyma are termed recesses, of which there are two. The costodiaphragmatic recess is formed by the reflection of costal and diaphragmatic pleurae. The costomediastinal recess is formed between the costal and mediastinal pleurae.

Technique

Chest Wall Structures and Pleural Line

PECTORAL MUSCLES RIBS INTERCOSTAL SPACE PLEURAL LINE
Longitudinal (Parasagittal)
FIG. 6.1

The patient should be supine and appropriately draped to allow for palpation of landmarks and for placing and manipulating the probe while maintaining patient privacy and comfort. Use a high-frequency linear probe (although all the relevant anatomy can be viewed by using a curved array probe, the resolution is much better with the linear probe, which is better for learning the anatomy), with the marker directed toward the head.

Place the probe on the midclavicular line over the second, third, or fourth intercostal space with the marker side pointing over the rib above and heel over the rib below (acoustic shadows from the ribs above and below on each side of the image).

From superficial to deep identify the following structures:

- pectoralis major
- pectoralis minor
- intercostal muscles and membranes
- hyperechoic pleural line (at the deep surface of the ribs)
- sonographic A- and B-lines

The pleura is about 0.2 mm thick, very close to the limit of sonographic identification. However, with careful examination, both the parietal and visceral pleurae can be depicted as two separate echogenic lines. In general, the parietal pleura is seen better compared with the visceral pleura and appears as a fine echogenic line. With high-definition ultrasound, a double line can be seen depicting

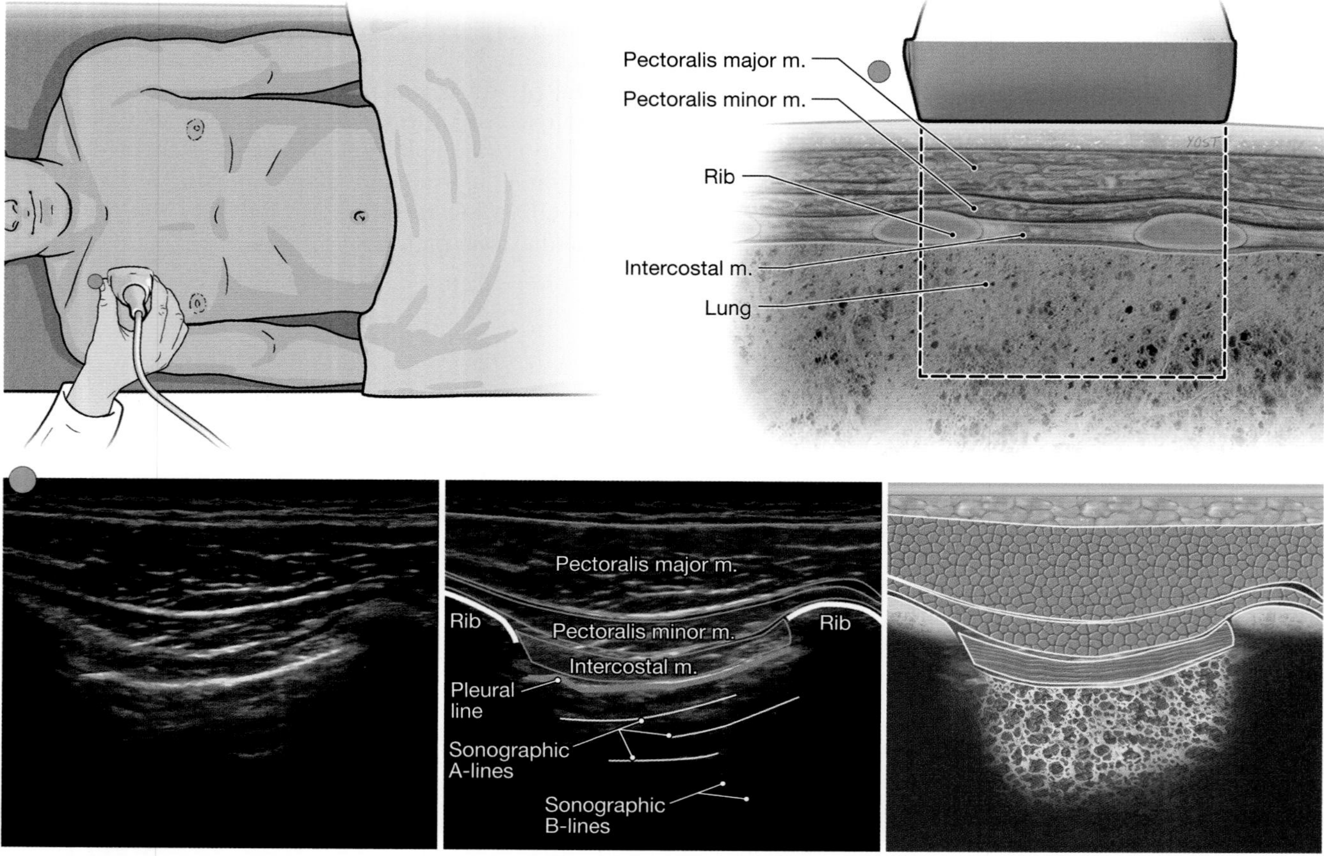

Figure 6.1 Normal longitudinal (parasagittal) view of an intercostal space and the pleural line.

the parietal pleura and endothoracic fascia. The visceral pleura, however, is more difficult to identify. It has been described as a delicate echogenic line, embedded in the near total reflection of ultrasound waves over the air-filled lung. Reflection and reverberation artifacts are the dominant imaging features of the visceral pleura and its surrounding structures. With careful observation, a back and forth shimmering movement referred to as the pleural sliding sign can be seen, in which the visceral pleura slides along the parietal pleura with respiration. The presence of pleural sliding virtually rules out pneumothorax at this location.

Occasional sonographic B-lines are also seen in normal individuals. These are thin hyperechoic comet-tail reverberation artifacts perpendicular to the pleural line, which move back and forth synchronously with pleural sliding. This is probably caused by differences in acoustic impedance of alveolar air versus interstitial fluid in the alveolar walls/interalveolar septae near the lung surface. Numerous, or coalescing thickened B-lines (lung rockets) indicate pulmonary edema and/or pneumonia.

Sonographic A-lines are equally spaced hyperechoic lines parallel to the pleural line and are reverberation artifacts (seen in normal lungs and in pneumothorax). Absence of pleural sliding indicates pneumothorax, and the location at which sliding stops is referred to as the *lung point* (the edge of the pneumothorax vs normal lung/pleural space). Absence of B-lines is also important in the diagnosis of pneumothorax. If any B-lines are seen, even in the absence of obvious pleural sliding, the probability of pneumothorax is greatly reduced.

Examination of pleural sliding in the left lung, especially for lung areas adjacent to the heart, is complicated by the presence of transmitted pulsations from the heart through the lungs. These are seen as rhythmic movements of the pleural line synchronized with the heartbeat and referred to as lung pulse. In general, the presence of lung pulse suggests that the visceral and parietal pleura are in apposition, and therefore there is no intervening pneumothorax in that location.

PECTORAL MUSCLES RIBS INTERCOSTAL SPACE PLEURAL LINE
Transverse
FIG. 6.2

Starting from the probe position described hereinbefore for Figure 6.1, rotate the probe by 90° counterclockwise so the marker points to the patient's right. Place the probe over an intercostal space

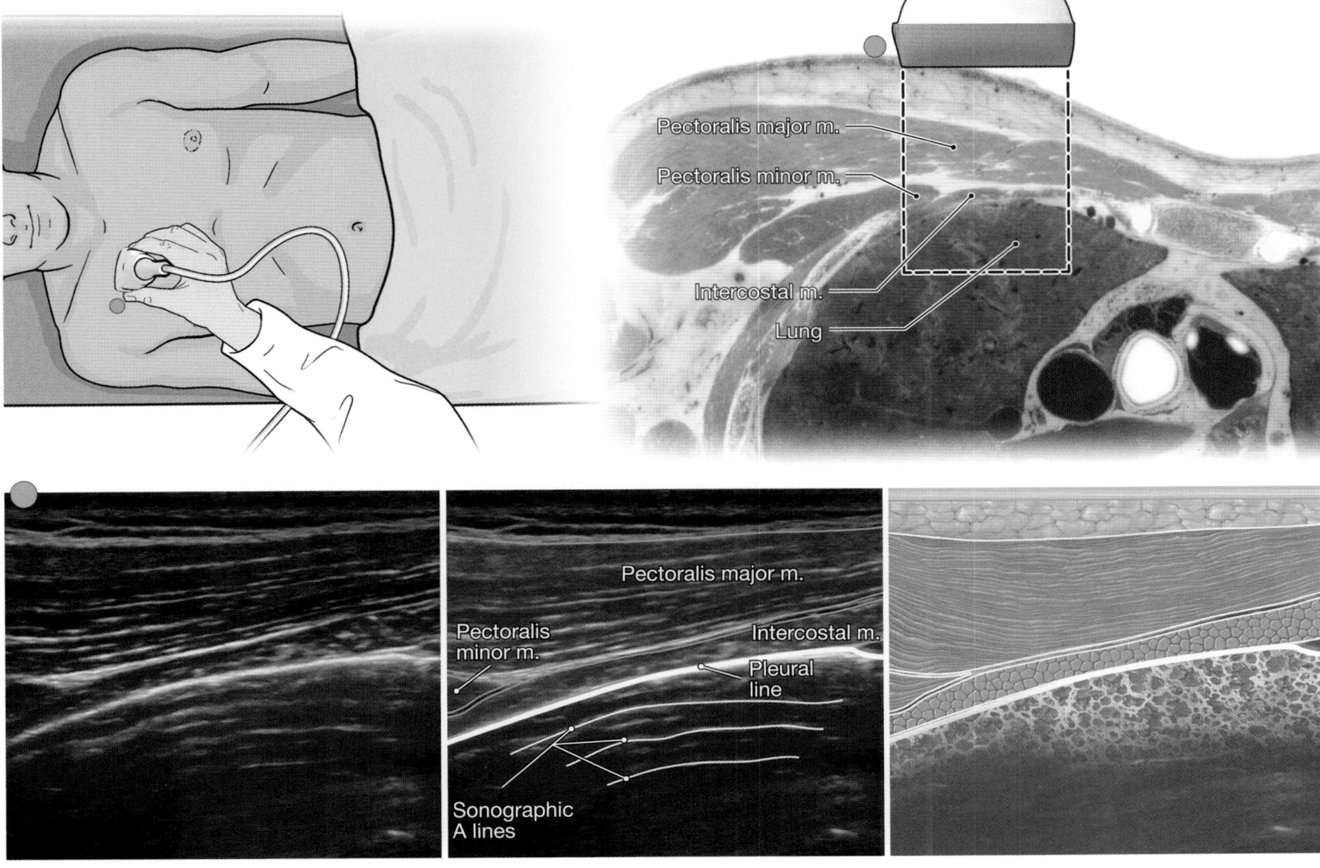

Figure 6.2 Normal transverse view of an intercostal space and the pleural line.

with no rib shadowing as in the sagittal view and identify the following structures:

- pectoralis major
- pectoralis minor
- intercostal muscles and membranes
- hyperechoic pleural line
- sonographic A-lines

Costal Cartilages and Pleural Line

PECTORALIS MAJOR
COSTAL CARTILAGES
INTERCOSTAL SPACE
PLEURAL LINE
Longitudinal (Parasagittal)
FIG. 6.3

The patient should be supine and appropriately draped to allow for palpation of landmarks and for placing and manipulating the probe while maintaining patient privacy and comfort. Use a high-frequency linear probe, and place it along the long axis of the torso approximately 1 cm lateral to the sternum and over the second and third or third and fourth costal cartilages (probe marker directed superiorly). Identify the skin, pectoral fascia, pectoralis major muscle, costal cartilages, intercostal space, and pleural line. Note that while costal cartilages produce some variable posterior shadowing, the pleural line and pleural sliding are completely visible behind both the costal cartilages as well as the soft tissues of the intercostal space.

Internal Thoracic Vessels

PECTORALIS MAJOR
STERNUM
INTERCOSTAL SPACE INTERNAL THORACIC ARTERY AND VEIN(S)
PLEURAL LINE
Transverse
FIG. 6.4

The patient should be supine and appropriately draped to allow for palpating the landmarks and placing and manipulating the probe while maintaining patient privacy and comfort. Use a high-frequency linear probe, and place it along the second, third, or fourth intercostal spaces with the probe marker directed laterally and the nonmarker side of the probe face over the edge of the body of the sternum. Identify the skin, pectoral fascia,

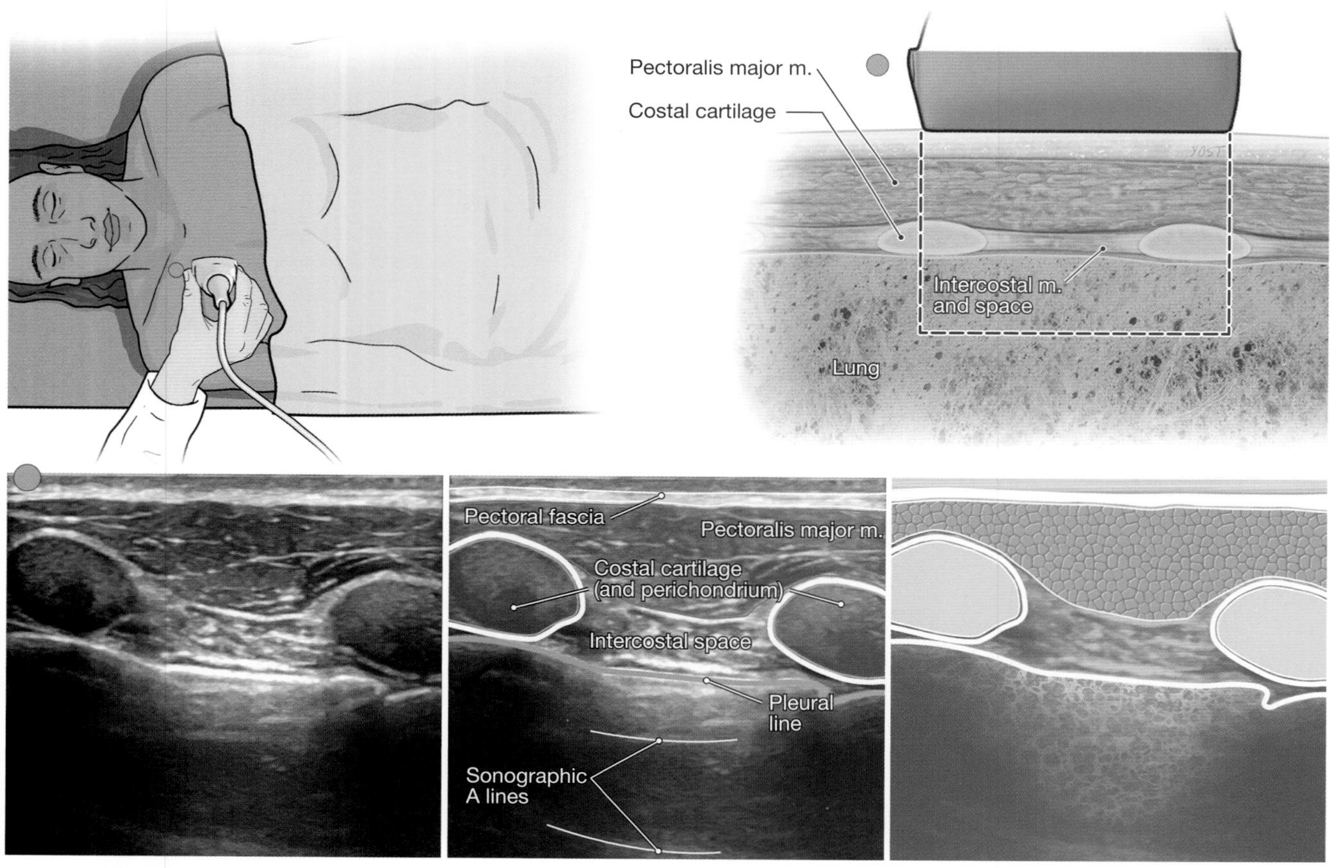

Figure 6.3 Longitudinal (parasagittal) view of costal cartilages, an intercostal space, and the pleural line.

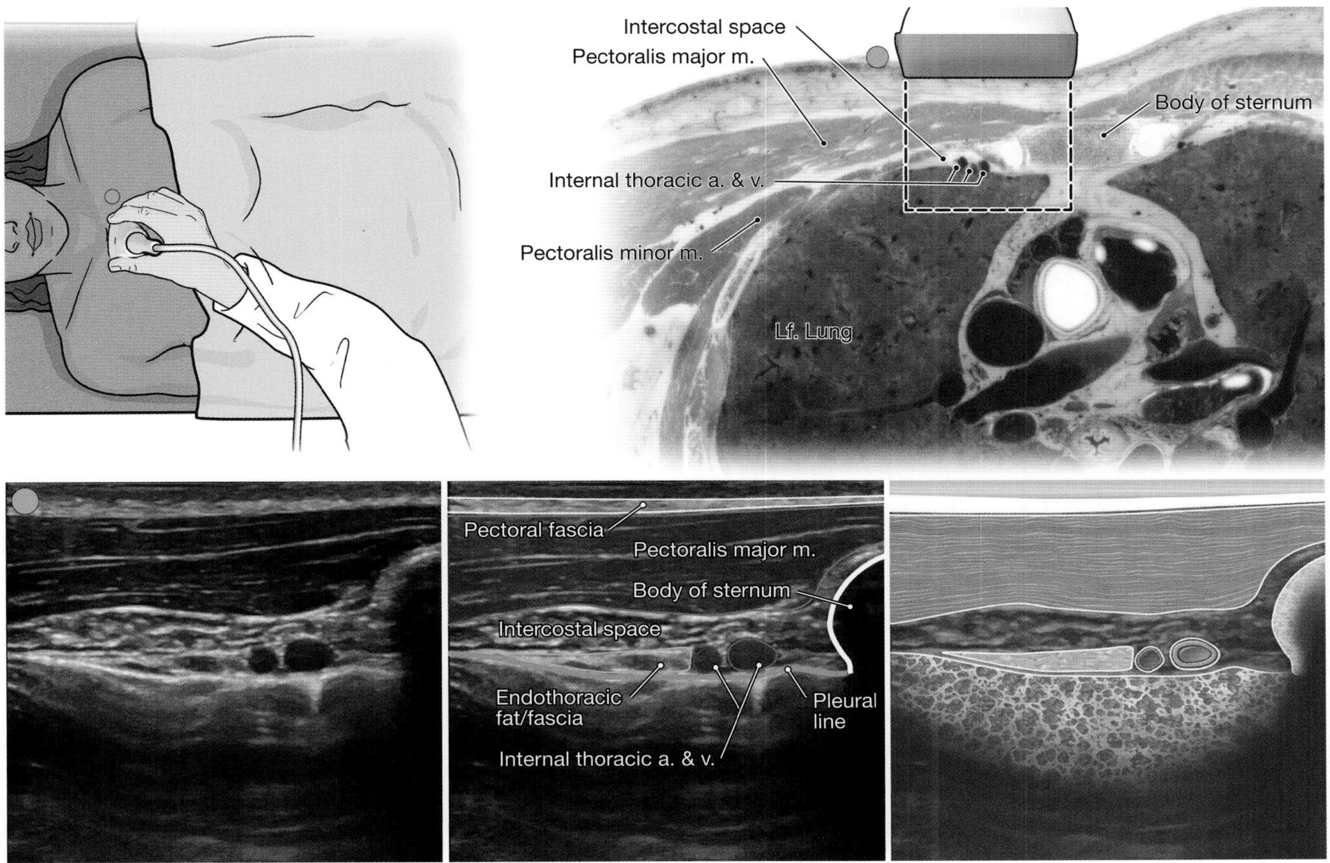

Figure 6.4 Transverse view of the sternum, an intercostal space, the internal thoracic artery and vein(s), and the pleural line.

pectoralis major muscle, sternum, intercostal space contents, internal thoracic vessels, and pleural line. The internal thoracic artery is readily identifiable by its pulsations and is accompanied by either one or two internal thoracic veins (both patterns are commonly seen).

PECTORALIS MAJOR COSTAL CARTILAGES INTERCOSTAL SPACE INTERNAL THORACIC ARTERY PLEURAL LINE
Longitudinal (parasagittal)
FIG. 6.5

Starting from the patient and probe position described hereinbefore, center the probe over the internal thoracic artery and rotate the probe by 90° (probe marker directed superiorly) until the artery can be seen throughout the image anterior to the pleural line. Identify the skin, pectoral fascia, pectoralis major muscle, costal cartilages, intercostal space, internal thoracic artery, and pleural line.

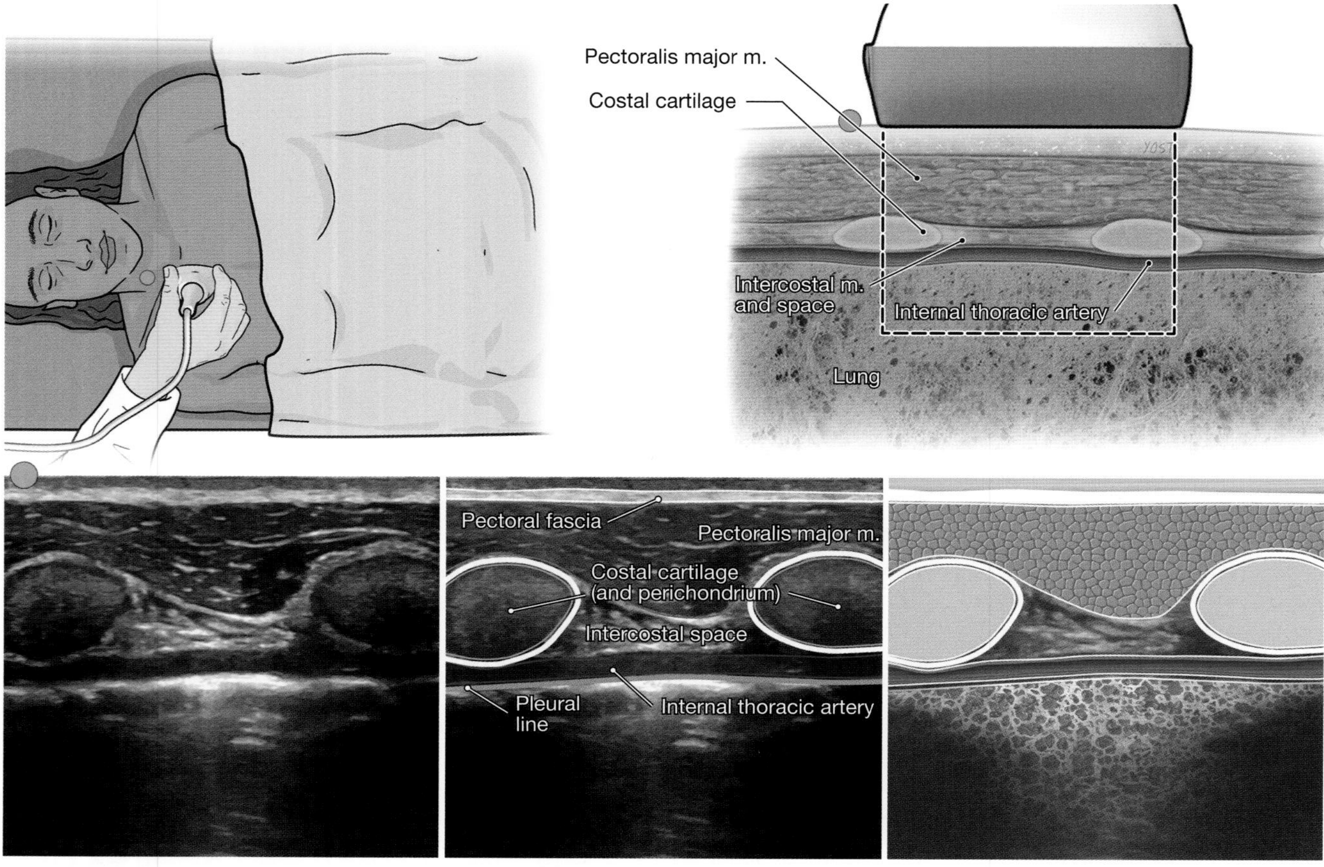

Figure 6.5 Longitudinal (parasagittal) view of costal cartilages, an intercostal space, the internal thoracic artery, and the pleural line.

CLINICAL APPLICATIONS

Ultrasound examination of the pleura, pleural line, and pleural sliding sign is used to screen for pneumothorax in thoracoabdominal trauma as part of the extended focused assessment with sonography for trauma examination.

The same techniques are also used in bedside examination for nontraumatic pneumothorax, pulmonary edema, pleural effusion, hemothorax, and hematomas. Ultrasound examination of the thorax can also detect rib fractures with fairly high accuracy, similarly, bone metastasis, and peripheral lung cancer infiltrating the chest wall.

Doppler ultrasound studies of the internal thoracic artery (and subclavian artery) can be used in noninvasive preoperative evaluation for coronary artery bypass grafting, and flow dynamics in the internal thoracic artery can be assessed noninvasively after bypass grafting, although this is a complex topic.

Breast

Review of the Anatomy

The breasts are located in the anterior part of the thorax at the pectoral region, in both females and males. They consist of the mammary glands, superficial fascia, nerves, vessels, and lymphatics. The female mammary gland is a modified sweat gland that is an accessory to reproduction. The glands contain variable volume of subcutaneous fat thus forming variable sizes and shapes depending on the genetics and environmental factors such as diet. During puberty, the mammary glands enlarge because of glandular and subcutaneous fat development. During pregnancy, the mammary glands undergo further development and new glandular tissue is formed. The mammary glands typically rest on top of the pectoral fascia covering the pectoralis major muscle. A small lateral portion of the mammary gland extends toward the axilla, forming the axillary tail (process) of Spence. The breast is attached to the inner surface of the skin by strong connective tissue bands, the suspensory ligaments of Cooper. Between the superficial fascia that covers the breast and the deep fascia that covers the pectoralis major is a potential space, the retromammary space. This space is responsible for the mobility of the female breast. The mammary gland extends from lateral border of the sternum to the midaxillary line between the second and sixth ribs. The gland contains a nipple that is typically found at the lever of the 4th intercostal space and 15 to 20 lobes of glandular tissue that a lactiferous duct opens at the tip of the nipple. Each lactiferous duct contains a lactiferous sinus that serves as a pocket to store milk during lactation. The male breast has no function. The blood supply of the breast is from mammary branches of the anterior perforating branches of the internal thoracic artery, branches from the lateral thoracic artery, pectoral branches from thoracoacromial artery, and lateral mammary branches from the posterior intercostal arteries. Its sensory innervation is from the anterior and lateral cutaneous branches of the 2nd to 6th intercostal nerves. The major lymphatic drainage of the breast is to the pectoral (anterior) lymph nodes that empty in the axillary lymphatics. A second group of lymphatics are the parasternal lymphatics found alongside the internal thoracic artery. A smaller group of lymphatics are the infraclavicular or deltopectoral lymphatics.

Technique

The patient should be supine with the palm of the hand on the side to be examined behind the head. This tenses the pectoralis major and minor muscles and somewhat flattens the breast tissue. In patients with large breasts, it is useful to place a pillow behind the shoulder so that the torso is rolled slightly toward the contralateral side. If breast tissue is still falling away from the anterior chest wall laterally, then the patient will need to be placed in some degree of contralateral decubitus for examination of the outer breast quadrants. The examiner should be either standing alongside the patient or seated alongside the patient at the level of the patient's torso. A number of different probes can be utilized in breast ultrasound (high-frequency linear probes, hockey-stick probes, curved array probes, etc.), but for our purposes we will use a high-frequency linear probe.

BREAST PECTORAL MUSCLES RIBS INTERCOSTAL SPACE PLEURAL LINE
Longitudinal (parasagittal)
FIG. 6.6

Place the probe marker (directed superiorly) on the breast with the nonmarker side just superior to the nipple-areolar complex, and apply light pressure through the probe, maintaining skin contact while not causing pain. Identify, from superficial to deep, the following layers/structures: skin; hypoechoic superficial fat (commonly referred to as premammary fat); hyperechoic mammary fibroglandular tissue, a usually thin layer of hypoechoic deep mammary fat (commonly referred to as retro-mammary fat); pectoralis major and minor muscles; ribs and intercostal spaces; and finally, the pleural line and underlying lung. The amount of fibroglandular tissue

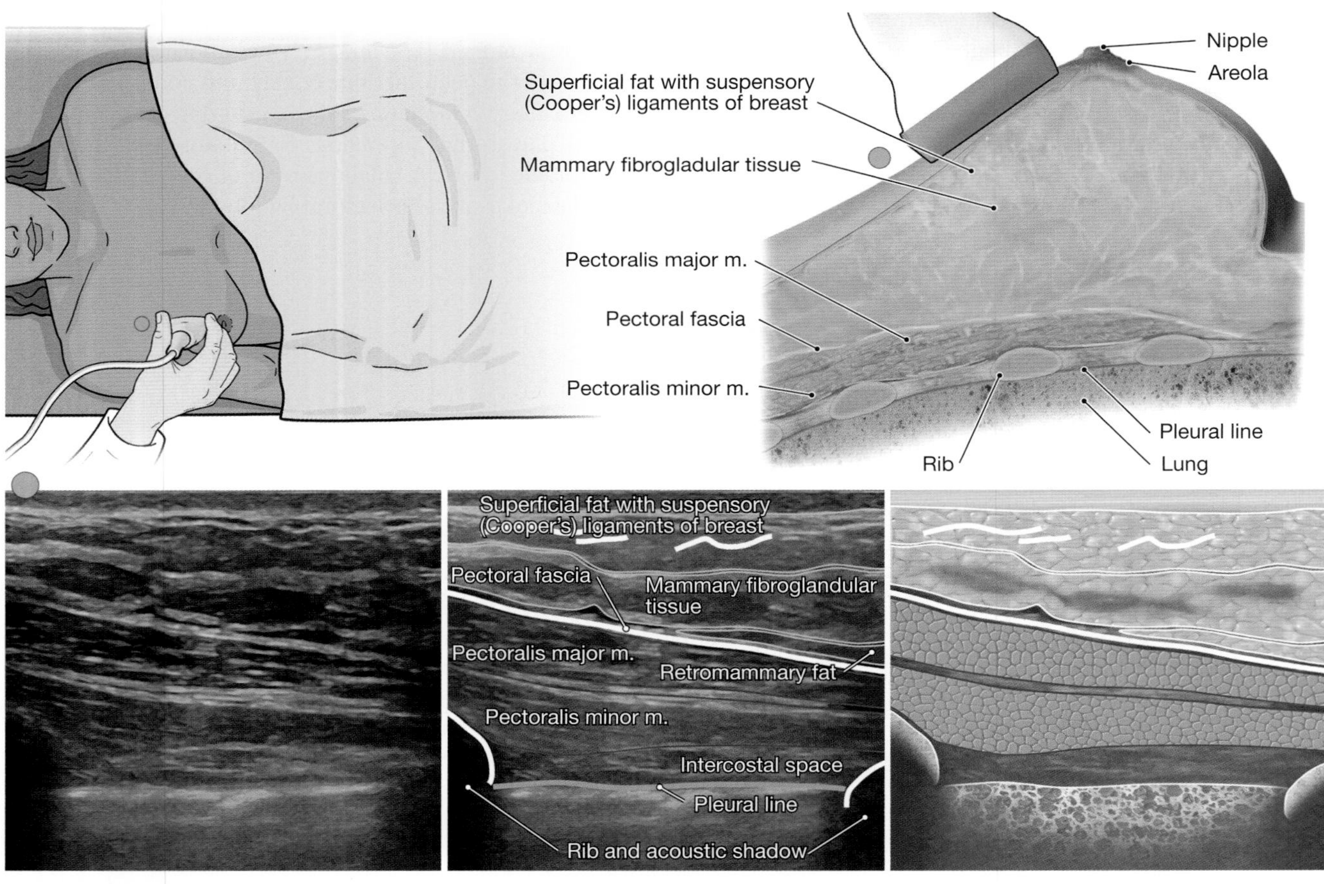

Figure 6.6 Longitudinal (parasagittal) view of the layers of the breast, pectoralis muscles, ribs, an intercostal space, and the pleural line.

varies among women and changes with puberty, aging, and menopause. In general, young women of the reproductive age have the greatest mass of fibroglandular tissue, and progressive fatty replacement of glandular tissue occurs with aging resulting in more or less complete fatty involution of breast tissue in postmenopausal women.

NIPPLE-AREOLAR COMPLEX
Longitudinal (parasagittal)
FIG. 6.7

In the superficial fat layer, look for thin echogenic lines extending from the fascia covering the fibroglandular tissue to the skin. These are the suspensory (Cooper) ligaments of the breast. The fibroglandular tissue may be more or less uniformly echogenic or there may be interspersed fatty islands. Pectoralis major muscle is seen throughout the chest deep to the retromammary fat, whereas pectoralis minor muscle is only seen in the upper part of the chest. Ribs, their acoustic shadows, tissues of the intercostal spaces, and the pleural line appear just as they did in the upper chest as described earlier in this chapter.

From the same position of the patient, apply a generous amount of gel over the nipple-areolar complex, and center the probe face over the nipple with the marker directed superiorly. Identify the nipple and the areola. Note that the sonographic density of the nipple and areolar complex frequently results in a variably dense acoustic shadow that obscures the breast and duct tissue deep to the nipple-areolar complex. Thus, in the clinical ultrasound examination of the breast in this area, care must be taken to view the tissues underlying the nipple and areola from various angles to insure that a mass is not hidden in the acoustic shadow.

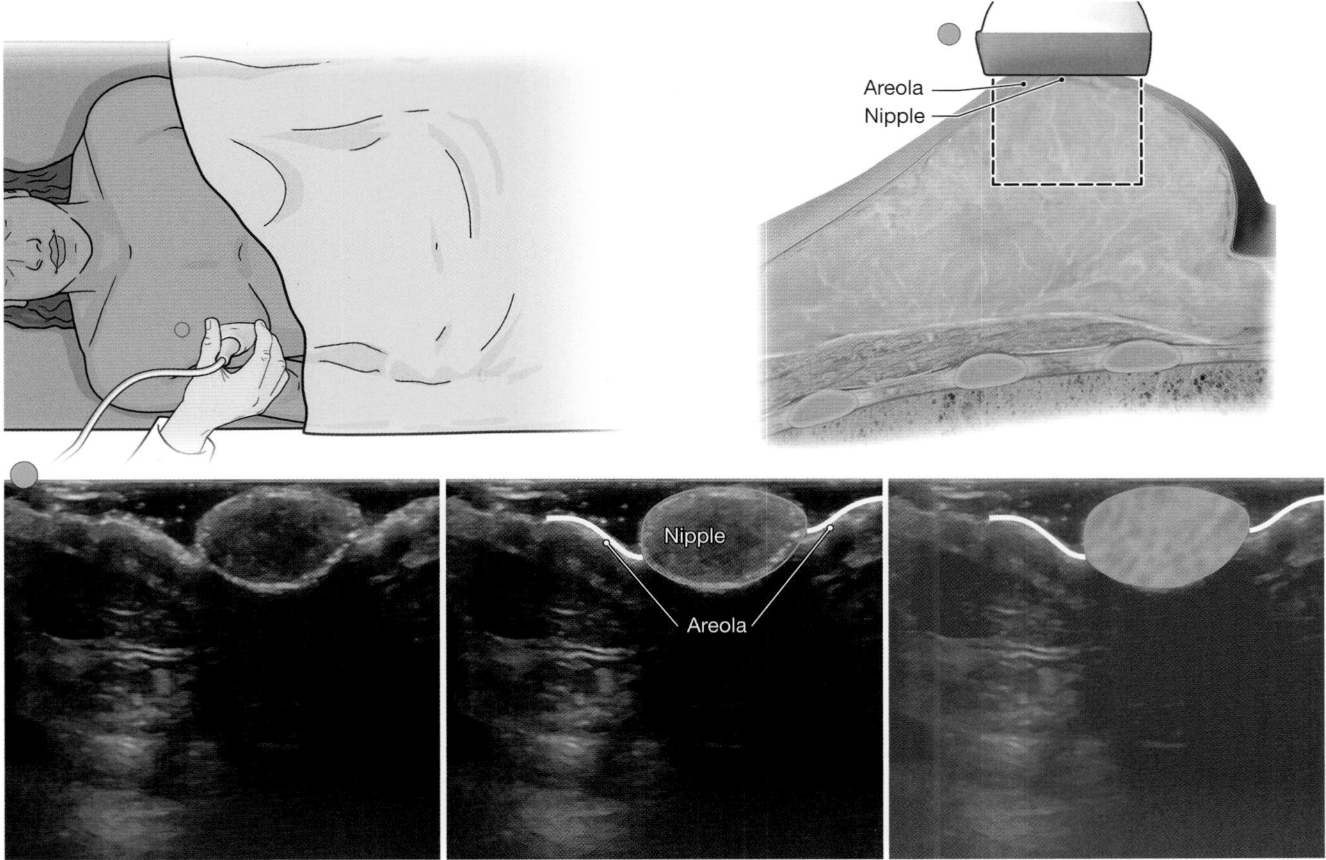

Figure 6.7 Longitudinal (parasagittal) view of the nipple and areola. Note the dense shadowing behind the nipple.

CLINICAL APPLICATIONS

Targeted breast ultrasound is commonly used for examining a specific area of breast where there is a palpable "lump," a suspicious finding from mammography or an area of asymmetrical (comparing similar regions of each breast to the other) breast density on mammography. Ultrasound needle guidance is also used for obtaining percutaneous biopsy specimens when appropriate.

Nontargeted or complete breast ultrasound may be utilized in younger women with increased risk of breast cancer because of either the patient's or family history. In young women with very dense breast tissue, lesions/masses can be hidden from view in mammographic images due to the overall increase in x-ray attenuation ("whiting out").

Multiple Choice Questions

1. A 19-year-old man is brought to the emergency department 35 minutes after being involved in a motor vehicle collision. Physical examination shows swelling, inflammation, and deformation of the chest wall caused upon impact with the steering wheel during the collision. A chest radiograph shows a fracture of the sternum at the manubriosternal joint. Which of the following ribs would most likely be involved in such an injury?

   A. First
   B. Second
   C. Third
   D. Fourth
   E. Fifth

2. A 19-year-old man is brought to the emergency department 35 minutes after being involved in a motor vehicle collision. Physical examination shows a wound in the neck just above the middle of the right clavicle and first rib. A chest radiograph shows collapse of the right lung and a tension pneumothorax. Injury to which of the following structures resulted in the pneumothorax?

   A. Costal pleura
   B. Mediastinal parietal pleura
   C. Diaphragmatic parietal pleura
   D. Cupula
   E. Endothoracic fascia

3. A 19-year-old man is brought to the emergency department 35 minutes after being involved in a motor vehicle collision. Physical examination shows a wound in the neck just above the middle of the right clavicle and the first rib. A chest radiograph shows collapse of the right lung and a tension pneumothorax. A chest tube is inserted and adequate local anesthesia of the chest wall before insertion of a chest tube is administered. Of the following layers, which is the deepest that must be infiltrated with the local anesthetic to achieve adequate anesthesia?

   A. Parietal pleura
   B. Visceral pleura
   C. Endothoracic fascia
   D. Intercostal muscles
   E. Subcutaneous fat

4. A 19-year-old man is brought to the emergency department 35 minutes after being involved in a motor vehicle collision. Physical examination shows a wound in the neck just above the middle of the right clavicle and the first rib. A chest radiograph shows collapse of the right lung and a tension pneumothorax. A chest tube is inserted, and adequate local anesthesia of the chest wall before insertion of a chest tube is administered. Between which layers will the chest tube have to be placed to relieve the pneumothorax?

   A. Between the mediastinal pleura and fibrous pericardium
   B. Between the visceral and parietal layers of the pericardium
   C. Between the serous and fibrous layers of the pericardium
   D. Between the endothoracic fascia and parietal pleura
   E. Between the parietal and visceral layers of the pleura

5. A 55-year-old woman is brought to the emergency department because of a 2-day history of sharp and localized pain over the thoracic wall during coughing. A chest radiograph shows pleural effusion. A chest tube is inserted to drain the effusion through an intercostal space. At which of the following locations is the chest tube most likely to be inserted?

   A. Between the internal and external intercostal muscles
   B. Inferior to the lower border of the rib
   C. Superior to the upper border of the rib
   D. At the middle of the intercostal space
   E. Between the intercostal muscles and the posterior intercostal membrane

6. A 45-year-old woman is brought to the emergency department because she was stabbed in her right anterior chest wall with a sharp instrument in a domestic dispute. Physical examination shows a puncture wound in the third right intercostal space at the midclavicular line and distended neck veins. There is hyperresonance on percussion and absent breath sounds over the right hemithorax. An ultrasound of the chest shows absent B-lines in the right hemithorax, but B-lines present in the left. Which of the following is the most likely diagnosis?

   A. Right tension pneumothorax
   B. Cardiac tamponade
   C. Atelectasis
   D. Pulmonary edema
   E. Pneumonia

7 Heart

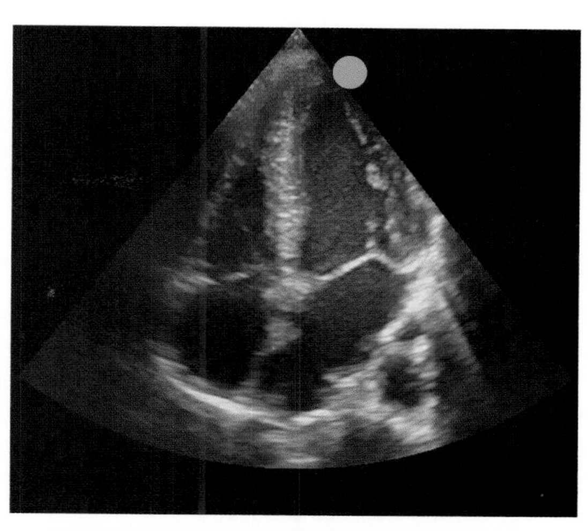

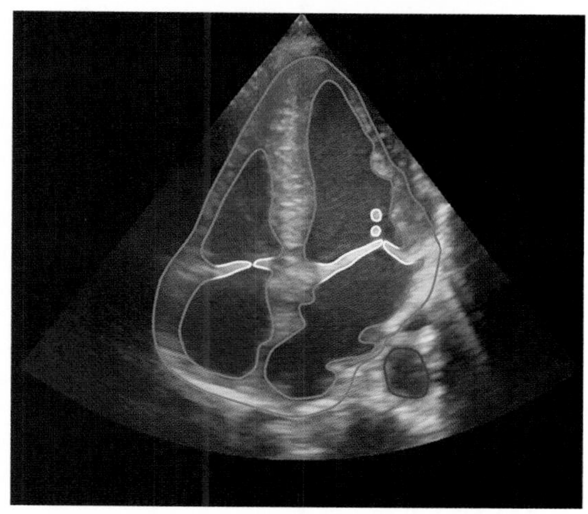

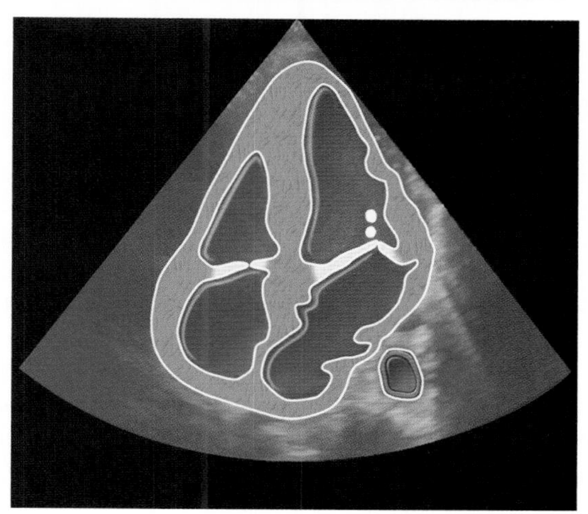

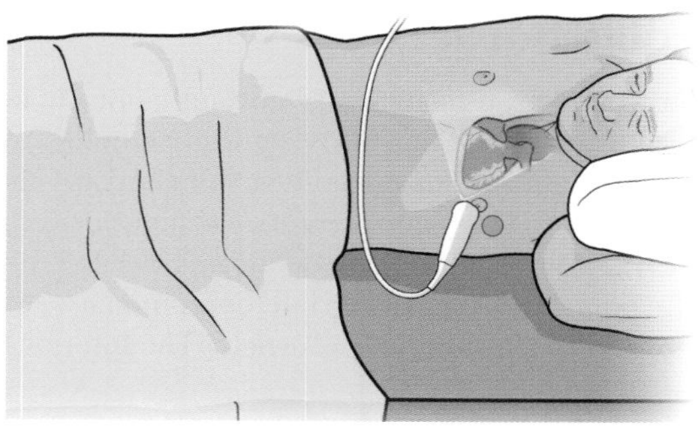

Review of the Anatomy

Pericardium

The pericardium is a fibroserous sac that encloses the entire heart and a portion of the great vessels and is composed of two layers, one fibrous and one serous. The fibrous pericardium is tough and dense, forming the outermost layer of the pericardial sac. The fibrous pericardium is attached to the deep surface of the sternum by the sternopericardial ligaments (composed of condensations of mediastinal areolar tissue), to the diaphragm (inferiorly), and to the adventitial layer of the aorta and pulmonary trunk.

The serous pericardium is composed of two layers of mesothelial cells, the visceral and the parietal. The parietal layer of the serous pericardium lines the interior surface of the fibrous pericardium. The visceral pericardium is most frequently referred to as the epicardium, which forms the outermost layer of the heart. The space between the visceral and the parietal serous pericardium is the pericardial cavity. The mesothelial lining of the serous pericardium secretes pericardial fluid. The function of the pericardial fluid is to allow the heart to move more efficiently by reducing the energy lost to friction.

The Heart

The heart is located within the pericardial sac. It weighs about 250 g in women and 300 g in men. The transverse diameter varies with inspiration and expiration but normally measures 8 to 9 cm in transverse diameter on a radiograph at end of a maximum inspiration in the standing position. Typically, the width of the normal heart is less than one-half width of the chest. The cardiac wall possesses three distinct layers, the endocardium, myocardium, and epicardium. The endocardium is composed of endothelial cells and forms the inner surface of the heart that comes into contact with the blood. The myocardium is composed of myocardial cells, which contract to expel blood. The epicardium is the visceral pericardium forming the outermost layer of the heart.

Cardiac Borders

The borders of the heart are important clinically because they are used as landmarks to diagnose pathologies of the heart. The right border of the heart demarcates the inferior vena cava (IVC), right atrium, and superior vena cava. The left border of the heart delineates the left ventricle and the pulmonary trunk. The left, or pulmonary, surface is composed mainly of the left ventricle. The inferior border demarcates the right ventricle. The right ventricle forms the sternocostal surface and part of the diaphragmatic surface of the heart. The apex of the heart is located in a healthy heart at the fifth intercostal space, ie, the point of maximal impulse of cardiac inspection/auscultation. The base of the heart is demarcated by the left atrium and a small portion of the right atrium.

Right Atrium

The right atrium has the thinnest wall of the four chambers of the heart. The right atrium is typically divided into two parts, the sinus venarum and the right atrium proper. The sinus venarum is the smooth-walled region of the right atrium, which contains the superior vena cava, the IVC, and the opening of the coronary sinus. The sinus venarum develops embryologically from the sinus venosus. The right atrium proper contains the crista terminalis, pectinate muscles, right auricular appendage, and interatrial septum.

The external surface of the right atrium is broad, triangular, and pyramidal in shape. There are two large orifices for the superior and inferior vena cavae on the right atrium. The superior vena cava is formed by the junction of the left and right brachiocephalic veins in the superior mediastinum. The IVC contains a small crescentic valve, the Eustachian valve. Rarely, this valve can be present as a fenestrated structure connected to the atrial vestibule (Chiari network). In some cases, a large fenestrated valve of the IVC can be misdiagnosed as a **thrombus** (blood clot).

The anterior cardiac vein also has an opening into the right atrium. The sulcus terminalis is a shallow groove in the roof of the right atrium, which extends between the right side of the orifice of the superior vena cava and that of the IVC. The sulcus terminalis externally corresponds to a muscular ridge, the crista terminalis, internally. The crista terminalis marks the line of junction of the right atrium with the right auricle. The auricles are appendages of the atria. The sulcus terminalis contains the sinoatrial nodal branch of the right coronary artery. The pectinate muscles are slender bands of muscle that arise from the crista terminalis and fan out through the wall of the right auricle. The roof of the atrium is smooth, in contrast with that of the auricle. The right auricular appendage contains small condensed pectinate muscles, which may potentially trap a venous thrombus and, if dislodged, result in a pulmonary embolism. The interatrial septum forms the medial wall of the right atrium. Within the septum is a depressed region, the fossa ovalis, bordered by a thicker rim of muscle, the limbus fossa ovalis. The fossa ovalis marks the line of fusion between the original embryonic septum secundum and the septum primum, closing the ostium secundum in the morphologic formation of the septum. In almost 20% of individuals, the area of fusion in the interatrial septum is incomplete and an oblique fissure of communication between the two atria is retained. This condition is known as *probe patency* of the foramen ovale and is usually of no physiologic significance. Finally, the right atrium opens into the right ventricles via the right atrioventricular (AV) valve (tricuspid valve).

Left Atrium

The left atrium is the most posteriorly located structure of the heart. It has thicker walls than the right atrium, and its endocardium is thicker than that of the right atrium because of higher pressures. The interior of the left atrium is smooth and possesses very few pectinate muscles, which are confined to the auricle. The left auricle is relatively long and thin, resembling a pointing finger. The left atrium receives four or five pulmonary veins, two from the left lung and three from the right lung. Several venae cordis minimae are also present within the walls of the left atrium. The left atrium receives oxygenated blood from the lungs and communicates with the left ventricle via the left AV valve (mitral).

Right Ventricle

The right ventricle is the most anterior of all the heart chambers and is almost in contact with the sternum. The right ventricle has thin walls and is separated into two parts, the inflow and outflow parts. The inflow portion contains the tricuspid valve, papillary muscles, interventricular septum, and trabeculae carneae. The tricuspid valve possesses three leaflets, the superior (also called anterior or anterosuperior), inferior (replaced the old terminology of posterior), and septal. The separation of the three leaflets may not be well-delineated. The leaflets are anchored to papillary muscles within the ventricle by slender, tough chordae tendineae. The chordae tendineae are connected to a large anterior papillary muscle, a small inferior (replaced the old terminology of posterior) papillary muscle, and septal papillary muscles. There may be several small septal papillary muscles arising from the interventricular septum, with short chordae tendineae passing to the septal leaflet of the valve. It is important to realize that the papillary muscles and their chordae tendineae do not open the tricuspid valve; in fact, the valve opens passively because of pressure differences between the right atrium and right ventricle when the right ventricle is relaxing (diastole). The papillary muscles and chordae tendineae keep the valve leaflets (and blood within the right ventricle) from being forced or "blown" upward into the right atrium when the right ventricle contracts (systole). Blood within the right ventricle is then expelled unidirectionally through the valve of the pulmonary artery.

The right ventricle contains thick, irregular-shaped bundles of muscle the trabeculae carneae of the right ventricle. One such bundle of muscle the moderator band (or septomarginal trabecula or septal band) is very prominent. This band of muscle passes from the muscular interventricular septum to the base of the anterior papillary muscle. The supraventricular crest (crista supraventricularis) separates the inflow from the outflow portions of the heart. The pulmonary semilunar valve has three semilunar-shaped leaflets the right, the left, and the non-adjacent (replaced the old terminology of anterior) that join one another at the commissures. Each leaflet is strengthened at the periphery by a rim of connective tissue known as the lunule and a thickened central portion of each leaflet called the nodule. The pulmonary trunk begins at the level of the pulmonary valve and after 3 to 5 cm bifurcates into the right and left pulmonary arteries. The conus arteriosus or infundibulum of the right ventricle is the horizontal mass of muscular tissue on which two-thirds of the pulmonary valve rests.

Left Ventricle

The wall of the left ventricle is approximately three times thicker than the wall of the right ventricle because of its need to propel blood to the systemic circulation. Traditionally, the left ventricle has been divided into the aortic vestibule and the ventricle proper. The aortic vestibule contains the smooth portion of the interventricular septum, the membranous septum, the aortic semilunar valve, and the aortic root. The aortic semilunar valves possess three semilunar leaflets, right (right coronary leaflet), left (left coronary leaflet), and the non-adjacent (replaced the old terminology of posterior or noncoronary leaflet). They also possess a lunule and nodule for each leaflet similar to the pulmonary valve. The ostia of the coronary arteries arise from depressions in the wall of the aorta, the aortic sinuses of Valsalva.

The left AV valve (mitral valve) rests between the left atrium and left ventricle. This valve is often called the bicuspid valve, although one may be able to distinguish an aortic (anterior) leaflet, a mural (replaced the old terminology of posterior) leaflet, and two smaller leaflets at the left and right ends of the valve orifice. However, the mitral valve typically has two leaflets, an aortic and a mural, attached via chordae tendineae to two papillary muscles, the inferior (replaced the old terminology of posteromedial) and the superior (replaced the old terminology of anterolateral). The chordae tendineae and papillary muscles keep the valve leaflets from being forced up into the atria during systole. Within the left ventricle there are muscular ridges, the trabeculae carneae of the left ventricle.

Cardiac Valves and Their Location

The position of the cardiac valves is as follows: The pulmonary semilunar valves are valve is typically located at the medial end of the left third costal cartilage. The aortic semilunar valve is located deep to the sternum at the level of the third intercostal space. The tricuspid valve lies behind the sternum to the right at the fourth intercostal space. The mitral valve is located deep to the sternum to the left at the fourth intercostal space.

Coronary Arteries

Right Coronary Artery

The right coronary artery arises from the anterior (right) aortic sinus of Valsalva. The artery passes between the pulmonary trunk and the edge of the right auricle and descends in the right coronary sulcus.

The first branch of the right coronary artery is the artery of the sinus node, which arises in approximately 60% of humans from the proximal portion of the right coronary artery, passing then up the medial wall of the right atrium to the junction of the superior vena cava and the right auricle, where it enters the sinus node. This artery, however, may arise from the proximal left coronary artery or be doubly supplied from both coronary arteries.

The second branch of the right coronary artery is the conal branch. The conal branch arises from the right coronary artery and passes to the left, around the right ventricle, at the level of the pulmonary semilunar valve. Close to the diaphragmatic surface of the heart, the right coronary artery typically gives off the right marginal branch, which supplies the inferior border of the right ventricle. The right coronary artery continues inferiorly in the AV groove and, in most cases, descends and terminates in the inferior (replaced the old terminology of posterior) interventricular groove as the inferior (replaced the old terminology of posterior) interventricular (descending) artery. This artery supplies the inferior one-third of the interventricular septum and a portion of the inferior wall of the left ventricle. In 80% of humans, the artery of the AV node arises from the right coronary near the inferior interventricular groove.

Left Coronary Artery

The left coronary artery is a short artery arising from the left aortic sinus of Valsalva and runs between the pulmonary trunk and ascending aorta before bifurcating into the anterior interventricular and circumflex arteries. The anterior interventricular artery in an abbreviated form is often clinically referred to as the left anterior descending (LAD) artery. This vessel, typically, gives off two or more large diagonal branches to the anterior surface of the left ventricle. Deeply penetrating septal branches arise from the deep surface of the anterior interventricular artery and enter the muscular interventricular septum, supplying the anterior two-thirds of the septum. The inferior one-third (replaced the old terminology of posterior) of the septum is supplied by similar branches from the inferior interventricular coronary artery. The circumflex coronary artery runs in the left AV groove toward the left border and around to the base of the heart. This vessel typically gives off the left marginal artery crossing the left border of the heart supplying the left ventricular free wall.

Cardiac Veins

The coronary sinus is a small confluence of veins approximately 2 cm long, which lies at the AV groove externally and between the opening of the IVC and the tricuspid valve internally to eventually empty into the right atrium. It receives the great cardiac vein, the middle cardiac vein, and occasionally the small cardiac vein and the oblique vein of the left atrium. The opening of the coronary sinus is guarded by the valve of the coronary sinus, the Thebesian valve.

The great cardiac vein lies in the anterior interventricular groove, accompanies the left anterior interventricular artery, and drains the anterior portion of the interventricular septum and the anterior aspect of both ventricles. The middle cardiac vein lies in the inferior interventricular groove, accompanies the inferior interventricular artery, and drains the interior (replaced the old terminology of posterior) part of the interventricular septum and the inferior aspect of both ventricles. The small cardiac vein lies in the AV groove next to the opening of the coronary sinus. It usually joins the right marginal vein or separately opens to the right atrium. It drains the marginal portion of the right ventricle and accompanies the right marginal artery. Not all venous drainage of the myocardium passes into the coronary sinus. The anterior cardiac veins drain directly into the right atrium. Other venous channels within the myocardium also empty directly into the chambers of the heart by small openings in the walls, especially within the right atrium; these are called smallest cardiac veins (Thebesian veins or venae cordis minimae).

Conduction Tissue of the Heart

Specialized cardiac muscle fibers compose the conduction tissue of the heart that sends electrical signals to the cardiac musculature, resulting in its contraction. The major specialized cardiac conduction muscle fibers are the sinoatrial and AV nodes, as well as the bundles of His and Purkinje fibers.

The sinoatrial node is located at the junction of the base of the superior vena cava with the right auricle. The AV node is situated deep to the musculature of the medial wall of the right atrium adjacent to the septal leaflet of the tricuspid valve. The bundle of His (common AV bundle) exits inferiorly from the AV node through the central fibrous body, curving inferior to the membranous septum to reach the superior margin of the muscular interventricular septum. The bundle of His passes for a short distance on the superior aspect of the interventricular septum and then divides into a broad left branch to the left ventricle and a narrow right branch, which passes into the right ventricle. A subendocardial network of specialized cardiac muscle cells (Purkinje fibers) arises from the left and right bundle branches. This network conveys the excitatory impulse from the branches of the common bundle (of His) to the myocardium of the ventricles.

Technique

Cardiac ultrasound (US) imaging, often referred to as **echocardiography**, has been integrated into the functional cardiac evaluation in cardiovascular disease. Although a very basic imaging modality, it provides vast amounts of information pertaining to cardiac structures and function. The two most common types of cardiac US imaging are transthoracic echocardiography and transesophageal echocardiography. In this chapter, we describe several different transthoracic approaches, namely, apical, IVC, suprasternal, parasternal long-axis (PLAX), parasternal short-axis (PSAX), and subxiphoid views.

Apical Views

APICAL 4-CHAMBER VIEW
FIG. 7.1

To obtain the apical 4-chamber view, place the patient in a supine position or in left lateral decubitis, which often greatly improves the image quality. Place the probe face lateral to the nipple line at the point of the cardiac apex or apical pulse. The transducer should be angled toward the right shoulder, and the probe marker should be directed toward the 2- or 3-o'clock position (wherein 12 o'clock is directly superior). Identify the interventricular septum separating the right and left ventricles. Identify the mitral and tricuspid valves. Observe the motion of the valves during the cardiac cycle. Note the point where the tricuspid valve meets the lateral free wall of the right ventricle, referred to as the tricuspid annulus plane. Observe how the tricuspid annulus plane moves toward the apex of the right ventricle during systole. This is referred to as tricuspid annulus plane systolic excursion or tricuspid annular plane systolic excursion. Look for left ventricular papillary muscles and tendinous cords as they move in and out of view during the cardiac cycle. Look for the descending thoracic aorta posterior to the left atrium. Note that the ventricles appear to sit on top of the atria. This is because the transducer is closest to the apex of the heart, so the ventricles are displayed in the near field whereas the atria are displayed in the far field.

APICAL 5-CHAMBER VIEW
FIG. 7.2

Starting from the position described hereinbefore for the apical 4-chamber view, tilt the probe

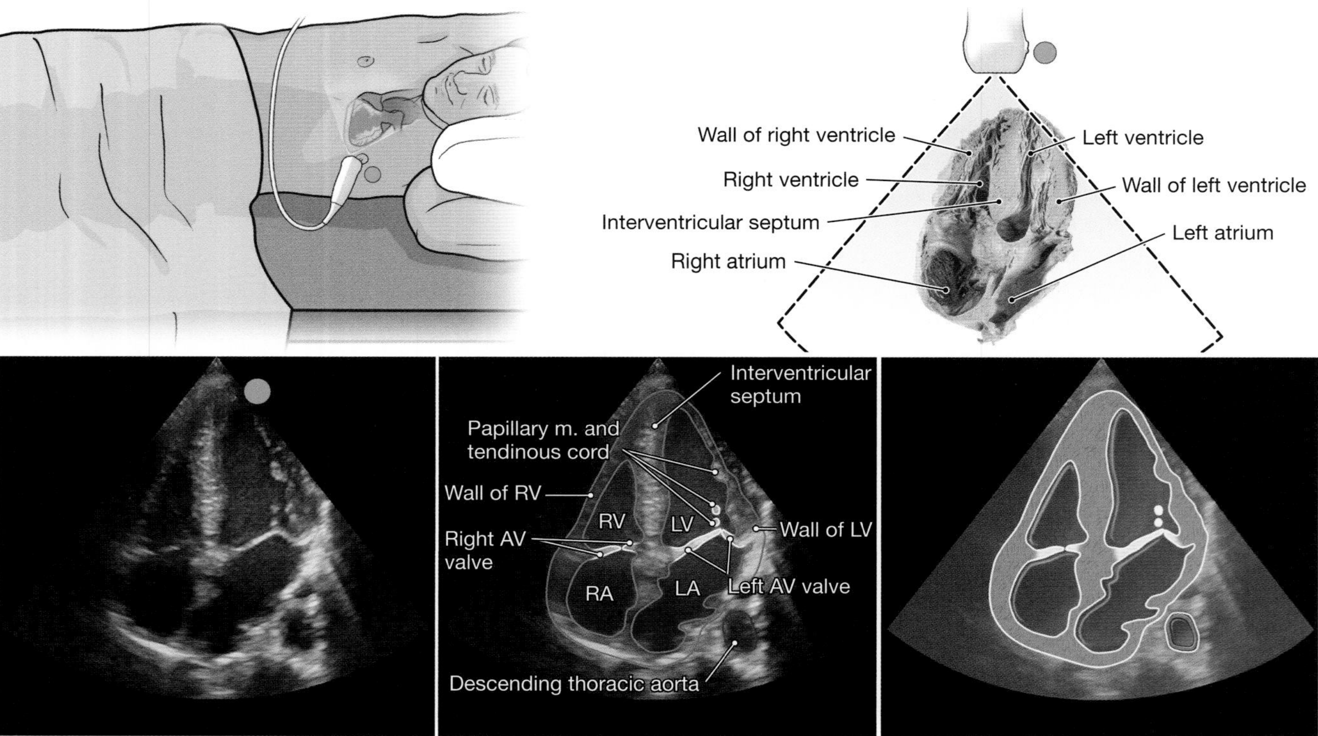

Figure 7.1 Apical 4-chamber view of the heart. LA, left atrium; LV, left ventricle; RA, right atrium; RV, right ventricle.

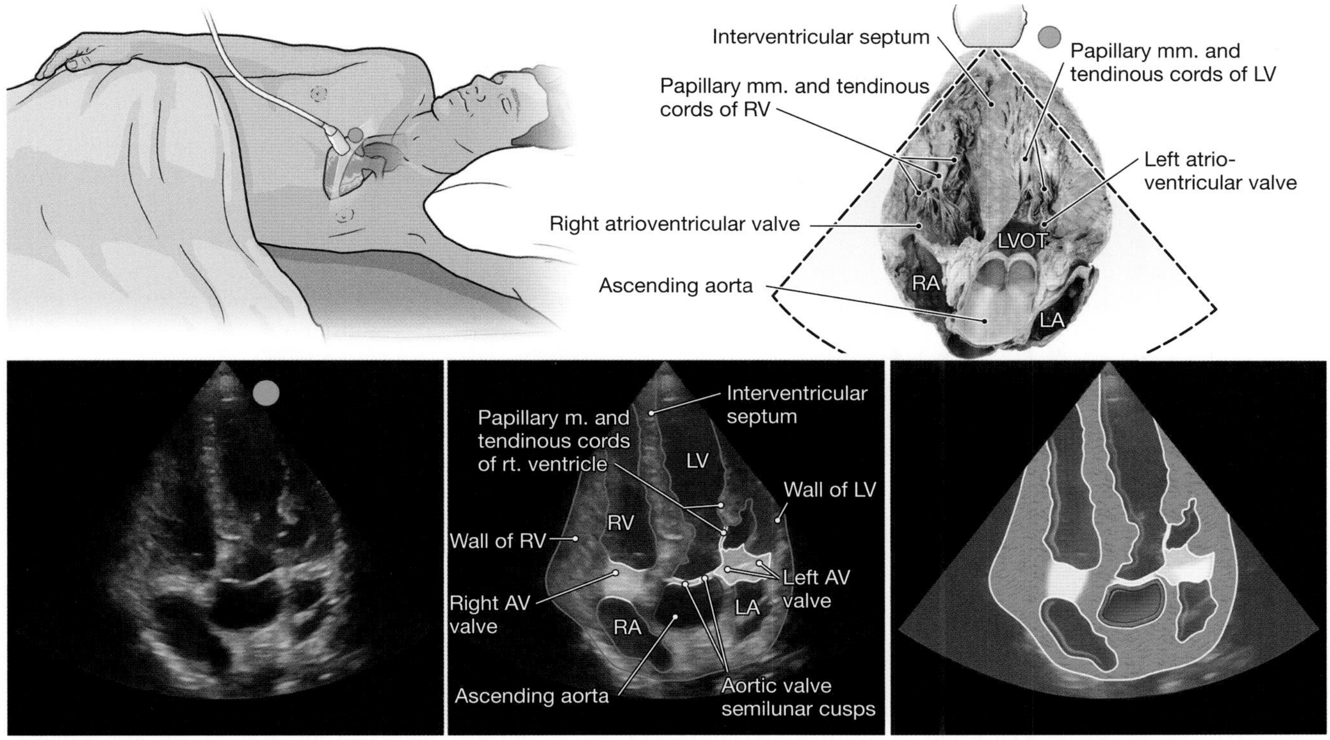

Figure 7.2 Apical 5-chamber view of the heart. LA, left atrium; LV, left ventricle; LVOT, left ventricular outflow tract; RA, right atrium; RV, right ventricle.

so that the US beam is directed increasingly anteriorly (tilting the handle of the probe increasingly closer to the surface of the examination table), until leaflets of the aortic valve and the ascending aorta come into view adjacent to the superior part of the interventricular septum. This is the apical 5-chamber view, in which the outflow tract of the left ventricle, the aortic valve and the ascending aorta comprise the "fifth chamber." Identify leaflets of the aortic valve and the adjacent sinuses of Valsalva. Other structures in this view are similar to those previously identified in the apical 4-chamber view although much of the left atrium is posterior to this imaging plane.

Inferior Vena Cava View

INFERIOR VENA CAVA VIEW
FIG. 7.3

With the patient in the supine position, place the probe (either microconvex phased array or curved array probe) longitudinally oriented (marker directed superiorly with the curved array probe) to the right of the midline under the right costal margin, aiming up toward the thorax. Ask the patient to take deep breaths as needed to identify the liver speckled pattern, portal vein branches and hepatic veins, the retrohepatic course of the IVC, and cardiac movement above the diaphragm wherein the IVC passes through the hiatus for the IVC to open into the right atrium. Observe inspiratory collapse and expiratory filling of the IVC. Note the hepatic veins approaching the IVC a short distance below its opening into the right atrium.

Suprasternal View

SUPRASTERNAL VIEW
FIG. 7.4

To obtain the suprasternal view, the patient should be in a supine position with the head hanging just over the top of the examination table/bed to extend the head/neck as much as possible without causing pain (especially in older patients). A pillow placed under the patient's upper back and shoulders may also be helpful for increasing head extension. Place the probe (microconvex phased array) in the suprasternal notch with the probe marker directed approximately toward the acromion of the left shoulder. This rotation of the probe face posteriorly toward the left helps align the ultrasound beam with the oblique orientation of the ascending aorta, the aortic arch, and the descending aorta, relative to the true coronal plane. Make fine adjustments of probe position and tilt until the aorta comes into the best view from the ascending aorta through the descending aorta. Identify the three arteries of the arch, the brachiocephalic artery, the left common carotid artery, and the left subclavian artery. Under the arch of the aorta, identify the right pulmonary artery.

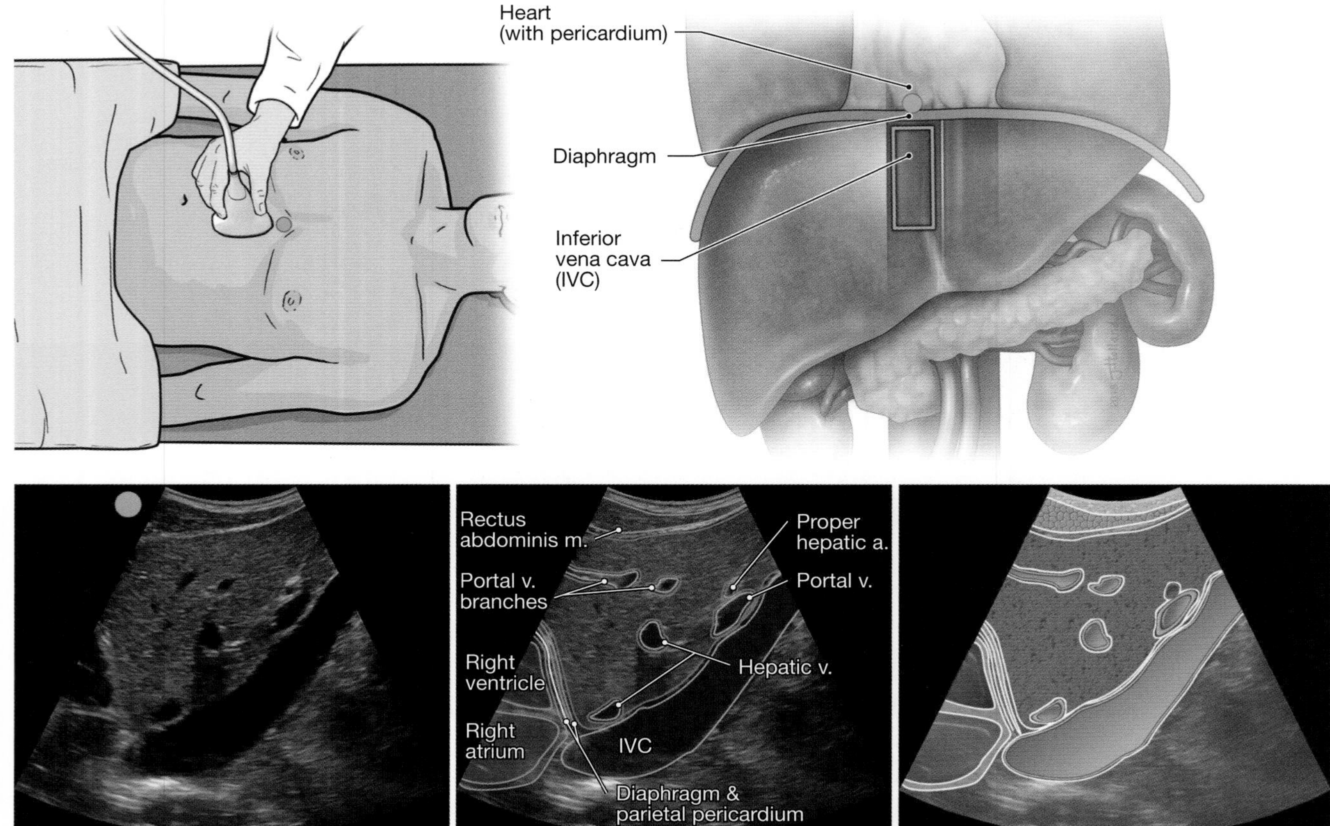

Figure 7.3 Inferior Vena Cava (IVC) view: longitudinal subcostal view of the course of the IVC posterior to the liver and approaching the right atrium (via caval hiatus of diaphragm).

Parasternal Long-Axis View

PARASTERNAL LONG-AXIS VIEW
FIG. 7.5

To obtain the PLAX view, the patient should either be supine or in left lateral decubitus (as needed for improved image quality). Place the probe face just to the left of the sternum in the third, fourth, or fifth intercostal space (most commonly fourth). When the screen marker is on the right side of the display, the marker side of the probe should be directed toward the right shoulder. The nonmarker side of the probe should be pointed toward the patient's right shoulder when the screen marker is on the left of the display image (so that the marker side of the probe is directed toward the 4-o'clock position). This orients the probe/US beam along the long axis of the left ventricle and displays an image as shown in Figure 7.5. Adjust probe position up or down one intercostal space at a time as needed, until an image of the heart as shown in Figure 7.5 can be best seen. In this view, the right ventricle is located more superficially to the top of the image, giving the impression that the right ventricle is sitting on top of the left ventricle. The right atrium is not visible. The posterior free wall of the left ventricle and adjacent posterior wall of the pericardium should be identified in the far field. The left atrium, mitral valve, inflow tract of the left ventricle, outflow tract of the left ventricle, aortic valve, and ascending aorta should be identified. The interventricular septum and outflow tract of the right ventricle should be seen in the near field. The descending thoracic aorta can often be seen just posterior to the left atrium near the position of the mitral valve annulus, and behind the posterior wall of the pericardium. The apex of the left ventricle should be beyond the edge of the display image to the left.

Parasternal Short-Axis View

PARASTERNAL SHORT-AXIS VIEW MID-VENTRICLE
FIG. 7.6

To obtain PSAX views, follow the previous instructions to obtain the "best" long-axis view and then rotate the probe 90° clockwise while keeping the probe in the same position/orientation otherwise. When the screen marker is on the right side of the display, the marker side of the probe should be directed toward the left shoulder. This orients the probe/US beam along the short axis of the

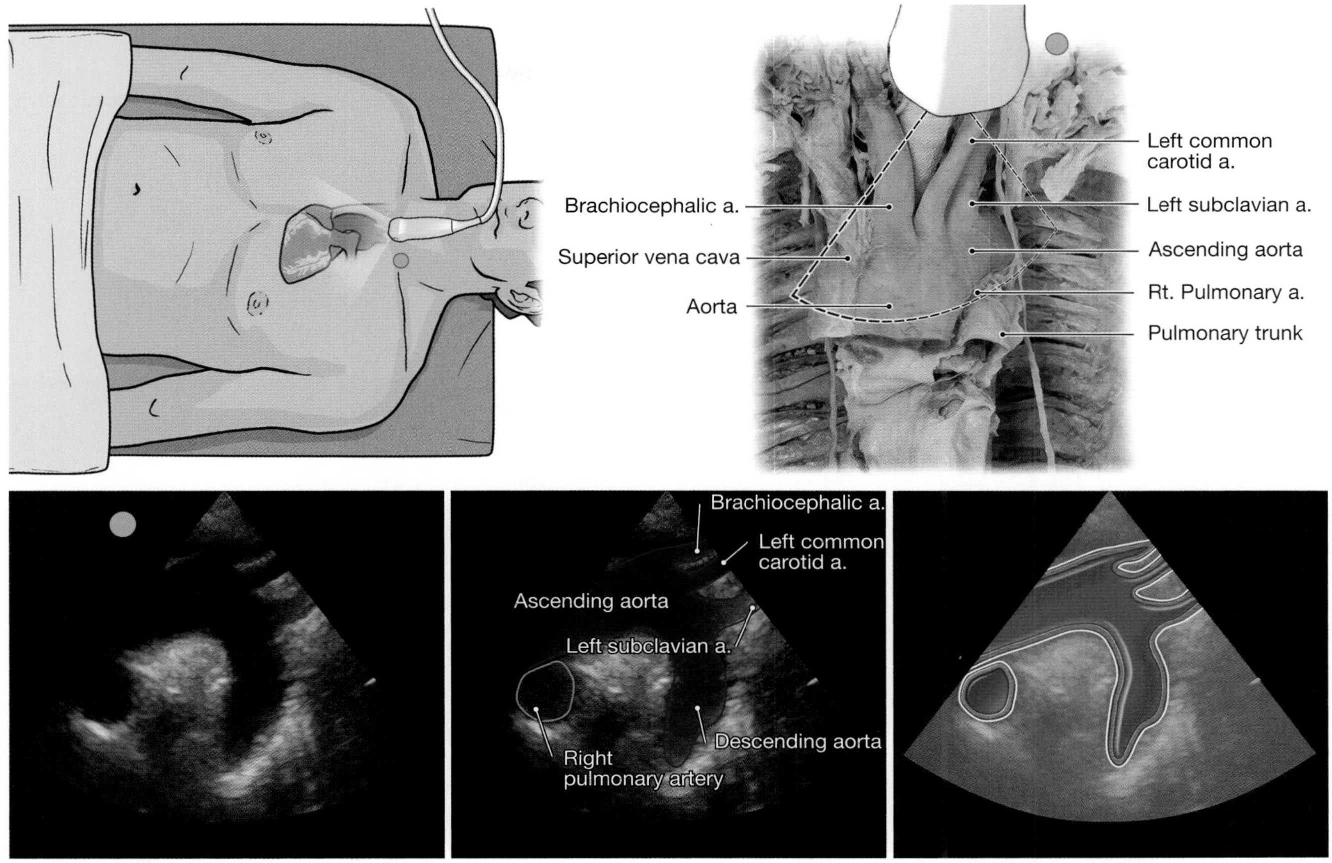

Figure 7.4 Suprasternal view of ascending aorta, aortic arch, brachiocephalic artery, left common carotid artery, left subclavian artery, descending thoracic aorta, and right pulmonary artery.

left ventricle, and the heart is seen in a plane perpendicular to the PLAX as displayed in Figure 7.6. Typically, the view obtained after rotating the probe from the PLAX into the PSAX, with the probe face remaining perpendicular to the chest wall, is the short-axis view at the mid-ventricle level. This is sometimes referred to as the "fish mouth" view due to the appearance of the aortic and mural leaflets of the mitral valve. Make fine adjustments to probe rotation until the left ventricle appears circular in the far field while the crescent-shaped right ventricle can be (partially) seen in the near field. Identify the interventricular septum (normally bowing toward the right ventricle), the left lateral wall of the left ventricle, the posterior wall of the left ventricle, and the posterior wall of the pericardium. Identify the aortic and mural leaflets of the mitral valve and observe their motion during the cardiac cycle. Look for the descending thoracic aorta behind the posterior wall of the pericardium.

PARASTERNAL SHORT-AXIS VIEW PAPILLARY MUSCLES
FIG. 7.7

Starting from the PSAX mid-ventricle view as described hereinbefore, maintain the probe position and rotation while carefully tilting the probe so that the US beam is progressively directed down and to the left, toward the apex of the ventricle (with the handle of the probe tilting toward the right shoulder). As the image moves below the mitral valve leaflets, look for the appearance of papillary muscles of the left ventricle, with one group near the junction of the posterior wall and interventricular septum (inferior papillary muscle) and the other group nearest to the lateral free wall of the ventricle (superior papillary muscle).

PARASTERNAL SHORT-AXIS VIEW AORTIC VALVE BASE OF THE HEART
FIG. 7.8

Continuing from the position described hereinbefore, now slowly tilt the probe so that the US beam is progressively directed superiorly to the right (away from the apex toward the base of the heart). Continue directing the beam toward the heart base as the mid-ventricle "fish-mouth" view returns into view and then beyond the mid-ventricle view until an image like the one shown in Figure 7.8 can be seen. Identify the aortic valve near the center of the image. In this view, the three leaflets of the aortic valve are evident as the aortic valve opens and closes. During closure of the aortic valve the aortic leaflets come together, and this gives the characteristic

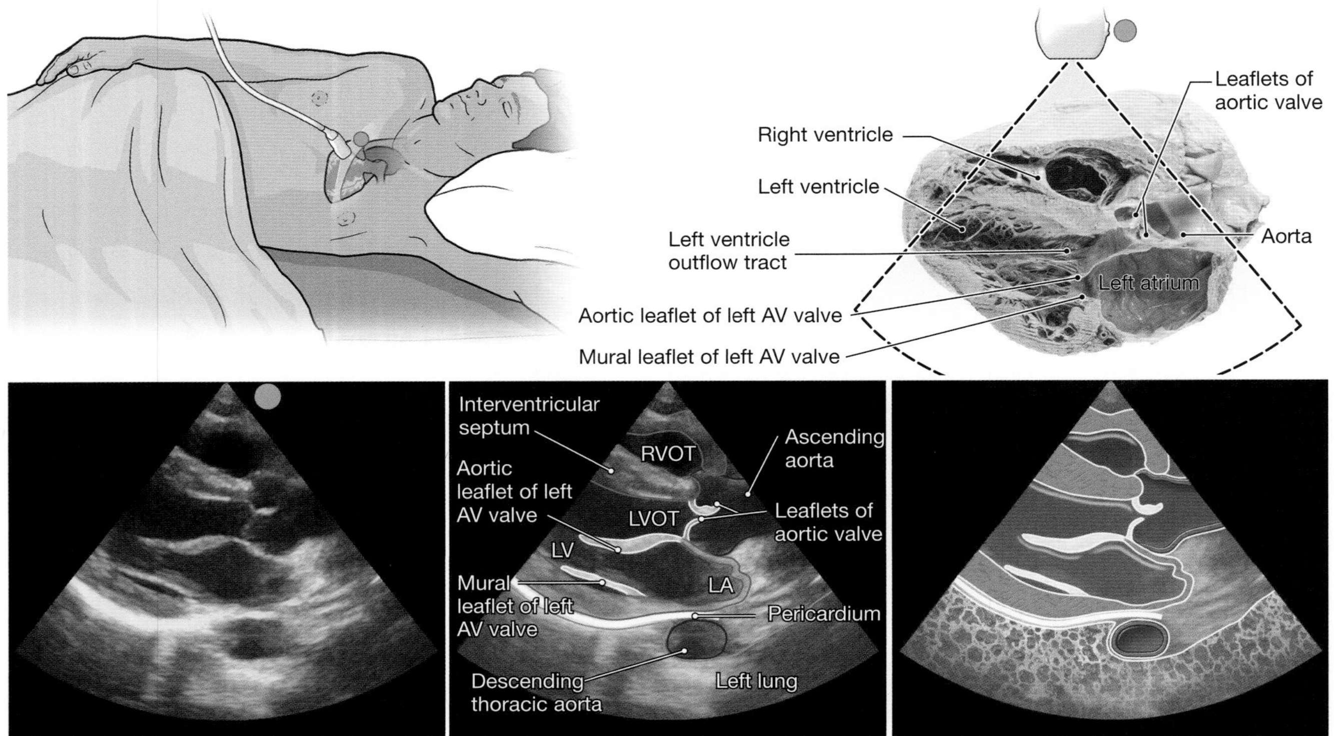

Figure 7.5 Parasternal long-axis view of the heart and pericardium. LA, left atrium; LV, left ventricle; LVOT, left ventricular outflow tract; MV, mitral valve; RVOT, right ventricular outflow tract.

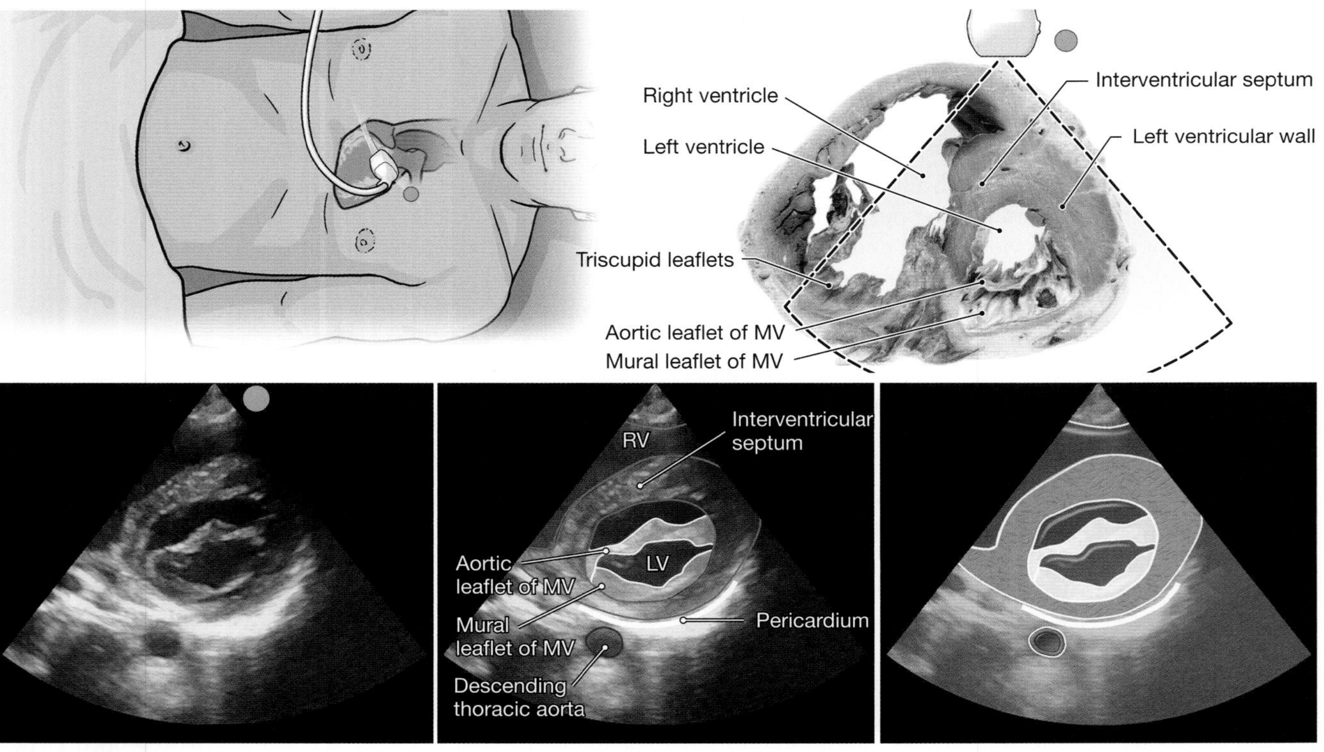

Figure 7.6 Parasternal short-axis view, mid-ventricle level. LV, left ventricle; RV, right ventricle.

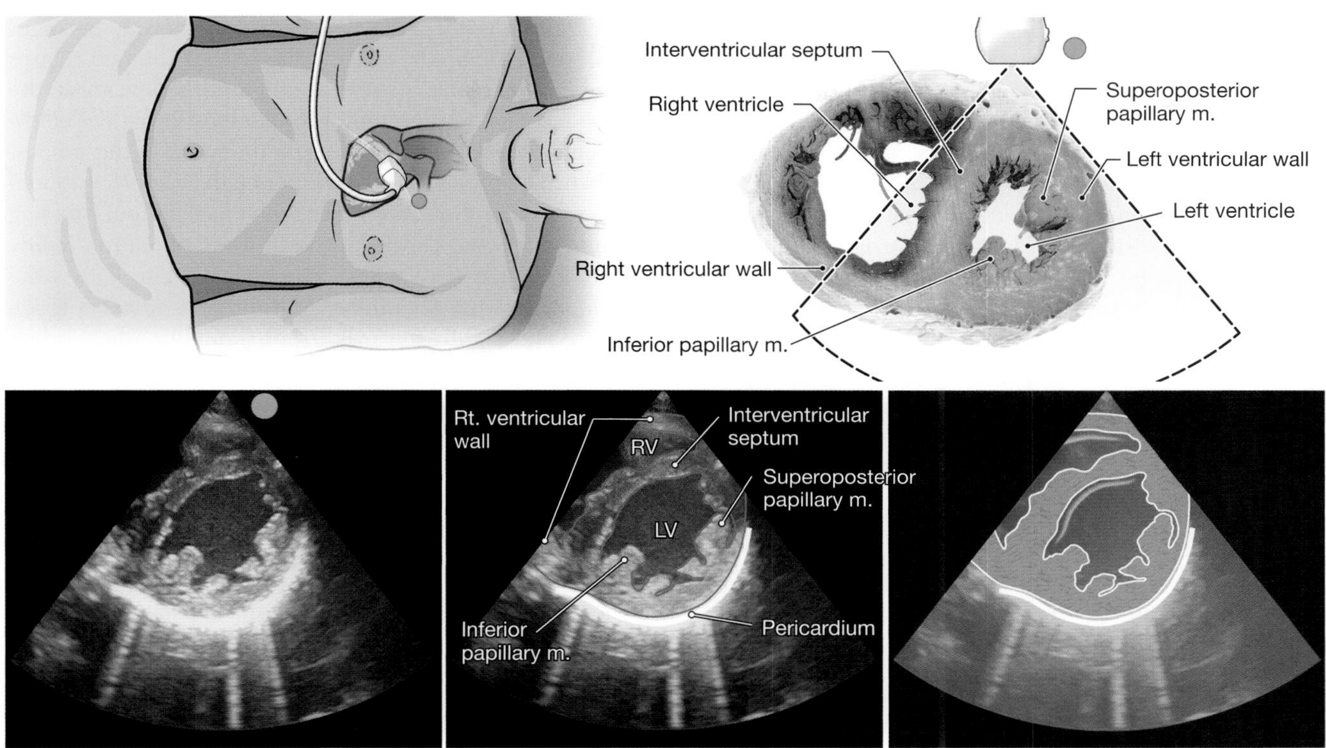

Figure 7.7 Parasternal short-axis view, level of papillary muscles. LV, left ventricle; RV, right ventricle.

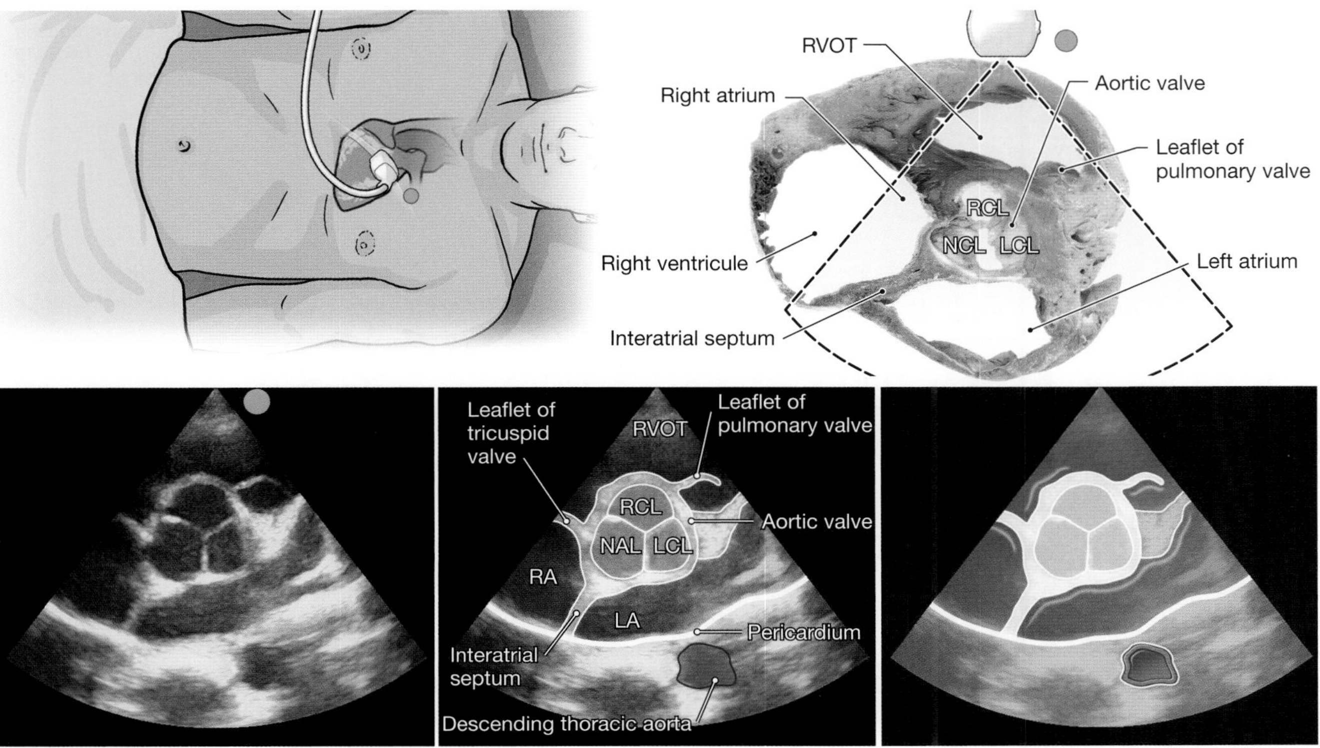

Figure 7.8 Parasternal short-axis view, level of aortic valve. LA, left atrium; RA, right atrium; RVOT, right ventricular outflow tract; LCL, left coronary leaflet; NAL, nonadjacent leaflet; RCL, right coronary leaflet.

appearance of the "Mercedes Benz" sign. The aortic valve possesses three leaflets, the right coronary leaflet, the left coronary leaflet, and the non-adjacent leaflet. The right coronary leaflet is the most anterior leaflet located adjacent to the right ventricle and pulmonary valve. The non-adjacent leaflet is located adjacent to the interatrial septum and the right atrium, and the left coronary leaflet is located in front of the left atrium. Identify the atria and interatrial septum, the septal leaflet of the tricuspid valve, and the right ventricular outflow tract. Often a leaflet of the pulmonary valve can be seen adjacent to the right coronary leaflet of the aortic valve. Beyond the plane of the pulmonary valve is the main pulmonary artery. Look for the descending thoracic aorta located posteriorly to the left atrium and behind the posterior wall of the pericardium.

Subxiphoid View

SUBXIPHOID 4-CHAMBER VIEW
FIG. 7.9

The subxiphoid 4-chamber view uses the liver as a sonographic window to view the heart and pericardium. If the patient can cooperate, flexing the knees to 90° and placing the soles of the feet on the bed relaxes the abdominal musculature. To obtain this view, place the probe face just to the right of the midline 2 to 4 cm below the xiphoid process, depending on the width of the subcostal arch. The probe should be far enough below the xiphoid process so that the sides of the probe face are not pressing against ribs/costal cartilages. Next, exert pressure directly posteriorly, and then with a scooping motion, flatten the probe against the abdominal wall directing the US beam upward and slightly toward the left shoulder. Adjust probe position and tilt until the liver, right and left ventricles, right and left atria, and pericardium can be identified. The right ventricle appears to be on the top of the picture because it is the closest to the probe. If needed, increase the depth setting until the pericardium adjacent to the free wall of the left ventricle can be clearly seen in the far field. If need be, ask the patient to take a deep breath, which brings the heart closer to the probe and improves the image quality.

Note: When a microconvex phased array (cardiac) probe is used, many US units automatically place the

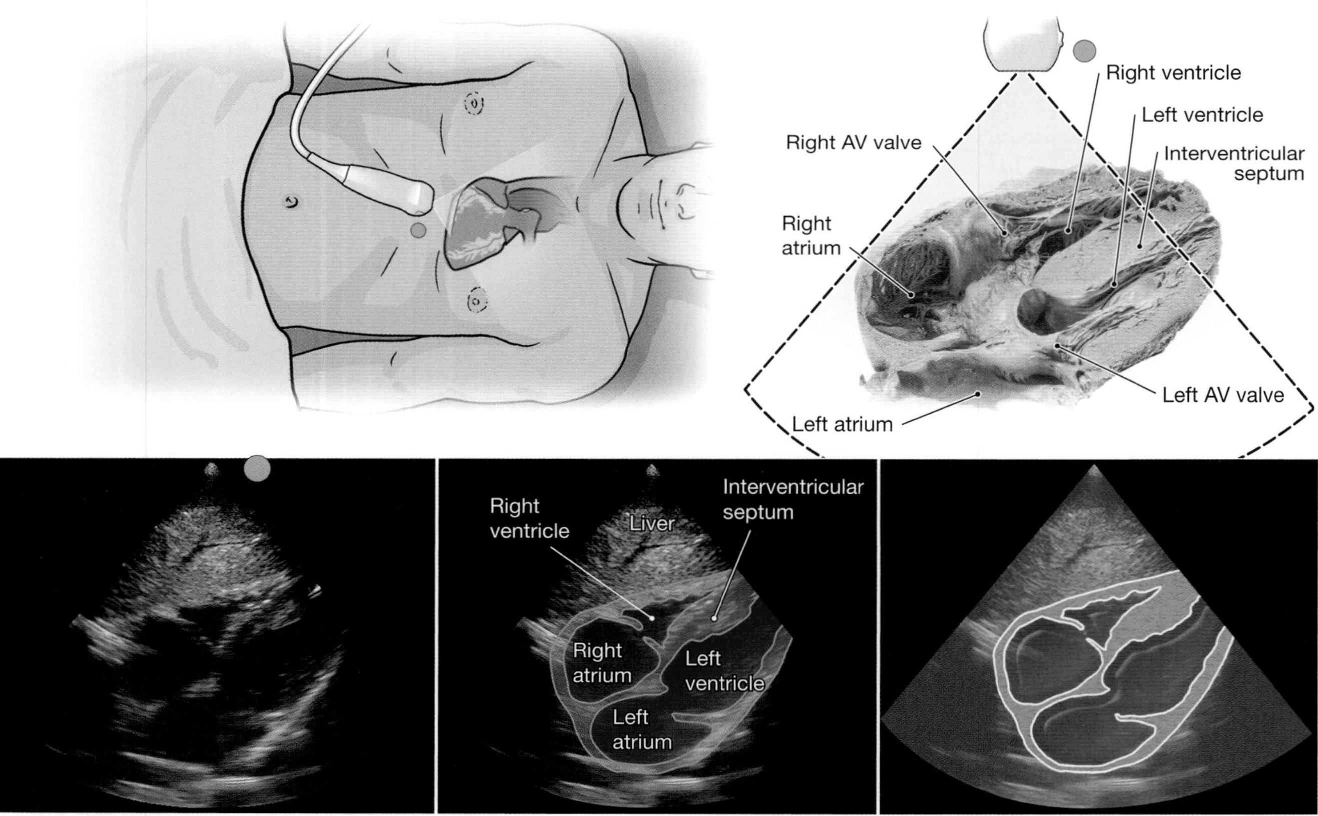

Figure 7.9 Subxiphoid 4-chamber view of the heart and pericardium.

screen marker dot to the right of the screen image rather than to the left of the screen image as in all other applications. If the screen marker dot is on the left of the image as usual, then the marker side of the probe should be directed toward the patient's right axilla to obtain display images as shown in Figure 7.1. If the marker dot is on the right of the screen image, then the marker side of the probe should be directed toward the patient's left flank to obtain the same image orientation on the display.

CLINICAL APPLICATIONS

Echocardiography is used to examine the pericardium, heart, and cardiac valves in a variety of conditions. The extended focused assessment with sonography for trauma (eFAST) examination is used in the setting of blunt and/or penetrating trauma of the thorax and abdomen. The subxiphoid 4-chamber view or the PLAX view are commonly used in the eFAST examination to determine whether there is free fluid accumulating in the pericardial space (hemopericardium or pericardial effusion). The **eFAST examination** and the potential findings are discussed in detail in Chapter 12.

Cardiac tamponade is the compression of the heart that occurs when the pericardial sac, which resists sudden distention, contains excessive fluid or blood. When an excess of fluid is present, the heart is unable to fill properly in diastole; therefore, cardiac output is compromised. In addition to observing fluid accumulation in the pericardial space, diastolic collapse of the right ventricle can be observed with US in the setting of cardiac tamponade.

The contraction of the ventricles can be observed in real time with US, allowing for detection of global or focal wall motion abnormalities such as those produced by coronary artery disease or ventricular failure. Doppler technologies are used to observe regurgitant flow across incompetent valves and to measure systolic flow velocity across stenotic valves. **Pericardiocentesis** is the removal of fluid from the pericardial sac so as to relieve the problem of tamponade. Although it can be performed using landmarks alone, US-guided pericardiocentesis allows for visualization of the effusion, as well as the needle path and guidewire during the procedure, and has been shown to reduce clinical errors such as pneumothorax. US can also be used for detecting the presence of atrial mural thrombi and cardiac tumors such as left atrial myxomas. The IVC view is used for measuring the diameter of the IVC and to quantify inspiratory collapse of the IVC, for estimation of central venous pressure. The suprasternal view can be used in the evaluation of thoracic aortic aneurysm and dissection, and in the evaluation of aortic valve regurgitation (Doppler flow velocity/direction).

7 Heart

Multiple Choice Questions

1. A 65-year-old man is brought to the emergency department 30 minutes after he had an episode of intense chest pain. He describes the pain as retrosternal, radiating to the left side of his neck and shoulder and down to the medial aspect of his left arm. There is no family history of heart disease. His temperature is 98.6 °F (37 °C), pulse is 100/min, respirations are 22/min, and blood pressure is 130/80 mm Hg. Physical examination also shows a slight rhythmic pulsation on the chest wall at the left fifth intercostal space near the midclavicular line. Which of the following structures is most likely responsible for this pulsation?

   A. Aortic arch
   B. Mitral valve
   C. Right atrium
   D. Left atrium
   E. Apex of the heart

2. A 60-year-old man is brought to the emergency department with his wife because of a 3-week history of progressively worsening difficulty in breathing. He has no prior history of hospitalizations or any major illness. Physical examination shows moderate respiratory distress. An ultrasound examination of his heart shows severe aortic valve prolapse. At which of the following locations is auscultation of this valve best performed?

   A. Directly over the middle of the manubrium
   B. Left fifth intercostal space, just below the nipple
   C. Right lower part of the body of the sternum
   D. Right second intercostal space near the lateral border of the sternum
   E. Left second intercostal space near the lateral border of the sternum

3. A 65-year-old man is brought to the emergency department 30 minutes after he had an episode of intense chest pain. He describes the pain as retrosternal, radiating to the left side of his neck and shoulder and down to the medial aspect of his left arm. There is no family history of heart disease. His temperature is 98.6 °F (37 °C), pulse is 100/min, respirations are 22/min, and blood pressure is 130/80 mm Hg. Electrocardiography shows myocardial infarction of the anterior right ventricular wall. Which of the following arteries is most likely to be occluded?

   A. Anterior interventricular artery
   B. Inferior interventricular artery
   C. Circumflex
   D. Marginal branch of the right coronary artery
   E. Conal branch of right coronary artery

4. A 42-year-old woman is brought to the emergency department because of a 2-day history of severe chest pain, dyspnea, tachycardia, cough, and fever. An ultrasound examination shows pericardial effusion, and a pericardiocentesis is performed via the infrasternal angle. The patient is agitated and constantly moves. The needle pierces the visceral pericardium and enters the heart. Which of the following cardiac chambers would be the first to be penetrated by the needle?

   A. Right ventricle
   B. Left ventricle
   C. Right atrium
   D. Left atrium
   E. The left cardiac apex

5. A 70-year-old man is brought to the emergency department because of 2-day history of high fever, chills, and chest pain. Physical examination shows a holosystolic murmur that radiates toward the axilla. Two sets of blood cultures are positive for *Staphylococcus aureus*. A transesophageal echo is performed and an ultrasound probe is placed in the mid-esophagus with the probe facing surface directed toward the vertebral column. Which of the following valves is immediately posterior to the probe facing surface?

   A. Mitral
   B. Aortic
   C. Tricuspid
   D. Pulmonary
   E. Valve of IVC (Eustachian)

6. A 70-year-old man is brought to the emergency department because of 2-day history of high fever, chills, and chest pain. Physical examination shows a holosystolic murmur that radiates toward the axilla. Two sets of blood cultures are positive for *Staphylococcus aureus*. A transesophageal echo is performed and an ultrasound probe is placed in the mid-esophagus with the probe facing surface directed toward the sternum. Which of the following structures is immediately posterior to the probe facing surface?

   A. Mitral valve
   B. Aortic valve
   C. Left Atrium
   D. Azygos vein
   E. Right atrium

8

Abdomen

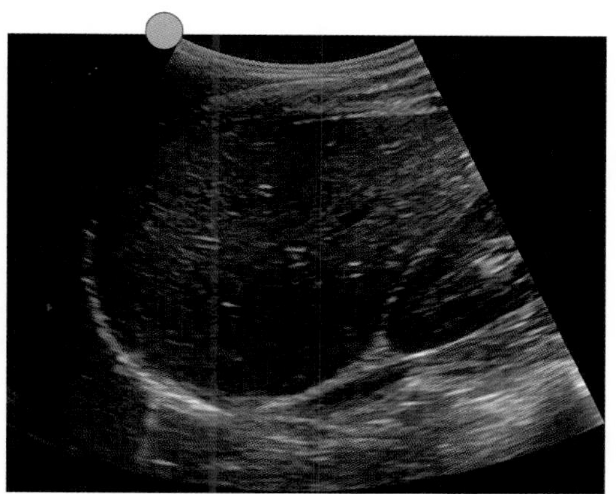

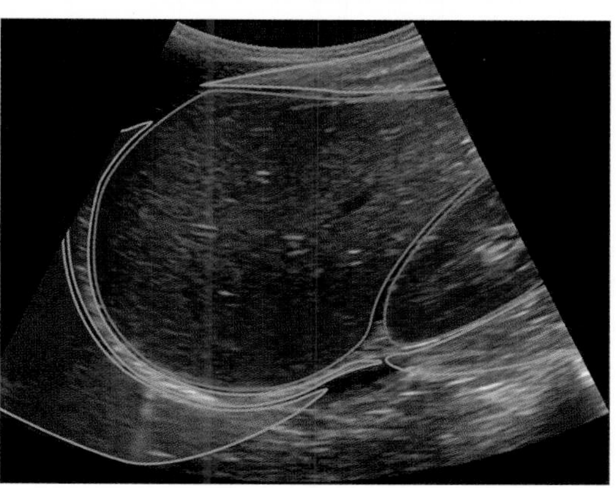

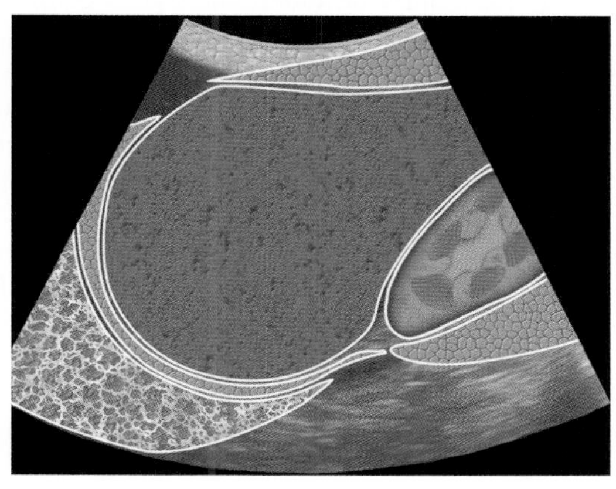

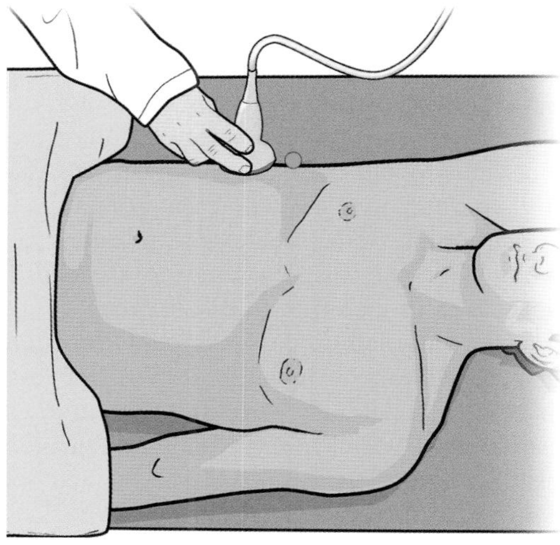

Abdominal Wall

Review of the Anatomy

Anterior Abdominal Wall

The abdominal wall is separated topographically into nine divisions by two longitudinal and two transverse planes. These divisions are the right hypochondriac, epigastric, left hypochondriac, right lumbar, umbilical, left lumbar, right inguinal (iliac), hypogastric (pubic), and left inguinal (iliac). In addition, the abdominal wall can also be segregated into right and left upper quadrants and right and left lower quadrants via vertical and horizontal planes that form four quadrants. The abdominal wall is composed of skin, subcutaneous tissue, fat, muscles, and their **aponeuroses** and deep fascia, extra-peritoneal fat, and parietal peritoneum.

Fasciae, Ligaments, and Muscles

The fascia of the anterior abdominal wall is composed of superficial and deep layers. The superficial layer is composed of a superficial fatty layer (Camper fascia), a deep membranous layer (Scarpa fascia), and a further layer of adipose tissue deep to membranous layer. **Camper fascia** lies over the inguinal ligament and merges with the superficial fascia of the thigh. It continues over the pubis and perineum as the superficial layer of the superficial perineal fascia. The deep membranous layer **Scarpa fascia** becomes continuous with the membranous layer of the superficial fascia of the perineum (**Colle fascia**).

The deep fascia continues over the spermatic cord at the superficial inguinal ring by conjoining with the external spermatic fascia. The deep fascia also connects with the deep fascia of the penis, known as **Buck fascia**, located over the penis, and extends over the pubis and perineum as the deep perineal fascia.

Another important fascial layer is the transversalis fascia that lies between the deep surface of the transversus abdominis muscle and the extraperitoneal fat. Anteriorly, it blends superiorly with the fascia that covers the inferior portion of respiratory diaphragm and inferiorly becomes continuous with the iliac and pelvic parietal fasciae. Posteriorly, it fuses with the anterior layer of the thoracolumbar fascia. Internally, it passes through the deep inguinal ring and continues as the internal spermatic fascia.

There are five bilaterally paired muscles in the anterolateral abdominal wall. Of these muscles, three are flat muscles, including the external abdominal oblique, internal abdominal oblique, and transversus abdominis. Two muscle groups are vertically oriented, the rectus abdominis and pyramidalis. The muscle fibers of the three flat muscles are oriented in a diagonal and perpendicular fashion to each other. These three flat muscles extend anteriorly and medially as well-fortified sheetlike aponeuroses. The fusion of the aponeuroses of the external abdominal oblique, internal abdominal oblique, and transversus abdominis muscles forms a midline avascular connective tissue white line known as the **linea alba**. The linea alba is positioned between the two rectus abdominis muscles and stretches from the xiphoid process to the pubic symphysis. A curved line along the lateral border of the rectus abdominis is called the linea semilunaris. A crescent-shaped line called the linea semicircularis or arcuate line forms the lower border of the posterior layer of the rectus sheath located inferior to the level of the iliac crest. The fusion of the aponeuroses of the external abdominal oblique, internal abdominal oblique, and transversus abdominis muscles form the **rectus sheath**. It surrounds the rectus abdominis and occasionally the pyramidalis muscle. It also contains the superior and inferior epigastric vessels and the ventral primary rami of thoracic nerves 7 to 12. Superior to the arcuate line, the anterior layer of the rectus sheath is formed by the aponeuroses of the external and internal abdominal oblique muscles and by the aponeuroses of the external, internal abdominal oblique, and transversus abdominis muscles inferior to the arcuate line. The posterior layer of the rectus sheath is formed by the aponeuroses of the internal abdominal oblique and the transverse muscles above the arcuate line. The rectus abdominis connects to the transversalis fascia below the arcuate line.

Inguinal Region

The inguinal (Hesselbach) triangle is bounded medially by the linea semilunaris, laterally by the inferior epigastric vessels, and inferiorly by the inguinal ligament. The superficial inguinal ring is a triangular opening in the aponeurosis of the external abdominal oblique muscle located lateral to the pubic tubercle. However, the deep inguinal ring is found in the transversalis fascia, located lateral to the inferior epigastric vessels. The **inguinal canal** starts at the deep inguinal ring and continues to the superficial ring where it terminates. This canal carries the spermatic cord or the round ligament of the uterus and the genital branch of the genitofemoral nerve. Both these structures travel through the deep inguinal ring and the inguinal canal. Although the ilioinguinal nerve is carried through a portion of the inguinal canal and the superficial inguinal ring, it does not travel through the deep inguinal ring. The anterior wall of the inguinal canal is created by the aponeuroses of the external and internal abdominal oblique muscles. The posterior wall is formed by the aponeurosis of the transversus abdominis muscle and transversalis fascia. The superior surface (roof) is formed by arching fibers of the internal abdominal oblique and transversus abdominis muscles. The inferior surface (floor) is formed by the inguinal and lacunar ligaments.

Nerves

The anterior and anterolateral abdominal wall is innervated by the anterior divisions of the 7th to 11th intercostal nerves, known as thoracoabdominal nerves. In addition, the inferior segment of the anterolateral wall is supplied by additional nerves including the subcostal, iliohypogastric, and ilioinguinal nerves. The subcostal nerve is the ventral ramus of the 12th thoracic nerve that innervates the muscles of the anterior abdominal wall. The iliohypogastric nerve emerges from the first lumbar nerve and innervates the internal oblique and transverse muscles of the abdomen. It subsequently branches into a lateral cutaneous branch to supply the skin of the lateral side of the buttocks and hips and an anterior cutaneous branch to supply the skin superior to the pubic symphysis. The ilioinguinal nerve arises from the first lumbar nerve and pierces the internal oblique muscle near the deep inguinal ring. It travels alongside the spermatic cord through the inguinal canal and superficial inguinal ring to innervate the internal abdominal oblique and transversus abdominis muscles. In addition, the ilioinguinal nerve contributes to giving off the femoral branch, which innervates the upper and medial parts of the anterior thigh, and the anterior scrotal nerve, which innervates the skin of the root of the penis (or the skin of the mons pubis) and the anterior portion of the scrotum (or the labium majus).

Vasculature

The superior epigastric artery emerges from the internal thoracic artery, enters the rectus sheath, and courses inferiorly on the posterior border of the rectus abdominis to eventually join with the inferior epigastric artery within the rectus abdominis. The inferior epigastric artery emerges from the external iliac artery superior to the inguinal ligament and enters the rectus sheath to ascend between the rectus abdominis and the posterior layer of the rectus sheath. The inferior epigastric artery subsequently joins with the superior epigastric artery and supplies collateral circulation between the subclavian and external iliac arteries. It also branches into the cremasteric artery, which travels alongside the spermatic cord. The superficial epigastric artery branches from the femoral artery and courses superiorly toward the umbilicus over the inguinal ligament to become continuous with branches of the inferior epigastric artery. The thoracoepigastric veins are longitudinal venous connections between the lateral thoracic vein and the superficial epigastric vein.

Lymphatic Drainage

Lymphatics in the area superior to the umbilicus empty into the axillary lymph nodes. The lymphatics in the area below the umbilicus empty into the superficial inguinal nodes. The superficial inguinal lymph nodes obtain lymph from the lower abdominal wall, buttocks, penis, scrotum, labium majus, and the lower parts of the vagina and anal canal. Their efferent vessels predominately gain access to the external iliac nodes and, ultimately, the lumbar (aortic) nodes.

Technique

Rectus Abdominis and Rectus Sheath

RECTUS ABDOMINIS
RECTUS SHEATH
Transverse
FIG. 8.1

With the patient in the supine position and properly draped, place the probe centered at the midline, midway between the xiphoid and the umbilicus. Identify the skin, hyperechoic anterior layer of rectus abdominis muscles, posterior layer of rectus sheath, and transversalis fascia. Identify the centered echogenic linea alba between the medial edges of the right and left rectus abdominis muscles. Trace the thin layer of hypoechoic extraperitoneal fat between the transversalis fascia and parietal peritoneum.

External Abdominal Oblique, Internal Abdominal Oblique, and Transversus Abdominus

EXTERNAL ABDOMINAL OBLIQUE INTERNAL ABDOMINAL OBLIQUE TRANSVERSUS ABDOMINIS
Transverse
FIG. 8.2

With the patient in the supine position and properly draped, place the probe about midway between the xiphoid process and the umbilicus, just lateral to the lateral edge of the rectus abdominis muscle at the linea semilunaris. Slide the probe medially until the rectus abdominis is

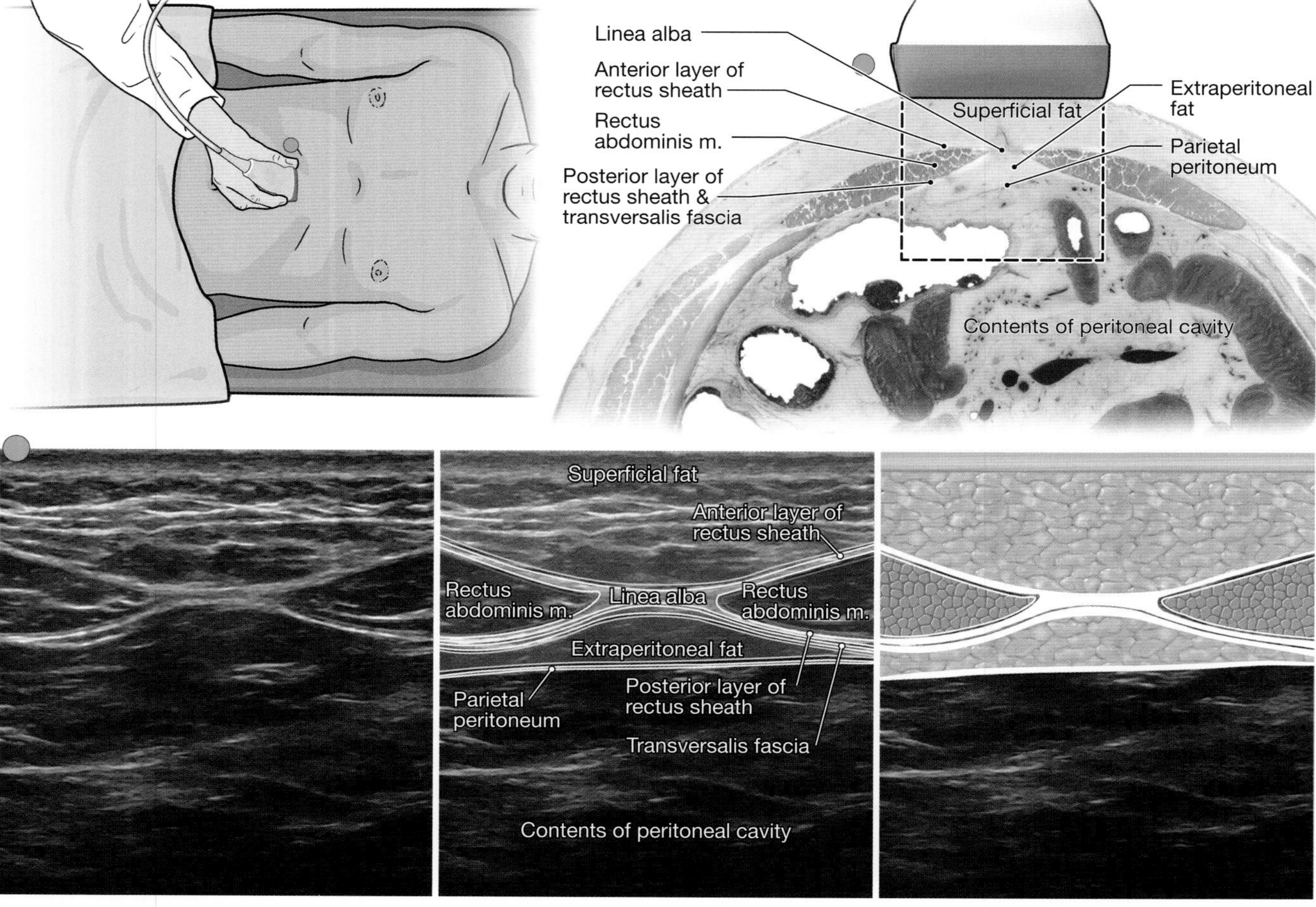

Figure 8.1 Normal transverse view, about midway between the xiphoid process and the umbilicus, of the rectus abdominis muscles, rectus sheath, linea alba, transversalis fascia, extraperitoneal fat, and parietal peritoneum.

identified, then slide back laterally until the rectus muscle disappears just off the screen image. Adjust the probe and tilt and angle until the three layers of the abdominal wall muscles are clearly visible. Adjust the probe as necessary and angle to visualize the hyperechoic transversalis fascia and parietal peritoneum at the deep surface of the transversus abdominis muscle. Note the hyperechoic reflection and shadowing from gas in the gastrointestinal track deep to the parietal peritoneum.

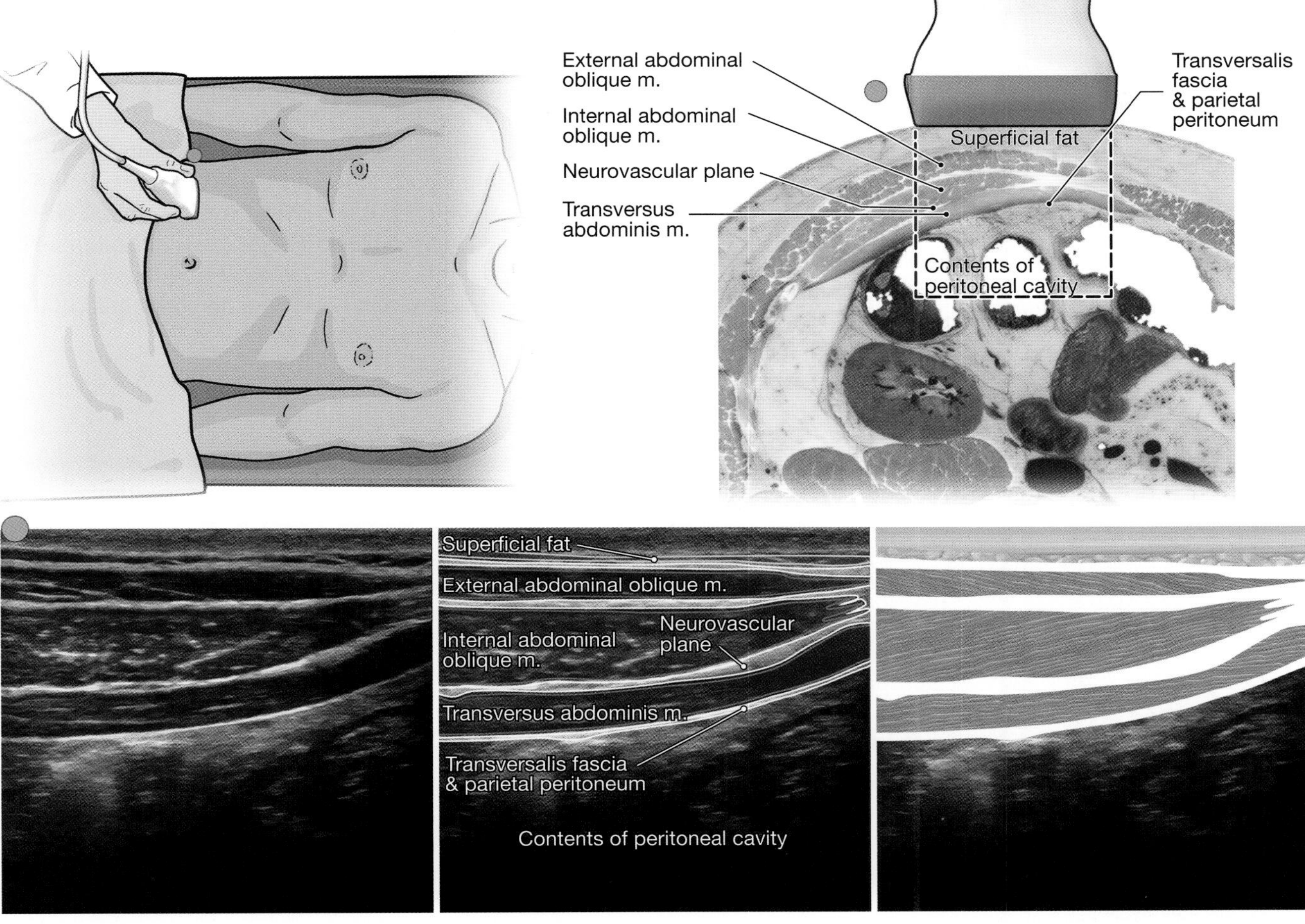

Figure 8.2 Normal transverse view, midway between the xiphoid process and umbilicus, of the external abdominal oblique, transversus abdominis, transversalis fascia, and parietal peritoneum.

CLINICAL APPLICATIONS

Hernias

Epigastric hernia is a type of hernia situated at the anterolateral abdominal wall in which extraperitoneal fat or portion of the greater omentum or portion of the small intestines protrude through a defect in the linea alba superior to the umbilicus. Complications of such herniation include strangulation or incarceration of the small intestines.

Spigelian hernia (lateral ventral hernia) is a type of hernia of the anterolateral abdominal wall situated at the semilunar line. The diagnosis of a Spigelian hernia is confirmed with ultrasound (US) or computed tomography scan. The clinical presentation is dependent on the composition of the hernial sac and the degree and type of herniation. The most common presenting symptom is pain. **Incisional hernia** is another subtype of the anterolateral abdominal wall hernia, wherein the abdominal viscera extends out of a defect in the abdominal wall resulting from surgery or trauma. These types of hernias commonly occur after open abdominal operations in about 5% to 15% of patients. It has also been found that the incidence of very large or giant hernias increases with increases in the obesity of the population and the complexity of abdominal surgeries.

Transversus Abdominis Plane Block

Transversus abdominis plane block (TAPB) is a US-guided block that is typically used for blocking T9 to T10 nerves. TAPB with US guidance is used for accurately guiding the needle bevel into a plane between the internal abdominal oblique and transversus abdominis muscles to provide local anesthetic for abdominal wall incisions medial to the block. This block is indicated for several surgical procedures such as hernia repair, open appendectomy, caesarian section, total abdominal hysterectomy, and radical prostatectomy.

Peritoneum, Gastrointestinal Tract, and Liver

Review of the Anatomy

Peritoneum and Peritoneal Cavity

The peritoneum is formed by a serous membrane, which consists of mesothelial cells. It has two parts, the parietal and the visceral peritoneum. The parietal peritoneum lies over the abdominal and pelvic walls and the inferior aspect of the diaphragm, whereas the visceral peritoneum drapes over the abdominal viscera.

The parietal and visceral layers of the peritoneum form a potential space enabling the free movement of the abdominal viscera. The peritoneal cavity in males is a closed cavity; however, in females the peritoneal cavity is open through the vagina, uterine tubes, and uterus wherein it contains a small amount of peritoneal fluid. The peritoneum is innervated by the phrenic, lower intercostal, subcostal, iliohypogastric, and ilioinguinal nerves, which causes it to be sensitive to pain, in contrast to visceral peritoneum, which is insensitive to pain.

The parietal and visceral peritoneum create peritoneal reflections across the abdominal viscera. These reflections are the lesser and greater omenta, mesentery proper, transverse and sigmoid mesocolon, and the mesoappendix.

The **lesser omentum** is a dual layer of peritoneum from the porta hepatis of the liver and continues to the lesser curvature of the stomach and the beginning of the duodenum. The hepatogastric and hepatoduodenal ligaments compose the lesser omentum. They also form the anterior wall of the lesser sac of the peritoneal cavity and transmit the left and right gastric vessels, which course within the two layers along the lesser curvature. The lesser omentum has a free right margin that accommodates the proper hepatic artery, bile duct, and portal vein.

The **greater omentum** suspends down from the greater curvature of the stomach, draping over the transverse colon and other abdominal viscera. It transmits the right and left gastroomental vessels along the greater curvature of the stomach and seals the neck of a hernial sac, preventing the coils of the small intestine from entering the space. The greater omentum attaches to the regions of inflammation and encases itself around inflamed organs, thus preventing serious diffuse peritonitis.

The greater omentum is often defined to encompass the following peritoneal ligaments: gastrosplenic, gastrophrenic, and gastrocolic. The splenorenal ligament is also considered by some authors as part of the greater omentum. The gastrosplenic ligament stretches from the left portion of the greater curvature of the stomach to the hilus of the spleen and contains the short gastric and left gastroomental vessels. The gastrophrenic ligament travels from the upper surface of the greater curvature of the stomach to the diaphragm. The gastrocolic ligament runs from the greater curvature of the stomach to the transverse colon. Finally, the splenorenal ligament travels from the hilum of the spleen to the left kidney and holds the splenic vessels and the tail of the pancreas.

The mesentery of the small intestine or mesentery proper is a doublefold of the peritoneum that supports the jejunum and the ileum from the posterior abdominal wall and carries nerves, blood vessels, and lymphatics to and from the small intestine. It forms a root that stretches from the duodenojejunal flexure to the right iliac fossa. It has a free border that surrounds the small intestine and includes the superior mesenteric and intestinal (jejunal and ileal) vessels, nerves, and lymphatics.

The transverse mesocolon adjoins the posterior surface of the transverse colon to the posterior abdominal wall. It combines with the greater omentum to form the gastrocolic ligament and encloses the middle colic vessels, nerves, and lymphatics. The sigmoid mesocolon links the sigmoid colon to the pelvic wall and encompasses the sigmoid vessels. The mesoappendix connects the appendix to the mesentery of the ileum and contains the appendicular vessels.

The phrenicocolic ligament travels from the left colic flexure to the diaphragm.

The falciform ligament is a peritoneal fold that adheres the liver to the diaphragm and the anterior abdominal wall. It also contains the round ligament of the liver and the paraumbilical vein, which adjoin the left branch of the portal vein with the subcutaneous veins at the umbilicus.

The round ligament of the liver (ligamentum teres) lies in the free margin of the falciform ligament and travels superiorly from the umbilicus to the inferior (visceral) surface of the liver, lying in the fissure that forms the left boundary of the quadrate lobe of the liver. Embryologically, it is a remnant of the left umbilical vein, which carries oxygenated blood from the placenta to the left branch of the portal vein in the fetus. (The right umbilical vein is obliterated during the embryonic period.)

The coronary ligament is a peritoneal reflection, which originates from the diaphragmatic border of the liver onto the diaphragm and encloses a triangular area of the right lobe. It has right and left extensions that create the right and left triangular ligaments.

The ligamentum venosum is an embryological remnant of the ductus venosus. It is fibrous in nature and is situated in the fissure on the inferior portion of the liver, which forms the left boundary of the caudate lobe of the liver.

The umbilical folds are five folds of the peritoneum below the umbilicus, including the median, medial, and lateral umbilical folds. The rectouterine fold courses from the cervix of the uterus, along the side of the rectum, to the posterior pelvic wall, which creates the rectouterine pouch (of Douglas). The ileocecal fold extends from the terminal ileum to the cecum.

Gastrointestinal Viscera

Stomach

The stomach is completely draped over by the peritoneum and is located in the left hypochondriac and epigastric regions. The stomach has a greater and lesser curvature, anterior and posterior walls, cardiac and pyloric openings, and cardiac and angular notches. It is divided into 4 sections: cardia, fundus, body, and pylorus.

The cardia is the part of the stomach surrounding the cardiac orifice. The *fundus* is the area of the stomach inferior to the apex of the heart at the left diaphragmatic dome, at the level of the fifth rib. The body occupies the major part of the stomach and is the area between the fundus and the pyloric antrum. The *pylorus* is further subdivided into the pyloric antrum and pyloric canal. The pyloric orifice is encompassed by the pyloric sphincter, which is a band of thickened circular smooth muscle that controls the rate of release of stomach contents into the duodenum. Constriction of the sphincter is regulated by sympathetic stimulation and relaxed by parasympathetic action. The stomach receives arterial supply from the right and left gastric, right and left gastroomental, and short gastric arteries. As the stomach experiences contraction, it is distinguished by the appearance of longitudinal folds of mucous membrane, known as **rugae**. The gastric canal, a grooved channel along the lesser curvature formed by the rugae, directs fluids toward the pylorus. The stomach also yields hydrochloric acid and a protein-digesting enzyme, pepsin, in its fundus and body. In addition, it synthesizes the hormone gastrin, which stimulates the release of gastric acid in the pyloric antrum via parasympathetic fibers from the vagus nerve.

Small Intestine

The small intestine extends from the pyloric aperture to the ileocecal junction. The process of complete digestion and absorption of contents of digestion and water, electrolytes, and minerals such as calcium and iron take place in the small intestine. The small intestine is divided into three regions: duodenum, jejunum, and ileum.

Duodenum

The duodenum is a C-shaped tube surrounding the head of the pancreas. Among the other three regions, the duodenum is the shortest (25 cm long or 12 fingerbreadths in length) but the widest portion of the small intestine. Other than the proximal portion of the duodenum, the remainder is retroperitoneal. The proximal region is connected to the liver by the hepatoduodenal ligament of the lesser omentum. The arterial supply of the duodenum is from branches of the celiac and superior mesenteric arteries.

The duodenum is divided into four parts:

1. ***Superior (first) part:*** This portion has a mobile section, known as the duodenal cap, into which the pylorus retracts.
2. ***Descending (second) part:*** This contains the juncture of the foregut and midgut, where the common bile and the main pancreatic ducts open. It also contains the greater papilla, where the terminal ends of the bile and the main pancreatic ducts are located, and the lesser papilla, which lies 2 cm above the greater papilla and marks the opening of the accessory pancreatic duct.
3. ***Transverse (third) part:*** This is the longest part, and it traverses the inferior vena cava (IVC), aorta, and vertebral column to the left. It is intersected anteriorly by the superior mesenteric vessels.
4. ***Ascending (fourth) part:*** This part of the duodenum ascends to the left of the aorta to the level of the second lumbar vertebra and stops at the duodenojejunal junction, which is fixed in position by the suspensory ligament of Treitz, a surgical landmark. This fibromuscular band is linked to the right crus of the diaphragm.

Jejunum

The jejunum is located in the proximal two-fifths of the small intestine, whereas the ileum is situated in the distal three-fifths. The jejunum is emptier, wider, and thicker walled when compared with that of the ileum. The jejunum has the valvelike tall, circular, and closely packed folds called the plicae circulares. It has no **Peyer patches**, which are collections of lymphoid tissue. The jejunum also possesses some luminous areas called windows between the blood vessels of its mesentery. When compared with the ileum, the jejunum has less conspicuous arterial arcades in its mesentery. However, it has longer vasa recta (straight arteries, or arteriae rectae).

Ileum

The ileum is longer than the jejunum and resides in the false pelvis in the right lower quadrant of the abdomen. It is distinguished by the presence of the Peyer patches in its distal portion, shorter plicae circulares and vasa recta, and more mesenteric fat and arterial arcades when compared with the jejunum. The ileocecal fold is the bloodless fold of Treves.

Large Intestine

The large intestine extends from the ileocecal junction to the anus and is nearly 1.5 m long. It is made up of the cecum, appendix, colon, rectum, and anal canal. The main role is to convert the liquid contents of the ileum into semisolid feces by absorbing water, salts, and electrolytes. It also stores and lubricates the feces with mucus.

Cecum

It is the blind pouch of the large intestine. It is located in the right iliac fossa and is often surrounded by peritoneum but without a mesentery.

Appendix

This is a narrow, hollow, muscular tube with a large collection of lymphoid tissue in its wall. The appendix hangs from the terminal ileum by a small mesentery, the mesoappendix, which encompasses the appendicular vessels. When inflamed, the appendix can be a cause of spasm and distention, leading to pain that is referred to the periumbilical region and moves down and to the right lower quadrant. The appendix has a base located deep to the **McBurney point**, which occurs at the junction of the lateral one-third of the line between the right anterior superior iliac spine and the umbilicus.

Rectum and Anal Canal

These extend from the juncture of the sigmoid colon to the anus. They are described as pelvic organs.

Colon

The colon has ascending and descending portions that are retroperitoneal and transverse and a sigmoid portion that is surrounded by peritoneum. The superior mesenteric artery and the vagus nerve supply the ascending and transverse parts of the colon, whereas the descending and sigmoid parts of the colon are supplied by the inferior mesenteric artery and the pelvic splanchnic nerves. The colon is characterized by the following:

- *Teniae coli:* These are three narrow bands of the outer longitudinal muscular coat.
- *Sacculations or haustra:* These are produced by the teniae, which are slightly shorter than the gut.
- *Epiploic appendages:* These are peritoneum-covered sacs of fat, connected in rows along the teniae.

Liver

The liver is the largest visceral organ and the largest gland in the human body. It plays an important role in the synthesis and secretion of bile to emulsify fats; detoxification (by filtering the blood to remove bacteria and foreign particles that have crossed the intestinal mucosa); storage of carbohydrate as glycogen (to later break down into glucose); synthesis and sequestration of lipids as triglycerides; plasma protein synthesis (albumin and globulin); production of blood coagulants (fibrinogen and prothrombin), anticoagulants (heparin), and bile pigments (bilirubin and biliverdin) from the breakdown of hemoglobin; storage for blood and platelets; and storage of certain vitamins, iron, and copper. In the fetus, the liver plays a pivotal role in the synthesis of red blood cells.

The liver is enclosed by peritoneum and is joined to the diaphragm by the coronary and falciform ligaments and the right and left triangular ligaments. It has an exposed area on the diaphragmatic surface, which is limited by layers of the coronary ligament but without peritoneum. The liver has a dual blood supply receiving oxygenated blood from the hepatic artery and deoxygenated, nutrient-rich, sometimes toxin-containing, blood from the portal vein. It also contains a group of vessels grouped together: the hepatic artery, branch of the portal vein, and bile duct, together commonly known as the portal tract (according to old terminology is also known as the **portal triad**). The liver is enclosed by a connective tissue sheath called the perivascular fibrous capsule. The liver is divided, based on hepatic drainage and blood supply, into the right and left lobes by the fossae for the gallbladder and the IVC. (These lobes correspond to the functional units or hepatic segments.)

Lobes of the Liver

The lobes of the liver include:

- *Right lobe:* It is divided into anterior and posterior segments, each of which is further subdivided into superior and inferior areas or segments.

- *Left lobe:* It is divided into medial and lateral segments, each of which is subdivided into superior and inferior areas (segments). It consists of the medial superior (caudate lobe), medial inferior (quadrate lobe), lateral superior, and lateral inferior segments. The quadrate lobe receives oxygenated blood from the left hepatic artery and drains the bile into the left hepatic duct, whereas the caudate lobe receives oxygenated blood from the right and left hepatic arteries and drains the bile into both the right and left hepatic ducts.

Fissures and Ligaments of the Liver

These include an H-shaped group of fissures:

- *Fissure for the round ligament* (ligamentum teres hepatis), located between the lateral aspect of the left lobe and the quadrate lobe.
- *Fissure for the ligamentum venosum*, located between the lateral aspect of the left lobe and the caudate lobe.
- *Fossa for the gallbladder*, located between the quadrate lobe and the major part of the right lobe.
- *Fissure for the IVC*, located between the caudate lobe and the major part of the right lobe.
- *Porta hepatis.* This transverse fissure is situated on the visceral surface of the liver between the quadrate and the caudate lobes and contains the hepatic ducts, hepatic arteries, branches of the portal vein, hepatic nerves, and lymphatic vessels.

Technique

LEFT LOBE OF LIVER
LEFT PORTAL VEIN
INFERIOR VENA CAVA EPIGASTRIC
Transverse
FIG. 8.3

With the patient in the supine position and properly draped, place the probe transversely to the right of the midline of epigastrium with the beam aimed slightly up. The liver appears with a speckled pattern and a hyperechoic halo (sometimes called "train-tracks" when portal branches are seen in their long axis) around the portal veins (periportal connective tissue/fat). Identify the caudate lobe separating the IVC and the left portal vein (and ascending branch of left portal vein). There is a hyperechoic line in the fissure between the caudate and left liver lobe demarcating the ligamentum venosum (the patient should be asked to take a deep breath and hold while you are scanning the liver).

INFERIOR VENA CAVA
HEPATIC VEINS
SUBCOSTAL
Transverse
FIG. 8.4

With the patient in the supine position, place the probe transversely under the right costal margin with the beam aimed up, following the IVC and adjusting the tilt and angle when hepatic veins are identified. To differentiate between the hepatic and portal veins, note that there is no halo or train tracks around hepatic veins entering the IVC. Attempt to identify the left, middle, and right hepatic veins.

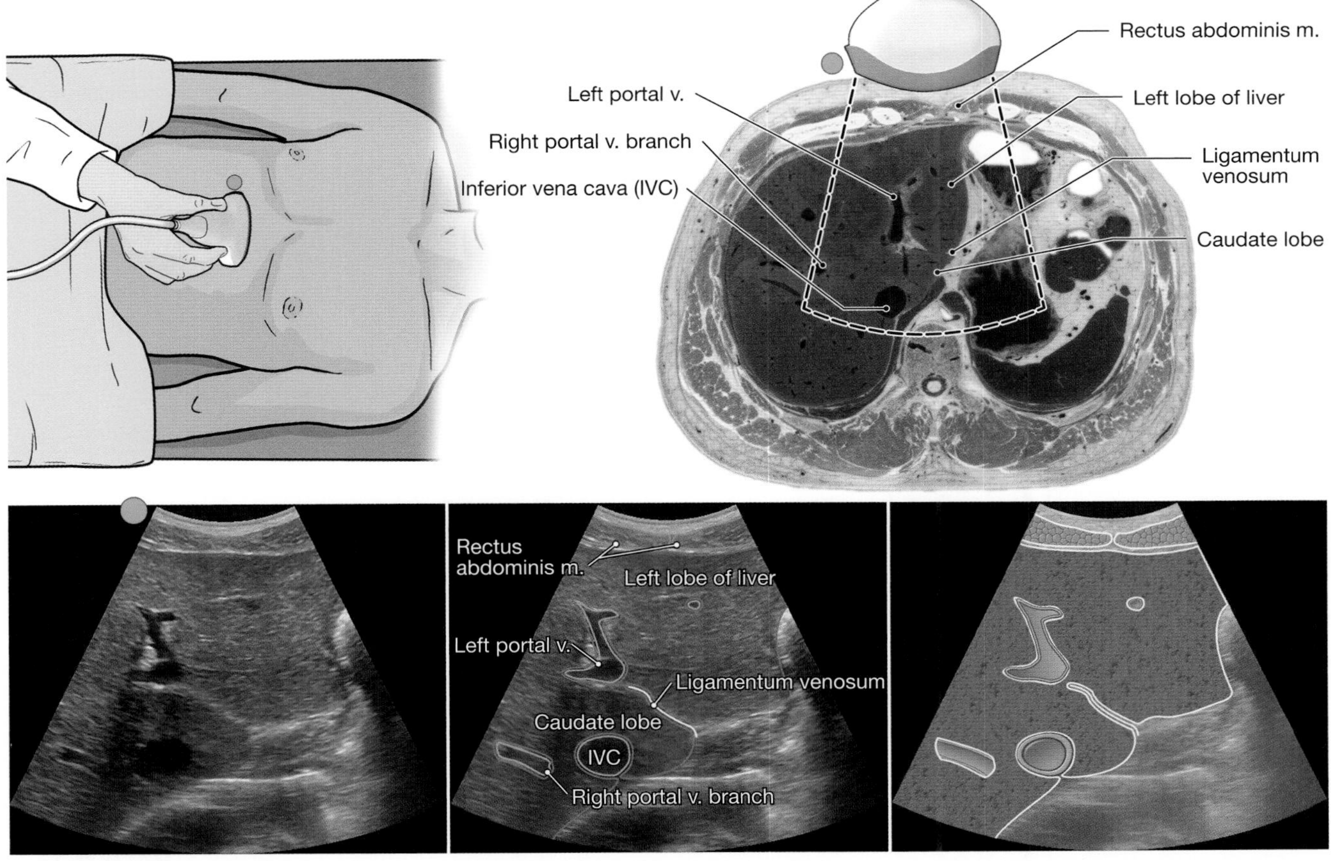

Figure 8.3 Epigastric transverse view of the left liver lobe, left portal vein and branches, caudate lobe, inferior vena cava, and ligamentum venosum.

LEFT LIVER LOBE CAUDATE LOBE PORTAL VEIN COMMON HEPATIC ARTERY SUBCOSTAL
Longitudinal (Parasagittal)
FIG. 8.5

With the patient in the supine position, place the probe in longitudinal orientation to the right of the midline under the costal margin. Adjust the probe and tilt/position it to identify the left lobe of the liver and caudate lobe. Identify the portal vein emerging from behind the neck of the pancreas as a continuation of the superior mesenteric vein below, accompanied by the common hepatic artery.

PORTAL TRIAD INFERIOR VENA CAVA AORTA SUBCOSTAL
Transverse (Oblique)
FIG. 8.6

With the patient in the supine position, place the probe slightly oblique to the transverse plane of the abdomen and parallel to the right side of the costal margin (marker should be pointing to the right, although some clinical protocols have the marker pointing to the left shoulder). Identify and follow the portal vein to the porta hepatis and adjust and tilt/angle to see the "Mickey Mouse" sign. This sign refers to the head being the portal vein, right ear the bile duct, and the left ear being the proper hepatic artery. The IVC should be seen posterior to the portal vein (omental foramen) and the aorta just to the left of the body of the lumbar vertebra.

PORTAL VEIN INFERIOR VENA CAVA SUBCOSTAL
Longitudinal (Oblique)
FIG. 8.7

With the patient in the supine position, place the probe under the right side of the costal margin oriented along the longitudinal axis of the body. Rotate the probe counterclockwise to oblique longitudinal orientation (the portal vein crosses obliquely from left to right) to lie along the long axis of the portal vein. Tilt up/down and left/right to identify the portal vein approaching and entering the liver. The IVC posteriorly has a vertical course, so it is not parallel to the portal vein for more than a few centimeters.

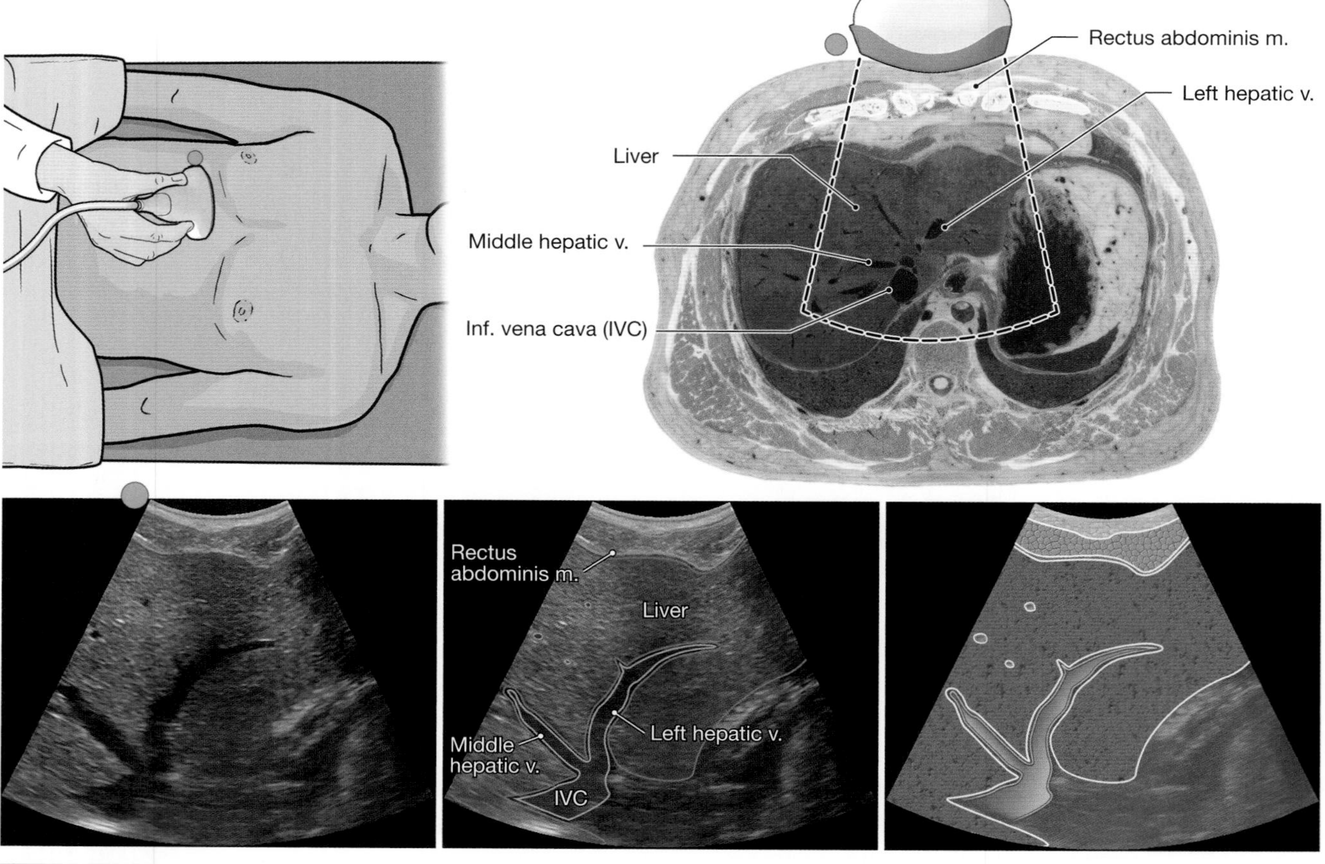

Figure 8.4 Subcostal transverse view of the inferior vena cava receiving the middle and left hepatic veins.

DIVISION OF PORTAL VEIN RIGHT AND LEFT PORTAL VEINS INFERIOR VENA CAVA SUBCOSTAL
Transverse
FIG. 8.8

With the patient in the supine position, place the probe to the right of the midline transversely to the axis of the body, aiming up under the costal margin. Ask the patient to take a deep breath and tilt/fan the probe to identify the IVC, tail of caudate lobe, and portal vein dividing into right and left branches. The portal veins have characteristic hyperechoic halo/train tracks surrounding them.

INFERIOR VENA CAVA LIVER RIGHT ATRIUM RIGHT VENTRICLE SUBCOSTAL
Longitudinal
FIG. 8.9

With the patient in the supine position, place the probe longitudinally oriented (marker directed superiorly with the curved array probe) to the right of the midline under the right costal margin, aiming up toward the thorax. Ask the patient to take deep breaths as needed to identify the liver speckled pattern, portal vein branches and hepatic veins, the retrohepatic course of the IVC, and cardiac movement above the diaphragm where the IVC passes through the hiatus for the IVC to open into the right atrium. Observe the inspiratory collapse and expiratory filling of the IVC. Note hepatic veins approaching the IVC a short distance below its opening into the right atrium. The portal vein is seen anterior to the IVC accompanied by the proper hepatic artery.

RIGHT LIVER LOBE MORISON POUCH RIGHT KIDNEY
Longitudinal (Intercostal Oblique)
FIG. 8.10

Place the patient in the supine position and place the palm of the right hand behind the head, abducting the arm and helping to open up intercostal spaces on the right. Place the probe along the midaxillary line at about the horizontal level of the xiphisternal junction with the probe marker directed superiorly. The probe face should be rotated until it is parallel to the intercostal spaces (the intercostal oblique orientation), which minimizes rib shadowing over the structures

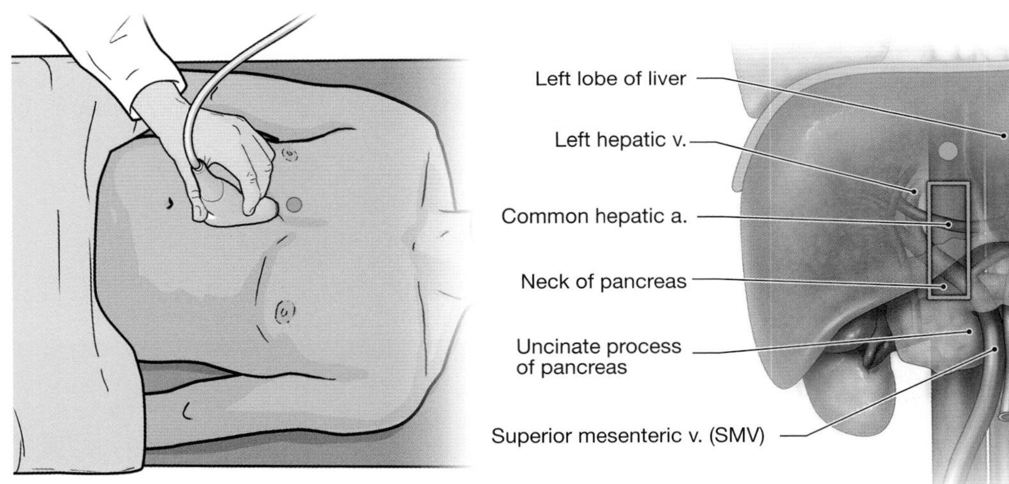

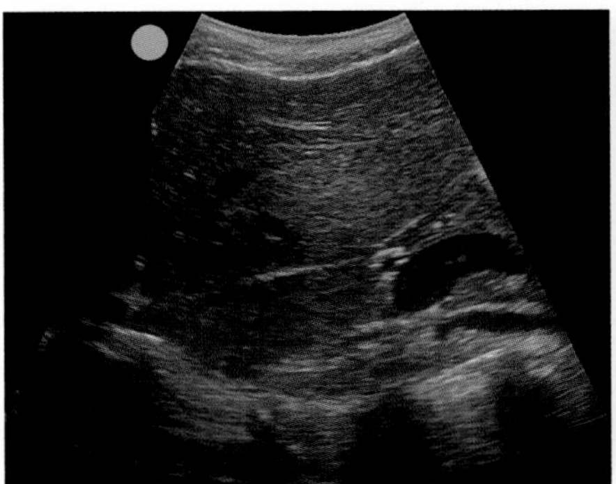

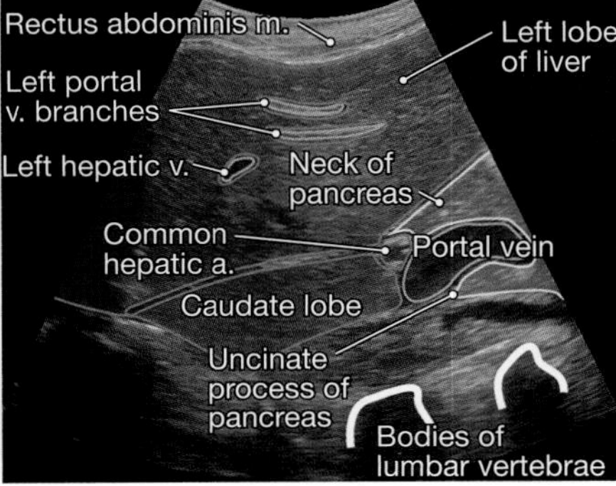

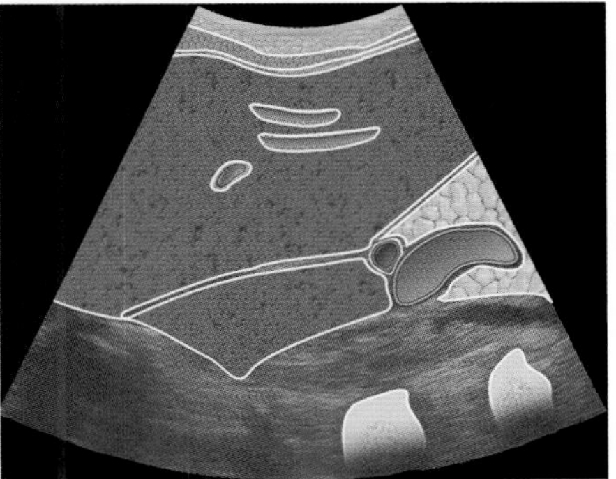

Figure 8.5 Subcostal longitudinal view of the left lobe of the liver, caudate lobe, the portal vein forming (from superior mesenteric vein being joined by the splenic vein), the surrounding neck and uncinate process of the pancreas, and the common hepatic artery.

of interest and brings the probe into closer alignment with the typical orientation of the right kidney. Identify the speckled appearance of the liver and the hyperechoic stripe representing the diaphragm over the curving superior surface of the liver. The probe face should be tilted posteriorly until the interface between the visceral surface of the liver and the right kidney can be viewed. The potential space at the hepatorenal recess is commonly referred to as the Morison pouch. This is the most dependent site in the peritoneal space above the transverse mesocolon; therefore, it is a common location for free fluid accumulation in the upper abdomen. The hepatorenal recess should be carefully and completely scanned for any anechoic fluid collections.

Next, slide the probe superiorly (1 or 2 intercostal spaces) until the superior surface of the liver, the diaphragm, and the lower part of the right hemithorax can be seen in the image. In the presence of a normally aerated lung, the hyperechoic diaphragm creates a mirror image artifact over the lung fields such that the speckled appearance of the liver is mirrored over the right hemithorax/pleural space. The presence of free fluid in the pleural space (hemothorax or pleural effusion) abolishes the mirror image artifact, and the space above the diaphragm appears anechoic, often with an atelectatic lung floating in and out of view with respiratory efforts. In addition, look carefully for any free fluid accumulation in the right subphrenic space, the potential space between the diaphragm and the superior surface of the liver.

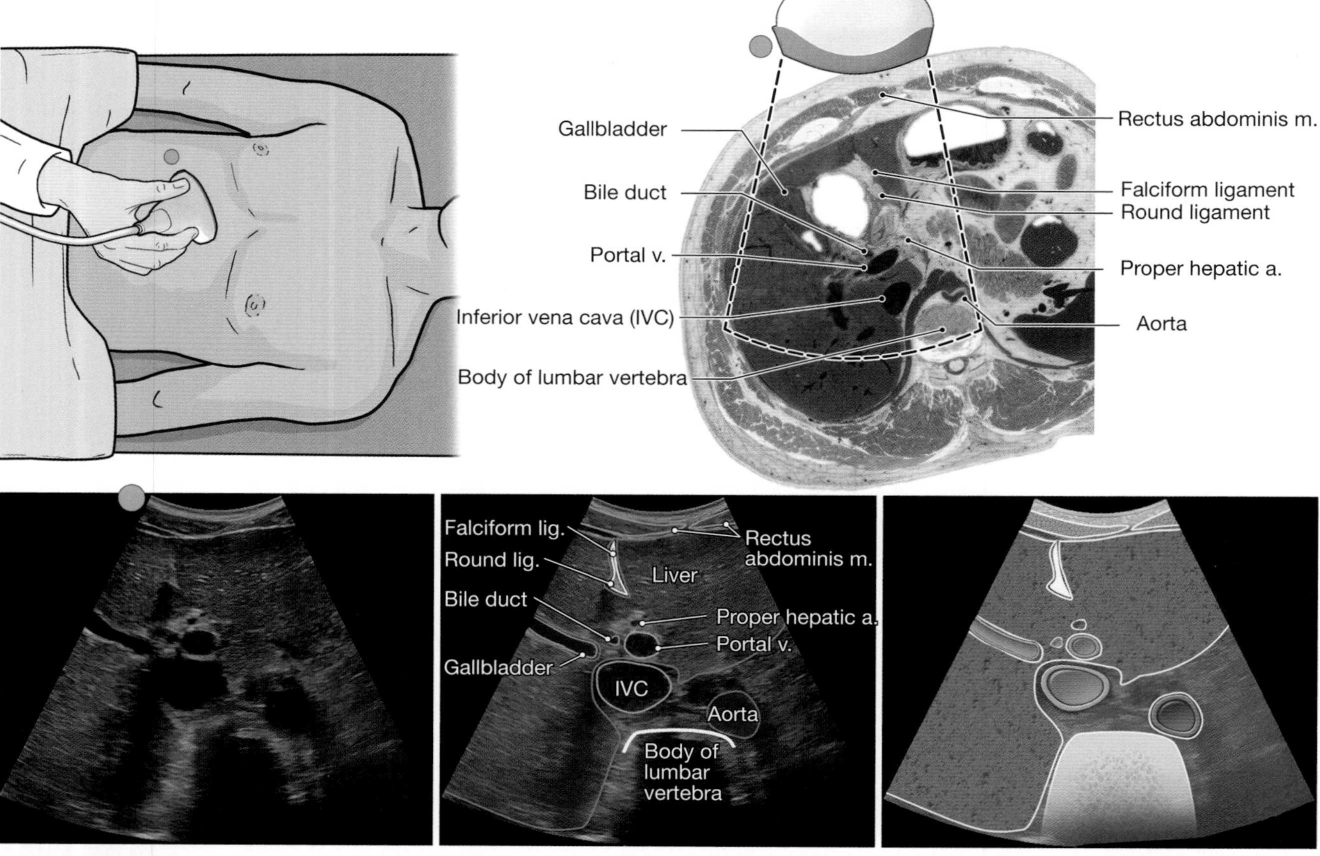

Figure 8.6 Transverse (oblique) subcostal view of the portal triad (portal vein, proper hepatic artery, and bile duct) entering/exiting the liver via the porta hepatis. The inferior vena cava is seen immediately posterior to the portal vein. The hyperechoic falciform ligament and round ligament of the liver (ligamentum teres hepatis) are seen at the border between the left lobe of the liver (segments 2 and 3) and the quadrate lobe (segment 4b).

CLINICAL APPLICATIONS

Meckel Diverticulum

Meckel diverticulum refers to an outpouching of the ileum. This tissue is derived from the unobliterated yolk stalk and is located 2 ft from the ileocecal junction. It is usually 2 inches in length, occurs in approximately 2% of the population, may contain two types of ectopic tissues (gastric and pancreatic), presents in the first 2 decades of life, and is found two times as frequently in boys as in girls. The diverticulum can be free or connected with the umbilicus through a fistula or a fibrous cord. Complications include ulceration, perforation, bleeding, and obstruction, which may require surgical intervention. In addition, it can mimic acute appendicitis because of similar presentation, which includes right lower quadrant abdominal pain, vomiting, and fever, which should be managed surgically if it causes severe pain, significant bleeding, or obstruction.

Acute Appendicitis

Acute appendicitis refers to acute inflammation of the appendix resulting from blockage of the lumen by **fecalith** (a hard, stony mass of feces that occurs in the intestinal tract). It presents as right lower quadrant pain (McBurney point) that starts in the periumbilical region, rebound tenderness, loss of appetite, nausea, vomiting, and fever. Rupture of the appendix can cause peritonitis leading to spread of the infection (septicemia) and death, if untreated. Appendicitis is managed surgically by appendectomy.

Liver Cirrhosis

Liver cirrhosis refers to a condition in which hepatocytes are progressively replaced by fibrous tissue surrounding the intrahepatic blood vessels and biliary radicles leading to the obstruction of blood through the liver. It can be caused by chronic alcoholism; infections such as hepatitis B, C, and D; and poisons. Liver cirrhosis can result in portal hypertension, causing esophageal varices, hemorrhoids, caput medusa spider naevi or spider angioma, ascites, pedal edema, jaundice, hepatic encephalopathy, splenomegaly, hepatomegaly, palmar erythema, testicular atrophy, gynecomastia, and pectoral alopecia. Additional symptoms include fatigue, nausea, loss of appetite, and weight loss. Management includes a low-sodium and low-protein diet and diuretics. Hepatocellular carcinoma is one of the most common cancers. Risk factors include liver cirrhosis due to viral hepatitis, alcoholism, and hemochromatosis. Hepatocellular carcinoma is diagnosed based on the number of cirrhotic nodules with the liver.

Liver Biopsy

Liver biopsy is performed percutaneously under US guidance using a needle in the right eighth or ninth intercostal space at the right midaxillary line. The patient is instructed to hold their breath in full expiration to collapse the costodiaphragmatic recess, thus lessening the possibility of damage to the lung and causing pneumothorax. Transjugular liver biopsy can be performed by inserting a catheter into the internal jugular vein on the right and passing it through the superior and inferior vena cavae and the right hepatic vein. A needle is then inserted through the catheter to the liver and a biopsy is taken.

Fatty Liver

This term characterizes a wide array of diseases with the most common being alcoholic and nonalcoholic fatty liver disease. Alcoholic liver disease relates to the excess of alcohol consumption, whereas nonalcoholic fatty liver relates to the insulin resistance and metabolic syndrome. In addition, viral hepatitis and certain medications can also cause triglyceride accumulation (**steatosis**). If steatosis is pronounced and chronic, it may cause fibrosis and eventually lead to liver cirrhosis. Recent studies place the prevalence of liver steatosis to approximately 15% of the general population. US can diagnose liver steatosis by identifying poor demarcation of intrahepatic architecture, revealing the loss of diaphragmatic demarcation, and showing that liver echogenicity is higher than that of renal cortex and spleen.

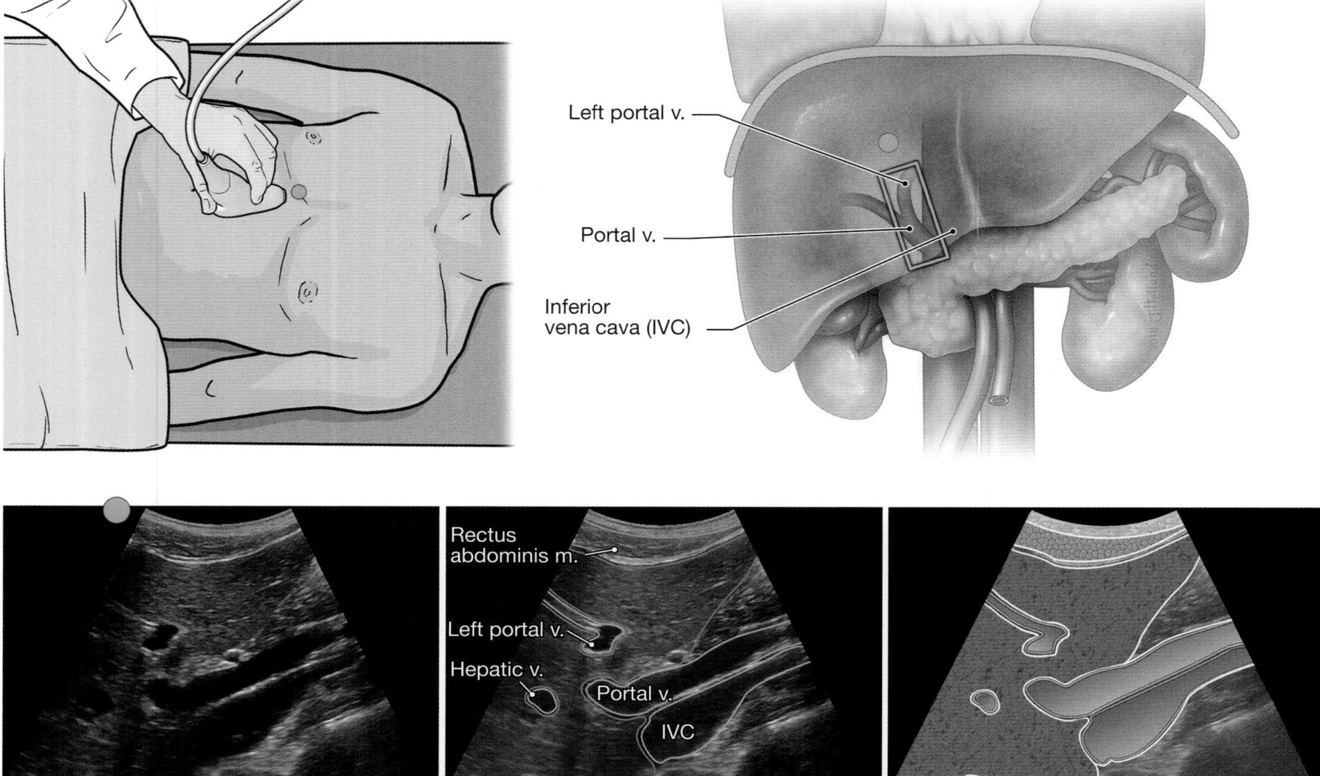

Figure 8.7 Longitudinal (oblique) subcostal view of the portal vein approaching and entering the liver at the porta hepatis. The inferior vena cava is seen posterior to the portal vein.

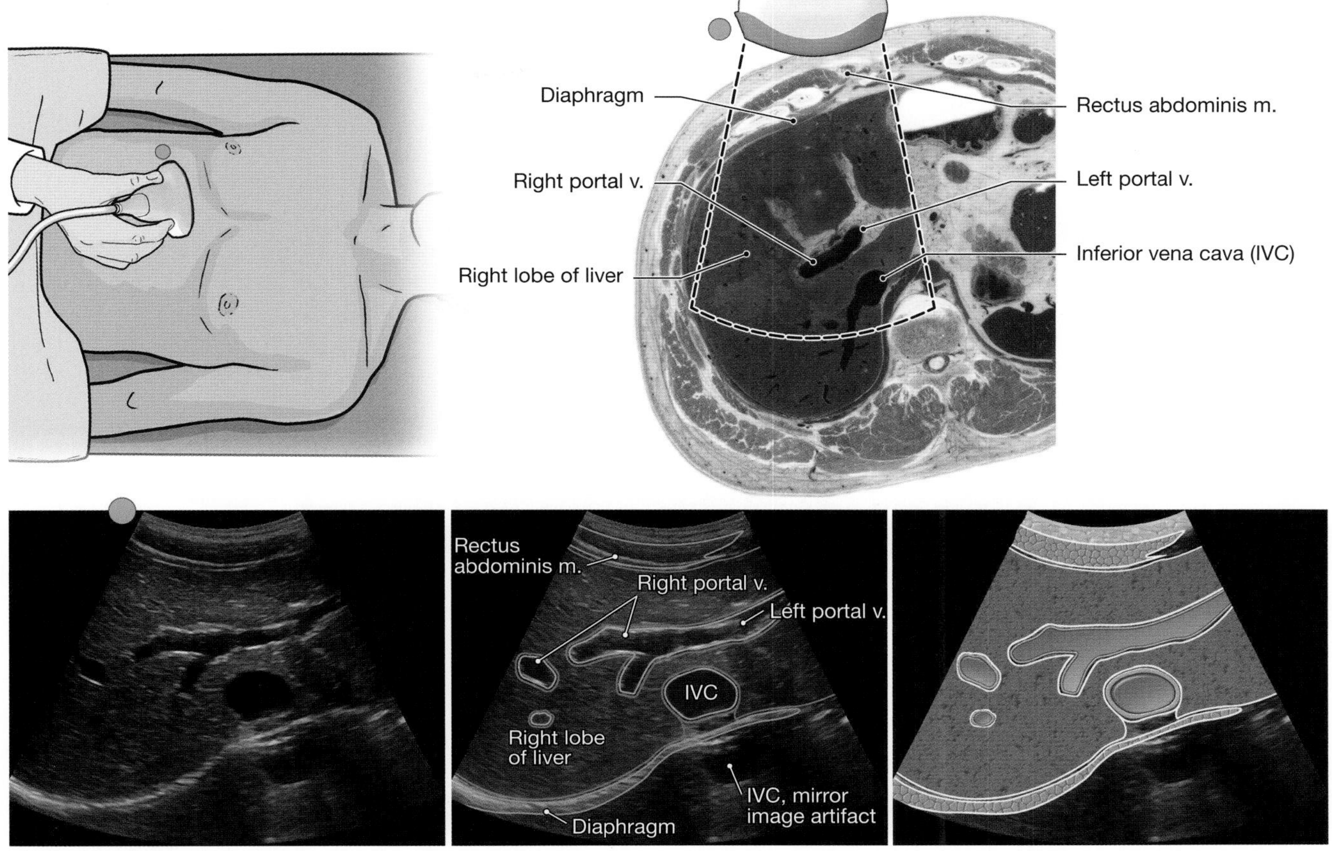

Figure 8.8 Transverse subcostal view of the portal vein dividing within the liver into right and left portal veins. The inferior vena cava is seen posterior to the dividing portal vein (separated by the "tail" of the caudate lobe).

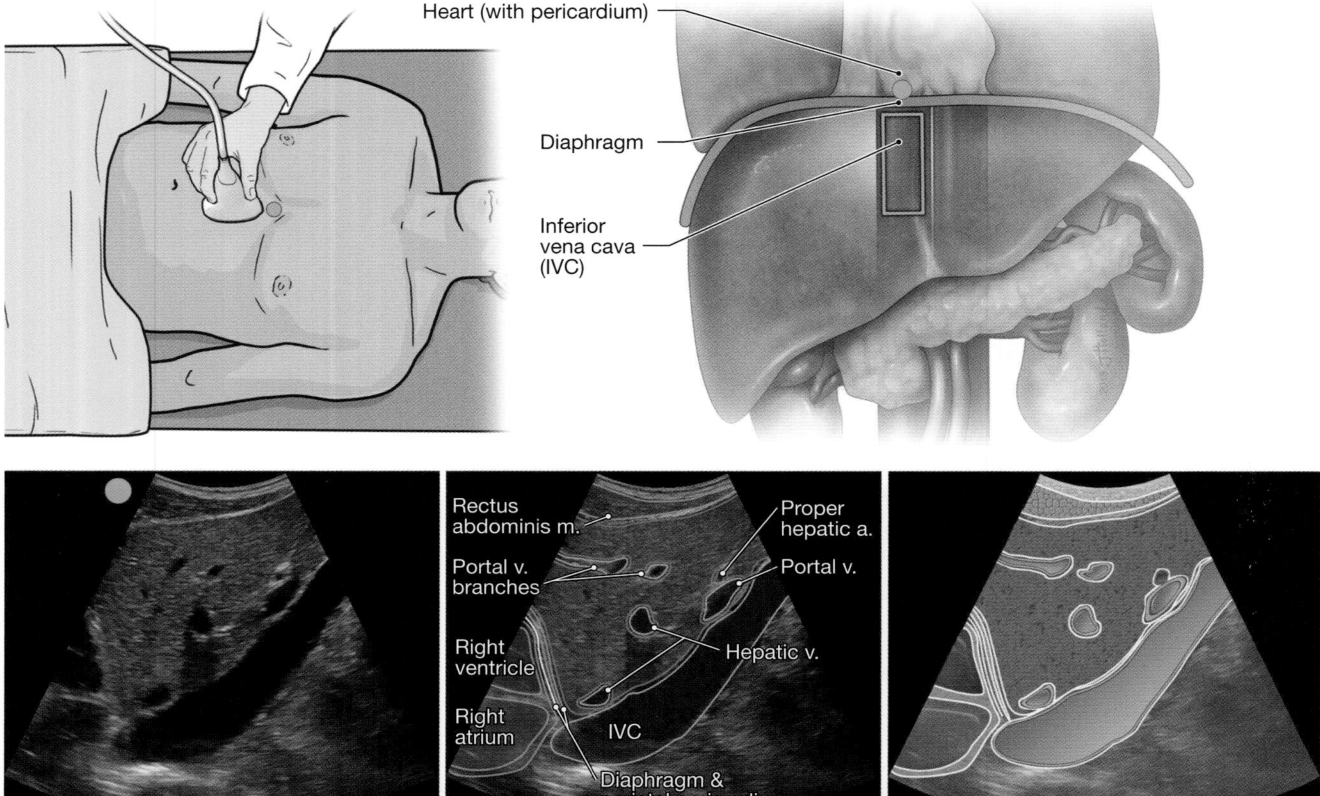

Figure 8.9 Longitudinal subcostal view of the course of the inferior vena cava posterior to the liver and approaching the right atrium (via caval hiatus of diaphragm).

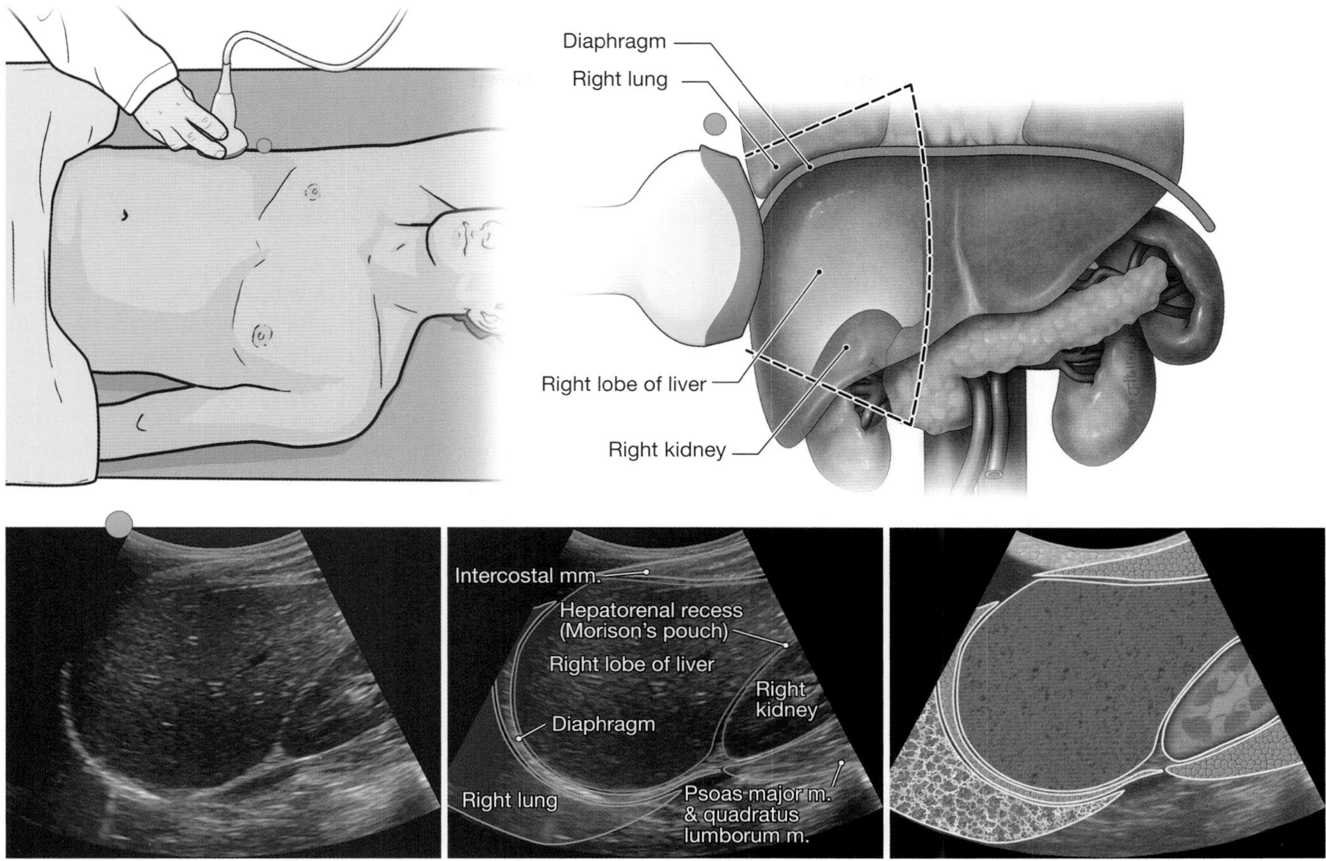

Figure 8.10 Longitudinal (intercostal oblique) view of the right hemithorax, diaphragm, right lobe of liver, Morison pouch, and right kidney.

Gallbladder

Review of the Anatomy

The gallbladder is situated where the lateral border of the rectus abdominis junctions with the right ninth costal cartilage. This is the site of **Murphy sign**, ie, tenderness due to acute inflammation of the gallbladder (acute cholecystitis). The gallbladder lies in a fossa between the quadrate and right lobes inferior to the liver and has a capacity of 30 to 50 m. It is located superior to the transverse colon and superolateral to the duodenum. Its structure can be divided into the neck, fundus, and body.

The neck of the gallbladder is the narrowest part and is continuous with the cystic duct, which contains spiral valves (Heister valves). The fundus is the round blind end situated on the midclavicular line at the tip of the right ninth costal cartilage in contact with the transverse colon. The body forms the major part of the gallbladder and is in contact with the upper part of the duodenum and the transverse colon. In some cases, an abnormal conical pouch (Hartmann pouch) might be present in the neck of the gallbladder (also known as ampulla of the gallbladder).

The gallbladder functions to receive bile, concentrate it by absorbing salts and water, store it, and release it during digestion. As the food reaches the duodenum, cholecystokinin is produced by the duodenal mucosa, which together with parasympathetic stimulation acts to contract the gallbladder, resulting in the expulsion of bile into the duodenum.

The gallbladder is supplied by the cystic artery, which comes from the right hepatic artery located in the cystohepatic triangle (of Calot), formed medially by the common hepatic duct, superiorly by the visceral surface of the liver and inferiorly by the cystic duct.

Technique

INTERCOSTAL VIEW GALLBLADDER LIVER
Longitudinal (Intercostal Oblique)
FIG. 8.11

There are several techniques for examining the gallbladder such as the subcostal, right subcostal oblique, and intercostal approaches. The intercostal and the subcostal ("subcostal sweep") views are described in the following. The intercostal view uses the liver as an **insonation window**, which minimizes bowel gas interference with the view. The subcostal view allows for easier transitions between the longitudinal and transverse views of the gallbladder without rib shadowing. Direct probe pressure on the gallbladder fundus can be help visualize the sonographic Murphy sign (see Clinical Applications in the following).

Intercostal View of Gallbladder

With the patient in the supine position and with the patient right hand behind the head (this is to expand the intercostal spaces on the right side), place the probe positioned with the marker side up toward right shoulder/axilla, at the horizontal level of the xiphoid process about 7 to 8 cm laterally. Align the probe with the intercostal spaces, aiming across the upper abdomen slightly posteriorly (if you tilt too far posteriorly the right kidney will come into view) to identify the anechoic lumen of the pear-shaped gallbladder. Slide the probe inferiorly to visualize as much of the gallbladder as possible. Often the bowel gas interferes with imaging the fundus, which is beyond the liver edge/costal margin. Note the veins in the liver and attempt to differentiate between hepatic veins and portal vein branches (hyperechoic halo/train tracks).

Subcostal View of Gallbladder

SUBCOSTAL VIEW GALLBLADDER LIVER
Longitudinal (Parasagittal)
FIG. 8.12

The subcostal "sweep" view of the gallbladder can be performed with the patient in the supine position or in left lateral decubitus position. Place the probe in a longitudinal (parasagittal) orientation under the right costal margin a short distance medial to the midclavicular line, with the probe marker directed superiorly and aiming the US beam up toward the patient thorax. Ask the patient to take a deep breath (this moves the liver edge and gallbladder fundus below the costal margin) and slide ("sweep") the probe laterally following the right costal margin. When the gallbladder becomes visible under the probe, stop sliding and adjust the tilt and angle of the probe to obtain the best possible longitudinal view of the gallbladder from the fundus to the neck. Identify the liver, portal vein branches, hepatic veins and IVC.

CLINICAL APPLICATIONS

Gallstones

Gallstones (cholelithiasis) are formed by the crystallization of bile constituents and are made of cholesterol crystals mixed with bile pigments and calcium. Bile crystallizes to form sand, gravel, and finally stones. A common presentation of gallstones is in fertile (multiparous) fat females who are older than 40 years (4 F). Stones in the fundus of the gallbladder might ulcerate through the wall of the fundus into the transverse colon passing naturally through the rectum. They might also ulcerate through the wall of the body into the duodenum and lodge at the ileocecal junction, leading to obstruction. Stones lodged in the bile duct interfere with bile flow to the duodenum, resulting in obstructive jaundice. Finally, stones lodged at the hepatopancreatic ampulla block the biliary and the pancreatic duct systems. In this case, the bile may enter the pancreatic duct system, causing aseptic or noninfectious pancreatitis.

Sonographic Murphy Sign

Sonographic Murphy sign refers to the subcostal view only wherein the probe is placed against the fundus with applied pressure. Once the patient expresses pain or maximal discomfort because of direct pressure on gallbladder only, then the sign is positive.

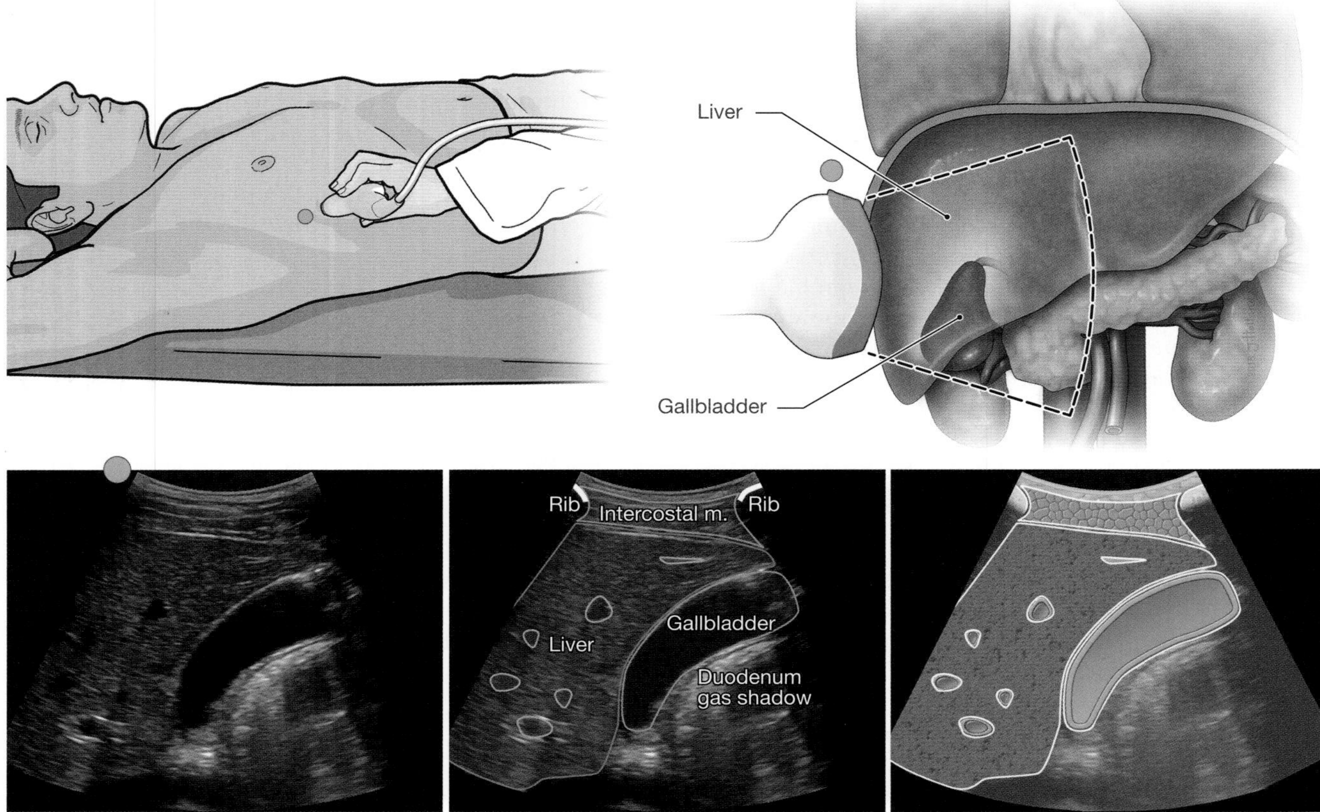

Figure 8.11 Intercostal (hepatic window) longitudinal view of the gallbladder.

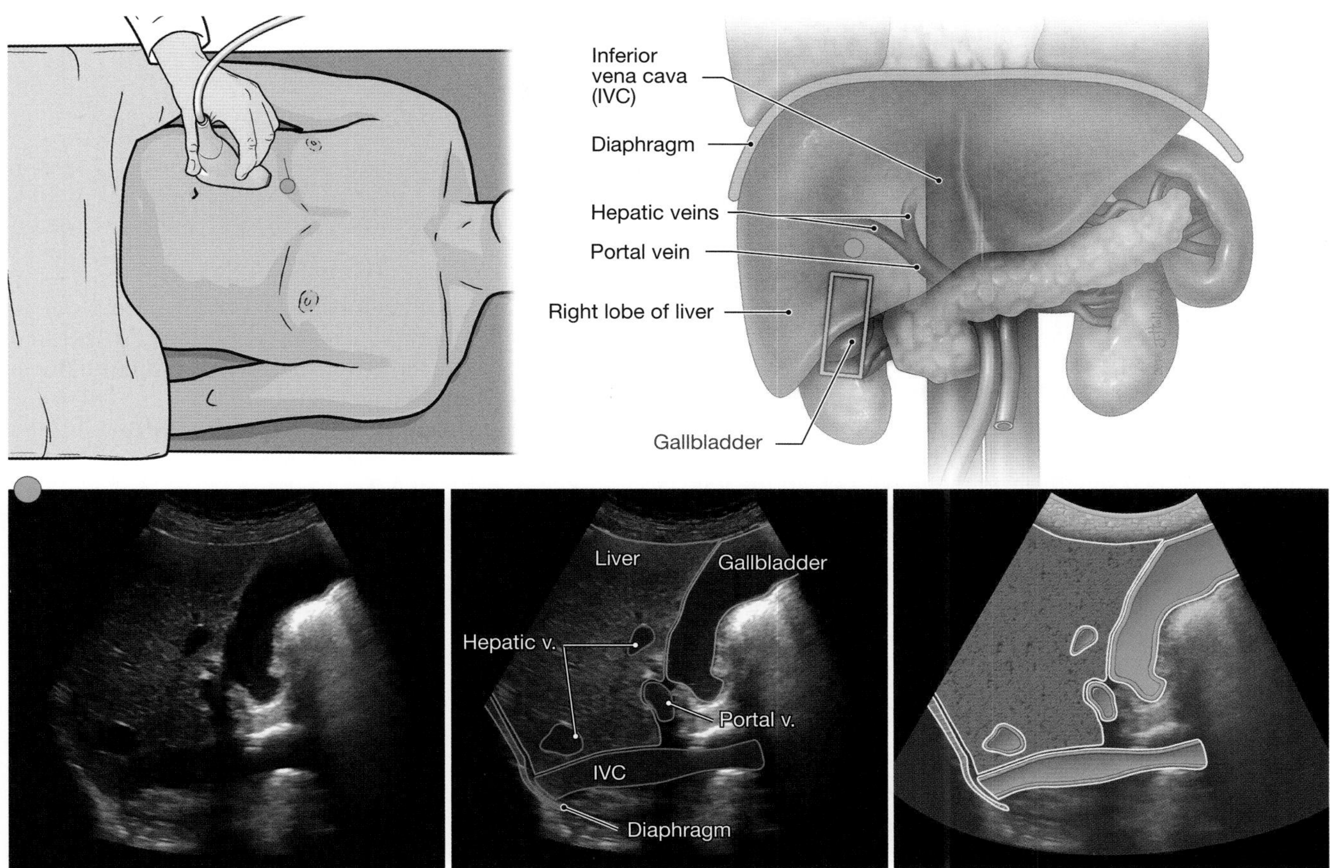

Figure 8.12 Subcostal longitudinal view of the gallbladder.

Spleen and Kidneys

Review of the Anatomy

Spleen

The spleen is a vascular lymphatic organ located below the diaphragm at 9th to 11th ribs, ie, at the left hypochondriac region. It is supported by the splenorenal and splenogastric ligaments and is covered by the peritoneum, except at the hilum. It is located superiorly to the upper pole of the left kidney (almost in contact with it) and the tail of the pancreas. More specifically, the splenorenal ligament contains the splenic vessels and the tail of the pancreas.

The splenic artery supplies blood to the spleen, which empties into the splenic vein. It is divided into two regions, namely, the white and red pulp. The white pulp is composed of lymphatic tissue around the central arteries and is the site of phagocytic activity. The red pulp is composed of venous sinusoids and splenic cords and is the site of filtration. As the blood filters through the spleen, worn-out and damaged red blood cells and platelets are removed by macrophages. Other functions of spleen include storing blood and platelets in the red pulp; immune response; and production of mature lymphocytes, macrophages, and antibodies in the white pulp. The spleen is also the site of hematopoiesis in early life.

Kidneys

The kidneys are bilateral retroperitoneal organs located along the T12 to L3 spinal level. The right kidney is lower when compared with the contralateral left kidney because of the large size of the liver and can be found at the level of the 12th rib. The left kidney is usually found at the level of the 11th and 12th ribs. The outer layer of the kidney contains thick fibrous capsule that is enclosed by the renal fascia along with the perinephric and pararenal fat. The nerves and vessels that supply the kidney along with the ureter enter the kidney on the medial side at the hilum.

The kidney can be divided anatomically into the cortex and medulla, which contain the nephrons. The outer cortex contains the renal corpuscles and is the location of the glomerulus and the glomerular capsule (Bowman capsule) and the proximal and distal convoluted tubules. The inner part of the kidney is the medulla and contains the loops of Henle and the collecting tubules. Several nephrons can be found in each kidney, which can be further divided into the renal corpuscle, the proximal convoluted tubule, Henle loop, and the distal convoluted tubule.

Each kidney is supplied by the **renal artery**, which contains segmental branches with several anatomical variations, and is drained by the renal vein. Urine exits the kidney from the collecting tubules into the minor and major calyces. The major calyces empty into the renal pelvis exiting as the ureter.

Ureters

The ureter is a retroperitoneal muscular organ that joins the kidney to the urinary bladder. It courses along the iliopsoas muscle and transverse processes of the lumbar vertebrae and anterior to the bifurcation of the common iliac artery. The ureter contains certain locations wherein there is a high chance for **renal calculi** obstruction, which include the ureteropelvic and ureterovesicular junctions. It is supplied by branches of the abdominal aorta, renal, common and internal iliac, and gonadal arteries. Sympathetic innervation to the ureter is provided by the lumbar splanchnic nerves, whereas parasympathetic innervation is provided by the pelvic splanchnic nerves.

Adrenal Gland

The **adrenal gland** is situated at the superior medial pole of the kidney. It is a retroperitoneal organ and is invested by a capsule and the renal fascia. The adrenal gland is asymmetrical with a pyramidal-shaped right adrenal gland and semilunar-shaped left gland. Branches from the inferior phrenic artery, the middle suprarenal artery (which is a direct branch of the aorta), and the inferior suprarenal artery (a branch of the renal artery) supply oxygenated blood to the adrenal gland. On the right, the suprarenal vein drains the gland, whereas venous drainage on the left is by the renal vein. Both venous drainages empty into the IVC.

The adrenal gland can be divided anatomically into a **cortex** and a **medulla**. The cortex has three separate layers, the most superficial layer being the zona glomerulosa, the middle layer the zona fasciculata, and the deepest layer the zona reticularis. Each layer of the adrenal cortex produces steroid hormones that are fundamental to maintaining homeostasis within the body. The zona glomerulosa consists of cells that produce aldosterone. The zona fasiculata cells synthesize cortisol and corticosterone. The zona reticularis secretes androgens, namely, dehydroepiandrosterone and androstenedione. The adrenal medulla has neural crest origin. The cells of the medulla are called neuroendocrine cells that play a significant role in the release of epinephrine and norepinephrine in response to sympathetic fiber stimulation.

Technique

SPLEEN LEFT KIDNEY
Longitudinal (Intercostal Oblique)
FIG. 8.13

With the patient in the supine position or rolled into the right lateral decubitus position, place the probe with the marker pointing toward the head in the posterior axillary line (as a starting point) aligned with the intercostal space. Note that decubitus positioning is not appropriate for some applications such as the focused assessment with sonography for trauma (FAST), whereby decubitus would cause fluid to drain to the right side. Fan/tilt/slide the probe, looking for grainy echotexture of the spleen as it moves with respirations. Adjust the probe to see the spleen and the hyperechoic diaphragm clearly. Then tilt to aim the beam more posteriorly (and/or slide probe posteriorly as possible) until the left kidney can be seen adjacent to the spleen (separated by the potential space of splenorenal recess). Adjust the position/tilt to get the best view possible of the left hemithorax, diaphragm, spleen, and left kidney. Note that the inferior pole of the kidney is often obscured by colon gas. Observe the mirror image artifact that causes the appearance of the spleen echotexture in the left pleural space (abolished by free fluid such as hemothorax or left pleural effusion). Place the patient in a right lateral decubitus position if there is substantial bowel gas shadowing.

LEFT KIDNEY
Longitudinal (Intercostal Oblique)
FIG. 8.14

Position the patient and the probe as shown in Figure 8.13. Slide the probe as far posteriorly as possible (it is already near the examination table surface) and adjust the tilt/angle/position to image as much of the left kidney as possible. It may be necessary to gently roll the patient into the right decubitus position to position the probe behind the posterior axillary line and image the kidney from posterior to the left colic flexure (gas shadowing), identifying the cortex and columns, renal pyramids, hyperechoic fat, and connective tissue of the renal sinus.

SPLEEN
Longitudinal (Intercostal Oblique)
FIG. 8.15

Position the patient and the probe as shown in Figure 8.13. Slide the probe superiorly and aim the beam slightly anteriorly to image the spleen in its long axis, observing its hyperechoic

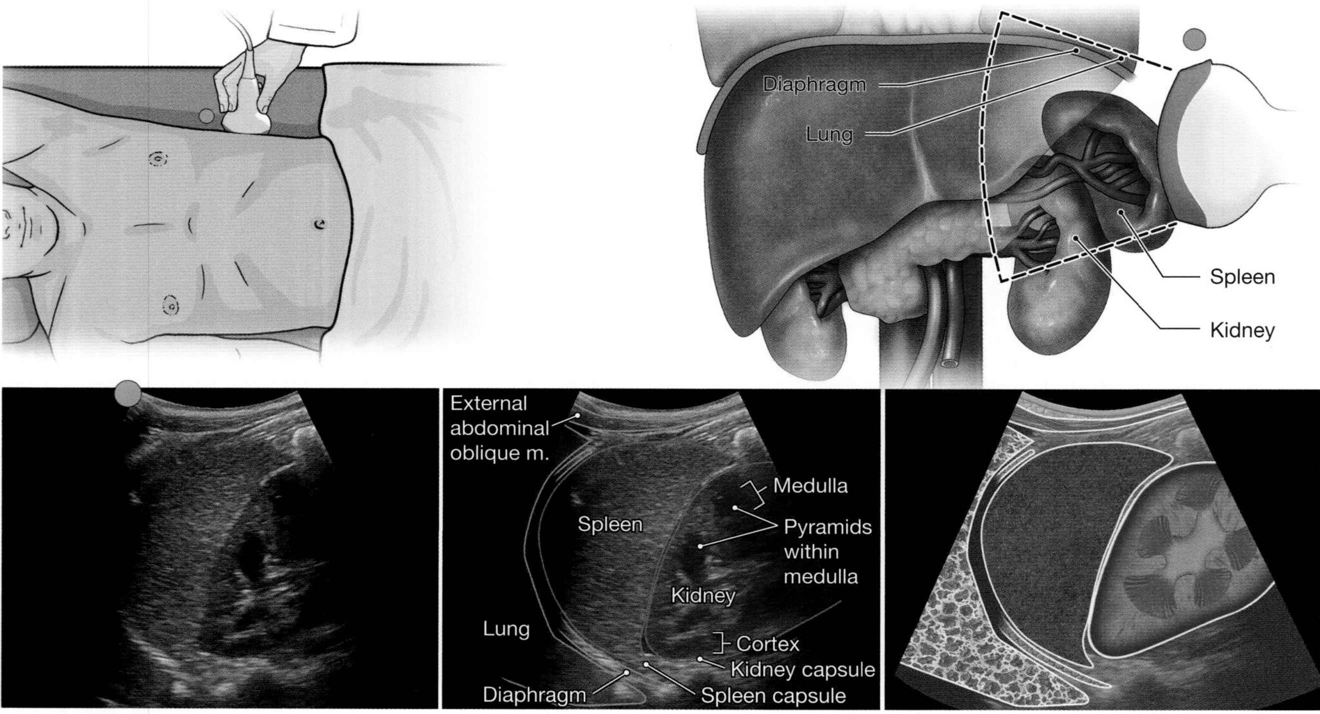

Figure 8.13 Longitudinal (intercostal oblique) view of the left hemithorax, spleen, and left kidney.

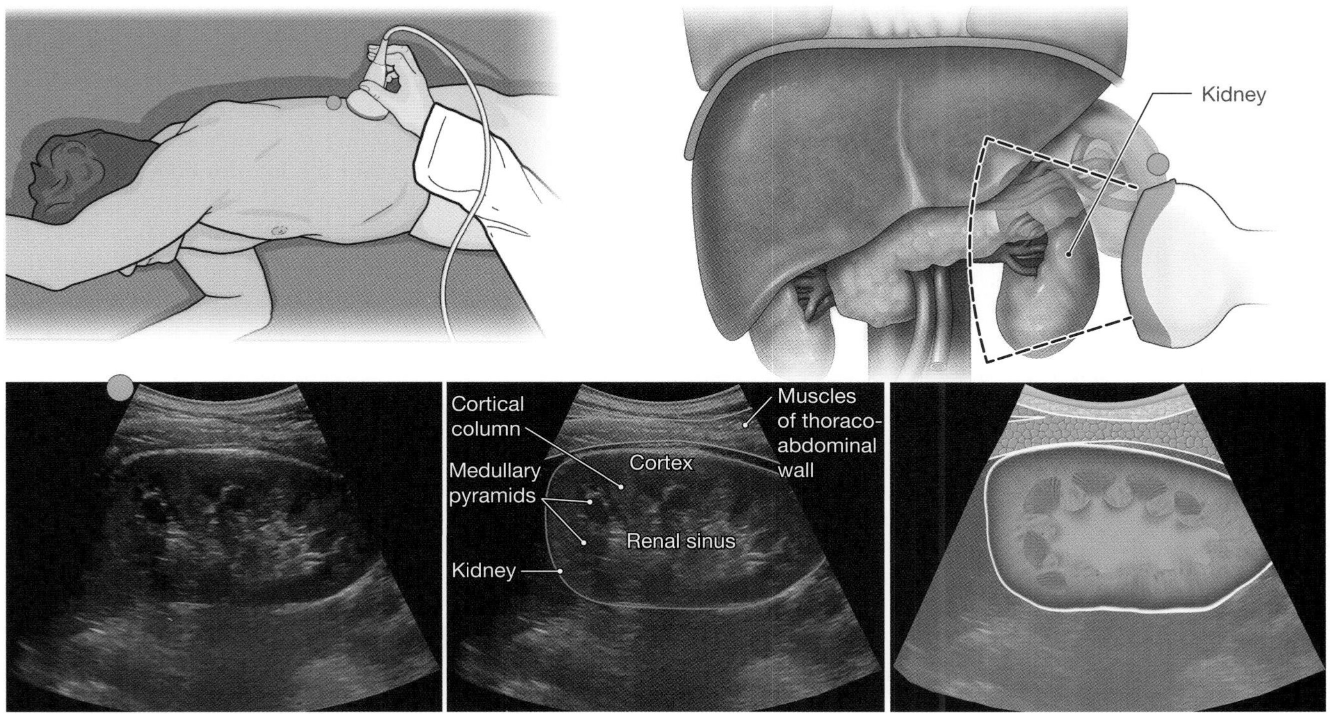

Figure 8.14 Longitudinal (intercostal oblique) view of the left kidney.

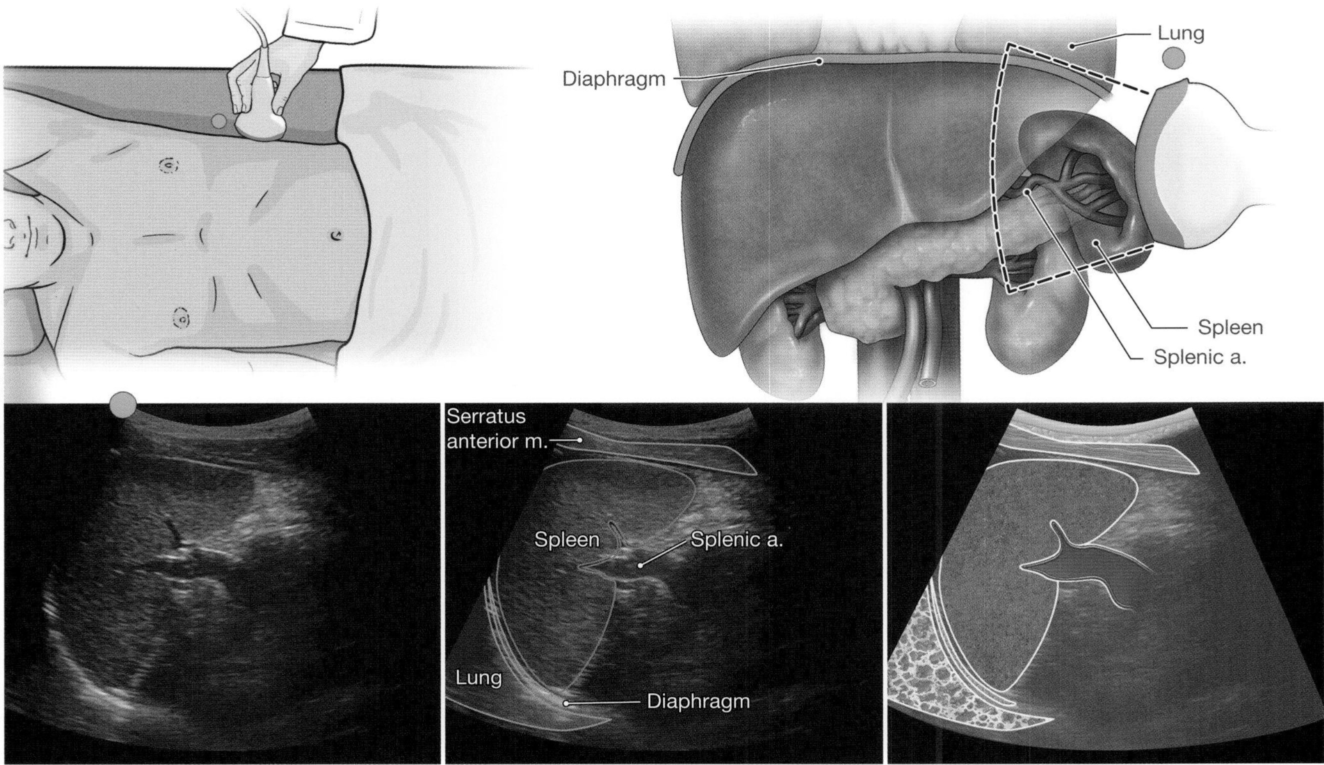

Figure 8.15 Longitudinal (intercostal oblique) view of the spleen.

grainy echotexture, the hyperechoic diaphragm along its superior surface, and respiratory movements of the spleen and diaphragm.

RIGHT KIDNEY
Longitudinal (Intercostal Oblique)
FIG. 8.16

With the patient in the supine position, place the probe midaxillary line approximately at the level of the xiphisternal junction, aligned with an intercostal space to minimize rib shadowing. Aim slightly posteriorly (toward the spine) to view the liver, the hepatorenal recess, and the right kidney. Slide the probe inferiorly (and realign with the intercostal space) until the right kidney can be seen from the superior pole to the inferior pole (gas shadowing may interfere with imaging of the inferior pole beyond the inferior edge of the right liver lobe). Identify Morison pouch, kidney capsule, psoas muscles, and vertebral bodies. A subcostal approach is also used to identify the kidney to avoid bowel gas by using the liver as an insonation window.

CLINICAL APPLICATIONS

Splenomegaly is the result of venous congestion due to portal hypertension or thrombosis of the splenic vein. It typically leads to sequestration of blood resulting in thrombocytopenia and easy bruising. Its symptoms include weight loss, night sweats, fever, diarrhea, and bone pain.

Splenic rupture most commonly occurs because of fractured ribs or severe trauma in the left hypochondrium, leading to severe bleeding. It is difficult to surgically repair a ruptured spleen, and splenectomy is performed to prevent death due to exsanguination. The spleen can be removed, as its functions are assumed by other reticuloendothelial organs.

Cancer of the lymphoid tissue is called **lymphoma**. **Hodgkin disease** is a type of malignant lymphoma, and its clinical features include painless, progressive enlargement of the lymph nodes, spleen, and other lymphoid tissue; night sweats; fever; and weight loss.

Urolithiasis is the condition in which renal calculi may present at any part of the urinary tract. About 70% to 80% of kidney stones (renal calculus or nephrolith) are formed of high levels of calcium and, as a result, are easily detectable with US when patients are suspected for nephrolithiasis because of renal colic. Based on the size and shape of kidney stones, severe colicky pain may be produced at the renal calyx or while traveling down through the ureter. In addition, hydronephrosis or obstruction of the ureters by a stone can be a surgical emergency. Another type of kidney stone is the Staghorn or coral calculi. These stones fill every part of the renal pelvis and calyces. Their composition is of magnesium ammonium phosphate, known as struvite, or calcium carbonate apatite. They are formed most commonly in females owing to recurrent infections. The clinical symptoms include fever, pain, hematuria, and abscess formation.

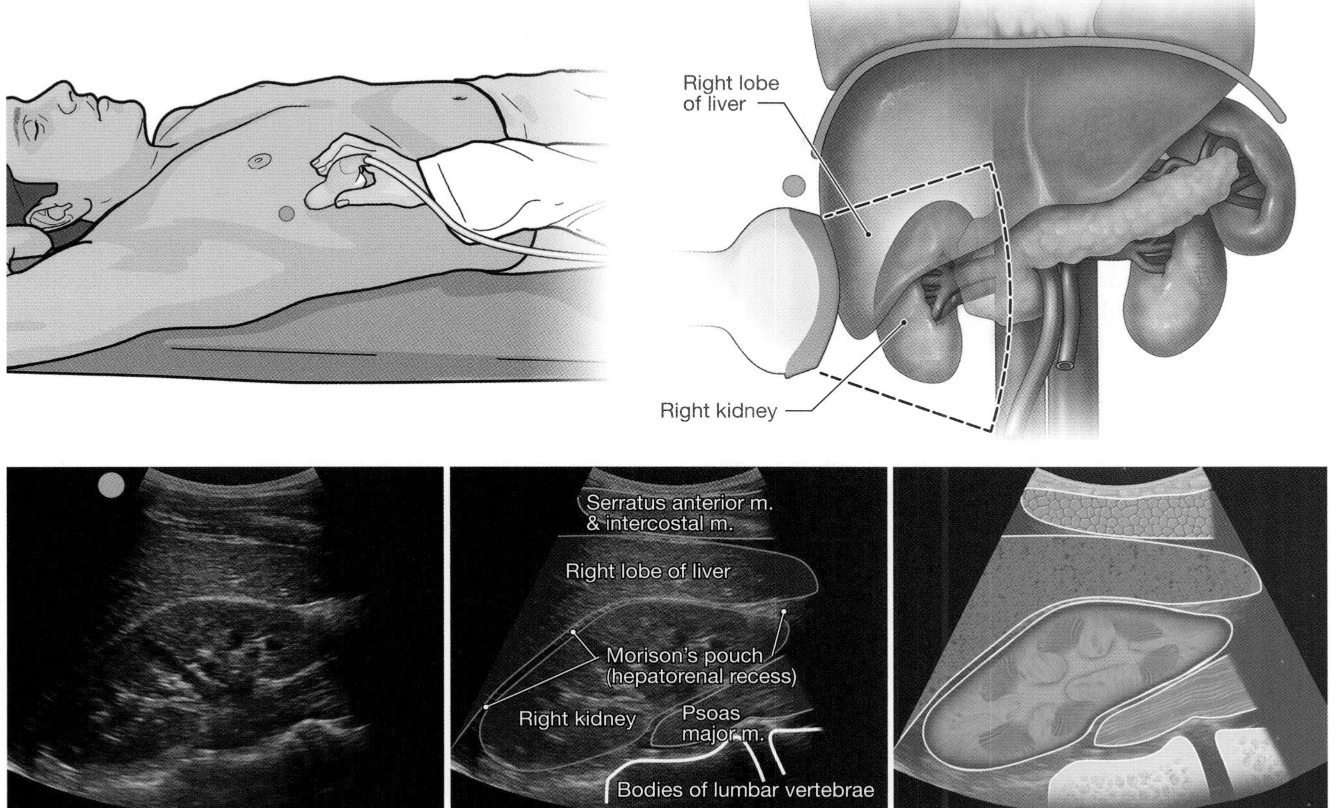

Figure 8.16 Longitudinal (intercostal oblique) view of the right kidney and right liver lobe.

Pancreas

Review of the Anatomy

The pancreas is located on the floor of the lesser sac in the left hypochondriac and epigastric regions, forming a portion of the bed of the stomach. It is situated in the retroperitoneal space, except a small portion of its tail, which is located in the splenorenal ligament. The head of the pancreas is situated in the C-shaped curvature of the duodenum. The uncinate process of the pancreas is the lower part of its head located to the left and posterior to the superior mesenteric vessels. It is both an exocrine gland that produces digestive enzymes involved in fat, protein, and carbohydrate digestion and an endocrine gland (islets of Langerhans) because it secretes insulin and glucagon, which are involved in the metabolism of glucose.

The blood supply of the pancreas is from branches of the splenic artery and the inferior and superior pancreaticoduodenal arteries. The pancreas consists of two ducts, the main pancreatic duct and the accessory pancreatic duct.

The main pancreatic duct (duct of Wirsung) starts in the tail, courses to the right along the pancreas, and drains the pancreatic juice, which contains enzymes. The bile duct and the main pancreatic duct join to form the hepatopancreatic ampulla (ampulla of Vater) as it enters the second part of the duodenum at the greater papilla. The accessory pancreatic duct (Santorini duct) starts in the lower part of the head of the pancreas to drain a portion of the body and head. It eventually empties at the lesser duodenal papilla superior to the greater papilla.

Technique

PANCREAS
ABDOMINAL AORTA
Longitudinal
(Parasagittal)
FIG. 8.17

With the patient in the supine position, place the probe in the longitudinal axis of the body just left of midline. You may need to start high in the epigastric area and slide inferiorly while applying pressure to the probe face to move bowel gas. Ask the patient to take a deep breath (asking the patient to drink a water load of two or three glasses may improve the imaging by displacing stomach gas) while you identify the left lobe of the liver and its edges and contours.

Tilt the probe to identify the pulsations of the abdominal aorta and adjust the beam angle until the aorta is roughly horizontal (rather than curving steeply up inferiorly with the lumbar curvature). Identify the celiac and superior mesenteric branches of the aorta. Anterior to the proximal part of the superior mesenteric artery, locate the splenic vein posterior to the body of the pancreas. The pancreas echo texture is variable, but generally similar to the liver with a slightly hypoechoic background with hyperechoic speckling. The left renal vein may be visible (physiologically compressed) in the space between the superior mesenteric artery and the anterior surface of the abdominal aorta.

HEAD OF PANCREAS
UNCINATE PROCESS
NECK OF PANCREAS
BODY OF PANCREAS
Transverse
FIG. 8.18

With the patient in the supine position, place the probe transversely across the midline. You may need to start high in the epigastric area and slide inferiorly while applying pressure to the probe face to move bowel gas. Ask the patient to take a deep breath (asking the patient to drink a water load of two or three glasses may improve the imaging by displacing stomach gas).

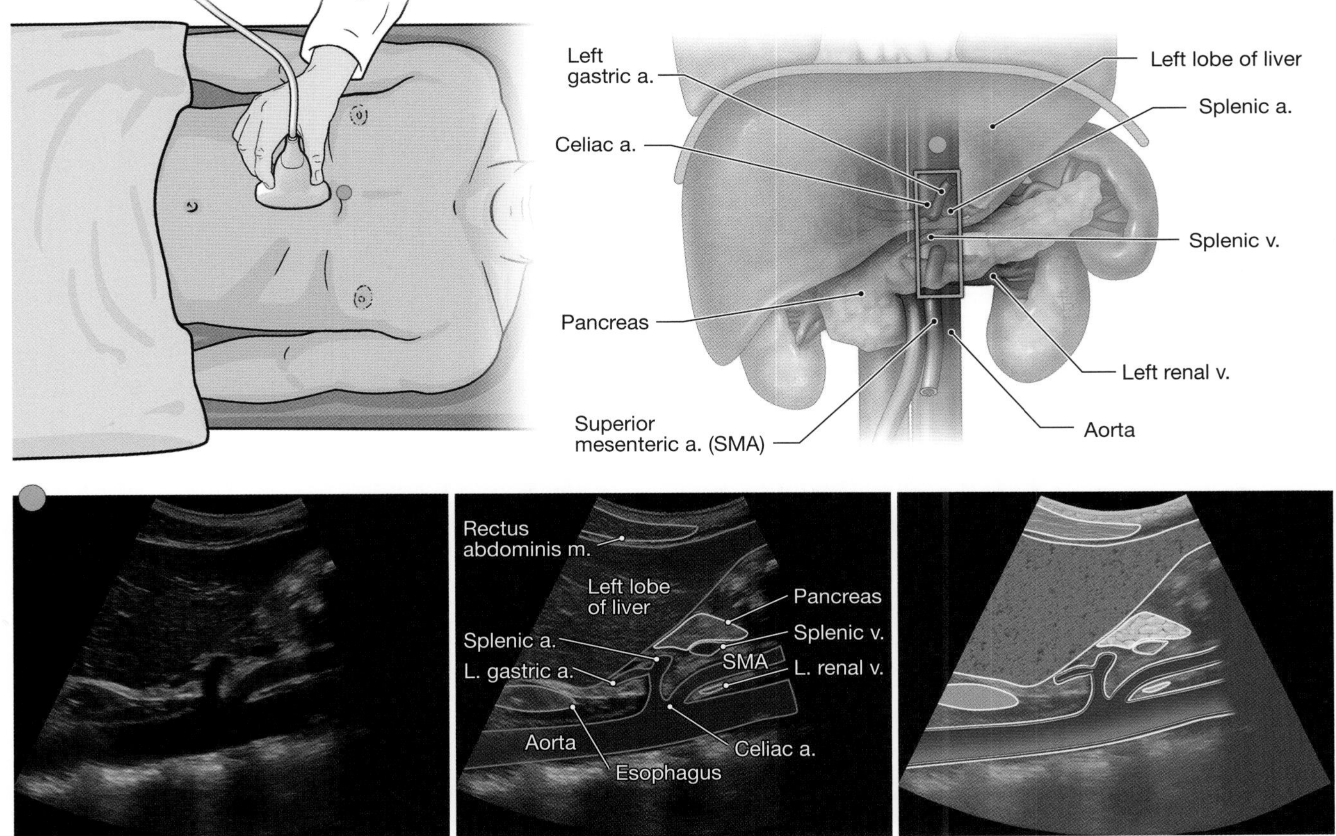

Figure 8.17 Longitudinal (parasagittal) view of the body of the pancreas in relationship to the left liver lobe, splenic vein, and abdominal aorta with its celiac and superior mesenteric branches.

With the probe in a transverse position across the midline, adjust the angle/tilt to look for the echotexture of the pancreas posterior to the left lobe of the liver and, more importantly, in relationship to abdominal vessels such as superior mesenteric and splenic veins at its posterior surface. Look for the superior mesenteric artery to the left of the superior mesenteric vein with a hyperechoic ring (surrounded by fat and connective tissue at the root of the mesentery), the head of the pancreas to the right of the superior mesenteric vein with the uncinate process extending posterior to the superior mesenteric vein, a pulsating aorta just along the left side of the vertebral body, and a left renal vein in the space between the aorta and the superior mesenteric artery (physiologically compressed in the space and expanding beyond) leading to the IVC to the right of the vertebral body. The neck of the pancreas is situated anterior to the superior mesenteric vessels and the body extends posteriorly out of view beyond the superior mesenteric vessels.

CLINICAL APPLICATIONS

Pancreatitis refers to inflammation of the pancreas and can be caused by gallstones or alcohol consumption. Its symptoms include severe and constant epigastric pain radiating to the back.

Pancreatic cancer can present as severe back pain and may invade into the surrounding organs. It usually presents late and is thus difficult to treat. Surgical resection called a pancreaticoduodenectomy (Whipple procedure) is possible in some cases. Cancer of the head can compress the bile duct, leading to obstructive jaundice. Cancer of the neck and body can cause obstruction of the portal vein or IVC as the pancreas is in proximity to these veins.

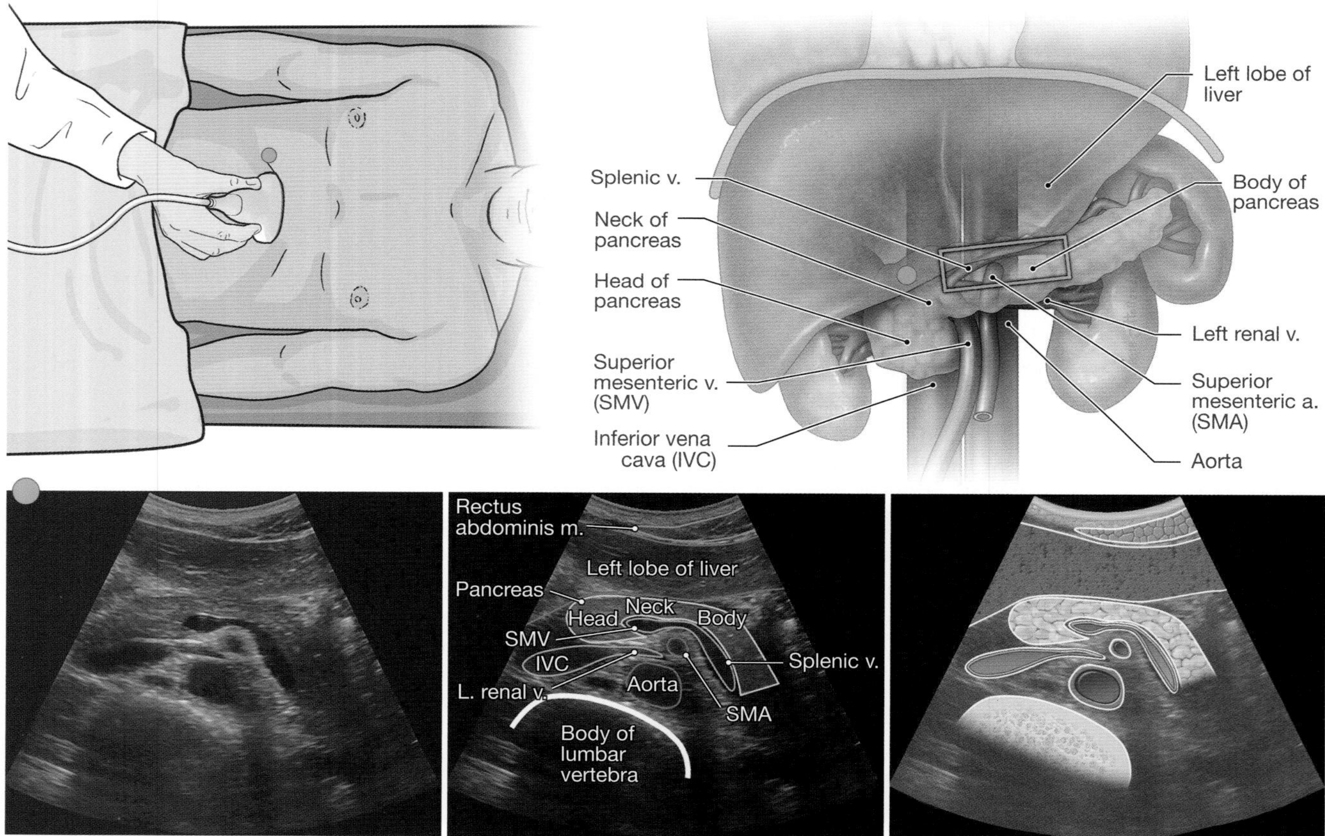

Figure 8.18 Transverse view of pancreas along with superior mesenteric artery and vein, splenic vein, left renal vein, inferior vena cava, and aorta.

Abdominal Vessels

Review of the Anatomy

Celiac and Mesenteric Arteries

The celiac trunk is a branch from the abdominal aorta, located at the anterior surface of the aorta just below the aortic hiatus of the diaphragm. The celiac trunk trifurcates into the left gastric, splenic, and common hepatic arteries.

The smallest branch from the celiac trunk is the left gastric artery. The left gastric artery travels superiorly toward the gastric cardia and communicates to the esophagus and liver with branches to the esophageal and hepatic arteries. The left gastric artery also runs along the lesser curvature of the stomach while forming a connection with the right gastric artery.

The splenic artery is a large, tortuous vessel that courses over the superior surface of the pancreas before entering the splenorenal ligament. This artery is the largest branch of the celiac trunk and usually has numerous terminal branches that include the short gastric arteries, the left gastroomental (gastroepiploic) artery, and pancreatic branches.

The short gastric arteries supply the fundus of the stomach and course through the splenogastric ligament. The left gastroomental artery supplies the stomach and the greater omentum by also passing through the splenogastric ligament to reach the greater omentum and course beside the greater curvature of the stomach. One of the pancreatic vessels, which branches off the splenic artery, includes the dorsal pancreatic artery.

After arising from the celiac trunk, the common hepatic artery travels toward the liver along the superior border of the pancreas. The common hepatic artery branches into the proper hepatic artery, the gastroduodenal artery, and occasionally the right gastric artery. The proper hepatic artery is located along the free edge of the lesser omentum. The proper hepatic artery divides into the left and right hepatic arteries. The right hepatic artery subsequently divides into the cystic artery at the cystohepatic triangle of Calot. The borders of the triangle of Calot are the cystic duct, the common hepatic duct, and the inferior border of the liver. The right gastric artery can arise from the common hepatic artery, but may occasionally originate from the proper hepatic artery. The right gastric artery travels to the pylorus of the stomach and along the lesser curvature of the stomach, where it forms an anastomosis with the left gastric artery. The gastroduodenal artery travels posterior to the first part of the duodenum. It is known to give off multiple branches, including the supraduodenal artery superiorly and various retroduodenal arteries inferiorly. In particular, the gastroduodenal artery divides into the right gastroomental artery and the superior pancreaticoduodenal artery.

The right gastroomental artery travels along the greater curvature of the stomach. It provides blood supply to the stomach and the greater omentum. The superior pancreaticoduodenal artery courses between the head of the pancreas and the duodenum. The superior pancreaticoduodenal artery divides into the anterior-superior pancreaticoduodenal artery and the posterior-superior pancreaticoduodenal artery.

Superior Mesenteric Artery

The superior mesenteric artery arises from the abdominal aorta posterior to the neck of the pancreas. It descends anterior to the uncinate process of the pancreas and the third part of the duodenum and enters the root of the mesentery posterior to the transverse colon and runs into the right iliac fossa. The superior mesenteric artery gives rise to five terminal branches: the inferior pancreaticoduodenal artery, the middle colic artery, the right colic artery, the ileocolic artery, and the intestinal arteries. The inferior pancreatoduodenal artery courses to the right and divides into two branches, the anterior-inferior pancreaticoduodenal artery and the posterior-inferior pancreaticoduodenal artery. The inferior pancreaticoduodenal artery (anterior and posterior) then anastomoses with respective branches of the superior pancreaticoduodenal artery.

The middle colic artery bifurcates into the right and left branches. The right branch anastomoses with the right colic artery, and the left branch also has connections with the ascending branch of the left colic artery. As these arterial connections occur, the marginal artery is formed running along the large bowel.

The right colic artery originates from the superior mesenteric artery and courses to the right behind the peritoneum. The right colic artery may frequently arise from the ileocolic artery. The right colic artery terminates into ascending and descending branches, which course along the ascending colon.

The ileocolic artery traverses inferiorly, posterior to the peritoneum toward the right iliac fossa. It then divides into the ascending colic artery, anterior and posterior cecal arteries, the appendicular artery, and ileal branches. The ascending colic artery forms an anastomosis with the right colic artery. Branches from the superior mesenteric artery (usually 12-15 in number) supply the jejunum and ileum. The intestinal arteries branch and anastomose to form a series of arcades in the mesentery.

Inferior Mesenteric Artery

The inferior mesenteric artery arises inferiorly to the superior mesenteric artery on the anterior surface of the aorta and courses to the left posterior to the peritoneum. Terminal branches of the inferior mesenteric artery supply the descending colon, the sigmoid colon, and the upper portion of the rectum. The inferior mesenteric artery trifurcates into the left colic artery, the sigmoid artery, and the superior rectal artery. The left colic artery courses to the left toward the descending colon and normally divides into ascending and descending branches. The sigmoid arteries (2-3 in number) course toward the sigmoid colon in its mesentery dividing into ascending and descending branches. The superior rectal artery descends into the pelvis and terminates into two branches. The branches of the superior rectal artery course along the sides of the rectum and connect with the middle and inferior rectal arteries.

Veins

Portal Vein

The **portal vein** is formed by the splenic vein and the superior mesenteric vein posterior to the neck of the pancreas. The portal vein is about 8 cm (3.2 in) long and collects venous blood from the abdominal part of the gut, spleen, pancreas, and gallbladder.

Inferior Mesenteric Vein

The inferior mesenteric vein does not directly drain into the portal vein. It can merge with the splenic or the superior mesenteric vein or at the junction of these two veins. The inferior mesenteric also receives venous drainage from the left gastric (or coronary) vein. This vein courses superiorly behind the bile duct and hepatic artery within the free margin of the lesser omentum, carrying deoxygenated blood and nutrients extracted from digestion. It carries three times as much blood as the hepatic artery and has a higher blood pressure than in the IVC.

Superior Mesenteric Vein

The superior mesenteric vein courses along the right side of the superior mesenteric artery. Some of the branches of the superior mesenteric vein also follow the tributaries of the superior mesenteric artery. The root of the superior mesenteric vein usually traverses the third part of the duodenum and the uncinate process of the pancreas. The termination of the superior mesenteric vein is located behind the neck of the pancreas. At this point, the splenic vein merges with the superior mesenteric vein to form the portal vein.

Splenic Vein

The splenic vein (formerly known as the lineal vein) originates from the merging of venous sinusoids in the spleen. The splenic vein also receives venous drainage from the short gastric, left gastroomental, and pancreatic veins.

Inferior Mesenteric Vein

The inferior mesenteric veins originate from the joining of the superior rectal and sigmoid veins. The inferior mesenteric vein receives venous drainage from the left colic vein. Often the inferior mesenteric vein drains into the splenic vein. However, the inferior mesenteric vein can drain directly into the superior mesenteric vein or at the merging point of the superior mesenteric and splenic veins.

Left Gastric (Coronary) Vein

The left gastric (coronary) vein usually spans over a short distance in the superior portion of the lesser curvature of the stomach, where it is nestled between the two lesser omental layers. The left gastric vein continues to travel toward the junction of the stomach and esophagus. At this point, the left gastric vein can join venous tributaries of the esophagus, which eventually empty into the azygous vein, thus formulating the systemic venous distribution of the left gastric vein. In addition, the left gastric vein drains into the portal vein directly as well as through an anastomosis with the right gastric vein, to form the portal venous portion of the left gastric vein.

Paraumbilical Veins

The paraumbilical veins are nested in the falciform ligament. These veins connect the left branch of the portal vein with small periumbilical subcutaneous veins. The periumbilical subcutaneous veins are radicles of the superior epigastric, inferior epigastric, thoracoepigastric, and superficial epigastric veins. The paraumbilical veins are usually closed but can become patent and dilated in portal hypertension.

Hepatic Veins

The hepatic veins (left, right, and middle) are valveless veins located in the intersegmental planes of the liver. These veins drain into the IVC; however, frequently the left and middle hepatic veins often merge before joining the IVC.

Technique

AORTA CELIAC ARTERY SUPERIOR MESENTERIC ARTERY
Longitudinal (Parasagittal)
FIG. 8.19

With the patient in the supine position, place the probe in the longitudinal axis of the body just left of midline. You may need to start high in the epigastric area and slide inferiorly while applying pressure to the probe face to move the bowel gas. Ask the patient to take a deep breath (asking the patient to drink a water load of two or three glasses may improve the imaging by displacing stomach gas). Identify the left lobe of the liver and its edges and contours. Tilt the probe face to identify the pulsations of the abdominal aorta and adjust the beam angle until the aorta is roughly horizontal (rather than curving steeply up inferiorly with the lumbar curvature). Identify the celiac and superior mesenteric branches of the aorta. Anterior to the proximal part of the superior mesenteric artery, locate the splenic vein posteriorly to the body of the pancreas. The pancreas echo texture is variable but generally similar to the liver, slightly hypoechoic background with hyperechoic speckling. The left renal vein may be visible (physiologically compressed) in the space between the superior mesenteric artery and the anterior surface of the abdominal aorta.

CELIAC ARTERY SPLENIC ARTERY COMMON HEPATIC BRANCHES
Transverse
FIG. 8.20

With the patient in the supine position, place the probe transversely with the marker pointing to the right. Identify the left lobe of the liver and the bodies of the lumbar vertebrae. Identify the aorta and the IVC along the vertebral body. Slide the probe and tilt/fan while watching for the celiac artery and the sweeping "gull-wing" appearance of its splenic and common hepatic branches. The splenic artery is useful for "following" along the body of the pancreas. The portal vein is seen immediately anterior to the IVC.

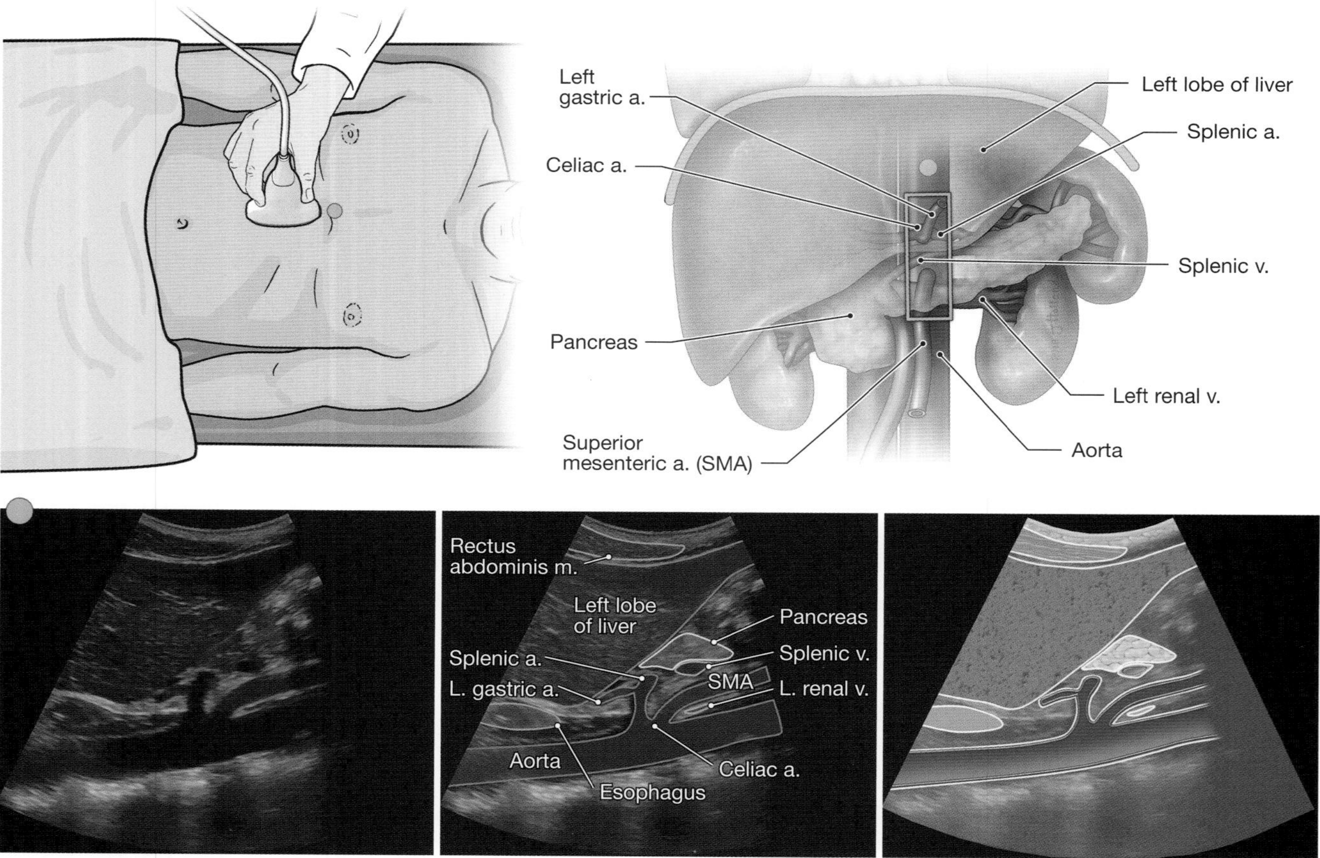

Figure 8.19 Longitudinal (parasagittal) view of the abdominal aorta along with its celiac and superior mesenteric branches.

SUPERIOR MESENTERIC ARTERY SUPERIOR MESENTERIC VEIN AORTA INFERIOR VENA CAVA
Transverse
FIG. 8.21

Continue from Figure 8.20 and tilt/fan and slide slightly inferiorly while watching for the next ventral branch of the aorta, the superior mesenteric artery. The celiac and the superior mesenteric branches of the aorta arise very close together, and only slight movements (sliding/tilting) of the probe go back and forth between them. After identifying the superior mesenteric artery, adjust the probe position until the superior mesenteric artery can be clearly seen surrounded by a hyperechoic ring (of fat/connective tissue at the root of the mesentery) just to the left of the superior mesenteric vein. Tilt/slide up and down to see the splenic vein joining the superior mesenteric vein from the left side, forming the portal vein behind the neck of the pancreas (superior to the position where the splenic vein joins the superior mesenteric vein is the portal vein). Look for the echotexture and identify the pancreatic head and uncinate process adjacent to the superior mesenteric vein. Carefully adjust the position of the probe to identify the right renal artery and the (physiologically compressed) left renal vein traversing the space between the superior mesenteric vein and aorta to join the IVC. In this image, the falciform ligament is clearly seen at the border between the left liver and quadrate lobes. The right crus of the diaphragm is also well seen in this image along the vertebral body, between the IVC and aorta.

SUPERIOR MESENTERIC VESSELS SPLENIC VEIN AORTA INFERIOR VENA CAVA
Transverse
FIG. 8.22

Place the probe in the same position as in Figure 8.21 and adjust the probe position to see the splenic vein joining the superior mesenteric vein. Keep as much of the splenic vein in view as possible. Follow the body of the pancreas to the left and posteriorly,

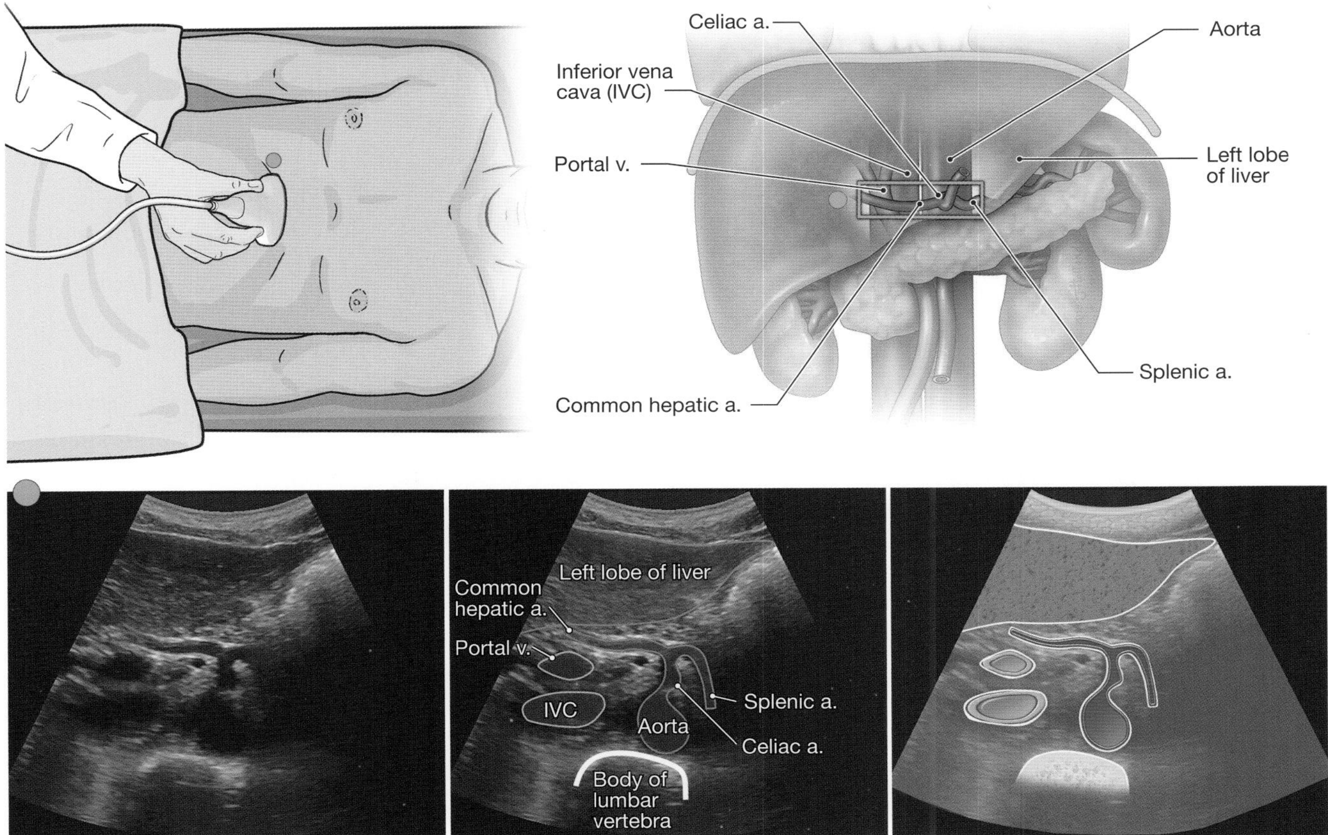

Figure 8.20 Transverse view of the celiac artery along with its splenic and common hepatic branches.

and identify the superior mesenteric vessels, the aorta, the IVC, and their relationships with the left renal vein.

ABDOMINAL AORTA INFERIOR VENA CAVA
Transverse
FIG. 8.23

Starting from the superior mesenteric artery in Figure 8.22, slide the probe inferiorly keeping the aorta and IVC in view to a position a few centimeters above the umbilicus. The bifurcation of the abdominal aorta occurs approximately at the level of the umbilicus. The aorta and IVC become progressively more superficial inferiorly, following the lumbar curvature of the spine. There is small intestine and gas shadowing, but as the vessels and the lumbar vertebrae become more superficial, it becomes easy to apply probe pressure to gently push the intestinal gas out of the way.

BIFURCATION OF ABDOMINAL AORTA
Transverse
FIG. 8.24

Continue from Figure 8.23 and follow the aorta inferiorly to about the level of the umbilicus (need to fill the umbilicus with gel to eliminate air shadowing and poor image quality when the probe is over the umbilicus). At this level, the aorta typically divides into the right and left common iliac arteries. After identifying the right and left common iliac arteries at their origin, slide the probe a few centimeters inferiorly and observe the left common iliac vein crossing horizontally behind the iliac arteries to join the more vertical right common iliac vein at the confluence of the IVC.

INFERIOR VENA CAVA
Longitudinal (Subcostal)
FIG. 8.25

With the patient in the supine position, place the probe in the longitudinal axis of the body just right of the midline under the right costal margin, aimed up toward the thorax (a deep breath by the patient may be helpful). Identify the liver speckled pattern and veins; note the inspiratory collapse and rhythmic transmitted pulsations of the IVC. The portal vein is seen anterior to the IVC, accompanied by the proper hepatic artery.

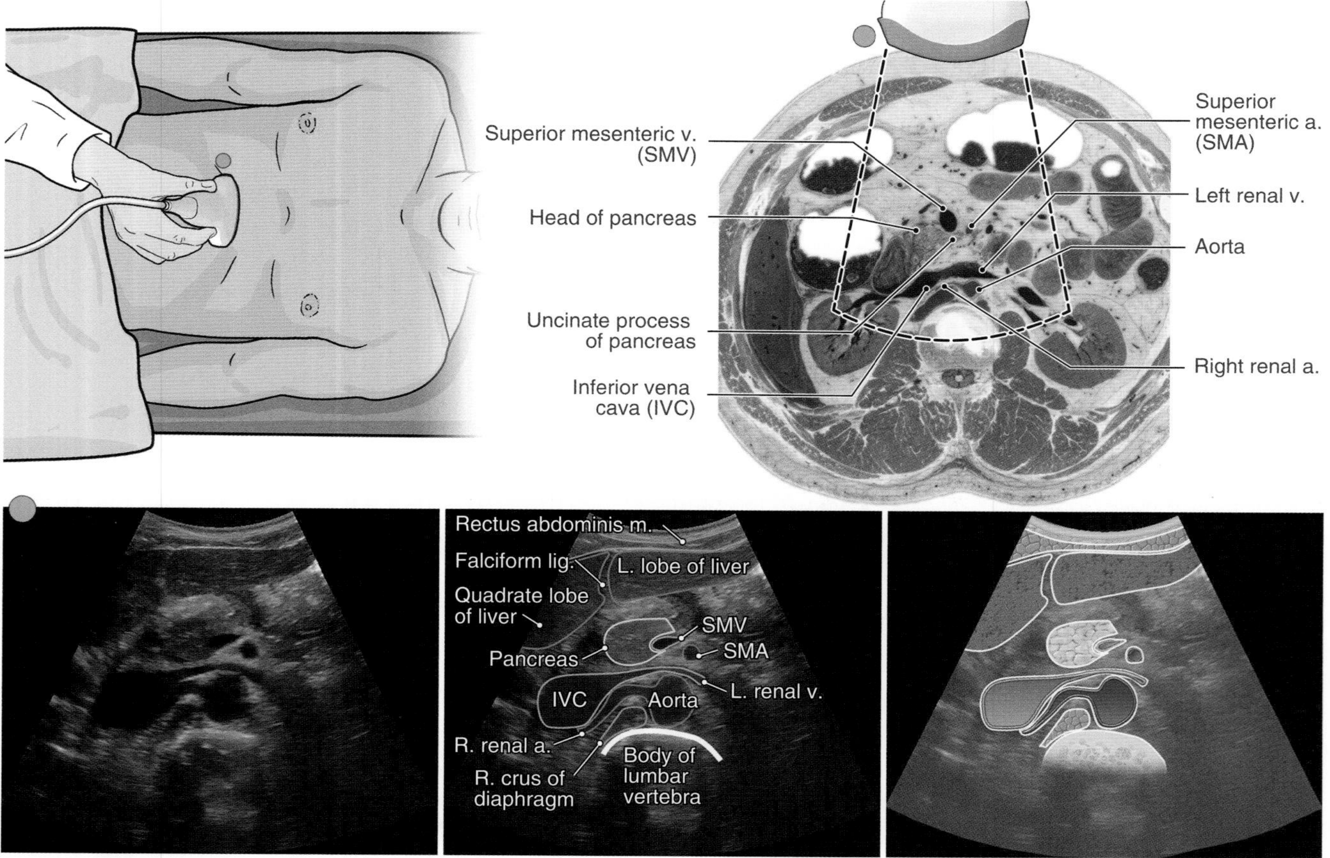

Figure 8.21 Transverse view of the superior mesenteric artery and vein, head and uncinate process of the pancreas, abdominal aorta, and inferior vena cava.

CLINICAL APPLICATIONS

Abdominal Aortic Aneurysm

Abdominal aortic aneurysm is defined as the dilatations of the abdominal aorta if greater than 50% of its proximal normal segment (>3 cm). Males are more commonly affected, and it is present in approximately 10% of the population over 65 years of age. Unfortunately, the majority of abdominal aortic aneurysms are asymptomatic and are diagnosed incidentally during routine examinations. However, the most common complication of abdominal aortic aneurysm is rupture, which presents with severe abdominal pain or back pain leading to hypovolemic shock with a high mortality rate. The most common causes leading to aneurysm are atherosclerosis, inflammation, chronic aortic dissection, different types of vasculitis, and Marfan and Ehlers-Danlos syndromes.

Splenic Artery Aneurysm

Splenic artery aneurysm is the most common aneurysm of the viscera. These focal dilatations of the splenic artery can be saccular or true aneurysms. These aneurysms are more common in females; however, rupture is more common in males. Their discovery is typically incidental, but are most commonly associated with atherosclerosis, different types of vasculitis, fibromuscular dysplasia, portal hypertension, and cirrhosis. The most common complication of splenic aneurysm is rupture (5% of cases), which presents with left upper quadrant pain. There is a double-rupture sign when the initial blood after the rupture collects at the lesser sac and provides a pseudohemodynamic stabilization, followed by sudden hypovolemic shock when the blood moves into the peritoneal cavity.

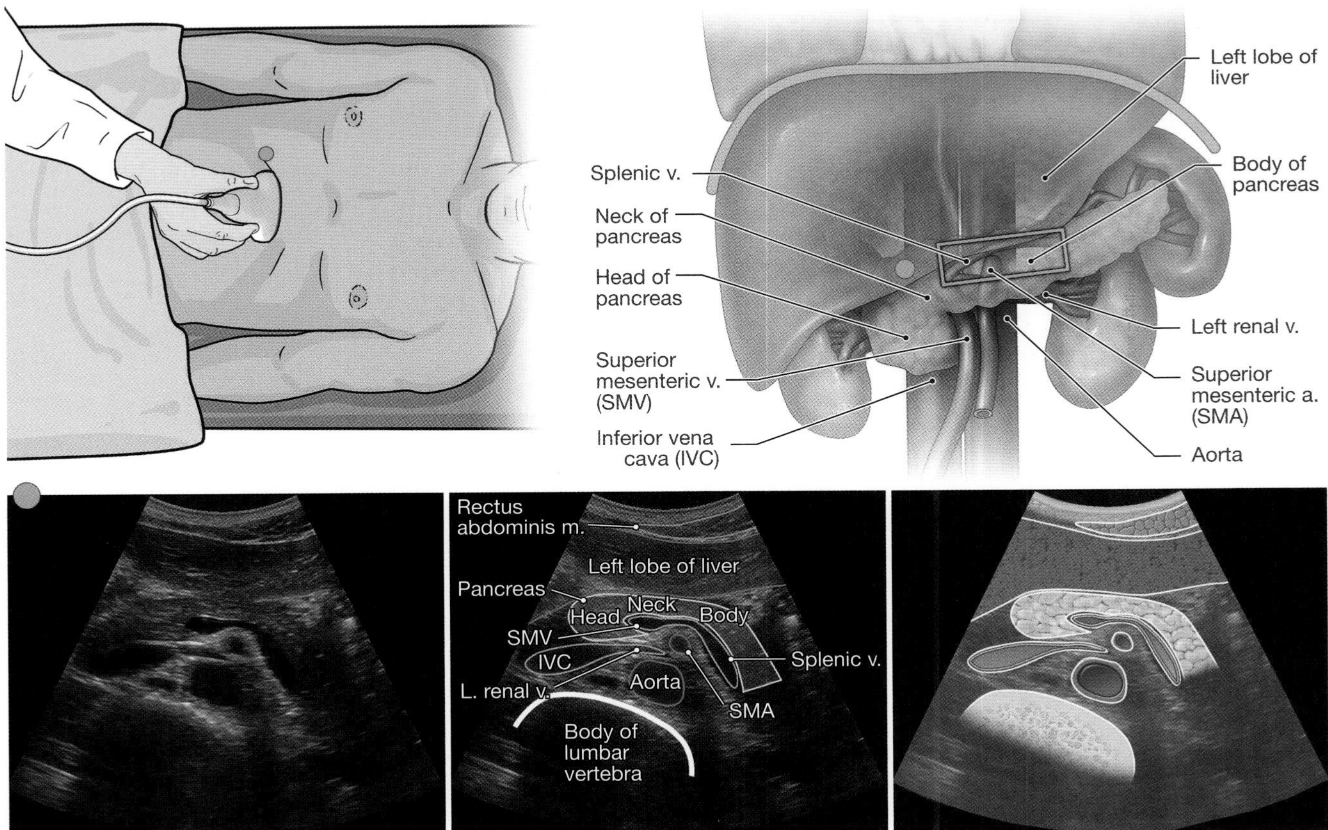

Figure 8.22 Transverse view of the superior mesenteric artery and vein, head, uncinate process, neck and body of the pancreas, splenic vein, abdominal aorta, and inferior vena cava.

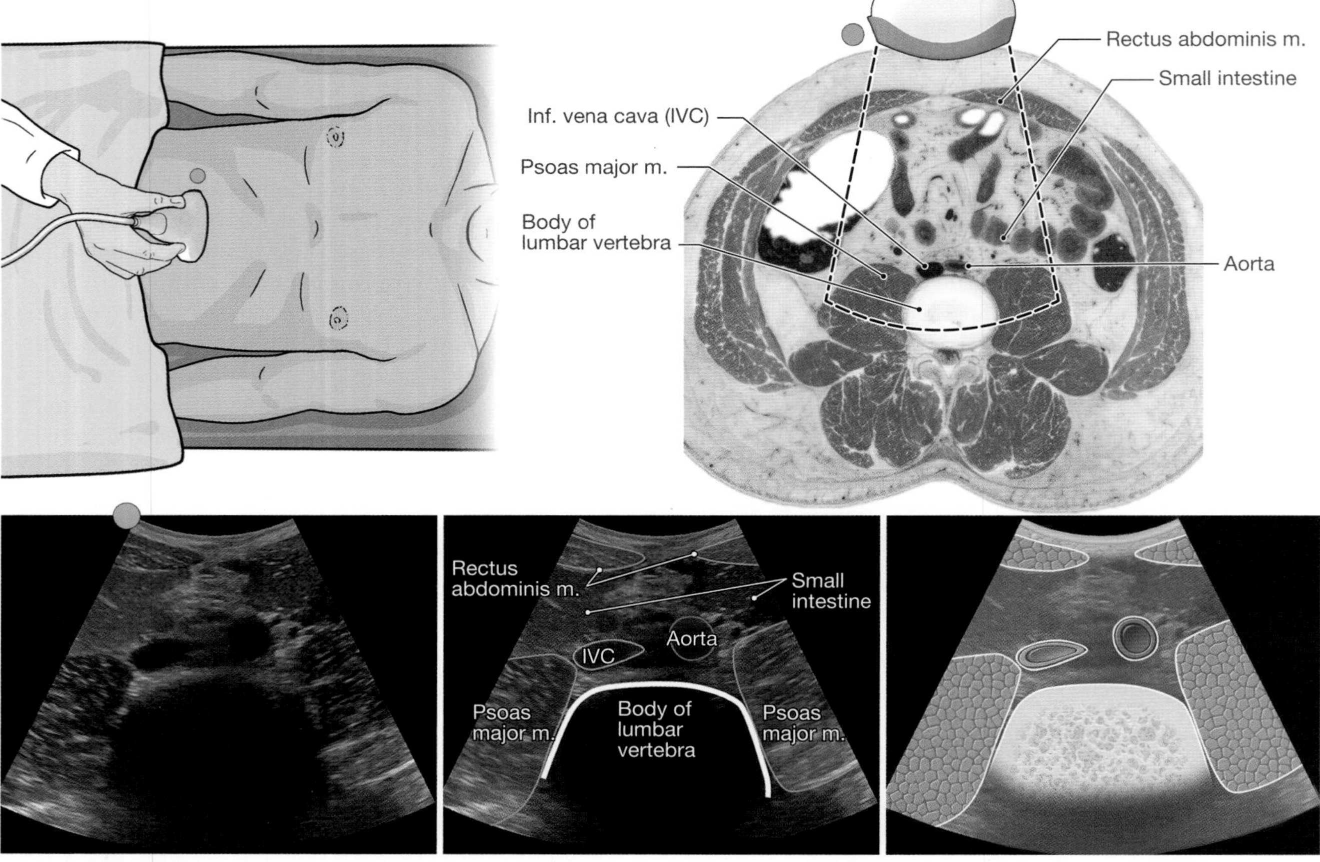

Figure 8.23 Transverse view, above the umbilicus, of the aorta and inferior vena cava in relationship to the lumbar vertebral body and psoas major muscles.

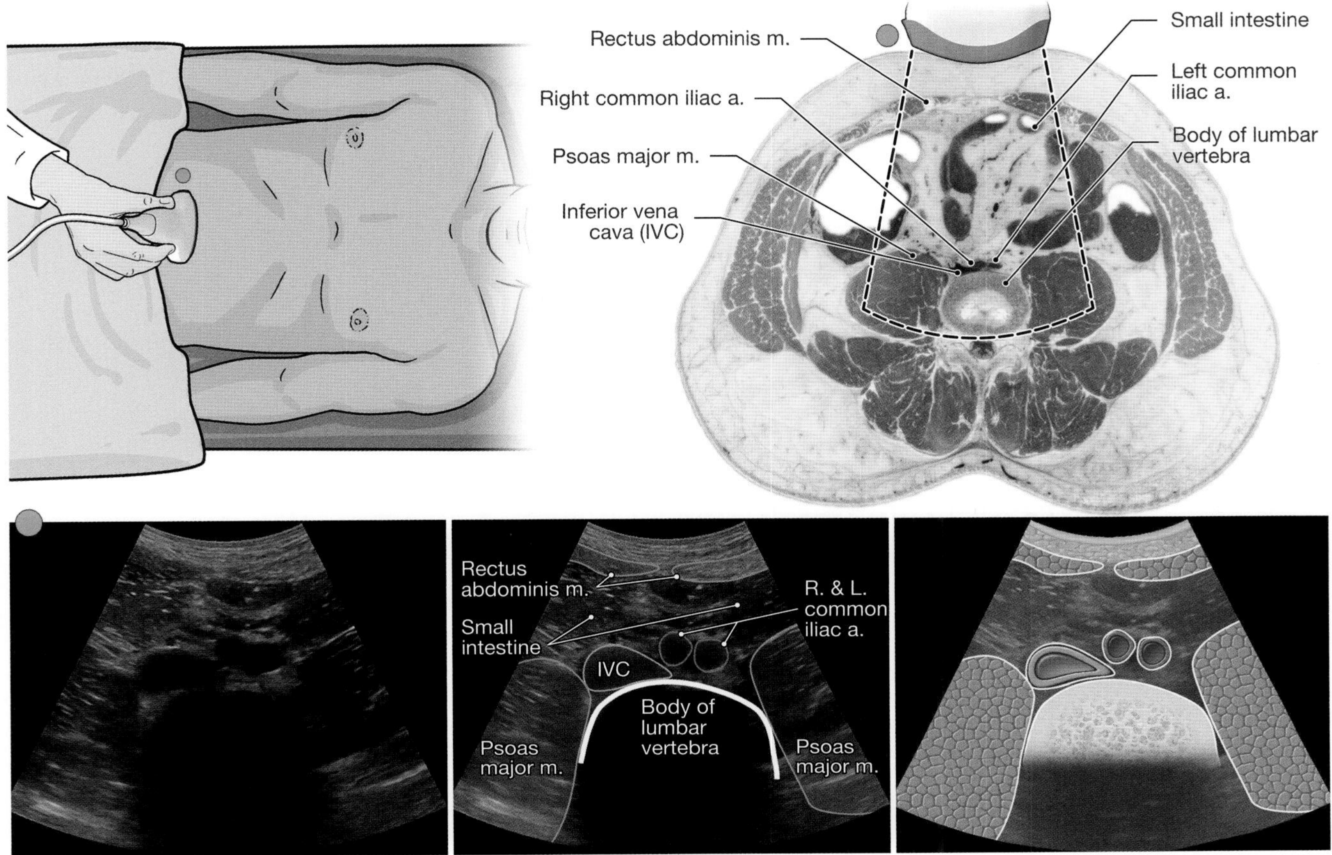

Figure 8.24 Transverse view of the bifurcation of the abdominal aorta into right and left common iliac arteries.

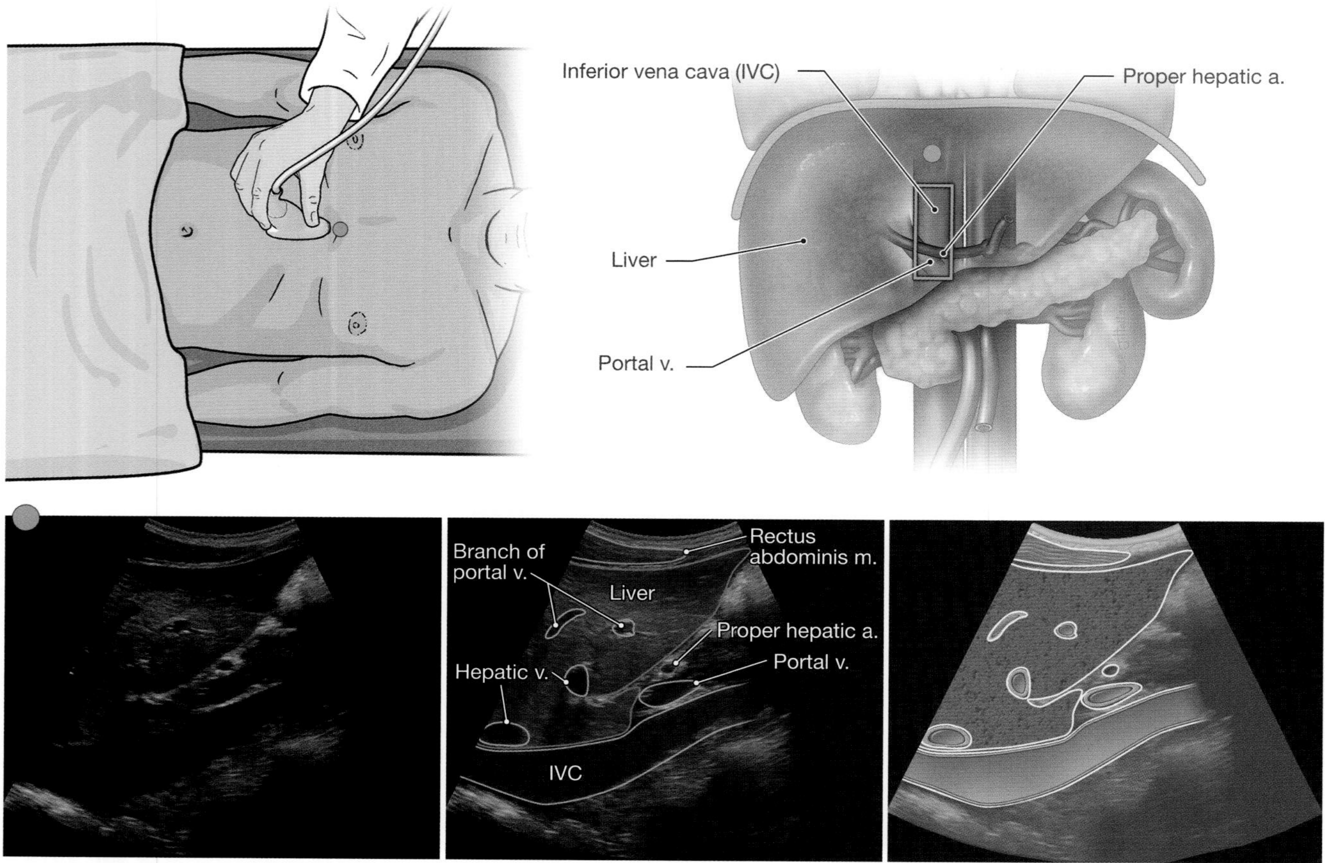

Figure 8.25 Longitudinal (subcostal) view of the course of the inferior vena cava posterior to the liver.

Multiple Choice Questions

1. A 70-year-old man is brought to the emergency department because of a 2-hour history of severe pain radiating from his lower back toward his pubic symphysis. Ultrasound examination shows a kidney stone obstructing his right ureter. At which of the following locations is the stone most likely lodged?

   A. Major calyx
   B. Minor calyx
   C. Pelvic brim
   D. Midportion of the ureter
   E. Between the pelvic brim and the urinary bladder

2. A 70-year-old man is brought to the emergency department because of a 2-hour history of severe pain radiating from his lower back toward his pubic symphysis. Ultrasound examination shows a kidney stone obstructing his right ureter. Which of the following nerves is most likely responsible for conducting the sensation of pain?

   A. Lateral femoral cutaneous
   B. Ilioinguinal
   C. Obturator
   D. Subcostal
   E. Iliohypogastric

3. A 45-year-old man is brought to the emergency department because of a 2-day history of abdominal pain, vomiting, and fever. The pain started as poorly localized to the epigastrium but became progressively sharp in nature and radiated to the right hypochondriac region. The pain now radiates to the right shoulder. Physical examination shows yellowing of the sclerae, soft and tender abdomen, and a positive Murphy sign. An ultrasound examination of his abdomen shows thickened gallbladder, with several echogenic gallstones and dilation of the biliary tree. Laboratory studies show elevated serum bilirubin, alanine aminotransferase (ALT), aspartate aminotransferase (AST), alkaline phosphatase (ALP), and gamma-glutamyl transferase (GGT) and increased prothrombin time. Endoscopic retrograde cholangiopancreatography shows an obstruction along the extrahepatic biliary tree with normal pancreatic duct flow. Which of the structures is most likely obstructed?

   A. The hepatopancreatic ampulla
   B. The cystic duct
   C. The common bile duct
   D. The left hepatic duct
   E. The infundibulum of the gallbladder

4. A 45-year-old man is brought to the emergency department because of a 2-day history of abdominal pain, vomiting, and fever. The pain started as poorly localized to the epigastrium but became progressively sharp in nature and radiated to the right hypochondriac region. The pain now radiates to the right shoulder. Physical examination shows yellowing of the sclerae, soft and tender abdomen, and a positive Murphy sign. An ultrasound examination of his abdomen shows thickened gallbladder, with several echogenic gallstones and dilation of the biliary tree. Laboratory studies show elevated serum bilirubin, alanine aminotransferase (ALT), aspartate aminotransferase (AST), alkaline phosphatase (ALP), and gamma-glutamyl transferase (GGT) and increased prothrombin time. A laparoscopic cholecystectomy is performed using the triangle of Calot as landmark. Which of the following are the boundaries of the triangle of Calot?

   A. Cystic artery, common hepatic duct, bile duct
   B. Gallbladder, hepatic duct, bile duct
   C. Inferior border of the liver, cystic duct, common hepatic duct
   D. Inferior border of liver, bile duct, common hepatic duct
   E. Cystic artery, inferior border of liver, bile duct

5. A 45-year-old man is brought to the emergency department because of a 2-day history of abdominal pain, vomiting, and fever. The pain started as poorly localized to the epigastrium but became progressively sharp in nature and radiated to the right hypochondriac region. The pain now radiates to the right shoulder. Physical examination shows yellowing of the sclerae, soft and tender abdomen, and a positive Murphy sign. An ultrasound examination of his abdomen shows thickened gallbladder, with several echogenic gallstones and dilation of the biliary tree. Laboratory studies show elevated serum bilirubin, alanine aminotransferase (ALT), aspartate aminotransferase (AST), alkaline phosphatase (ALP), and gamma-glutamyl transferase (GGT) and increased prothrombin time. A laparoscopic cholecystectomy is performed using the triangle of Calot as landmark. Which of the following structures would most likely be identified and ligated within the triangle?

   A. Cystic artery
   B. Right hepatic artery
   C. Bile duct
   D. Cystic duct
   E. Right hepatic duct

6. A 45-year-old man is brought to the emergency department because of a 2-day history of abdominal pain, vomiting, and fever. The pain started as poorly localized to the epigastrium but became progressively sharp in nature and radiated to the right hypochondriac region. The pain now radiates to the right shoulder. Physical examination shows yellowing of the sclerae, soft and tender abdomen, and a positive Murphy sign. An ultrasound examination of his abdomen shows thickened gallbladder, with several echogenic gallstones and dilation of the biliary tree. Laboratory studies show elevated serum bilirubin, alanine aminotransferase (ALT), aspartate aminotransferase (AST), alkaline phosphatase (ALP), and gamma-glutamyl transferase (GGT) and increased prothrombin time. A laparoscopic cholecystectomy is performed using the triangle of Calot as landmark. During laparoscopic cholecystectomy the scope is passed into the greater sac through a small port in the anterior abdominal wall. Which organ is the surgeon unable to view directly?

   A. Ileum
   B. Jejunum
   C. Pancreas
   D. Stomach
   E. Transverse colon

7. A 68-year-old woman comes to the emergency department because of cramping mid-abdominal pain, abdominal distension, and vomiting for the past 24 hours. Physical examination shows positive Murphy sign and right upper quadrant ultrasound shows gallstones with gallbladder thickening. An x-ray of the abdomen shows air in the gallbladder and biliary tree. In which of the following sites will an ultrasound examination show a gallstone lodged?

   A. Cystic duct
   B. Bile duct
   C. Duodenum
   D. Jejunum
   E. Ileum

8. A 60-year-old man comes to the emergency department with severe abdominal pain. He has a history of peptic ulcer disease and recently started a course of NSAIDs for arthritic pain in his knees. Physical examination of the abdomen shows a nondistended firm abdomen with guarding and rebound tenderness. An ultrasound of the abdomen shows intraperitoneal fluid. A diagnosis of a perforated peptic ulcer is made. Which of the following sites is least likely to contain a collection of fluid under ultrasound examination in this patient?

   A. Hepatorenal pouch (of Morison)
   B. Rectouterine pouch of (Douglas)
   C. Right paracolic gutter
   D. Greater sac
   E. Omental bursa

9. A 55-year-old man comes to the emergency department because of 1-week history of pain at the right upper quadrant. Physical examination shows pain radiation to the right side of his back beneath his scapula. There is no icterus. An ultrasound of the abdomen shows cholecystitis with a large gallstone located at the area of the right upper quadrant. In which of the following structures the gallstone is most likely located?

   A. Bile duct
   B. Hartmann pouch
   C. Left hepatic duct
   D. Pancreatic duct
   E. Right hepatic duct

10. A 20-year-old woman is brought to the emergency department by her husband because of a sudden, sharp pain in the left lower quadrant. Physical examination shows severe abdominal tenderness, abdominal pain, amenorrhea and vaginal bleeding. She says that her last menstrual period was 10 days ago. A pregnancy test is negative. A CT scan shows a ruptured left fallopian tube, which has resulted in approximately 150 mL blood and fluid in the pelvis. During an ultrasound examination, in which of the following spaces would fluid most likely accumulate?

   A. Right subphrenic space
   B. Hepatorenal pouch (of Morison)
   C. Paracolic gutters
   D. Vesicouterine pouch
   E. Rectouterine pouch of (Douglas)

9

Female Pelvis

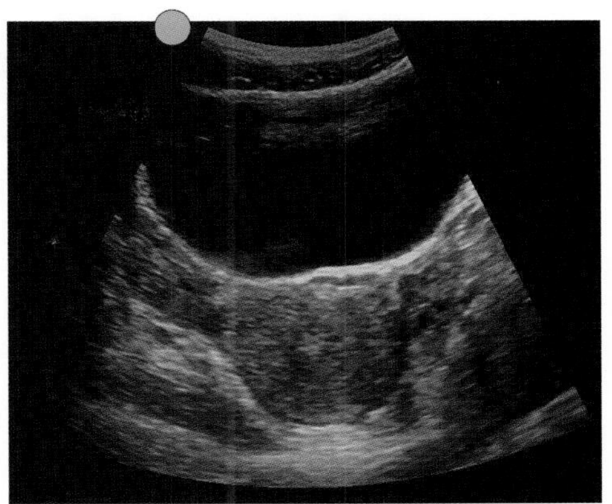

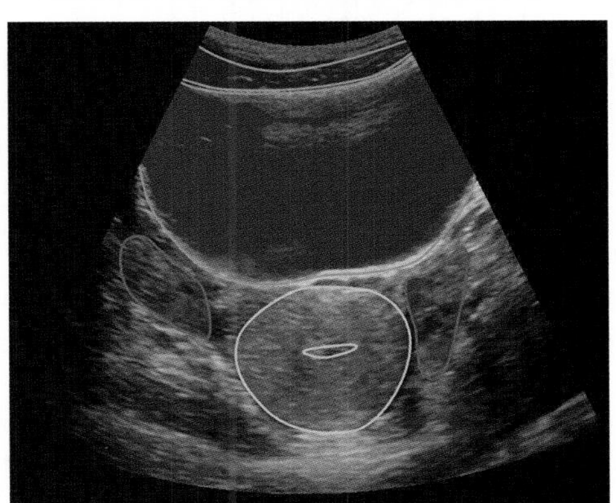

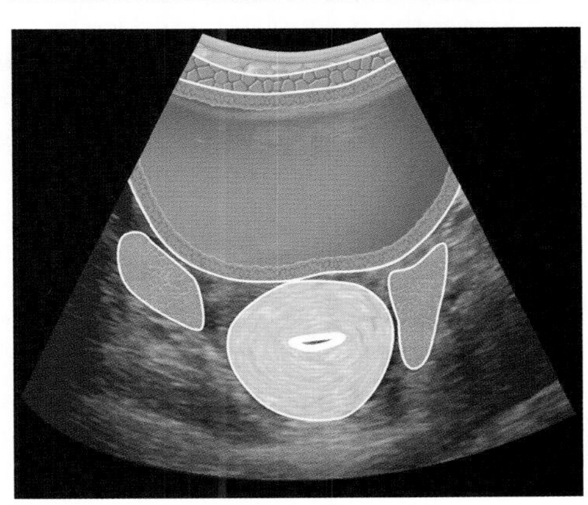

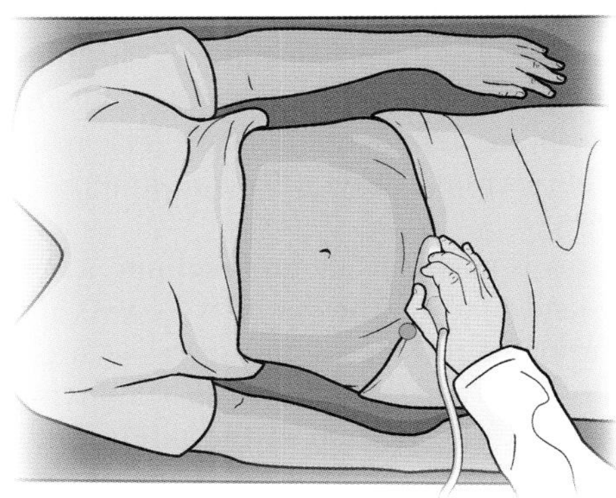

Review of the Anatomy

The general anatomical presentation of the pelvis is described in Chapter 10. This chapter focuses specifically on the elements of the female pelvis. However, there are some differences noted while comparing the pelvises of males and females. In females, the pelvis is typically smaller, denser, and less thicker than in males. In comparison, the female pelvic cavity is less deep and wide, the **pubic arch** (also known as the subpubic angle) is bigger in size, and the greater sciatic notch is broader. When detailed, the pelvic inlet in males has a heart-shaped appearance, whereas the female pelvis is described as having an oval-shaped inlet. The pelvic outlet, however, is also bigger in females because of the outward protuberance of the ischial tuberosities. Finally, the obturator foramen is described as being triangular or egg-shaped in females compared with a more rounded shape found in males.

In females, the **ureter**s and the ovarian vessels are found traveling together along the pelvic brim (linea terminalis) and are crossed superficially by the uterine arteries. As a result of this anatomical arrangement, there is a potential risk of injury to the ureters while performing an oophorectomy or hysterectomy. In males, the ureters enter the bladder at the posterolateral surface by coursing behind and inferiorly to the ductus deferens and anteriorly to the seminal vesicles. In females, the urethra is short in length, roughly 4 cm, and is observed passing through the pelvic floor into the perineum and opening into the vestibule of the vagina.

Uterus

The uterus is a muscular organ and the largest female reproductive organ. It is supported and kept in place by numerous ligaments such as the round, broad, and cardinal ligaments, as well as the pubocervical, and uterosacral (rectouterine) ligaments (described as follows). The uterus occupies the space between the bladder and the rectum at the level of the pelvic midline. The uterus allows for implantation of the fertilized oocyte and sustains life for the developing fetus until delivery. The main arterial source is the uterine artery, with contributions from the ovarian artery.

The uterus is anatomically grouped into a cervix, isthmus, body, and fundus. The cervix is located at the most inferior portion of the uterus and serves as a connection between the vagina and the uterus. The isthmus is a tapered (approximately 1 cm) portion of the uterus between the body and the cervix. The body, which is the largest segment of the uterus, contains the uterine cavity. The fundus is a rounded structure located at the upper region of the uterus. The uterine cavity joins with the cervical canal, which opens into the vaginal canal. The normal position of the uterus is **anteverted** (the cervical canal is turned anteriorly at approximately right angles to the vaginal canal) and **anteflexed** (the uterine cavity is bent slightly forward relative to the cervical canal). When the urinary bladder is filled, it displaces the uterus posteriorly, opening the angle between the vaginal and cervical canals.

Ligaments

There are various prominent peritoneal ridges or ligaments found within the pelvis of females, including the broad ligament of the uterus; round ligament of the uterus; ovarian ligament; suspensory ligament of the ovary; lateral, cardinal, or transverse cervical ligament; pubocervical ligament; pubovesical ligament; and uterosacral ligament.

The broad ligament of the uterus originates at the lateral border of the uterus and reaches the lateral pelvic wall. It comprises two layers of peritoneum and functions to hold the uterus in position. Many structures are found within the ligament, including the uterine tube, vessels, round ligament of the uterus, ovarian ligament, uterovaginal nerve plexus, lymphatics, and lower ureter. The broad ligament is subdivided into the mesovarium, mesosalpinx, and mesometrium. The mesovarium extends from the front of the ovary to the posterior border of the broad ligament; it is important to note that the mesovarium does not contain the ovary. The mesosalpinx aids in suspending the fallopian (uterine) tube. The mesometrium is inferior to the mesosalpinx and mesovarium and is a major contributor to the broad ligament.

The round ligament of the uterus runs within the (anterior/superior) layer of the broad ligament. It serves to hold the uterus anteverted and anteflexed by supporting the fundus of the uterus forward. The ligament attaches to the uterus anteriorly below the fallopian tubes. The round ligament passes through the inguinal canal at the deep inguinal ring and exits at the superficial inguinal ring. Both the ovarian ligament and suspensory ligament attach to the ovary. The ovarian ligament is found below the uterine tubes and attaches from the ovary to the uterus. It consists of a fibromuscular cord coursing within the broad ligament. The suspensory ligament of the ovary, however, is a band of peritoneum, which attaches the ovary to the pelvic wall. It carries the ovarian vessels, nerves, and lymphatics.

The cardinal ligament (of Mackenrodt) extends from the cervix and vagina to the pelvic walls, traveling inferior to the base of the broad ligament. The cardinal ligament is composed of fibromuscular pelvic fascia and functions to provide support to the uterus.

The pubocervical ligament is composed of bands of connective tissue and connects the posterior border of the pubis to the cervix of the uterus. The pubovesical ligament travels from the neck of the bladder to the pelvic bone, whereas the uterosacral ligament, a firm fibromuscular band of pelvic fascia, attaches to the lower portion of the sacrum and extends to the cervix and the upper portion of the vagina.

The uterosacral ligament maintains the anatomical position of the cervix upwards and posteriorly. Occasionally, the uterosacral ligament may create a fold of peritoneum, known as the rectouterine fold. This fold extends across the isthmus of the uterus and attaches laterally to the rectum at the posterior wall of the pelvis.

At the pelvic inlet, the inferior portions of the abdominal peritoneum drapes over the pelvic viscera. In females, the abdominal peritoneum covers the fundus and body of the uterus and extends laterally over the uterine tubes to the pelvic walls, forming the broad ligament of the uterus. The peritoneum spanning the anterior/inferior aspect of the uterus reflects onto the urinary bladder forming a relatively shallow space called the vesicouterine pouch. The peritoneum covering the posterior/superior aspect of the uterus and uterine cervix descends to the superior border of the posterior vaginal fornix and then reflects onto the anterior surface of the rectum, forming a deep potential space known as the rectouterine pouch (of Douglas). The rectouterine pouch is the deepest peritoneal space in the supine position.

Ovaries

The ovaries are the female reproductive organs covered by germinal epithelial, which is closely related to embryologic peritoneum. The ovaries are not invested within the broad uterine ligament. Each ovary is suspended by **mesovarium**, which attaches the ovaries to the posterior/superior layer of the broad ligament. The suspensory (infundibulopelvic) ligament is anchored at the pelvis sidewall and connects to the ovaries and thus, also maintains the position of the ovaries along with the mesovarium. The ovarian ligament attaches the ovaries to the uterus. The ovaries are bordered by the external and internal iliac vessels on the lateral walls of the pelvis. The ovarian arteries are the main arterial supply to the ovaries and form an anastomosis with the uterine artery. The ovarian arteries can be found within the suspensory (infundibulopelvic) ligament. Venous blood from the ovaries is collected by the left and right ovarian veins; the right ovarian vein drains into the inferior vena cava, whereas the left ovarian vein drains into the left renal vein.

Uterine Tubes (Fallopian Tubes)

The uterine tubes project laterally from the junction of the fundus and body of the uterus and open into the peritoneal cavity adjacent to the ovaries. The uterine tubes have fringelike appendages called fimbriae at the termination near the ovaries. The uterine tubes can be divided into four parts: infundibulum, ampulla, isthmus, and uterine part. An oocyte is expelled into the abdominal cavity from the ovaries during ovulation and is transferred to the uterus via the uterine tubes. The transport of oocytes is due to sweeping motions of the uterine tube fimbriae, the muscular contraction of the uterine tubes, and the ciliary motions of cilia lining the inner epithelial cells of the uterine tubes.

Vagina

The vaginal canal extends inferiorly from the cervix and terminates at the vaginal vestibule in the perineum. It serves to excrete menstrual products and receives the penis and the ejaculate during intercourse. The vestibule is partially surrounded by the hymen, which is a membranous fold that degenerates after first coitus. The vagina receives its blood supply from the vaginal branches of the uterine and internal iliac arteries. It is supported in the pelvis by the levator ani, the urogenital diaphragm, and the perineal body. The nerves innervating the upper three-fourths of the vagina comes from the uterovaginal plexus, whereas the lower one-fourth is innervated by the deep perineal branch of the pudendal nerve. Internal iliac nodes drain lymphatics from the upper three-fourths of the vagina, whereas the superficial inguinal nodes drain the lymphatics from the lower one-fourth portion of the vagina.

Technique

Transabdominal (Suprapubic) Views of Abdomen/Pelvis

SUPRAPUBIC FEMALE PELVIS
Longitudinal (Sagittal/ Parasagittal)
FIG. 9.1

This examination is best done when the patient's urinary bladder is full. If the bladder is not at least partially full, bowel as shadowing can interfere substantially with ultrasound (US) examination in this area. A full bladder displaces loops of bowel superiorly and provides an excellent acoustic window for US examination of pelvic structures behind the bladder.

With the patient in the supine position and properly draped, the heel of a curved array probe (nonmarker side) should be placed just over (or just above) the pubic symphysis with the marker side directed toward the head. Adjust the probe position and tilt until pelvic landmarks and structures can be identified. Urine, like all fluids, appears anechoic, and the bladder wall appears hyperechoic. In longitudinal view, a full bladder is roughly triangular with the apex pointing superiorly.

Posterior to the bladder, identify the **fundus** and body of the uterus, the hyperechoic endometrial stripe, and the cervix. The **myometrium** typically has a hypoechoic speckled appearance. Note the shape and position of the uterus, which changes with a full bladder. The endometrium appears as a hyperechoic stripe, which varies in thickness with the phase of the menstrual cycle. A thin hyperechoic vaginal stripe can often be identified extending inferiorly from the uterine cervix posterior to the bladder.

Identify the locations of the potential spaces, the rectouterine and vesicouterine pouches.

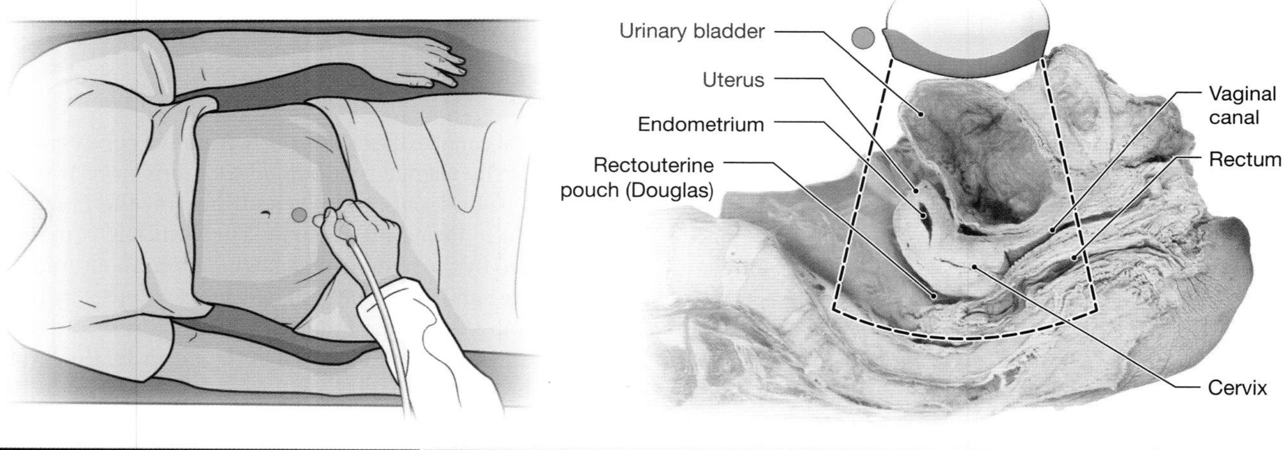

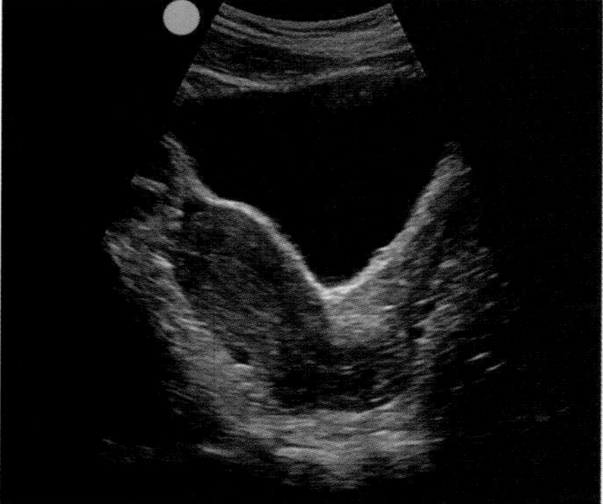

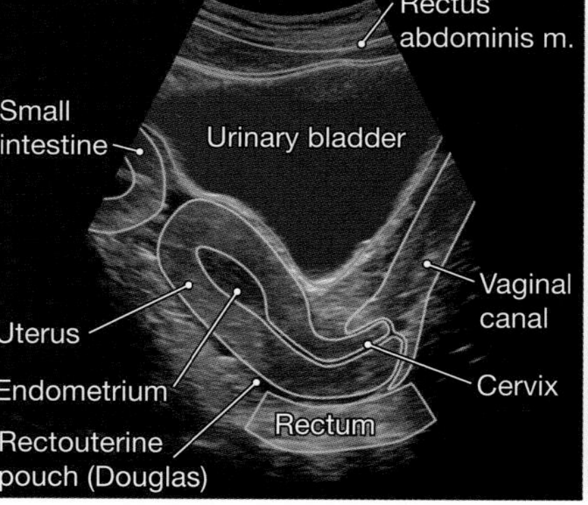

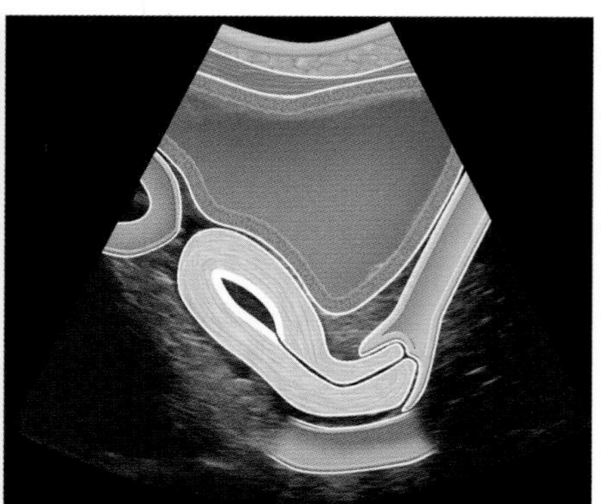

Figure 9.1 Normal longitudinal (sagittal/parasagittal) suprapubic view of the female pelvis.

SUPRAPUBIC FEMALE PELVIS
Transverse
FIG. 9.2

After completing the suprapubic examination of the pelvis in the longitudinal plane, rotate the probe 90° counterclockwise so that the marker side is directed to the right, and position the probe face just superior to the pubic symphysis. Adjust the probe position and tilt until pelvic landmarks and structures can be identified. In transverse view, a full bladder is roughly rectangular.

Identify the **bladder**, uterus, and **endometrial stripe.** Scan carefully superiorly and inferiorly along the uterus and uterine cervix. Attempt to identify the right and left ovaries, which are commonly found alongside the body of the uterus and posterior/inferior to the external iliac vessels. Ovaries are often described as having a "chocolate-chip cookie" US appearance, where the "chips" are anechoic/hypoechoic ovarian follicles and the "cookie" is the more echogenic ovarian stroma.

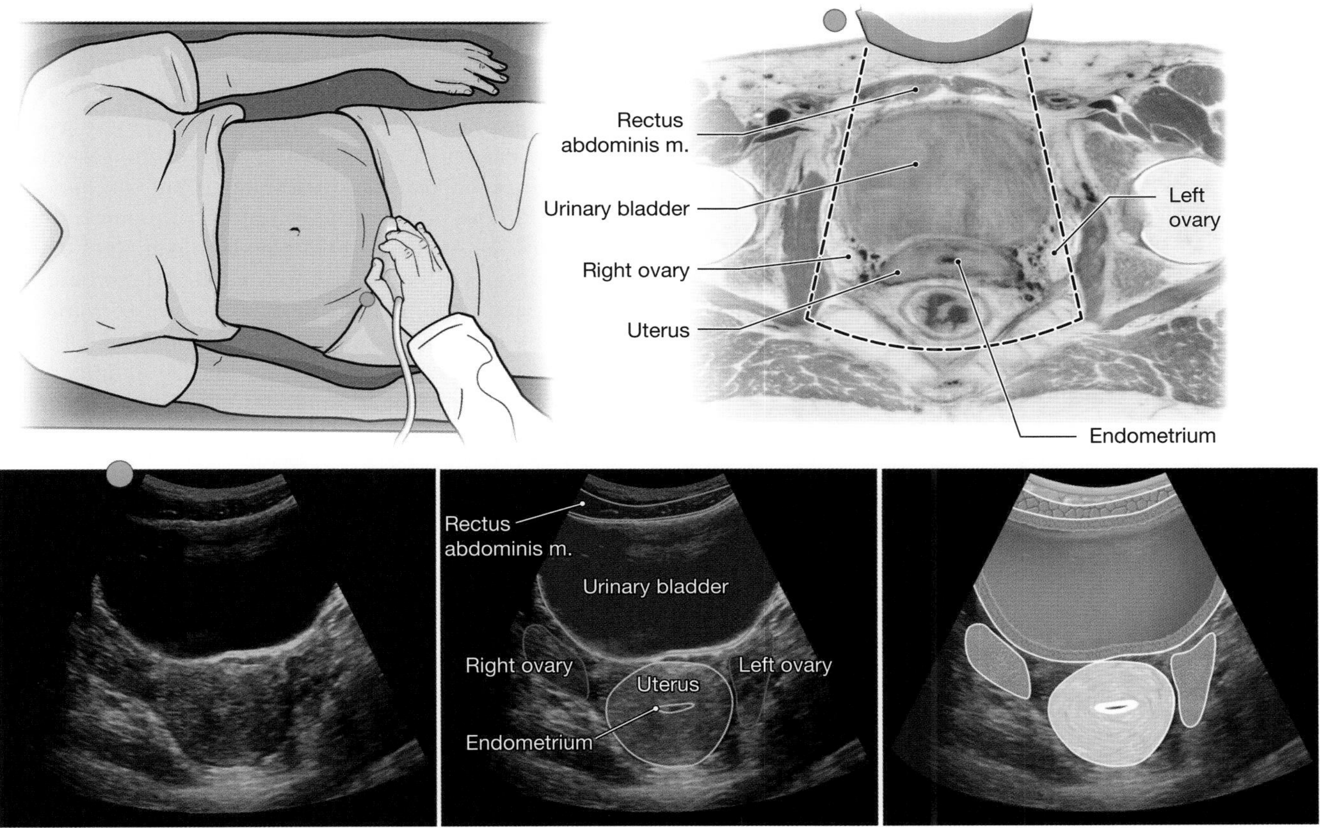

Figure 9.2 Normal transverse suprapubic view of the female pelvis.

CLINICAL APPLICATIONS

Focused Assessment With Sonography for Trauma Examination for Detection of Intraperitoneal Bleeding

In a supine patient, free intraperitoneal fluid or large amounts of blood from the abdominal viscera typically accumulate in the following locations: hepatorenal space (Morison pouch), splenorenal space, and pelvis, in the pouch of Douglas in females and the retrovesical pouch in males. Chapter 12 describes the Focused Assessment with Sonography for Trauma examination performed to identify these spaces with examples of fluid accumulation.

Ectopic Pregnancy

Ectopic pregnancy is defined as the pregnancy in which the embryo is implanted outside the normal intrauterine location. This accounts for approximately 2% of all pregnancies in the United States, which increases to 18% in patients with first-trimester bleeding. The most common ectopic locations include the fallopian tube, abdomen, ovary, uterine interstitium, prior surgical scar, and cervix. Approximately 95% of all ectopic pregnancies take place within the uterine tubes. A US examination shows an extraovarian adnexal mass and an empty uterus.

Fibromyoma (Leiomyoma)

Fibromyomas or **leiomyoma**s are the most common benign tumors of the uterus. These are primarily composed of smooth muscle and connective tissue. They are the most common cause of dysmenorrhea, pain, bleeding, and heavy menstrual cycles. They are commonly identified by US and surgically removed.

Endometriosis and Endometrial Cancer

Endometriosis is a mass of endometrial tissue such as stroma and glands that appears as a cyst and occurs in different extraendometrial locations such as uterine walls and ovaries. The majority of the adnexal masses, however, are benign masses. The most common type of uterine cancer in approximately 90% of the cases is an **endometrial cancer**. It develops from the endometrium of the uterus. The symptoms are similar to endometriosis, such as vaginal bleeding, pain, and pelvic cramping. A US examination can detect both endometriosis and endometrial cancer. In contrast, ovarian tumors are typically assessed with endovaginal ultrasonography with color Doppler specifically identifying vascularized tissue, thick septations, and solid parts of the tumor.

Multiple Choice Questions

1. A 55-year-old woman is brought to the emergency department because of an enlarged and painful abdomen. She has chronic renal failure for the past 3 years. An ultrasound examination shows ascites in the peritoneal cavity. An ultrasound-guided needle is placed through the posterior vaginal fornix to drain the fluid. Which of the following spaces/pouches will the needle enter to drain the fluid?

   A. Uterovesical pouch
   B. Pararectal space
   C. Paravesical space
   D. Rectouterine pouch
   E. Superficial perineal pouch

2. A 38-year-old woman is admitted to the hospital for a scheduled tubal ligation. Two days after the procedure, she has high fever and shows symptoms of hypovolemic shock. An ultrasound examination of her pelvis shows a large hematoma adjacent to the external iliac artery. Which of the following arteries is most likely injured during this procedure?

   A. Ovarian
   B. Ascending branch of uterine
   C. Descending branch of uterine
   D. Superior vesical
   E. Inferior vesical

3. A 39-year-old woman undergoes bilateral oophorectomy with ligation of the ovarian vessels. Three years ago, she had a prophylactic bilateral mastectomy because of a recent BRCA1 diagnosis. Both her mother and older sister have been diagnosed with breast cancer. Which of the following structures is most likely at risk of injury when the ovarian vessels are ligated?

   A. Uterine artery
   B. Pudendal nerve
   C. Internal pudendal artery
   D. Vaginal artery
   E. Ureter

4. A 42-year-old woman comes to the physician because of a 6-month history of heavy painful menstrual bleedings. She has extremely heavy periods and abdominal pain, which has resulted in anemia. An ultrasound examination shows several large uterine leiomyomas. A hysterectomy is performed, and the uterine artery is identified and ligated. Which of the following adjacent structures is most susceptible to iatrogenic injury during ligation of this artery?

   A. Obturator nerve
   B. Internal iliac artery
   C. Lumbosacral trunk
   D. Ureter
   E. Internal iliac vein

10

Male Pelvis

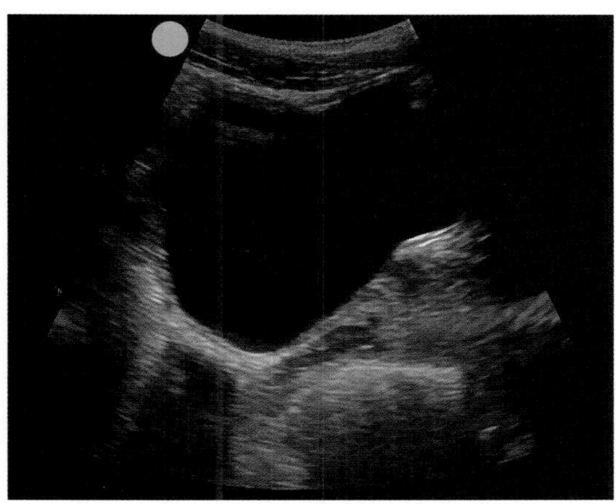

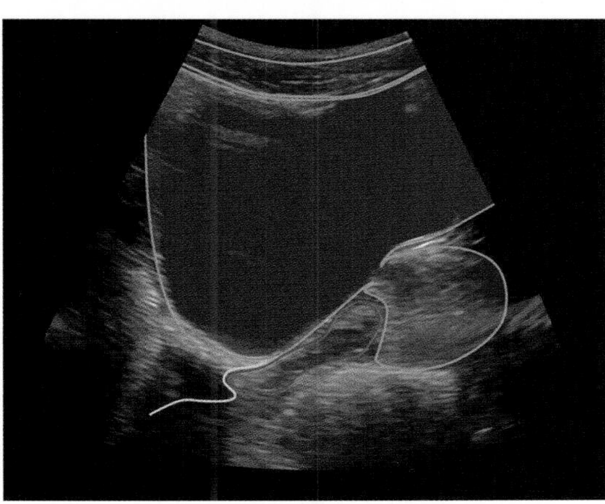

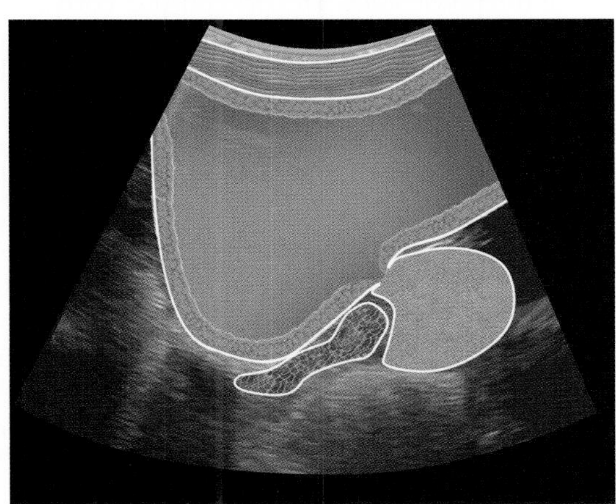

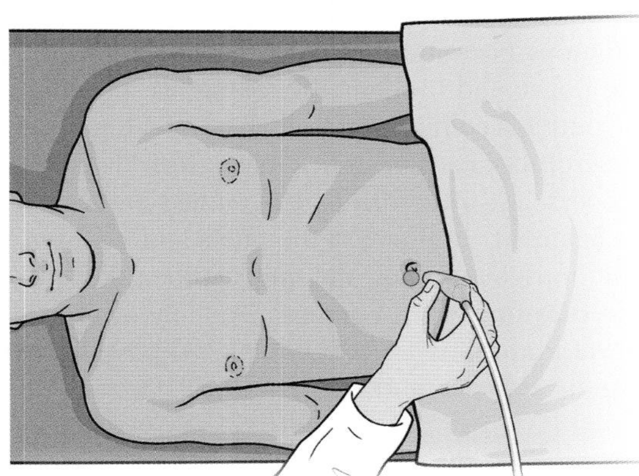

Review of the Anatomy

The pelvis (Latin for "basin") is a bowl-shaped bony structure positioned superior to the lower limbs and inferior to the abdomen. The bones of the pelvis are the **os coxae** (two hip bones), **sacrum**, and **coccyx**. The pelvis is divided by the linear terminalis (pelvic brim) into the lesser pelvis above and the greater below. The pelvic outlet is situated in the lesser pelvis and is sealed by the musculature of the pelvic floor, the coccygeus, and the levator ani. The pelvis sits in an angled position, with the vertical axis in line with the anterior superior iliac spine and pubic tubercles, and the horizontal axis containing the coccyx and the upper margin of the pubic symphysis. Thus, the pelvic cavity is parallel to the curvature of the sacrum.

The pelvis is also subdivided into an inlet and an outlet portion. The pelvic inlet, also known as the upper pelvic aperture, is the upper border of the pelvic cavity and is made up of three main parts, the sacral, iliac, and pubic portions. It has an almost entirely bony margin (linea terminalis) along the sacral promontory, ala of sacrum, arcuate line, pectineal line, pubic crest, and pubic symphysis. The sacrum, along with the anterior border of the ala of sacrum, makes up the sacral portion, forming the posterior border of the pelvic inlet. The iliac portion corresponds to the lateral border of the pelvic inlet, which is confined by the arcuate or iliopectineal line of the ilium. Finally, the pubic portion of the pelvic inlet is the upper border and includes the superior margin of the public symphysis. The pelvic inlet is mostly narrow and heart-shaped in males. At the pelvic inlet, the pelvic viscera is covered by the inferior aspect of the abdominal peritoneum. In males, peritoneum covering the urinary bladder reflects onto the anterior surface of the rectum, giving rise to the rectovesical pouch, a pocket that contains peritoneal fluid and some parts of the small intestine. The rectovesical pouch is also the most dependent area of the peritoneal cavity when positioned in a supine orientation.

The pelvic outlet is a diamond-shaped aperture that leads into the perineum. It has bony (ischiopubic rami) and ligamentous (sacrotuberous) margins secured in position by the pelvic and urogenital diaphragms. Specifically, the pelvic outlet is confined laterally by the ischial tuberosities and sacrotuberous ligaments, posteriorly by the sacrum and coccyx, and anteriorly by the pubic symphysis, arcuate pubic ligament, and rami of the pubis and ischium.

The musculature of the pelvic floor, known as the **pelvic diaphragm**, is composed mainly of the right and left levator ani muscles and completed posteriorly by the coccygeus muscles and their perineal fascia. The pelvic diaphragm acts to support the entire pelvic viscera, flexes the anorectal junction during excretion, and helps in voluntary micturition (urination). The levator ani is composed of the following muscles: pubococcygeus, puboanalis, iliococcygeus, puboperinealis, and puboprostaticus (in males) and pubovaginalis (in females).

The pelvic walls are made up of bone (os coxae and sacrum), ligaments (sacrospinous and sacrotuberous), and muscles (obturator internus and piriformis). There are foramina in the pelvic walls, the greater and lesser sciatic foramina posteriorly and the obturator foramen anteriorly. The majority of the obturator foramen is enclosed by the obturator membrane, but a small obturator canal remains open anterosuperiorly.

The joints of the pelvis include the lumbosacral, sacroiliac, sacrococcygeal joints, and the pubic symphysis. The lumbosacral joint is located between the L5 vertebra and the base of the sacrum. The joint is accompanied by the intervertebral disc and bolstered by the iliolumbar ligaments. The sacroiliac joint is situated between the articular surfaces of the sacrum and ilium. It is a combined synovial and cartilaginous joint, surrounded by cartilage and held by the anterior, posterior, and interosseous sacroiliac ligaments. The sacrococcygeal joint is positioned between the sacrum and coccyx. It is a cartilaginous joint reinforced with the anterior, posterior, and lateral sacrococcygeal ligaments. Finally, the pubic symphysis, a cartilaginous or fibrocartilaginous joint, is found between the pubic bones in the median plane.

In males, the pelvic ligaments observed include the puboprostatic ligament, which is a condensation of the pelvic fascia and attaches from the prostate gland and continues to the pelvic bone. The inferior pubic or arcuate pubic ligament is found in both males and females. This ligament stretches across the inferior aspect of the pubic symphysis to connect with the medial surface of the inferior pubic rami.

Ureters and Urinary Bladder

The **ureters** are muscular conduits for urine extending from the kidneys to the urinary bladder. The ureters are made of smooth muscles and transitional epithelium and propel urine via peristaltic waves. The ureters cross the pelvic brim superior to the common iliac artery bifurcation after which they descend laterally into the pelvic wall. The ureters travel medial to the umbilical artery and the obturator vessels and posteroinferiorly to the ductus deferens and anterior to the seminal vesicles before flowing into the posterolateral surface of the bladder. Through its course, there are three points of constriction—at the ureteropelvic junction, when it travels across the pelvic brim; at the point where it crosses the common iliac artery; and at its entrance into the bladder.

The ureters enter the bladder at the base on a slant. They possess a slitlike orifice that functions as a valve, whereas the intramural portion of the ureters has circular fibers operating as a sphincter. Thus, when the bladder becomes distended, the valve and the sphincter work to prevent the reflux of urine back into the ureters.

The **urinary bladder** is situated in the midline of the pelvis anteriorly, and the rectum occupies the midline of the pelvis posteriorly. It is made up of bundles of smooth muscles known as the detrusor muscle and is located inferior to the peritoneum. As the bladder fills, it extends toward the pelvic brim. Anatomically, the apex of the bladder is located anteriorly, and the fundus of the bladder forms the posteroinferior triangular aspect. There is a triangular section (bladder trigone) at the urinary bladder's fundus, where the bladder mucosa is tightly bound to the underlying smooth muscle layer that lines the base of the bladder. The bladder trigone is surrounded by two openings of the ureters and the internal urethral orifice that has the internal sphincter. The neck of the bladder, which is at the fundus, leads into the urethra. The arterial blood supply for the bladder comes from the superior and inferior vesical arteries. The vesical plexus (or prostatic) drains the venous blood toward the internal iliac vein. The vesical and prostatic nervous plexuses innervate the bladder. The parasympathetic pelvic splanchnic nerves (S2-S4) function to contract the bladder and the detrusor muscle and relax the internal urethral sphincter to initiate emptying of the bladder. The sympathetic nerves relax the bladder walls and constrict the internal urethral sphincter.

The urinary bladder empties into the urethra, which propels the urine to the exterior. In males, the urethra also functions for the passage of semen. The urethra passes through the prostate, the deep perineal pouch (membranous part), and the penis (penile or spongy urethra), thus containing three parts: prostatic, membranous, and spongy.

The process of micturition is initiated via the bladder filling, which causes the detrusor muscles to stretch. Initially, the sympathetic nerves are activated, which prevents emptying by relaxing the bladder and constricting the internal urethral sphincter. Second, the general visceral afferents from the bladder wall, due to the stretch receptors, enter the spinal cord via the pelvic splanchnic nerves (S2-S4). This signals the parasympathetic preganglionic fibers to synapse in the inferior hypogastric plexus and the postganglionic fibers to initiate bladder contraction and relaxation of the internal urethral sphincter. The general somatic efferent fibers in the pudendal nerve allow for voluntary relaxation of the external urethral sphincter, allowing the bladder to void. The external urethral sphincter contracts at the end of urination.

Testes

The testes are the male reproductive organs responsible for the production of spermatozoa and sex hormones. They are covered by a membranous structure known as the tunica albuginea, which is located under a visceral layer called the tunica vaginalis. Their development occurs in the retroperitoneum, after which they descend into the scrotum.

The blood supply of the testes is from the testicular artery, which arises from the abdominal aorta, and the venous blood leaves through the pampiniform venous plexus. Lymphatic drainage from the testes is to the lumbar (aortic) nodes, whereas the lymph from the scrotum drains to the superficial inguinal nodes.

The **epididymis** is a convoluted duct extending from the testicle to the vas deferens. Its main purpose is to store sperm and allow for its maturation before release. The epididymis is made up of a head, body, and tail. It is in the head and body of the epididymis where the spermatozoa are stored and undergo maturation.

The **ductus deferens** enters the pelvis at the deep inguinal ring lateral to the inferior epigastric artery. As it travels, it overlaps the medial aspect of the umbilical artery and obturator neurovascular bundle. It then travels superior to the ureter, posterior to the bladder, and becomes dilated to be the ampulla at its terminal junction. The ductus deferens contains fructose, a nutrient source to spermatozoa. The superior hypogastric plexus (sympathetic) and the pelvic splanchnic nerves (parasympathetic) innervate the ductus deferens.

Seminal Vesicles

The **seminal vesicles** consist of lobulated glandular structures, which originate from the diverticula of the ductus deferens. They are found inferolateral to the ductus deferens ampullae. The seminal vesicles, which extend superiorly from the prostate gland between the bladder and the rectum, join the ductus deferens near their end, forming the ejaculatory ducts. The ejaculatory ducts pass through the prostate gland and open into the prostatic urethra at the seminal colliculus. The ductus deferens and the ejaculatory ducts perform peristaltic contractions of its muscular layers to push the spermatozoa with seminal fluid toward the urethra. The **seminal fluid** secreted by the seminal vesicles contributes to the quality of the semen and is rich in fructose, choline, and other proteins that provide nutrients to the spermatozoa. The ducts of the seminal vesicles join with the ductus deferens forming the ejaculatory ducts.

Prostate

The **prostate** is situated immediately inferior to the bladder, posterior to the pubic symphysis, and anterior to the rectum. It has a base at the bladder neck where the urethra exits the bladder and enters the prostate and an apex resting on the pelvic floor.

The prostate is anatomically divided into five lobes: the anterior, middle, posterior, and the right and left lateral lobes. Glandular tissue is the main component of the prostate, together with smooth muscle and fibrous tissue. The prostate also contributes to the semen and secretes **prostate-specific antigen**, prostaglandins, and other proteins. The secretions of the prostate add alkalinity to the ejaculate and produce the distinctive odor of semen. The prostatic ducts receive semen from the ejaculatory ducts, which empty into a groove between the urethral crest and the prostatic urethra called the prostatic sinus.

Urethral Crest

The urethral crest is found on the posterior aspect of the prostatic urethra with several openings bilaterally to receive seminal fluid from the prostatic ducts. The seminal colliculus, also referred to as verumontanum, is an enlargement of the urethral crest that serves as an opening for the ejaculatory ducts and the prostatic utricle.

Penis

The penis consists of a root and a body. The root for the penis can be felt posterior to the scrotum by palpating the two crura and the bulb of penis. The root of the penis is supported by two ligaments the suspensory and the fundiform. The body of penis is entirely covered by skin and the tip of the body is covered by the glans penis. There are three components of vascular erectile tissue that surrounds the body of the penis, a paired corpora cavernosa and a midline corpus spongiosum. A bilayer fibrous structure encloses these erectile tissues, the tunica albuginea. The glans penis is composed of the distal part of corpus spongiosum and is covered by a skin fold, the prepuce. The prepuce contains a midline ventral fold, the frenulum. The margin of the glans penis is the corona. Its midline opening is the external urethral orifice demarcated by a dilated part of the urethra, the fossa navicularis. The arterial supply of the penis is derived from the dorsal arteries of the penis, the deep arteries of the penis, and the bulbourethral artery, all branches of the internal pudendal artery. The venous drainage is by the deep dorsal vein of the penis, this drains the cavernous structures into the prostatic venous plexus and the superficial dorsal veins that drain the superficial structures of the penis, such as the skin and cutaneous tissues.

Erection and Ejaculation

Erection is a process influenced by the parasympathetic nervous system and muscular contraction. The parasympathetic fibers from the pelvic splanchnic nerves cause arterial dilation of the erectile tissue, leading to enlargement of the corpora cavernosa and corpus spongiosum. Contraction of the bulbospongiosus and ischiocavernosus muscles allows for maintained erections. ***P**oint* for **p**arasympathetics (erection) and ***S**hoot* for **s**ympathetics (ejaculation) is a useful mnemonic to remember these associations.

Stimulation of the sympathetic fibers causes contraction of the smooth muscles of the ejaculatory tract, thus resulting in ejection of semen. **Ejaculation** is initiated by stimulation of the glans penis, which causes contractions of the bulbospongiosus muscles compressing the urethra to expel the ejaculate. Sympathetic stimulation prevents retrograde ejaculation into the urinary bladder by contracting the sphincter of the bladder.

Technique

Transabdominal (Suprapubic) Views of Abdomen/Pelvis

SUPRAPUBIC MALE PELVIS
Longitudinal (Sagittal/ Parasagittal)
FIG. 10.1

This examination is best performed when the patient's urinary bladder is full. If the urinary bladder is not at least partially full, bowel gas shadowing can interfere substantially with ultrasound (US) examination in this area. A full bladder displaces loops of bowel superiorly and provides an excellent acoustic window for US examination of pelvic structures behind the bladder.

With the patient in the supine position and properly draped, the heel of a curved array probe (nonmarker side) should be placed just over (or just above) the pubic symphysis with the marker side directed toward the head. Adjust the probe position and tilt until pelvic landmarks and structures can be identified. Urine, like all fluids, appears anechoic, and the bladder wall appears hyperechoic. In longitudinal views, full bladders are roughly triangular with the apex pointing superiorly. Posterior to the bladder, identify the honeycomb appearance of seminal vesicles and the prostate. Scanning carefully across the prostate from the right to the left and back again, attempt to identify the urethral opening into the prostate at the bladder neck.

SUPRAPUBIC MALE PELVIS
Transverse
FIG. 10.2

After completing the suprapubic examination of the pelvis in the longitudinal plane, rotate the probe 90° counterclockwise so that the marker side is directed to the right and position the probe face just superior to the pubic symphysis. Adjust the probe position and tilt

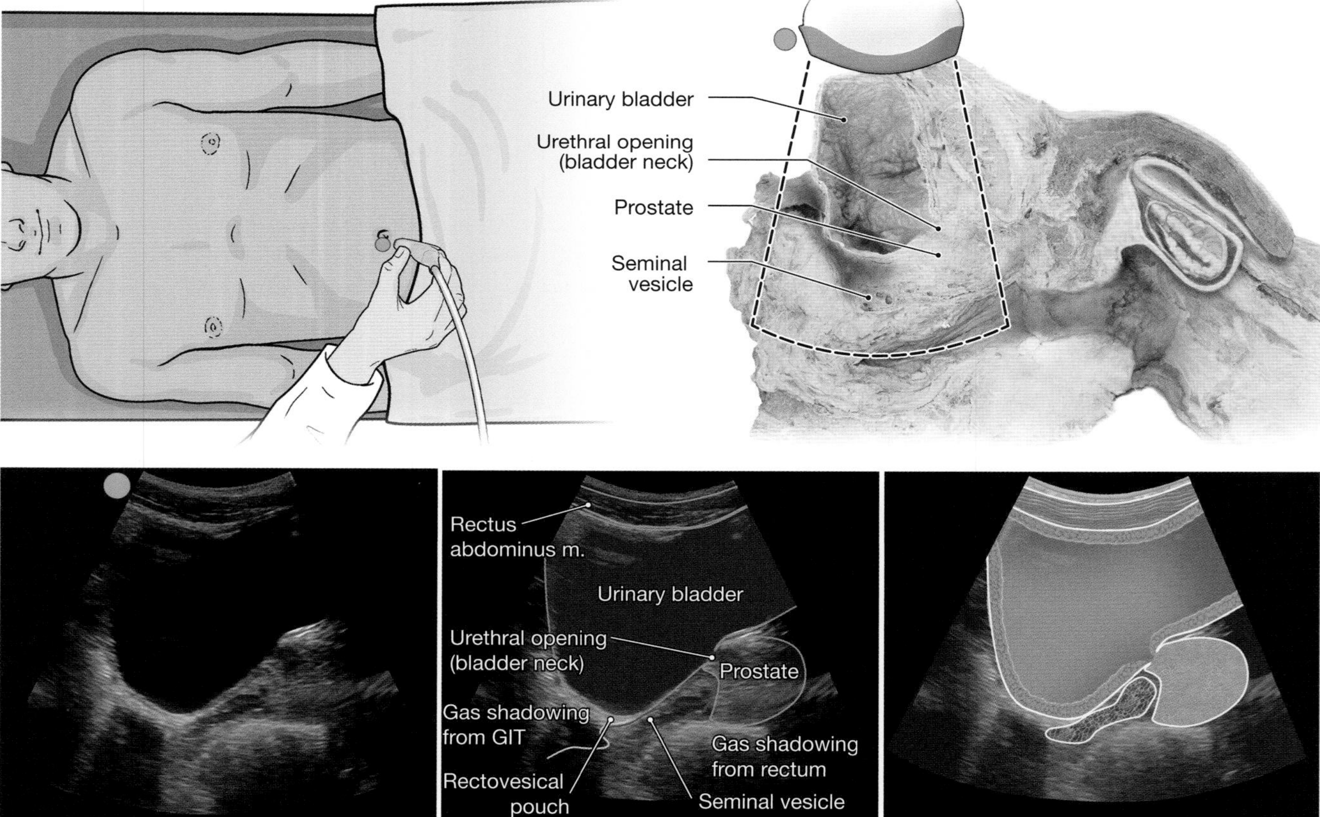

Figure 10.1 Normal longitudinal (sagittal/parasagittal) suprapubic view of the male pelvis. GIT, gastrointestinal tract.

until pelvic landmarks and structures can be identified. In transverse views, full bladders are roughly rectangular. By scanning carefully superiorly and inferiorly, identify the bladder and the hypoechoic "bow-tie" appearance of the seminal vesicles posterior to the bladder.

Penis

CORPORA CAVERNOSA
CORPUS SPONGIOSUM
Transverse
FIG. 10.3

The patient should be in the supine position with the penis supported on a towel draped over the scrotum. Use a generous amount of gel and place a high-frequency linear probe transversely on the dorsum of the penis (marker directed to the patient's right). You may also need to angle/tilt the probe back and forth to visualize the penile anatomy near the mid-line due to edge-shadowing artifact from parts of the tunica albuginea, where the right and left corpora cavernosa meet. Identify the right and left corpora cavernosa and the corpus spongiosum. Observe the "spongy" echotexture of the erectile tissue. Locate and identify the deep artery of each corpus cavernosum. Identify the hyperechoic tunica albuginea surrounding the three erectile bodies. The parts of tunica albuginea which are approximately perpendicular to the path of the US beam are relatively easy to identify while those parts which are parallel to the beam are difficult or impossible to see (without substantially changing the angle of the ultrasound path).

CORPUS CAVERNOSUM
CORPUS SPONGIOSUM
Longitudinal
FIG. 10.4

Starting from the patient and probe position above, center the probe over the right or left corpus cavernosum and rotate the probe 90° clockwise so that the probe is aligned with the long axis of one of the corpora cavernosa with the marker directed superiorly/proximally. Identify the corpus cavernosum, the corpus spongiosum, and associated tunica albuginea. Sliding the probe a short distance from side-to-side attempt to identify the deep artery of the corpus cavernosum in its longitudinal axis as an anechoic stripe with hyperechoic "train-track" walls.

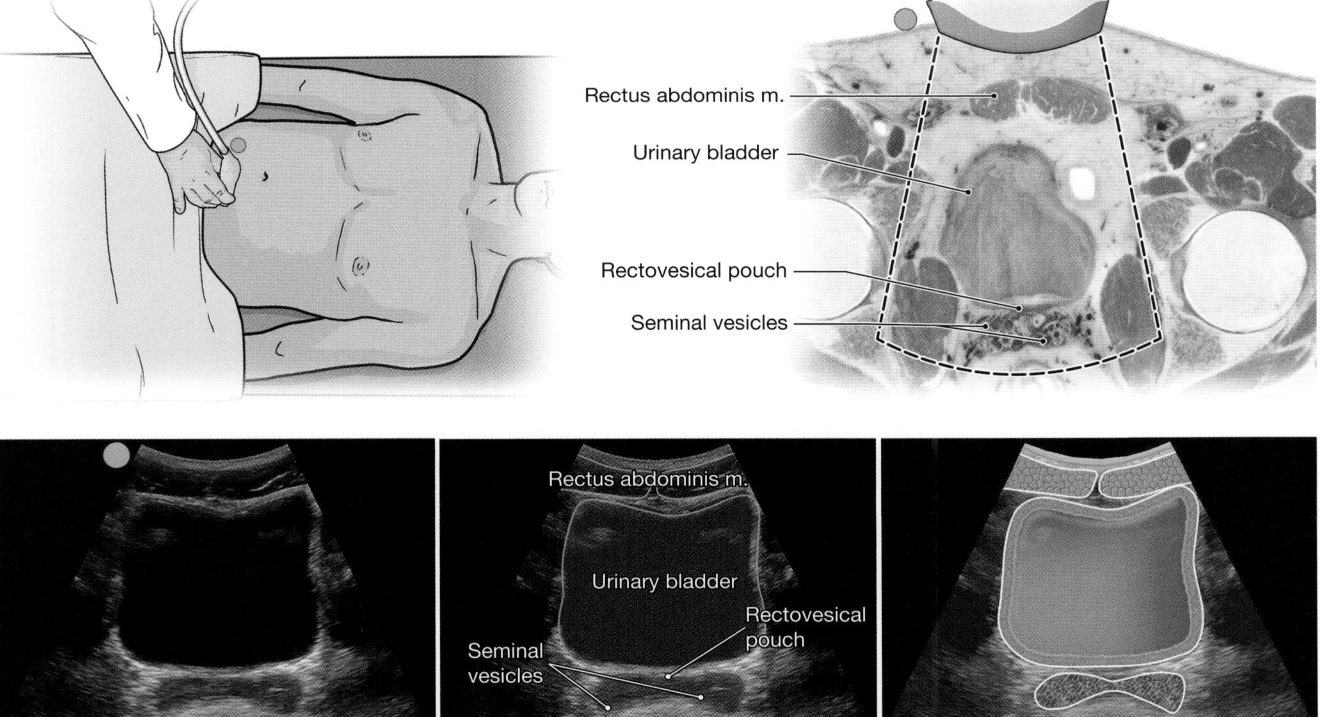

Figure 10.2 Normal transverse suprapubic view of the male pelvis.

Scrotum and Testes

TESTIS HEAD OF EPIDIDYMIS
Longitudinal
FIG. 10.5

The patient should be supine with a folded towel under the scrotum to elevate, support, and immobilize the scrotum/testes (if needed, the patient can also assist in immobilizing the testes). The patient should also hold a towel to keep the penis draped against the lower abdominal wall. Place the probe along the longitudinal axis of the right or left testicle with the marker directed superiorly. The probe should be centered over the testis with the US beam directed through the testis in approximately the sagittal (parasagittal) plane. Slide the probe up and down while fanning the probe back and forth from the parasagittal plane toward the coronal plane (probe handle toward the patient's inner thigh) until the head of the epididymis can be identified just above the superior pole of the testis. Identify the head of the epididymis, the epididymal sinus, the testis along with its tunica albuginea, and as possible, the visceral and parietal layers of the tunica vaginalis testis (at least a small fluid accumulation, physiological hydrocele, is needed to distinguish these two layers). The individual layers of the scrotal wall and spermatic fascia are difficult to resolve/identify with US. Note the homogeneous echotexture of the testicular stroma. The head of the epididymis is normally isoechoic or slightly hypoechoic relative to testis.

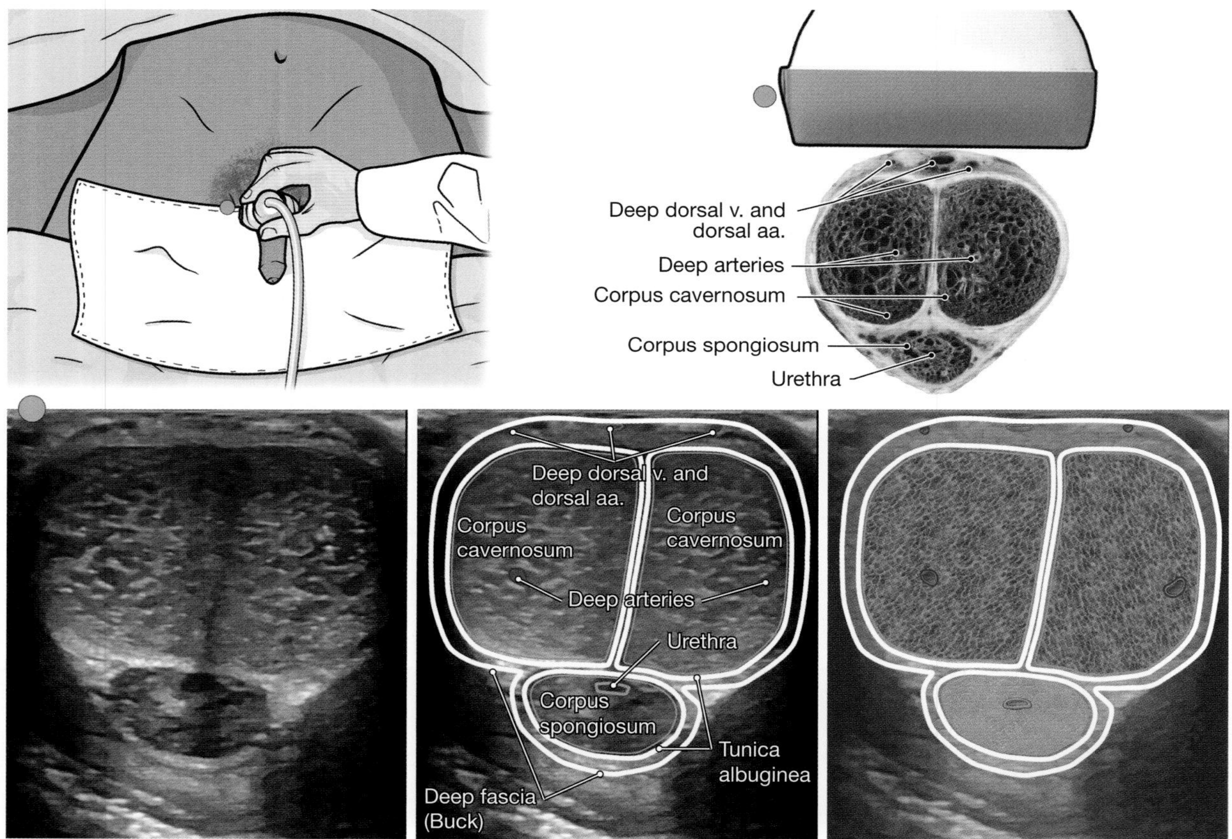

Figure 10.3 Transverse view of penis including the corpora cavernosa, the corpus spongiosum, and associated tunica albuginea.

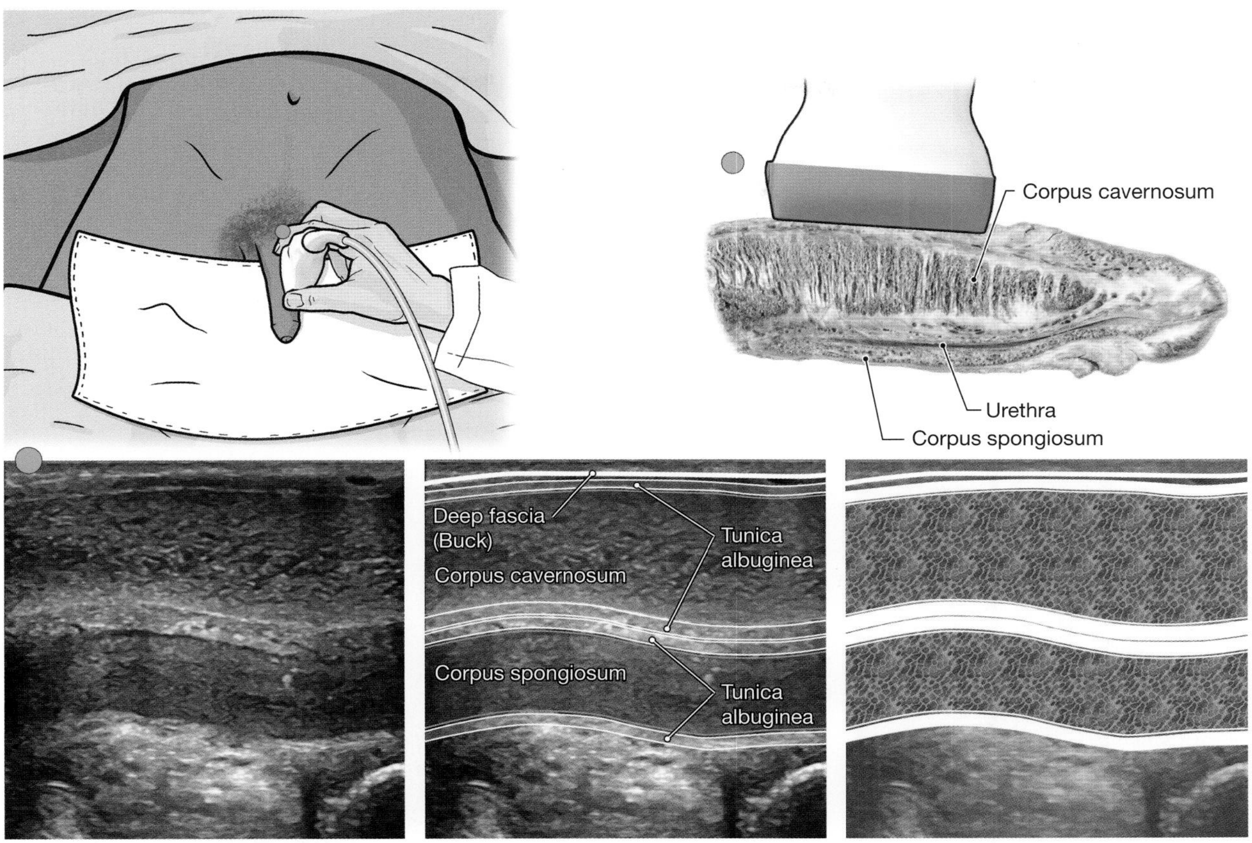

Figure 10.4 Longitudinal view of the penis including a corpus cavernosum, the corpus spongiosum, and associated tunica albuginea.

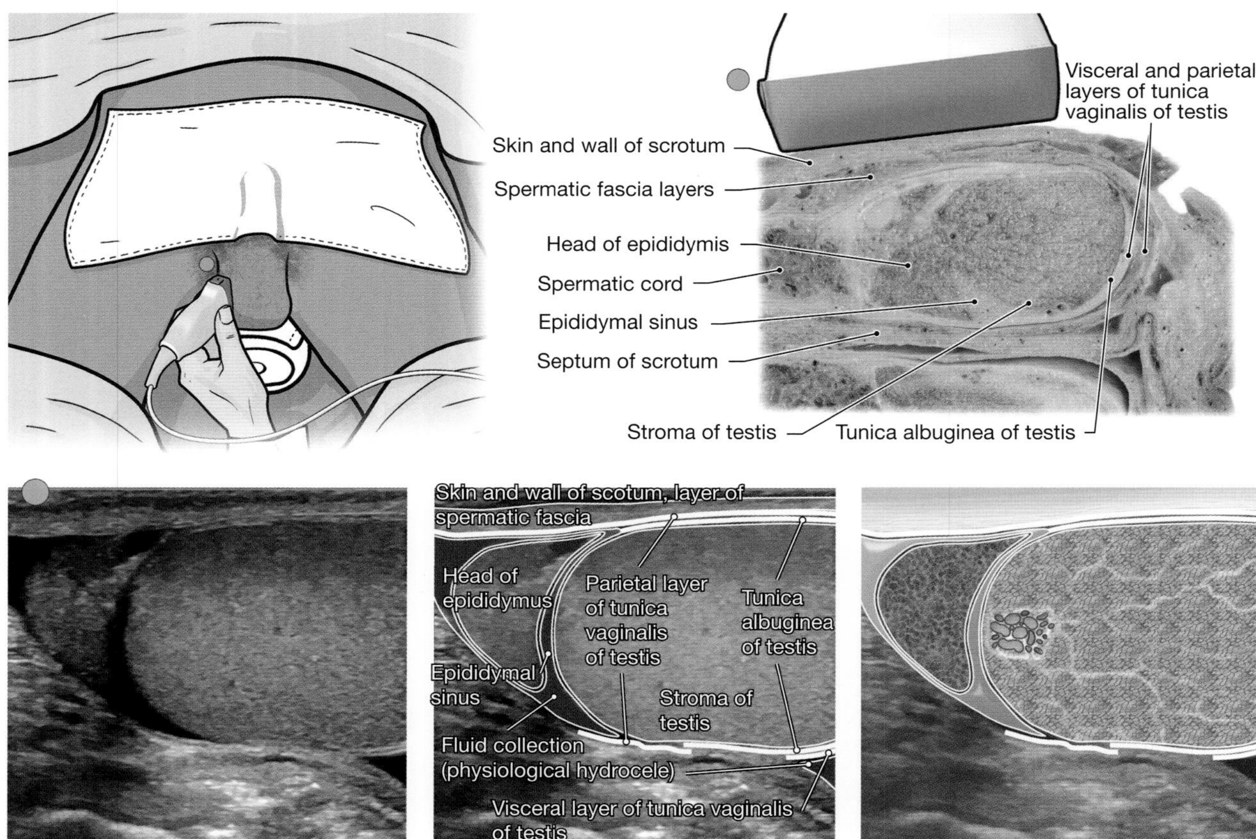

Figure 10.5 Longitudinal view of the right hemiscrotum including the testis, the head of epididymis, tunica albuginea testis, and the visceral and parietal layers of the tunica vaginalis.

CLINICAL APPLICATIONS

Focused Assessment with Sonography for Trauma Examination for Detection of Intraperitoneal Bleeding

In the supine patient, free intraperitoneal fluid or large amounts of blood from the abdominal viscera typically accumulate in the following locations: hepatorenal space (Morison pouch), splenorenal space, and in the pelvis in the pouch of Douglas in females and the retrovesical pouch in males. Chapter 12 describes the Focused Assessment with Sonography for Trauma examination performed for identifying these spaces with examples of fluid accumulation.

Ruptured Urinary Bladder

Fractures of the pelvis or injuries at the inferior portion of the anterior abdominal wall may rupture a distended urinary bladder. Urine may escape extraperitoneally or intraperitoneally. In instances in which the rupture takes place at the superior portion of the urinary bladder, this results into extravasation of urine into the peritoneal cavity. Posterior rupture of the urinary bladder results in extravasation of urine extraperitoneally into the perineum.

Bladder Thickening

Bladder thickening is relative to the degree of urinary bladder distention. It ranges from >3 mm when distended to >5 mm when nondistended. If the bladder is well-distended, then diffuse bladder wall thickening is due to urinary bladder obstruction, neurogenic bladder, and infections (cystitis). Focal urinary bladder thickening is typically due to malignancy such as transitional cell carcinoma.

Suprapubic Catheter Placement

Suprapubic catheter placement refers to the procedure in which a drainage tube is inserted into the urinary bladder under US guidance. This is because the placement of a urethral catheter is either contraindicated or unsuccessful. Typical indications for suprapubic catheter placements include urinary retention, severe benign prostatic hyperplasia, morbid obesity, urethras strictures, and trauma, among others.

Penis

US of the penis is used in the diagnosis and management of erectile dysfunction, suspected penile fracture, Peyronie disease (fibrous calcifying plaques in the tunica albuginea, which typically cause curvature of the erectile bodies), priapism (persistent painful erection), penile masses, and urethral stricture. Erection-inducing drugs and Doppler flow are often used along with US in the investigation of erectile dysfunction.

Testes

Testicular US is used in the diagnosis and management of acute testicular pain, testicular trauma, testicular or other scrotal masses, hydrocele, varicocele, and infertility/hypogonadism. Doppler flow studies are used in testicular trauma, suspected testicular torsion, evaluation of suspected epididymitis, orchitis or epididymo-orchitis, the workup of infertility/hypogonadism, and the evaluation of intrascrotal masses.

10 Male Pelvis

Multiple Choice Questions

1. A 25-year-old man comes to the physician because of a 2-month history of a painless, swelling in his right scrotum. Physical examination shows a nontender, palpable mass on the right testis. An ultrasound examination of the right scrotum shows a 3 × 3 cm intratesticular mass. A radical orchiectomy is performed. Biopsy of the mass shows testicular seminoma. Which of the following lymph nodes will most likely receive metastatic cells first?

   A. External iliac
   B. Superficial inguinal
   C. Deep inguinal
   D. Internal iliac
   E. Lumbar

2. A 24-year-old woman is brought to the emergency department with a report of having been sexually assaulted 24 hours earlier. She says that a man she had met at a campus party walked her to her apartment, where he assaulted and raped her, including vaginal penetration. She did not report the assault to the police but confided in a friend, who encouraged her to seek medical care. In collecting samples of an evidence-collection kit, two sterile dry cotton-tipped swabs are used simultaneously to collect sample. Fluids from her vagina are collected for DNA and fructose examination. Which of the following organs is most likely responsible for fructose production?

   A. Kidneys
   B. Prostate gland
   C. Testis
   D. Seminal vesicles
   E. Bulbourethral (Cowper) glands

3. A 75-year-old man comes to the physician because of a 6-month history of progressive dysuria, nocturia, and urinary urgency. Laboratory studies show high levels of prostate-specific antigen, and transurethral biopsy shows prostate cancer. A radical prostatectomy is performed. Postoperatively, he experiences urinary incontinence secondary to paralysis of the external urethral sphincter. Which of the following nerves was most likely injured during the operation?

   A. Parasympathetic preganglionic
   B. Pelvic splanchnic (S2-S4)
   C. General somatic efferent from the pudendal
   D. Sympathetic fibers from superior hypogastric plexus
   E. General visceral afferent

4. A 40-year-old man comes to the physician because of a 6-week history of a painful left scrotum. Physical examination shows a grossly enlarged left scrotum, which is tender to palpation. Ultrasonography of the scrotum shows a complex echoic mass connected to the testis. A diagnosis of scrotal abscess is made. Which of the following lymph nodes are most likely to be tender and swollen?

   A. External iliac
   B. Internal iliac
   C. Lateral aortic/lumbar
   D. Sacral
   E. Superficial inguinal

11

Neck, Face, and Eye

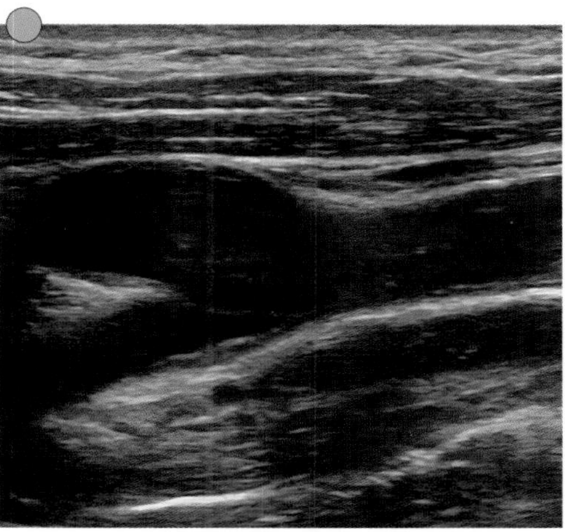

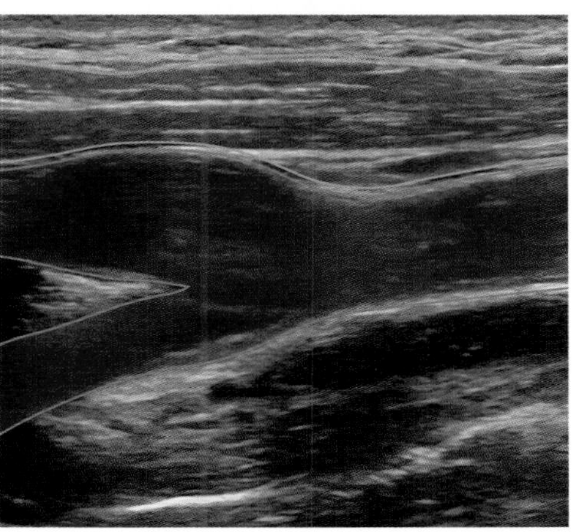

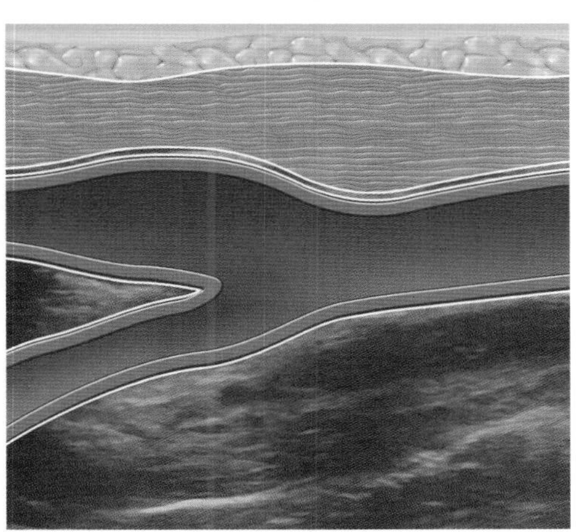

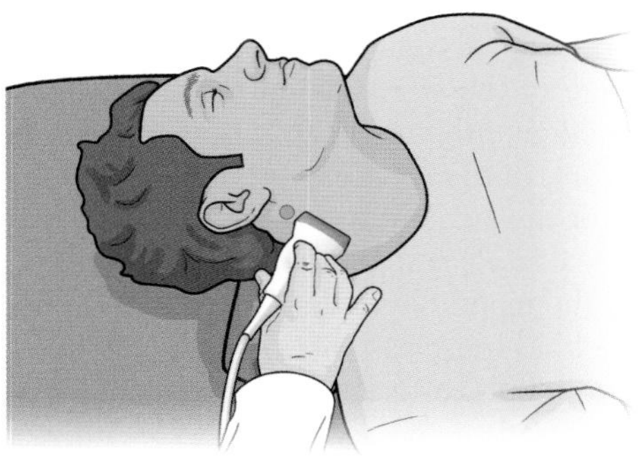

Neck

Review of the Anatomy

The neck is a compact region that is an intersection among the head, thorax, and upper limb. Classically, the neck has been geometrically divided into multiple triangles to aid in the study of its anatomy. Although not all these triangles are used clinically, some are useful for descriptive purposes. We will divide and describe the major structures of the neck by considering the anatomy within the posterior and anterior cervical triangles. The nuchal or posterior aspect of the neck will not be considered in this description.

Fasciae

The fasciae of the neck can be simplified into two layers:

1. *Superficial cervical fascia:* This layer is located in a subcutaneous location.
2. *Deep cervical fascia:* These fasciae subdivide the deeper layers of the neck. Each of these layers contributes to the column of fascia known as the carotid sheath, which envelopes the carotid artery, internal jugular vein, and vagus nerve in the neck.

The *superficial investing fascia* envelopes the outer perimeter of the neck splitting to encase the sternocleidomastoid and trapezius muscles. The *prevertebral fascia* covers the cervical vertebrae and their attached muscles such as the longus and scalene muscles. The *pretracheal* and *buccopharyngeal layers* surround the larynx/trachea, thyroid gland, and pharynx/esophagus and form the visceral cervical fascia. Primarily, for the convenience of description, the neck is divided into various triangles. We will focus on the two larger divisions, the posterior and anterior triangles and their contents.

Posterior Cervical Triangle

The posterior cervical triangle is bounded interiorly by the posterior edge of the sternocleidomastoid, posteriorly by the anterior edge of the upper trapezius, and inferiorly by the middle third of the clavicle.

The roof of this geometric region is the investing layer of deep cervical fascia and part of the platysma muscle as it travels from the mandible to the fascia over the pectoralis major and deltoid muscles. The muscular floor of this triangle covered by prevertebral fascia from anterior to posterior is composed of the scalenes, the levator scapulae, the splenius capitis, and a small portion of the semispinalis capitis. The inferior belly of the omohyoid muscle also crosses superficial to these aforementioned muscles on its way from the scapula to the hyoid bone. The inferior belly of the omohyoid divides the posterior cervical triangle into an upper occipital and a lower subclavian triangle. In addition, the small upper portion of the serratus anterior muscle is found here. Finally, the accessory nerve (spinal accessory nerve), the posterior lymphatic chain, and the emergence of brachial plexus are found in this triangle.

Muscles

The following muscles are located in the posterior cervical triangle:

- **Trapezius:** This muscle arises from the midline from near the external occipital protuberance, along the spinous processes and associated ligaments inferiorly to the 12th thoracic vertebrae. This muscle then travels laterally to attach to the scapula and lateral clavicle. Its upper fibers elevate the scapula.
- **Sternocleidomastoid:** This muscle arises from the manubrium of the sternum and medial aspect of the clavicle. This muscle then ascends to attach to the mastoid process of the temporal bone.
- **Scalenes:** These muscles arise from the cervical vertebrae and descend to attach to the first and second ribs. Functionally, the scalene muscles (anterior, middle, and posterior) are used for elevating the first and second ribs as is seen in forced inspiration.
- **Levator scapulae:** This muscle attaches medially to the transverse processes of the upper four cervical vertebrae and laterally to the superior angle of the scapula. On contraction, this muscle elevates and retracts the scapula.
- **Splenius capitis:** This muscle originates from the spinous processes and associated ligaments of the cervical and upper thoracic spinous processes and travels superiorly to insert onto the mastoid process and superior nuchal line. Bilateral contraction results in the extension of the neck.
- **Semispinalis capitis:** This muscle attaches superiorly between the superior and inferior nuchal lines and inferiorly from the transverse and articular processes and associated ligaments of the lower cervical and upper thoracic vertebrae.

- **Serratus anterior:** This muscle arises typically from the upper eight ribs and inserts onto the vertebral border of the scapula.

Vessels

The major blood vessels of the posterior triangle are the subclavian artery and vein. The subclavian artery as it crosses over the first rib lies between the anterior and middle scalene muscles. The subclavian vein, however, travels just anterior to the anterior scalene muscle.

Lymphatics

Lymphatics, including nodes, are found scattered throughout the posterior cervical triangle, including along the superficially located accessory nerve (see the following text). At the base of the posterior cervical triangle (eg, middle third of the clavicle), the lower deep cervical lymph nodes traveling with the internal jugular vein are referred to as the supraclavicular nodes of Virchow and, if enlarged, may signal malignancies of the viscera.

Nerves

Cutaneous Nerves

Four cutaneous nerves derived from the cervical plexus (C1-C4) emanate from the posterior border of the sternocleidomastoid muscle at a so-called nerve point found at the junction of the upper third and lower two-thirds of this muscle.

- **Lesser occipital nerve:** This branch, derived from C2 and C3, ascends along the posterior border of the sternocleidomastoid toward the skin of the auricle and occiput.
- **Great auricular nerve:** This nerve, derived from C2 and C3, ascends superficial to this muscle toward the ear and skin over the parotid region.
- **Transverse cervical nerve:** This nerve, derived from C2 and C3, travels anteriorly and superficial to the sternocleidomastoid toward the midline of the neck.
- **Supraclavicular nerve:** This branch, derived from C3 and C4, travels inferiorly and terminates as three branches that cross the medial, middle, and lateral aspects of the clavicle to supply regional skin.

Accessory Nerve

One important superficial nerve of the posterior triangle is the accessory nerve or the 11th cranial nerve. This nerve innervates only two muscles in the body, the sternocleidomastoid and trapezius muscles. After innervating the deep surface of the sternocleidomastoid muscle, the accessory nerve emerges from the posterior border of this muscle at approximately the junction between its upper third and lower two-thirds and then descends to the trapezius muscle just superficial to the levator scapulae muscle.

Brachial Plexus

The proximal parts (rami and trunks) of the brachial plexus formed by ventral rami of C5 to T1 are found in the posterior cervical triangle and are bordered by the anterior and middle scalene muscles. Between these two muscles, the proximal brachial plexus is just posterior to the subclavian artery.

Phrenic Nerve

In the neck, the phrenic nerve (C3, C4, and C5), which supplies the diaphragm, descends almost vertically along the superficial surface of the anterior scalene muscle to travel between the subclavian artery and the vein. Injury to this nerve may impair respiration. Irritation of this nerve results in spasm of the ipsilateral diaphragm (eg, hiccups).

C3 and C4

Branches of C3 and C4 may also travel through the posterior cervical triangle to terminate in the trapezius muscle or communicate with the accessory nerve. These nerves can be motor to the trapezius; however, the exact nature of such branches is debated.

Dorsal Scapular Nerve

This proximal branch of the C5 contribution to the brachial plexus exits the middle scalene muscle and travels posteriorly to the rhomboid muscles and sometimes the levator scapulae.

Long Thoracic Nerve

Either a portion or the entire long thoracic nerve, which arises from the upper three rami contributing to the brachial plexus, exits the middle scalene muscle to travel anteroinferiorly to terminate in the serratus anterior muscle.

Anterior Cervical Triangle

The anterior cervical triangle contains not only the main blood supply for the head, but also many cranial nerves and viscera such as the larynx and thyroid gland. The topography of the anterior cervical triangle includes:

- **Hyoid:** This U-shaped bone composed of a body and greater and lesser horns (cornu) does not articulate to surrounding bones but is rather suspended by muscles and ligaments at the C3 vertebral level. Its greater and lesser horns allow for attachment of muscles and ligaments.

- **Thyroid cartilage:** The thyroid cartilage is one of the nine cartilages of the larynx and the largest of these. This structure sits anterior to the C4 and C5 vertebrae. The thyroid cartilage is connected superiorly to the hyoid bone via the thyrohyoid membrane and inferiorly to the cricoid cartilage by the cricothyroid ligament.
- **Cricoid cartilage:** This ring-shaped cartilage of the larynx lies anterior to the sixth cervical vertebrae and marks the transition from larynx to trachea and pharynx to esophagus.

Muscles

The anterior cervical triangle is bordered by the anterior aspect of the sternocleidomastoid and the lower border of the mandible and the midline. Conveniently, muscles of the anterior cervical triangle can generally be divided into those that are superior to and those that are inferior to the hyoid bone. The infrahyoid muscles include from lateral to medial the omohyoid (discussed earlier in this chapter), the sternohyoid, the sternothyroid and thyrohyoid, and the cricothyroid. These muscles are named for their connections inferosuperiorly and, in general, assist in the movement of the hyoid bone and thyroid cartilage, which is one of the nine cartilages of the larynx (voice box). These muscles may also assist in depressing the mandible. The cricothyroid is a muscle of the larynx that modifies the pitch of the voice. The very thin platysma muscle covers these muscles in its descent from the lower jaw to the fascia of the pectoral and deltoid regions.

Suprahyoid muscles include the anterior and posterior bellies of the digastric, the mylohyoid, geniohyoid, stylohyoid, and hyoglossus. Each of these muscles, as many of their names imply, have some connection to the hyoid bone. The digastric muscle arises from the temporal bone (posterior belly) and inserts onto the mandible (anterior belly). An intermediate tendon connects these two bellies and is tethered to the hyoid bone by a thickening of fascia. The mylohyoid and geniohyoid arise from the internal aspect of the mandible and the stylohyoid from the styloid process of the temporal bone. The hyoglossus arises from the lateral aspect of the hyoid bone and inserts into the tongue. This muscle depresses the tongue within the oral cavity. Collectively, these muscles help elevate the hyoid bone and indirectly attached larynx. The mylohyoid muscle serves as the main component of the floor of the oral cavity.

A deeper group of muscles are located over the anterior aspect of the vertebral column and are together referred to as the prevertebral muscles. These include the scalenes (discussed earlier), the longus cervicis, and longus capitis muscles. These muscles together help flex the cervical spine and craniocervical junction.

Nerves

Cervical Branch of the Facial Nerve

This small branch of the cranial nerve VII supplies the platysma muscle.

Cervical Plexus

The cervical plexus is composed of fibers from the first four cervical ventral rami and includes cutaneous branches (described earlier in this chapter in the posterior cervical triangle)—the ansa cervicalis, the phrenic nerve and the branches to the accessory nerve from C2 to C4 (described hereinbefore), and direct muscular branches to the prevertebral muscles.

Ansa Cervicalis

Fibers from C1 to C3 unite and form a loop known as the ansa cervicalis that normally courses just anterior to the internal jugular vein. The superior root formed by C1 and C2 fibers that run with the hypoglossal nerve and the inferior root is derived from the second and third cervical nerves. This motor nerve supplies the infrahyoid muscles. A branch of C1 innervates the thyrohyoid and geniohyoid muscles by traveling along the hypoglossal nerve.

C2 and C3

These branches may also innervate the sternocleidomastoid muscle and, as the C3 and C4 fibers that terminate in the trapezius muscle, have an equivocal function.

Cervical Branches to the Scalenes and Prevertebral Muscles

Proximal branches from the ventral rami of cervical spinal nerves innervate the anterior, middle, and posterior scalenes, as well as the longus cervicis and capitis and rectus capitis and lateralis muscles.

Nerve to Mylohyoid

A branch of the third division (V3) of the trigeminal nerve (cranial nerve V) or mandibular nerve innervates the mylohyoid and anterior belly of the digastric muscle and is therefore known as the nerve to the mylohyoid.

Vagus Nerve

The vagus nerve has several branches in the neck. These include a pharyngeal nerve that supplies all muscles of the pharynx and soft palate and a superior laryngeal nerve that divides into an internal and external branch. The internal branch is a sensory nerve to the mucosa of the larynx superior to the vocal cords, and the external branch supplies primarily the cricothyroid muscle. The recurrent laryngeal nerves ascend symmetrically in a groove between the trachea and esophagus but have different courses inferiorly between the left and the right sides. On the left side, this nerve loops around the aortic arch, and on the right side, it loops more proximally around the subclavian artery. Other branches of the vagus nerve in the neck usually include two cardiac nerves destined for the thorax.

Hypoglossal Nerve

As its name implies, the hypoglossal nerve, cranial nerve XII, innervates the muscles of the tongue. Specifically, this nerve supplies the intrinsic muscles of the tongue and three extrinsic muscles that include the styloglossus, hyoglossus, and genioglossus. Primarily, these muscles retract, depress, and protrude the tongue, respectively.

Glossopharyngeal Nerve

Developmentally, the glossopharyngeal nerve, cranial nerve IX, is the cranial nerve of the third pharyngeal arch. In the neck, this nerve innervates the stylopharyngeus muscle and provides sensory innervation including taste to the posterior one-third of the tongue and supplies much of the pharyngeal mucosa. The typical complaint of a sore throat is mediated via the glossopharyngeal nerve. An additional branch travels to the carotid sinus and relays changes in blood pressure to the brainstem. Carotid sinus massage stimulates this branch with a resultant decrease in the heart rate/blood pressure.

Sympathetic Trunk

Generally, each spinal nerve of the body has an associated sympathetic ganglion. However, in the neck, these ganglia are usually combined to form superior, middle, and stellate ganglia. The superior ganglion is located just posterior to the internal carotid artery and connects with the upper 4 spinal nerves via 4 gray rami communicans, small branches that connect adjacent spinal nerves in the neck and carry postganglionic fibers. Cranially, the superior cervical ganglion has an extension known as the internal carotid nerve that travels with the internal carotid artery intracranially. An external carotid branch travels from the superior ganglion along the branches of the external carotid artery.

The middle and stellate ganglia connect to the fifth and sixth and seventh and eighth cervical spinal nerves, respectively. The middle cervical ganglion is located adjacent to the cricoid cartilage at the sixth cervical vertebrae. The stellate ganglion is formed by the fusion of the inferior cervical and the first thoracic ganglia and rests on the neck of the first rib just medial to the vertebral artery. Each cervical sympathetic ganglion issues a cardiac branch (postganglionic) that travels to the thorax for the innervation of its viscera.

Accessory Nerve

After leaving the skull base, this nerve descends obliquely across the anterior surface of the transverse process of the atlas posterior to the digastric and stylohyoid muscles to enter the deep aspect of the superior part of the sternocleidomastoid muscle.

Vessels

Common Carotid Artery

The left and right common carotid arteries originate from the aorta and brachiocephalic artery, respectively. As these vessels ascend in the anterior triangle of the neck, they are enclosed with the laterally placed internal jugular vein and posteriorly placed vagus nerve in the carotid sheath. The common carotid arteries generally bifurcate into the laterally placed internal carotid and medially placed external carotid artery at the level of the C4 vertebrae or at the superior edge of the thyroid cartilage. At the proximal internal carotid artery, an enlargement is seen and is referred to as the carotid sinus. Pressure receptors are found in this structure. Near the carotid bifurcation, a chemoreceptor, the carotid body, is present.

The *internal carotid artery* travels on to enter the cranium and, therefore, does not supply structures in the neck. The *external carotid artery* supplies multiple branches to the exterior of the head and neck. Other arteries include:

- *Superior thyroid artery:* The first branch of the external carotid artery is the superior thyroid artery, which descends to the superior pole of the thyroid gland after first providing a superior laryngeal branch that enters the larynx via the thyrohyoid membrane.
- *Lingual artery:* The lingual artery, as its name implies, is destined to supply the tongue. This artery travels deep to the hyoglossus muscle.
- *Facial artery:* The facial artery extends from the external carotid artery, through or by the submandibular gland, over the mandible just anterior to the masseter muscle where its pulse is palpable, and terminates as the angular artery traveling toward the medial canthus of the orbit.
- *Ascending pharyngeal artery:* This vessel arises and travels superiorly toward the pharynx.
- *Occipital artery:* This vessel arises from the posterior aspect of the external carotid artery and travels to the scalp over the posterior head.
- *Posterior auricular artery:* This vessel also arises from the posterior external carotid artery and travels to the posterior scalp.

- *Maxillary artery:* This is one of the two terminal branches of the external carotid artery and soon after its origin travels deep to the neck of the mandible into the infratemporal fossa where it provides multiple branches that supply, for example, meningeal branches, branches to muscles of mastication and vessels to the maxillary sinus, the nasal cavity, and hard and soft palates.
- *Superficial temporal artery:* This artery and the maxillary are the two terminal branches of the external carotid artery. The superficial temporal artery travels cephalad through the parotid gland, anterior to the external auditory meatus, where its pulse can easily be palpated, and supplies the anterolateral scalp. Along its course, this vessel also provides branches to the face.

Internal Jugular Vein

The internal jugular vein is the primary venous outlet from the cranium and, as described earlier, travels in the anterior triangle of the neck within the carotid sheath. This vessel joins with the subclavian vein to form the brachiocephalic vein. Within the neck, the main tributaries include pharyngeal branches, a common facial vein that receives the facial and lingual veins, and the superior and middle thyroid veins that drain the thyroid gland. The internal jugular vein can be cannulated for central venous access. A superficial landmark for this is to locate the interval between the sternal and clavicular heads of the sternocleidomastoid muscle.

Anterior Jugular Vein

This vessel, when present, travels on either side of the midline beginning just inferior to the chin and typically drains into the external jugular vein.

Subclavian Artery

As mentioned earlier, this vessel travels from the thorax through the superior thoracic aperture (ie, root of the neck) and between the first rib and clavicle. While on the first rib, the subclavian artery is maintained between the anterior and middle scalene muscles. Three portions can therefore be described. The first part is medial to the anterior scalene and gives rise to the vertebral artery, internal thoracic artery, and thyrocervical trunk. The second and the most superior part is posterior to the anterior scalene and gives rise to the costocervical trunk. The third part of this vessel may give rise to the dorsal scapular artery if this does not arise from the transverse cervical artery (discussed later in this chapter).

Vertebral Artery

The first branch of the subclavian artery is the vertebral artery. These vessels are important not only in supplying approximately one-third of the blood to the brain but also in supplying branches to the cervical spinal cord and adjacent muscles. This vessel begins by usually entering the transverse foramen of the sixth cervical vertebrae and then travels through the transverse foramina of the remaining cervical vertebrae to enter the cranium thereafter.

Thyrocervical Trunk

This vessel is usually the second branch of the subclavian artery and generally provides three branches:

- *Inferior thyroid artery:* This is usually the first branch of the thyrocervical trunk and travels medially to supply the inferior pole of the thyroid and parathyroid glands. The terminal branches of the inferior thyroid artery are in intimate contact with the recurrent laryngeal nerve. An ascending cervical branch also extends from the inferior thyroid artery and travels parallel to the phrenic nerve on the anterior scalene muscle to supply muscular, vertebral, and spinal branches.
- *Transverse cervical artery:* This vessel travels through the posterior cervical triangle to the trapezius and rhomboid muscles.
- *Suprascapular artery:* This vessel also traverses the posterior triangle closer to the clavicle than the transverse cervical artery and terminates in the supraspinatus and infraspinatus muscles.

Internal Thoracic Artery

This vessel arises usually just opposite to the origin of the thyrocervical trunk and descends into the thorax to supply anterior intercostals arteries and smaller branches to, for example, the thymus and sternum. Descriptions of its continuation will be discussed in the section on the thorax.

Costocervical Trunk

This branch of the second part of the subclavian artery divides into two branches:

- A descending branch known as the *highest intercostal artery* that supplies the first two posterior intercostals spaces and
- An ascending branch known as the *deep cervical artery* that ascends along the semispinalis cervicis muscle of the deep back muscles to form an anastomosis with a branch of the occipital artery

Dorsal Scapular Artery

If the transverse cervical artery does not give rise to a deep branch, a dorsal scapular artery is usually found and arises from the third part of the subclavian artery. This vessel then travels posteriorly to supply primarily the rhomboid muscles.

Lymphatics: Thoracic Duct

The thoracic duct is the primary lymphatic channel in the body and drains the entire body with the exception of the upper right half of the thorax, right upper limb, and right half of the head. This vessel begins in the abdomen and courses primarily in the thorax. Its termination is into the junction of the left subclavian vein and left internal jugular vein (venous angle); therefore, a portion of this structure is found in the left neck. At approximately the seventh cervical vertebrae in the neck, the thoracic duct takes an outward curve between the carotid and vertebral arteries before emptying into the venous angle.

The major lymphatic vessels and nodes are found concentrated along the internal jugular vein and are referred to as the deep cervical chain. One of the larger of these is located in the angle created as the common facial vein drains into the internal jugular vein and is known as the *jugulodigastric node.* This node is a surgical landmark for identifying the common facial vein, which can be accessed for placing venous catheters into the internal jugular vein. Superficial nodes of the neck include submental, submandibular, anterior jugular, and external jugular groups.

11 Neck, Face, and Eye

Technique

THYROID LATERAL LOBE COMMON CAROTID ARTERY INTERNAL JUGULAR VEIN
Transverse
FIG. 11.1

Place the patient in a supine position with the neck extended over a small bolster and head turned to the side opposite the one being examined. Position the probe low in the neck with a transverse orientation. Navigate from midline trachea and thyroid lateral lobes, then slide the probe laterally until the pulsating common carotid artery can be identified in contact with the lateral aspect of the thyroid lobe deep to the sternocleidomastoid and infrahyoid muscles (eg, omohyoid muscle, which "slips" between the sternocleidomastoid and common carotid artery/internal jugular vein). The oval internal jugular vein (deforms/effaces with probe pressure) is typically immediately lateral to the common carotid artery. The internal jugular vein changes its size (pulsates with respiratory movement and noticeably enlarges with Valsalva and collapses on Valsalva release, and valves may be seen). Tilt/fan the probe to look for the vagus nerve in the groove between the posterior surfaces of the common carotid artery and internal jugular vein. Note the reflection and acoustic shadow of the cervical transverse process posterior to the common carotid artery and internal jugular vein (and longus colli). The anterolateral projection at the lateral extent of the transverse process is the anterior tubercle of the transverse process.

COMMON CAROTID ARTERY CAROTID SINUS INTERNAL CAROTID ARTERY
Longitudinal
FIG. 11.2

Place the patient in a supine position with the neck extended and head turned to the side opposite the one being examined. Starting from the previous image, center the probe over the common

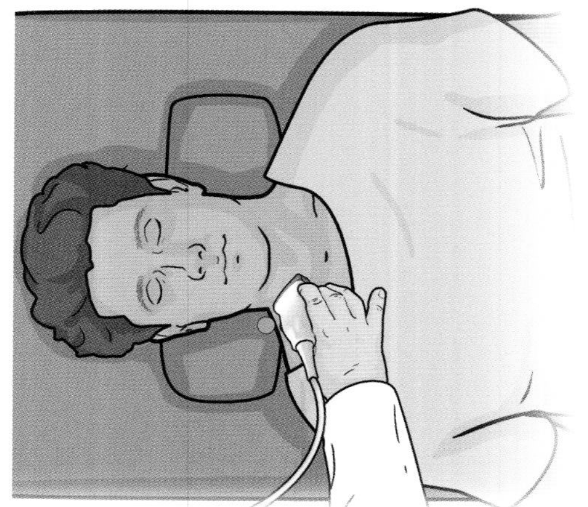

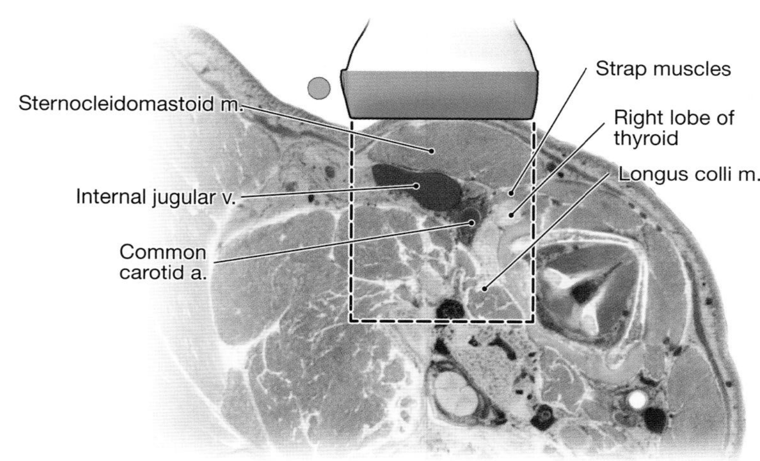

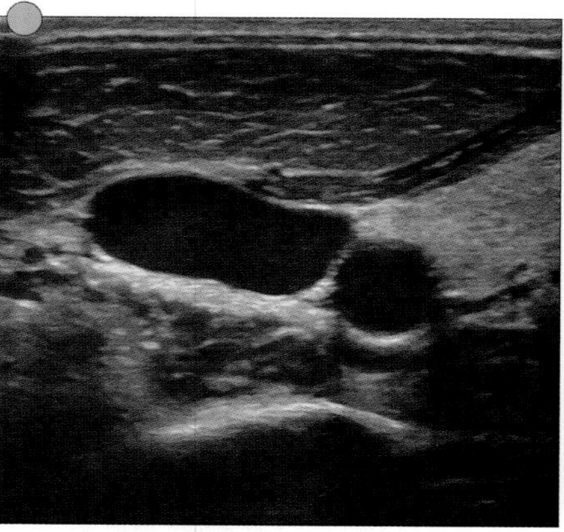

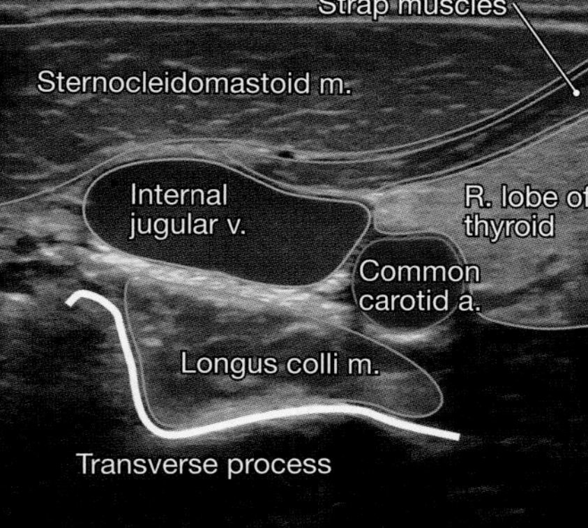

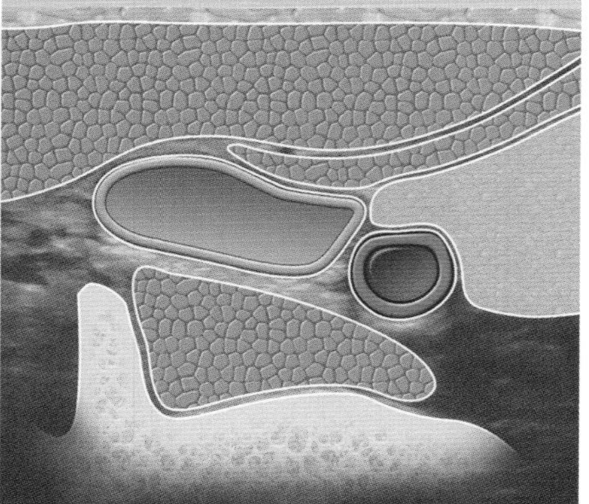

Figure 11.1 Transverse view of the lateral lobe of the thyroid gland, common carotid artery, and internal jugular vein.

carotid artery and carefully rotate 90° clockwise to view the common carotid artery in its longitudinal axis. Slide the probe superiorly, keeping the common carotid artery in view until the expansion at the carotid sinus can be identified. Continue to slide the probe superiorly a short distance until the full extent of the carotid sinus can be seen (the superior, marker end of the probe may need to be rotated slightly posteriorly while keeping the inferior heel of the probe stationary over the common carotid artery to identify, from inferior to superior, the common carotid artery, carotid sinus, and internal carotid artery).

INTERNAL CAROTID ARTERIES EXTERNAL CAROTID ARTERIES
Transverse
FIG. 11.3

Place the patient in a supine position with the neck extended and head turned to the side opposite the one being examined. Center the probe over the carotid sinus and slowly rotate approximately 90° counterclockwise. Then slide the probe superiorly until beyond the carotid bifurcation and both internal and external carotid arteries can be identified (in some patients, probe movement may be limited by contact against the angle of the mandible: patience and careful movement of the probe, patient head rotation, etc., usually allows visualization of both the internal and external carotid arteries in transverse).

The internal carotid artery is larger than the external carotid artery and is located posterolaterally to it. The external carotid artery branches in the neck may be seen (superior thyroid artery) with careful observation and can be distinguished based on flow dynamics (use of the spectral Doppler is beyond the scope of this text). The internal jugular vein is located lower in the neck (lateral to the external carotid artery, then lateral to the internal carotid artery), although in this image, the internal jugular vein has slipped between the internal and the external carotid arteries because of the probe pressure. The internal jugular vein flattens/deforms/effaces with probe pressure, but arteries do not. Note the transverse process with anterior and posterior tubercles and the hyperechoic honeycomb appearance of the vagus nerve.

COMMON CAROTID ARTERY CAROTID SINUS INTERNAL CAROTID ARTERY EXTERNAL CAROTID ARTERY
Longitudinal
FIG. 11.4

From the preceding transverse image, determine the path an ultrasound (US) beam would have to follow to pass through both internal and external carotid arteries when the probe is rotated into the longitudinal axis (look at the previous image and draw an imaginary line from the skin

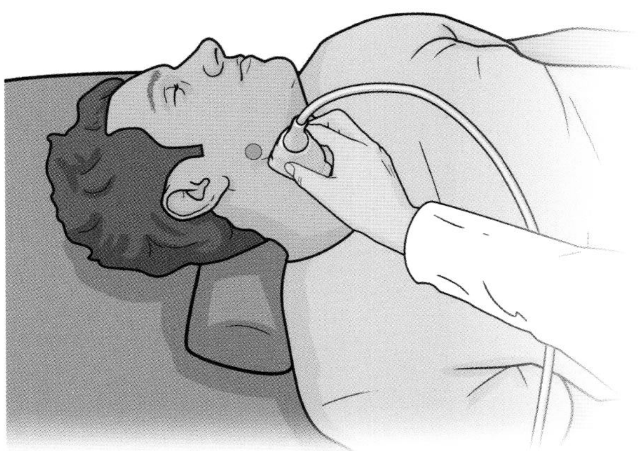

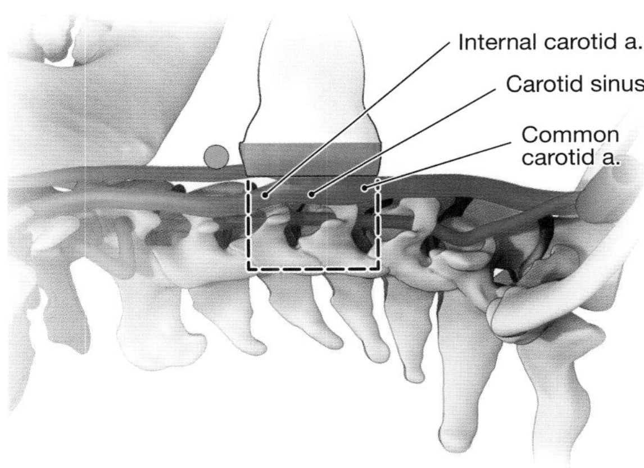

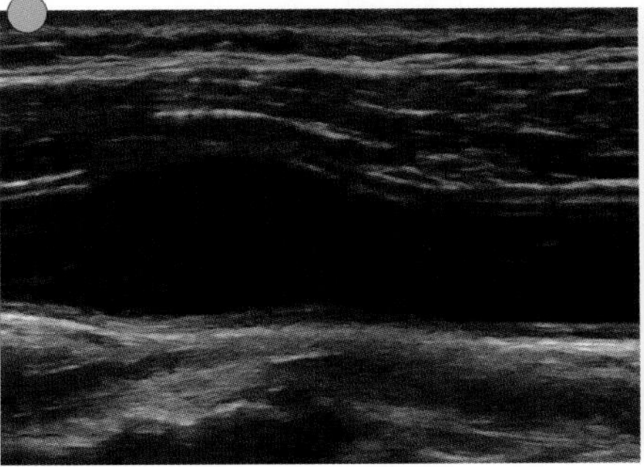

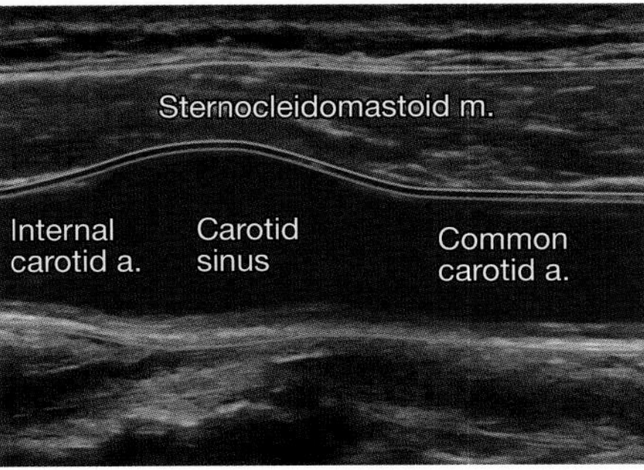

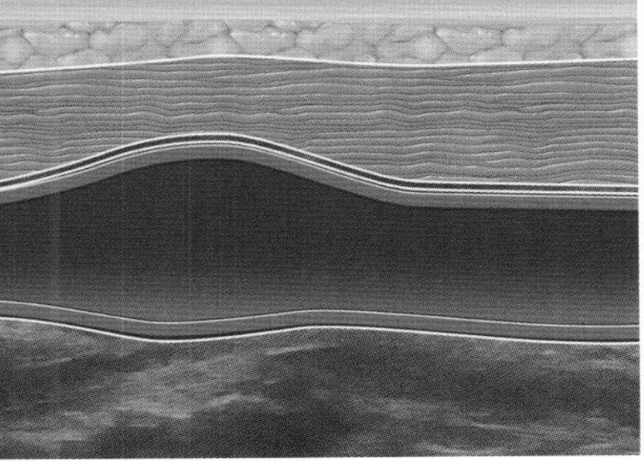

Figure 11.2 Longitudinal view of the common carotid artery, carotid sinus, and internal carotid artery.

surface through the sternocleidomastoid, the internal carotid artery, and then the external carotid artery). In this case, the angle needed to image both vessels is steep from posterolateral to anteromedial. The probe should be rotated into the longitudinal axis and the beam aimed along that imaginary line. Tilt/fan and adjust the probe's position until the common carotid artery, sinus, and internal and external carotid arteries can be seen within the image. Note that because the beam is traveling from posterolateral to anteromedial, the probe face is closest to the internal carotid artery. As a result, the internal carotid artery appears near to midfield of the image, and the external carotid artery, which is further from the probe face, appears deeper in the image (this mirror image orientation can be confusing early on). A similar image (mirror image in fact) could potentially be obtained by aiming the US beam along the same line but from anteromedial to posterolateral, although the contour of the neck and anterior edge of the sternocleidomastoid might render that image more difficult to obtain. One or the other is inevitably easier to obtain based on the relative positions of external / internal carotid arteries in each patient.

VERTEBRAL ARTERY
Longitudinal
FIG. 11.5

Place the patient in a supine position and extend the neck, head turned away from the examination side, and begin with a longitudinal view of the common carotid artery (Figure 11.2), maintaining the same probe tilt and orientation. Slowly slide the probe face a short distance posteriorly along the neck, watching carefully for the reflections/acoustic shadows of cervical transverse processes to appear. Carefully adjust the probe tilt/angle/position until the anechoic vertebral artery can be seen between two transverse processes ("river under the bridge"). Keeping the vertebral artery segment in view, carefully slide the probe inferiorly until the artery can be seen "diving" toward the transverse

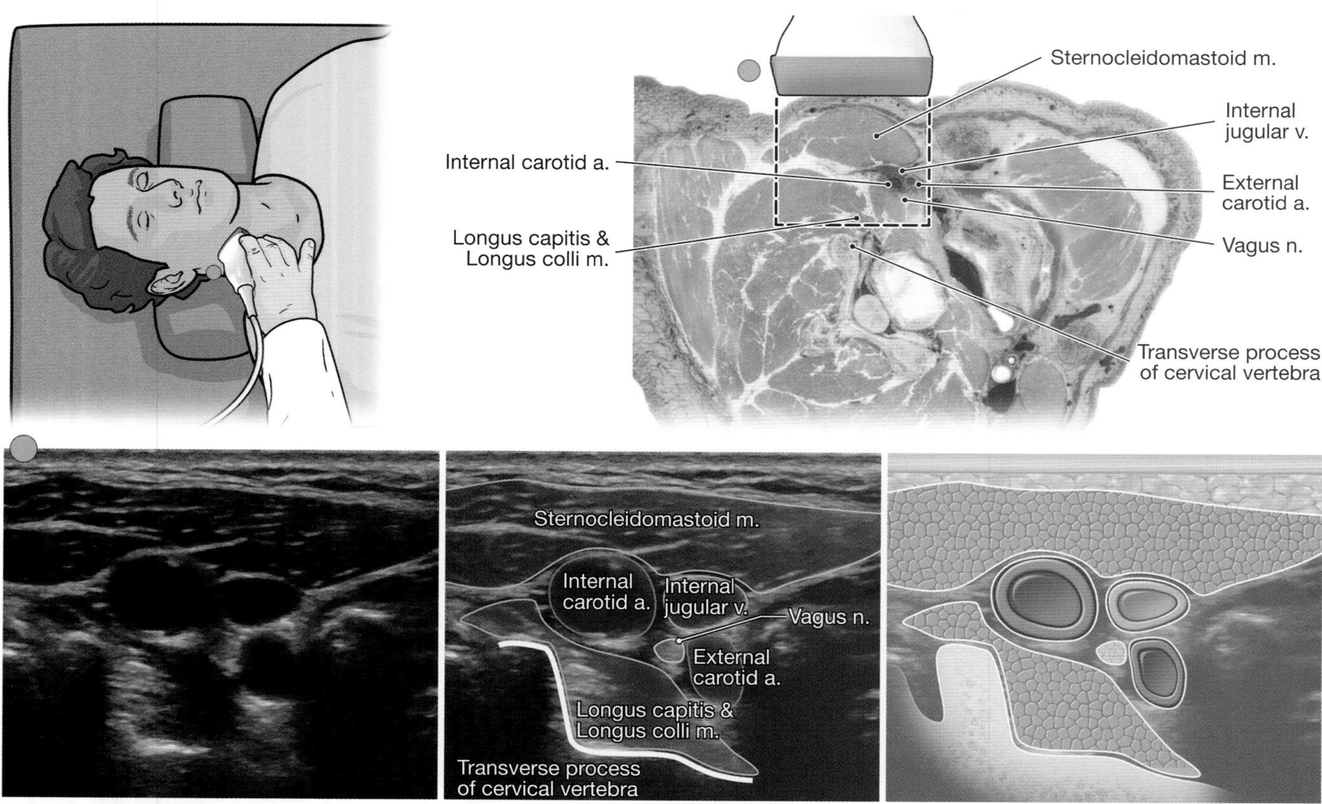

Figure 11.3 Transverse view of internal and external carotid arteries just superior to the bifurcation of common carotid artery.

foramen of CV6. In most patients, the vertebral artery can easily be followed further inferiorly to its origin from the subclavian artery. The vertebral vein may be seen anterior to the artery in the spaces between adjacent transverse foramina (acoustic shadows of transverse processes prevent US imaging of the vertebral vessels within the transverse foramina).

DEEP CERVICAL LYMPH NODE
Transverse
FIG. 11.6

Place the patient in a supine position with the neck extended over a small bolster. Orient the probe transversely with the common carotid artery and internal jugular vein in view (see Figure 11.1). Slowly slide the probe superiorly, keeping the common carotid artery and internal jugular vein in view. Watch for the appearance of occasional small, ovoid, hypoechoic lymph nodes with a linear hyperechoic band/stripe in the center (fat tracking into the hilum along the blood vessels and the efferent lymphatic vessel). Deep cervical nodes are seen at intervals along the anterior (medial), posterior (lateral), and superficial surfaces of the internal jugular vein.

The US image shows the typical hypoechoic appearance of a lymph node with a hyperechoic stripe/band in the center (fat tracking into hilum along blood vessels and the efferent lymph vessel), seen at the medial aspect of the internal jugular vein.

JUGULODIGASTRIC LYMPH NODE STERNOCLEIDOMASTOID POSTERIOR BELLY OF DIGASTRIC INTERNAL JUGULAR VEIN
Transverse
FIG. 11.7

To obtain a US image of the jugulodigastric lymph node, the patient should be supine with the head turned to the side opposite the one being examined. It may be helpful to extend the neck over a small bolster. Place the probe

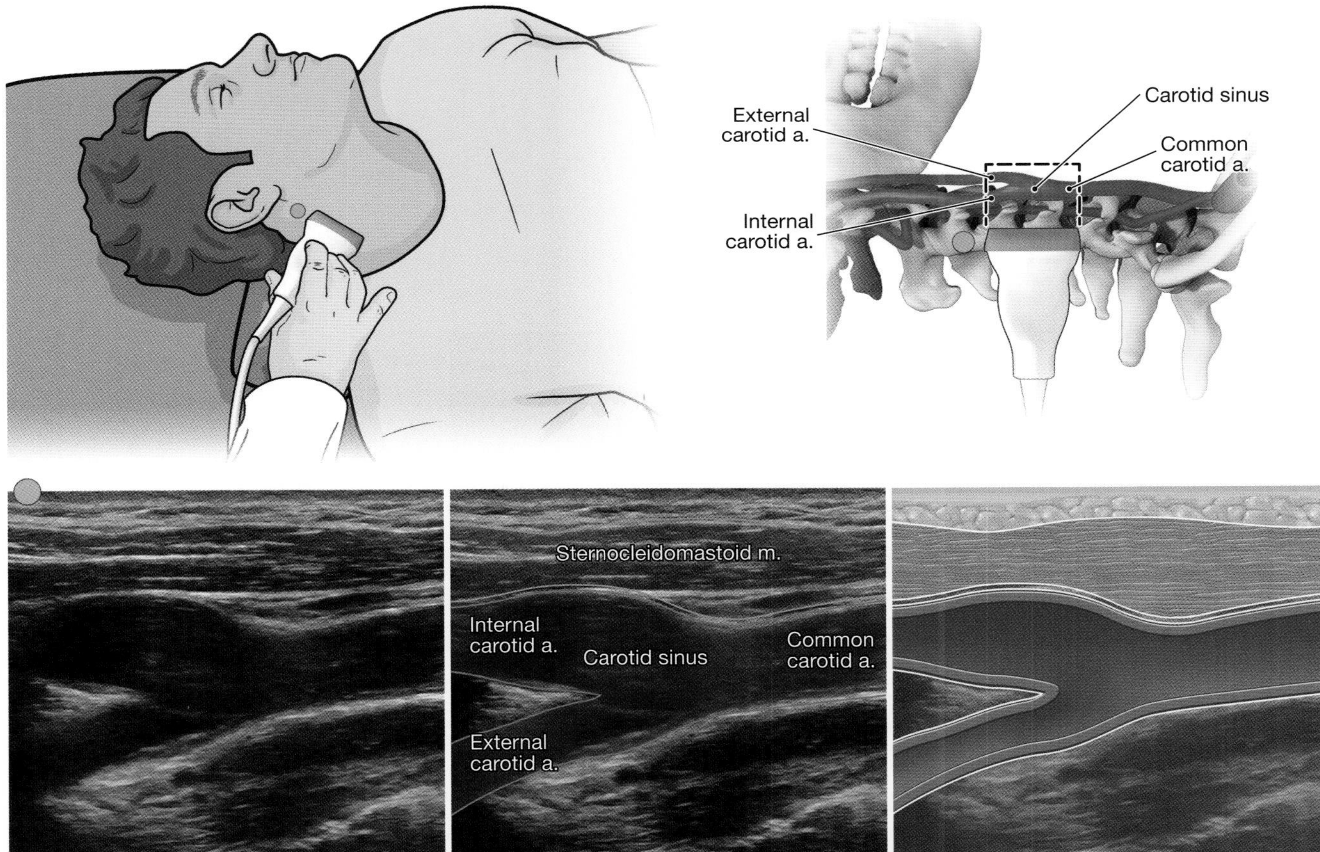

Figure 11.4 Longitudinal (parasagittal oblique) view of the common carotid artery, carotid sinus, internal carotid artery, and external carotid artery.

transverse to the neck (probe marker directed anteriorly) with the marker side of the probe face just over the ramus of the mandible a very short distance above the mandibular angle and the remainder of the probe face over the sternocleidomastoid muscle just below its origin from the mastoid process. Identify the ramus of the mandible and the sternocleidomastoid muscle. Slide the probe a few centimeters inferiorly and then back superiorly to observe the posterior belly of the digastric muscle as it appears deep to the sternocleidomastoid muscle and moves diagonally across the US image from posterosuperior (mastoid process) to anteroinferior (hyoid bone). Identify the internal jugular vein deep to the sternocleidomastoid and adjust the probe position (superiorly or inferiorly) until the posterior belly of digastric is in the anterior-most part of the image. Tilt and fan the probe as needed until the typically large jugulodigastric node can be seen as an oval or elliptical hypoechoic structure with an interior hyperechoic band (fat tracking into the hilum with nodal blood supply and the efferent lymphatic vessel), just anterior to the internal jugular vein, near the posterior belly of digastric muscle. Identify the internal and external carotid arteries near the internal jugular vein, a short distance above the bifurcation of common carotid artery.

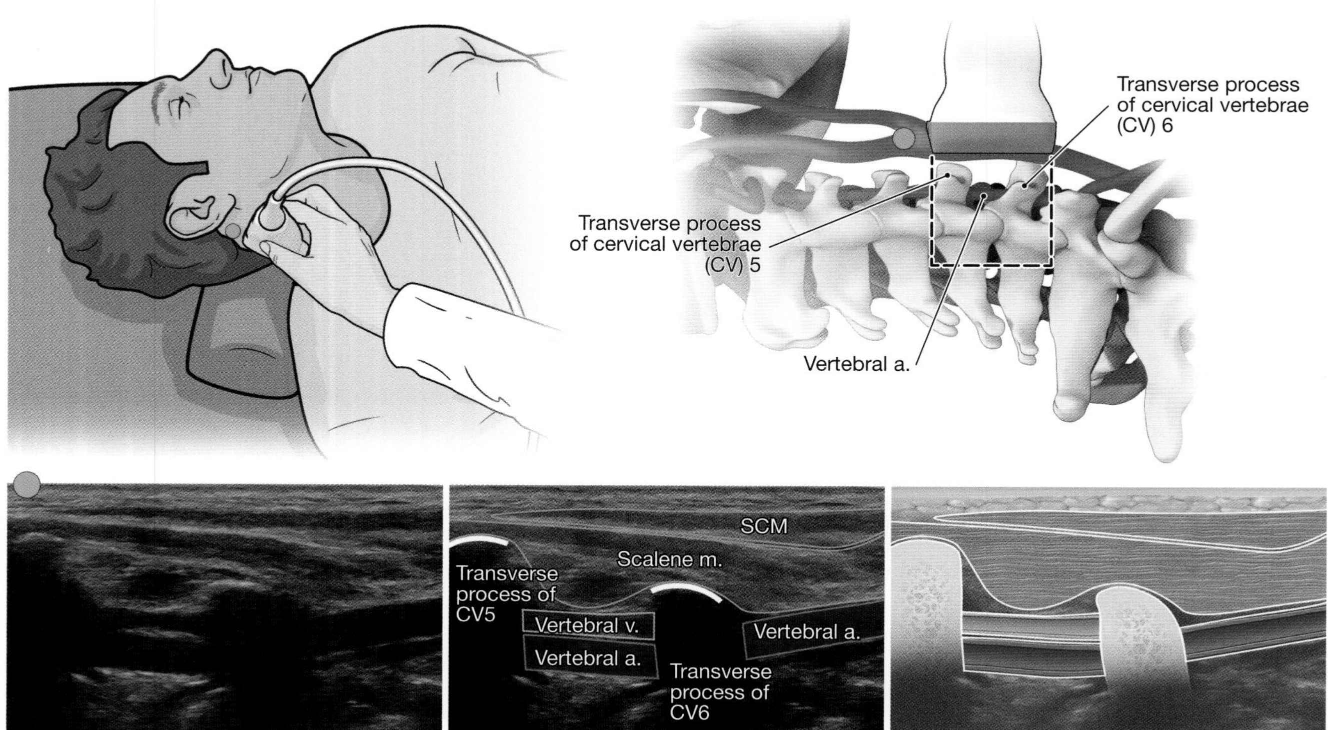

Figure 11.5 Longitudinal view of the vertebral artery entering the transverse foramen of the sixth cervical vertebra and then between the sixth and fifth transverse foramina.

CLINICAL APPLICATIONS

For patients who are in hypovolemic shock or very ill, establishing a vascular access is one of the priorities after airway breathing is ensured. In cases in which peripheral venous access is not possible, central venous access is performed to allow fluid resuscitation, measurement of hemodynamics, and delivery of medications and nutritional support.

The most common access point for central venous catheterization is the internal jugular vein. Other veins can also be used, such as the femoral vein. US is used for identifying the internal jugular vein through a supraclavicular approach visualizing the internal jugular vein at the lateral border of the clavicular head of the sternocleidomastoid. The vein can also be visualized between the two heads of the sternocleidomastoid muscle. The carotid arteries can be evaluated by color Doppler US for the detection of carotid artery stenosis and atherosclerotic plaques. Carotid US can accurately describe the location and internal characteristics, as well as the surface details of the carotid arteries. Specifically, the intima-media thickness is a measurable index for the degree of atherosclerosis in carotid arteries and is associated with increased risk factors for stroke. Similarly, the color Doppler can visualize the blood flow in the carotid vessels and identify stenotic segments. Specifically, when examining the vertebral artery, the flow direction is an important aspect in the diagnosis of proximal stenosis of the subclavian artery. The flow in the vertebral artery may be reversed in case of subclavian steal syndrome because of proximal stenosis of the subclavian artery.

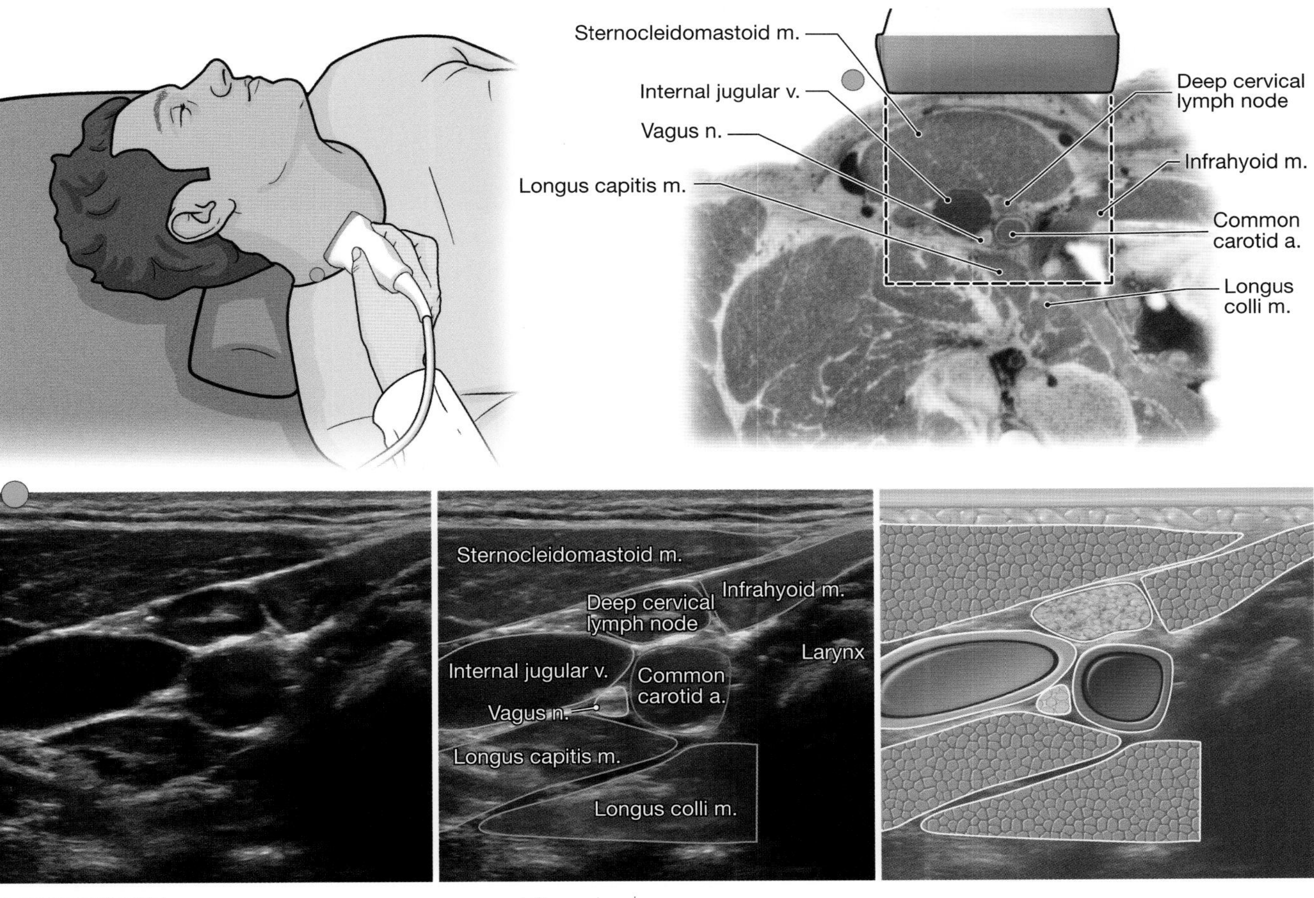

Figure 11.6 Transverse view of the deep cervical lymph node, internal jugular vein, and common carotid artery.

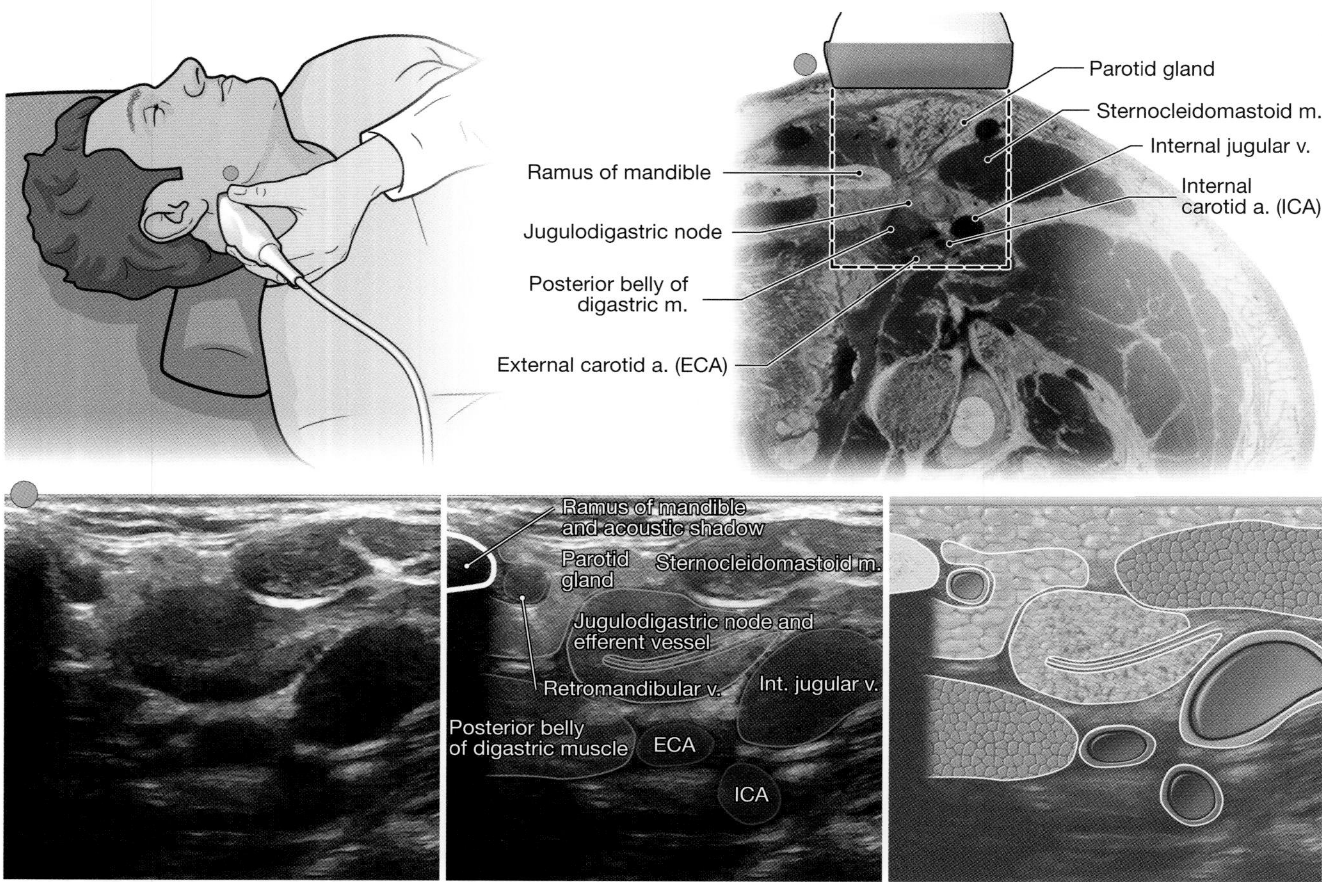

Figure 11.7 Transverse view of the jugulodigastric lymph node, sternocleidomastoid muscle, posterior belly of digastric muscle, internal jugular vein, external carotid artery and internal carotid artery.

Viscera of the Neck

Review of the Anatomy

The viscera of the neck include the submandibular gland, larynx, trachea, pharynx, esophagus, thyroid, and parathyroid glands.

Submandibular Gland

This second largest salivary gland is found overlying the posterior belly of the digastric and stylohyoid muscles. A smaller and deeper portion will also be found on the superior surface of the mylohyoid muscle. Sometimes, the gland connects with the parotid or sublingual gland through a glandular process. The duct of the submandibular gland (Wharton duct) runs from its deep aspect or glandular hilum at the level of the mylohyoid muscle toward the medial aspect of the sublingual gland. The facial artery usually grooves or traverses the superficial portion of this gland on its way to the face. The lingual artery and vein run at its medial side. Autonomically, the submandibular gland receives its innervation via a branch of the facial nerve, cranial nerve VII.

Sublingual Gland

The sublingual gland is found at the floor of the mouth covered by the oral mucosa (small ducts open at the base of the sublingual fold) between the geniohyoid, intrinsic muscles of the tongue, hypoglossal muscle (medially), and the mylohyoid muscle. Its medial side is wrapped around the terminal part of the submandibular duct. It receives postganglionic parasympathetic fibers from the submandibular ganglion.

Larynx/Trachea

The larynx (voice box) is composed of nine cartilages, three paired and three unpaired. The larger unpaired cartilages are the thyroid, cricoid, and epiglottis. The smaller paired cartilages are the arytenoids, corniculates, and cuneiforms. The epiglottis protects the inlet of the larynx, and the remaining cartilages provide support and, as related to the arytenoids, rotate and thereby cause tension or relaxation of the vocal cords. The recurrent laryngeal nerve innervates all muscles of the larynx with the exception of the cricothyroid muscle, which is innervated by the external laryngeal branch of the superior laryngeal nerve. The larynx terminates at the sixth cervical vertebrae and becomes the trachea, which continues inferiorly in the midline just anterior to the esophagus in the neck.

Pharynx/Esophagus

The pharynx, a thin, skeletal semicylindrical muscle, begins at the base of the skull and descends to the sixth cervical vertebrae, where it becomes the narrowed esophagus. The pharynx is common to the air we breathe and the food we eat. It is composed of an inner mucosa, a pharyngobasilar fascia, and skeletal muscles that are divided into semicircular fibers known as the pharyngeal constrictors and longitudinal muscles such as the stylopharyngeus. The pharynx is coated posterolaterally by the buccopharyngeal fascia. This fascia is in intimate contact posteriorly with the prevertebral fascia. The fascial plane between these two fasciae extends inferiorly to the superior mediastinum; therefore, infections that penetrate the posterior wall of the pharynx can extend into the mediastinum and result in mediastinitis or endocarditis.

The pharynx is common to the nasal and oral cavities and larynx and collects and propels food toward the esophagus. The pharynx is innervated by the pharyngeal plexus primary motor input of which is via the vagus nerve. The sensory and sympathetic input to this plexus found primarily on the posterior aspect of the middle pharyngeal constrictor muscle is via the glossopharyngeal and cervical sympathetic trunk, respectively.

The pharynx is divided into a naso, oro, and laryngo (hypo) pharynx as it passes posterior to these regions. Important structures found in the nasopharynx include the pharyngeal tonsil and the medial opening of the Eustachian tube. The oropharynx contains the lingual and palatine tonsils, and the laryngopharynx houses the piriform recess, which is a common site for foreign objects (eg, pills) to become entrapped.

Thyroid Gland

The thyroid gland contained in its own fibrous capsule is composed of left and right lateral lobes that are united across the midline by the isthmus that overlies the second through the fourth tracheal rings. The thyroid gland regulates the metabolic rate in the body by secreting thyroxine and thyrocalcitonin. It is covered superolaterally by the sternothyroid muscle and may have a cephalad extension called the pyramidal lobe, which is generally from the left lateral lobe. Remnants of the thyroglossal duct may also be found to extend from such a pyramidal lobe superiorly through the hyoid bone and even to the foramen cecum of the tongue. Cysts may develop along this duct and necessitate surgical removal. Its arterial supply is from the superior and inferior thyroid arteries, and its drainage is from the superior, middle, and inferior thyroid veins.

Parathyroid Glands

Normally located on the posterior aspect of the thyroid gland, the parathyroids are divided into two superior and two inferior glands. These structures maintain serum calcium levels and are derived from the fourth and the third pharyngeal arches, respectively. The inferior parathyroids may sometimes be found in the thorax.

Technique

SUBMANDIBULAR SALIVARY GLAND
Longitudinal (Oblique Parasagittal)
FIG. 11.8

Place the patient in a supine position with the neck extended over a small bolster. Orient the probe approximately parallel to the inferior margin of the body of the mandible near the angle. Adjust the probe position until the fine-grained hyperechoic submandibular gland can be identified. Slide the probe medially and laterally and anteriorly and posteriorly to locate the gland in relationship to the posterior free edge of mylohyoid. The largest mass of the gland is superficial (inferior) to mylohyoid, but a small part of the gland conveying the submandibular duct curves up over the posterior free edge of mylohyoid to enter the oral cavity. In the US image shown, the gland was actively secreting and the anechoic fluid within the duct is clearly seen at the superior edge of mylohyoid surrounded by a small amount of glandular tissue.

SUBMANDIBULAR SALIVARY GLAND
Longitudinal (Oblique Coronal)
FIG. 11.9

Place the patient in a supine position with the neck extended over a small bolster. Orient the probe perpendicular to the inferior edge of the body of the mandible, with the marker side resting on the inferior edge of the mandible. The remainder of the probe should be faced against the skin of the neck and the beam aimed superiorly toward the oral cavity. Identify the fine-grained hyperechoic appearance of the submandibular gland and the reflection and acoustic shadow of the body of the mandible. Slide the probe anteriorly and posteriorly along the edge of the mandible, and identify the thin sheet of mylohyoid muscle at the gland's deep surface and the hypoechoic oval of intermediate tendon of digastric between mylohyoid and the deep surface of the gland. Look for pulsations of the facial artery deep to and within the substance of the gland, usually near the posterior

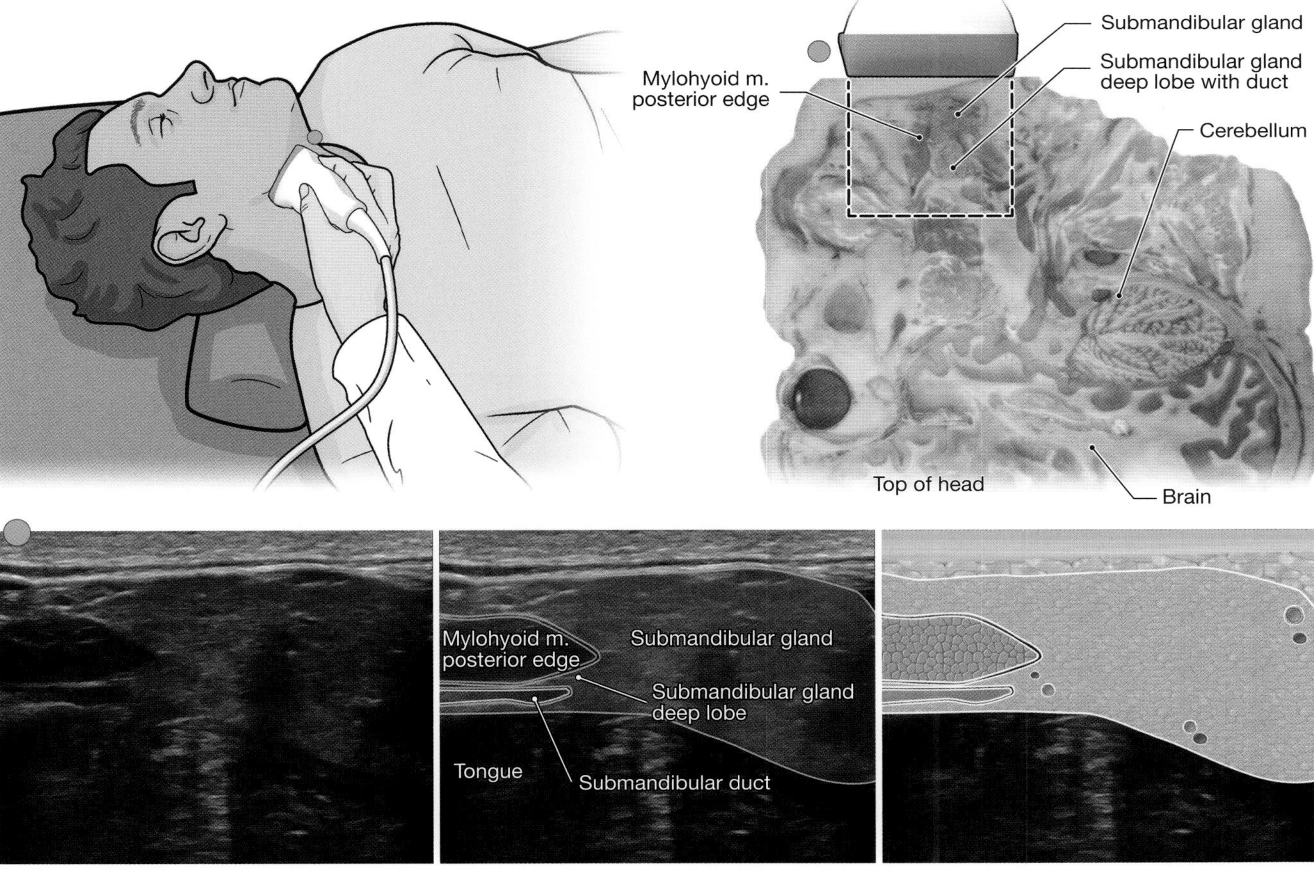

Figure 11.8 Longitudinal (oblique parasagittal) view of the submandibular salivary gland and submandibular duct in relationship to the posterior-free edge of mylohyoid muscle.

aspect of the gland. The tortuosity of the artery is seen as multiple sections of the artery in cross-section.

SUBLINGUAL SALIVARY GLANDS
Longitudinal (Coronal)
FIG. 11.10

Place the patient in a supine position with the neck extended over a small bolster. Orient the probe transversely (marker right) with the probe face against the skin of the neck just posterior to the inferior surface of the mental region of the mandible, with the beam aimed superiorly into the floor of the mouth. Identify from superficial (inferior) to deep (superior) the right and left anterior bellies of digastric (the reflections and acoustic shadows of the inferior margins of the mandibular bodies are just beyond the image edges on either side) and the thin sheet of the mylohyoid muscle, geniohyoid, and genioglossus muscles, with the right and left sublingual glands occupying the fatty spaces just lateral to the geniohyoid/genioglossus. Tilt/fan the probe face to see the ovoid glands, which are slightly hypoechoic to the surrounding fat/connective tissue.

THYROID GLAND TRACHEA
Transverse
FIG. 11.11

Place the patient in a supine position with the neck extended over a small bolster. Place the probe transversely over the skin of the neck few centimeters above the sternal notch. Adjust the probe's position until the lateral lobes of the thyroid gland (hyperechoic grainy appearance with multiple small anechoic vessels seen throughout) and the thin isthmus (anterior to the trachea) can be identified. The trachea appears

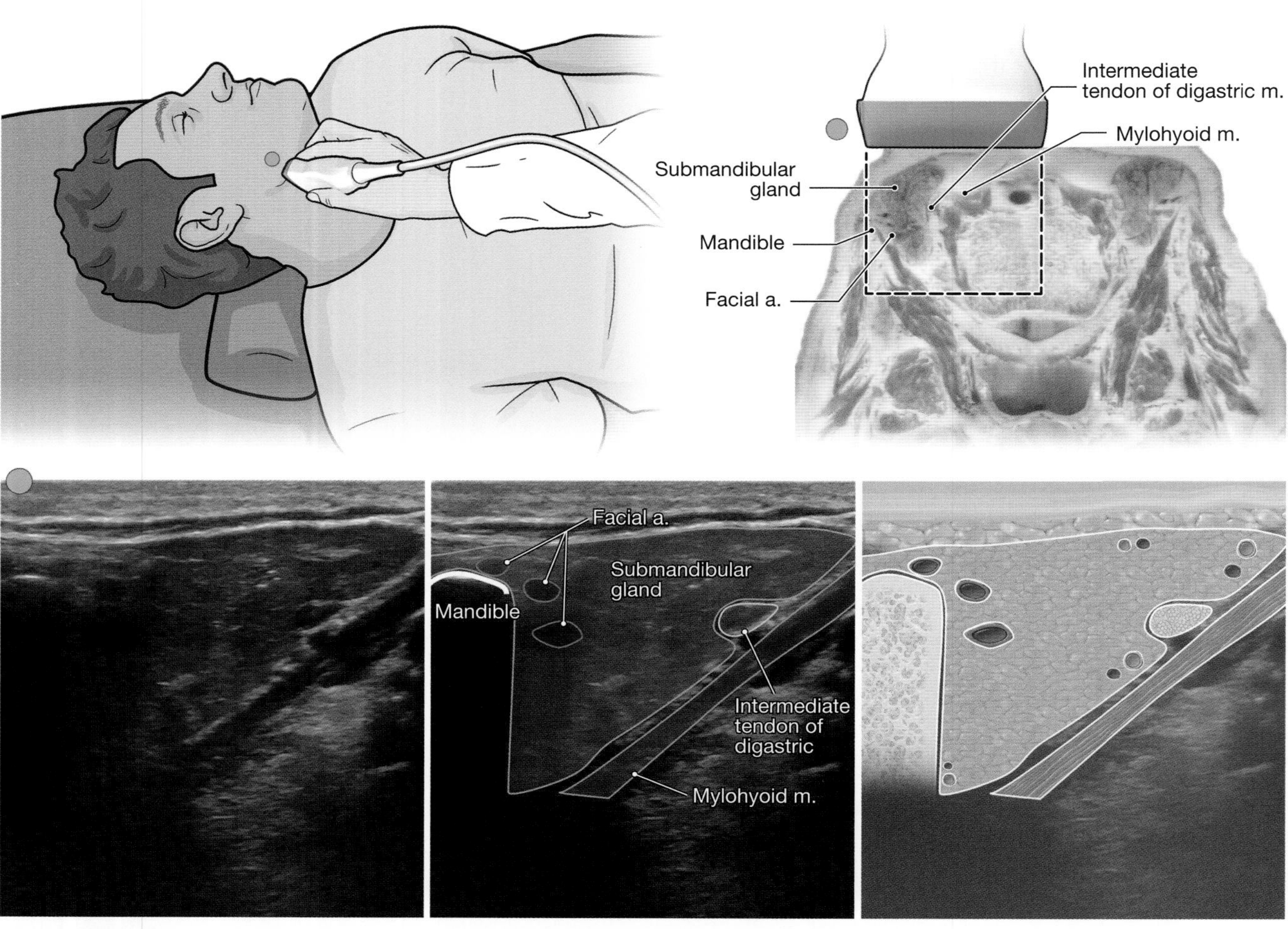

Figure 11.9 Longitudinal (oblique coronal) view of the submandibular salivary gland, mandible, mylohyoid muscle, intermediate tendon of digastric muscle, and facial artery.

hypoechoic with a bright reflection anteriorly where the US beam leaves the aqueous region of thyroid mucosa and enters the tracheal air column (air-mucosa interface), and multiple thin hyperechoic bands are seen (reverberation artifact). Thin infrahyoid (strap) muscles are seen at the superficial surface of the thyroid isthmus and lateral lobes. The medial edges of sternocleidomastoid may be seen superficial to the infrahyoid muscles on either side of the image (only the right sternocleidomastoid is seen in this image). The esophagus is seen clearly in this image just to the left of the trachea (common position) at the posteromedial aspect of the left thyroid lobe. It typically has a bullseye appearance with concentric hypoechoic/hyperechoic rings. Ask the patient to swallow and see a hyperechoic "flash" of air artifact.

LATERAL THYROID LOBE COMMON CAROTID ARTERY INTERNAL JUGULAR VEIN
FIG. 11.12

Place the patient in a supine position with the neck extended over a small bolster. The probe slides laterally (from previous midline thyroid) until several structures can be identified: from medial to lateral, deep to sternocleidomastoid muscle (and in this location deep to omohyoid and sternohyoid muscles); lateral lobe of the thyroid gland; common carotid artery; internal jugular vein; and anterior scalene muscle (from medial to lateral, useful landmarks for navigating, such as to scalene interval for brachial plexus). The omohyoid muscle (inferior belly) can be identified between the deep surface of the sternocleidomastoid muscle and the internal jugular vein.

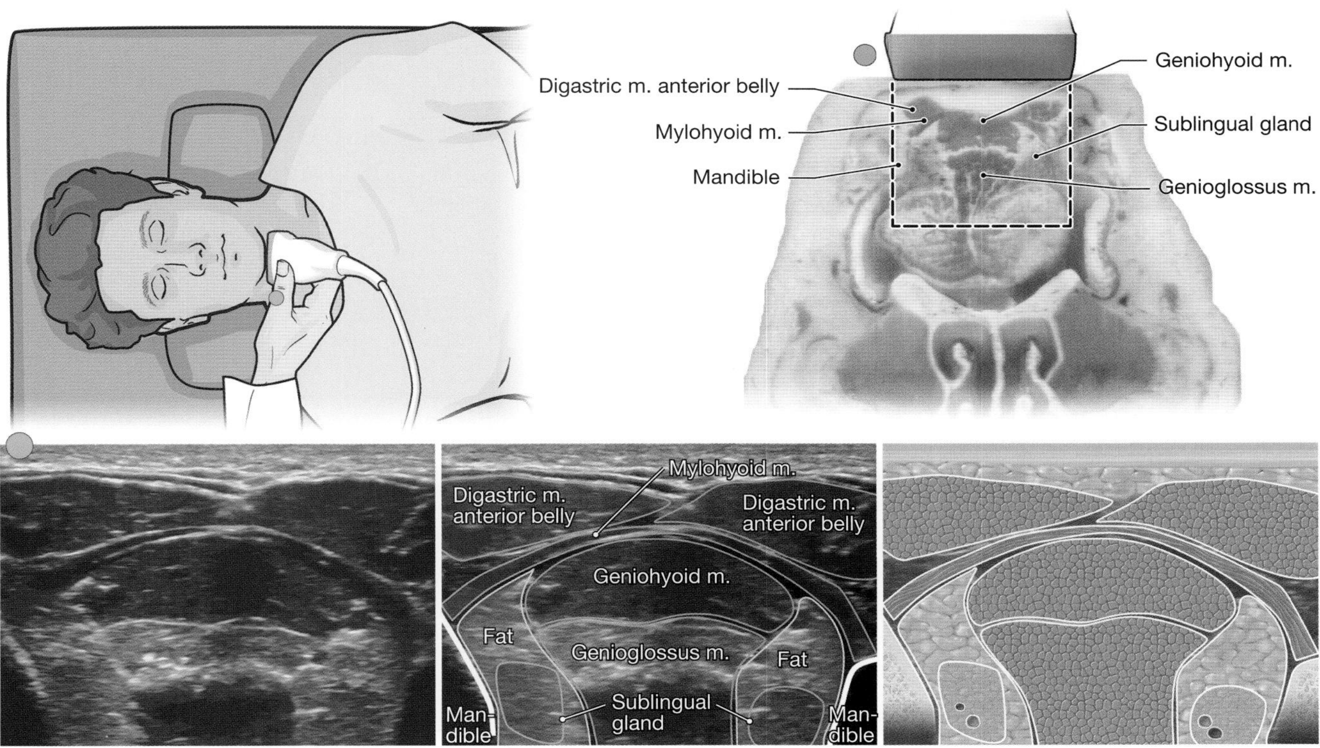

Figure 11.10 Longitudinal (coronal) view of the sublingual salivary glands, anterior bellies of digastric, mylohyoid, geniohyoid, and genioglossus muscles.

CLINICAL APPLICATIONS

Salivary stones are most often located in the submandibular gland (60%-90% of cases) and may be multiple, causing **sialolithiasis**. Sialolithiasis can cause partial or total obstruction of the salivary duct. Salivary stones or sialoliths when present in the distal part of the submandibular duct (Wharton duct) may be palpable in the floor of the mouth.

An autoimmune disease, **Sjögren syndrome,** affects women more than 40 years of age and is characterized by intense lymphocytic and plasma cell infiltration and destruction of salivary and lacrimal glands resulting in dry mouth and eyes. The most common malignant neoplasms occurring in salivary glands are mucoepidermoid carcinoma and adenoid cystic carcinoma.

Thyroid nodules are the most common finding on US examination (up to 50%). Approximately, 60% to 70% of these nodules are benign in nature and are benign follicular nodules or thyroiditis. Malignancy occurs in 5% to 7% of all thyroid nodules (papillary, follicular anaplastic, and medullary carcinomas); however, the lifetime risk of thyroid cancer is less than 1% in the United States.

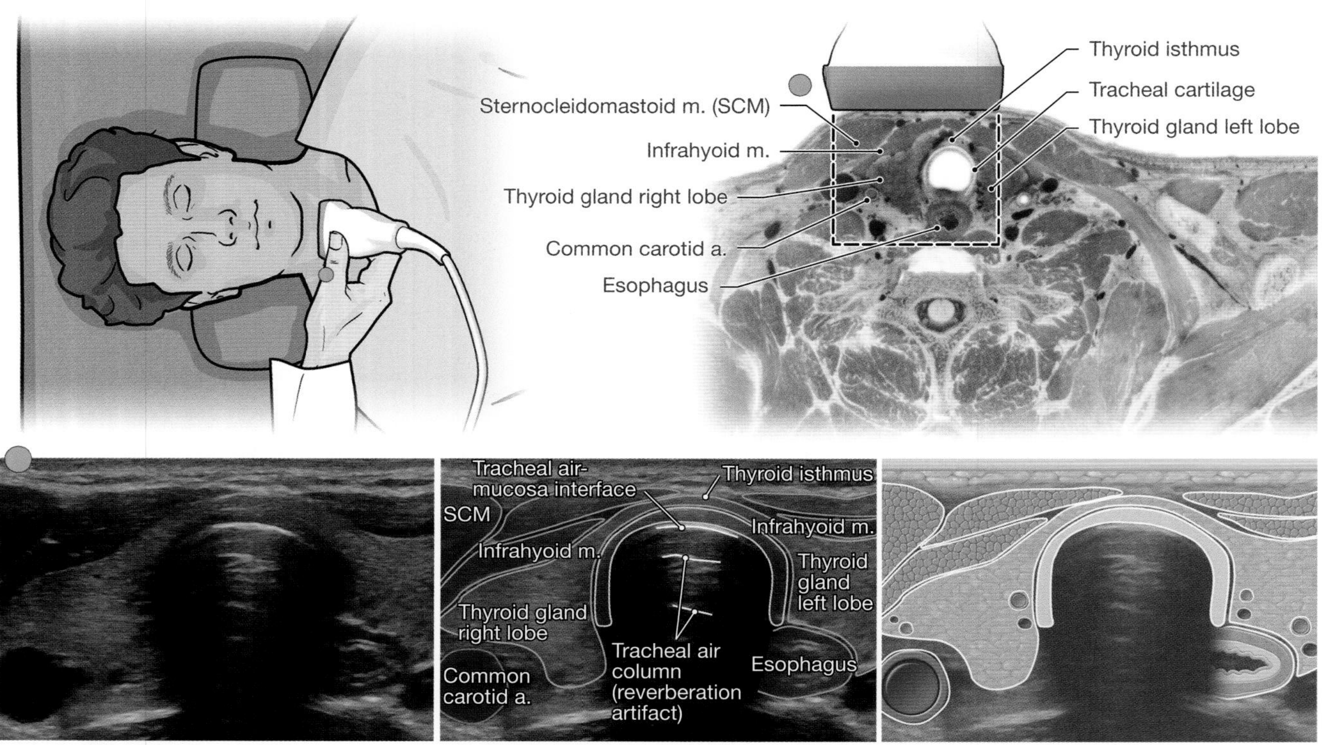

Figure 11.11 Transverse view of the thyroid gland lobes, thyroid isthmus, trachea, esophagus, and strap muscles.

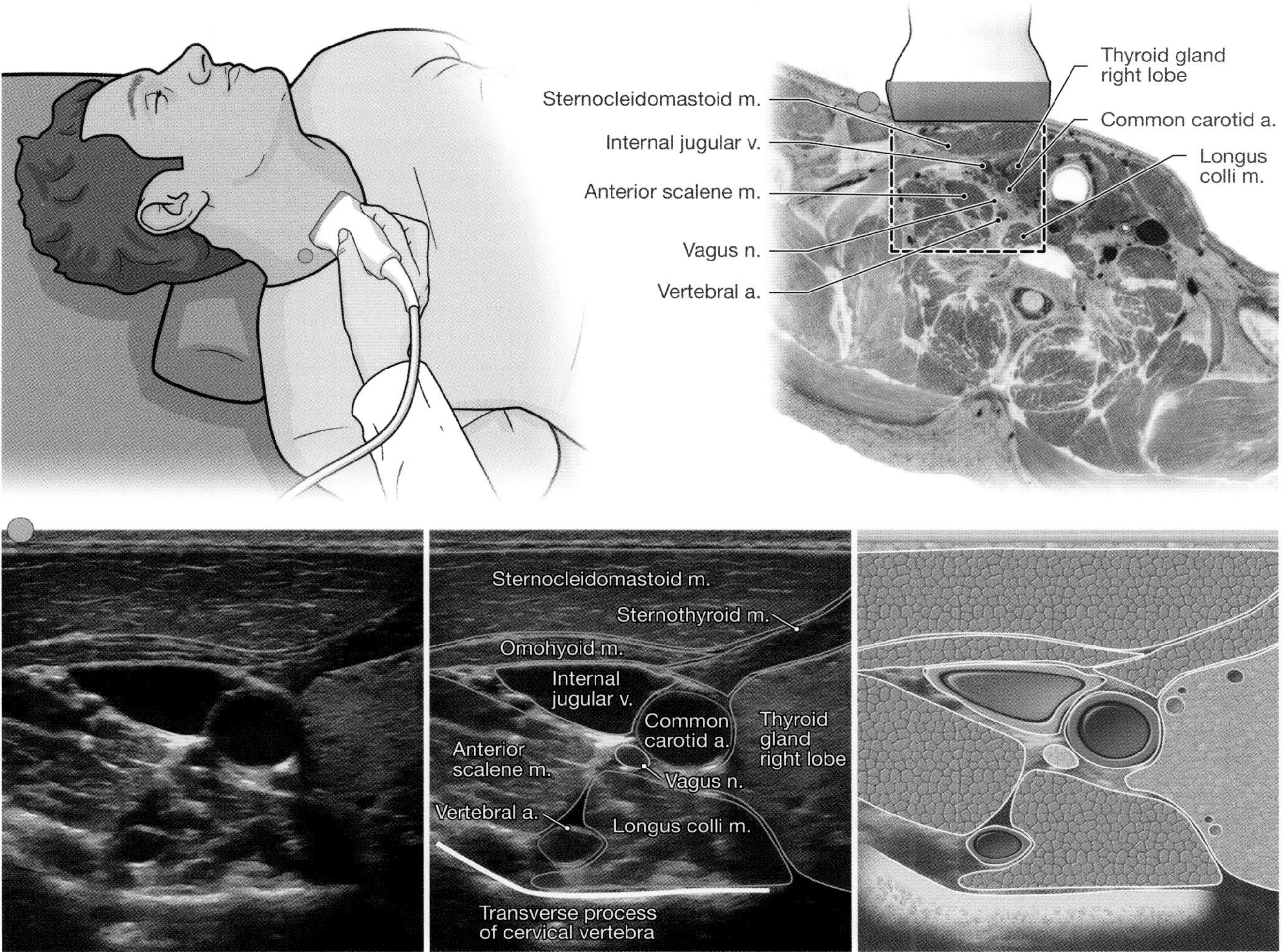

Figure 11.12 Transverse view of the right thyroid lobe, common carotid artery, internal jugular vein, vagus nerve, sternocleidomastoid, sternothyroid, omohyoid, and anterior scalene muscles.

Face

Review of the Anatomy

In general, the face is the region of the anterior head superiorly to the frontal bone, posteriorly to but not including the pinnae and inferiorly to the lower edge of the mandible. Not only are multiple sense organs (eye, nasal, and oral cavities) located here, but also the muscles that uniquely allow humans to communicate emotion (ie, muscles of facial expression). Portions of glands (parotid and lacrimal) and muscles of mastication are also found on the face.

Fasciae/Connective Tissue

The face differs from the rest of the body in that its subcutaneous fat is completely separated from the underlying muscles by investing fascia, which envelops the muscles. This superficial musculoaponeurotic system is a continuous, organized, fibrous network connecting the facial muscles with the dermis in the area of the forehead, parotid, zygomatic, infraorbital, nasolabial fold, and lower lip regions or the so-called facial ligaments. Additional defined fascial/connective tissue layers of the face include the following:

- **Galea aponeurotica:** this flattened tendon of the scalp connects the frontalis and occipitalis muscles and terminates on the zygomatic arch.
- **Deep cervical fascia:** continues cephalically to cover the parotid gland and masseter muscle:
  - *Parotid fascia:* splits into a deep and superficial layer to encapsulate the parotid gland. The deep layer forms a thickening known as the stylomandibular ligament that inserts onto the angle of the mandible. This ligament separates the parotid and submandibular glands. The parotid fascia extends cephalically to the zygomatic arch.
  - *Masseteric fascia:* continuous with the deeper layer of the temporal fascia and, specifically, its deeper lamina that attaches onto the lateral aspect of the zygomatic arch.

Muscles

Although some animals have muscles that move the overlying skin, a human is unique in having a concentration of such muscles under the skin of the face. These muscles are used for conveying facial expressions/emotions and close/open the orifices (eye, nasal, and oral cavities) and are all innervated by the facial nerve. Some of the larger muscles of facial expression are listed in Table 11.1. The last two muscles in the table (temporalis and masseter) are not muscles of facial expression but rather muscles of mastication that have a superficial position on the face. Therefore, they are not innervated by the facial nerve but by the mandibular division of the trigeminal nerve, which innervates all the muscles of mastication.

Vessels

The major arterial blood vessels of the face are derived from the external carotid artery. Smaller branches of the internal carotid artery are also found on the face around the outer orbit. In general, the same named veins travel with these external carotid branches. The following describe the arterial branches:

- **Facial artery:** the facial artery extends from the external carotid artery, through or by the submandibular gland, over the mandible just anterior to the masseter muscle where its pulse is palpable, and terminates as the angular artery traveling toward the medial canthus of the orbit. After crossing the mandible, the facial artery provides several branches:
  - *Inferior labial:* supplies the lower lip
  - *Superior labial:* supplies the upper lip and the nasal septum
  - *Lateral nasal:* supplies the ala and dorsum of the nose
  - *Angular:* supplies the orbicularis oculi and the lacrimal sac
- **Superficial temporal artery:** one of the two terminal branches of the external carotid artery. Provides small branches to the parotid gland and anterior ear and then courses into the scalp as a terminal frontal and parietal branch. Larger branches before this termination include the following:
  - *Transverse facial branch:* travels superficial to the masseter superior to the zygomatic arch. Supplies the parotid gland and the masseter muscle.
  - *Zygomatico-orbital branch:* travels to the lateral angle of the orbit and supplies the orbicularis oculi muscle.
- **Supraorbital artery:** a branch of the ophthalmic artery. On the face, it supplies the regional muscles and anastomoses with the angular artery and frontal branch of the superficial temporal arteries.

TABLE 11.1 Large Muscles of Facial Expression

Muscle	Origin	Insertion	Action
Frontalis	Epicranial aponeurosis	Skin of eyebrows and root of the nose	Horizontally wrinkles the skin of the forehead (ie, raises the eyebrows)
Corrugator supercilii	Medial superciliary arch	Skin over medial eyebrow	Vertically wrinkles the skin between the superciliary arches
Orbicularis oculi	Orbital rim	Skin overlying orbital rim, tarsal plates	Both parts (orbital/palpebral) close the eyelids
Procerus	Fascia of nasal bones and adjacent cartilages	Skin between superciliary arches	Horizontally wrinkles skin over the nasion
Nasalis	Maxillary bone	Ala of nose	Transverse portion constricts ala and alar portion widens the ala
Depressor septi nasi	Incisive fossa of maxillary bone	Ala and septum of nose	Widens nasal aperture
Levator labii superioris alaeque nasi	Frontal process of maxillary bone	Skin of ala and upper lip	Elevates ala and upper lip
Levator labii superioris	Maxillary bone	Skin of upper lip	Elevates upper lip
Zygomaticus minor	Zygomatic bone	Upper lip	Elevates upper lip
Zygomaticus major	Zygomatic bone	Angle of mouth	Elevates upper lip
Orbicularis oris	Maxillary bone	Skin of lips	Closes mouth
Levator anguli oris	Maxillary bone	Angle of mouth	Elevates angle of mouth
Risorius	Masseteric fascia	Angle of mouth	Draws angle of mouth laterally
Depressor anguli oris	Oblique line of mandible	Angle of mouth	Depresses angle of mouth
Depressor labii inferioris	Oblique line of mandible	Skin of lower lip	
Mentalis	Incisive fossa of mandible	Skin of chin	Elevates and protrudes lower lip
Buccinator	Mandible, maxillary bone, and pterygomandibular raphe	Angle of mouth	Tenses skin over cheek and maintains food between occlusal surfaces of the molar teeth
Temporalis	Bones and fascia of the temporal fossa	Coronoid process and distally along anterior ramus to the retromolar triangle of mandible	Retracts and elevates mandible
Masseter	Zygomatic bone and its arch	Angle of mandible	Elevates

- **Supratrochlear artery:** a terminal branch of the ophthalmic artery. Supplies the skin of the medial orbital region.
- **Dorsal nasal artery:** a terminal branch of the ophthalmic artery. Supplies the lacrimal sac and dorsum of the nose.
- **Lacrimal artery:** a branch of the ophthalmic artery. On the face, it supplies the lacrimal gland and the upper eyelid.
  - *Zygomaticofacial artery:* a branch of the lacrimal artery that supplies the skin over the cheek.
  - *Zygomaticotemporal artery:* a branch of the lacrimal artery that supplies the skin over the temporal fossa (ie, lateral forehead anterior to the hairline).
- **Infraorbital artery:** a branch of the maxillary artery that on the face supplies the skin and the associated muscles in the infraorbital, lateral nasal, and superior labial regions.
- **Buccal artery:** a branch of the maxillary artery that supplies the buccinator muscles and the skin and mucous membrane of the cheek.
- **Mental artery:** a branch of the inferior alveolar artery, which is a branch of the maxillary artery. It exits the mental foramen to supply adjacent skin and soft tissues.
- **Lymphatic vessels/nodes:** in general, lymphatic drainage from the conjunctiva, eyelids, central forehead, and lateral cheek pass to the anterior auricular and superficial and deep parotid nodes. Drainage from the external nose, cheeks, upper lip, and lateral parts of the lower lip drain directly into the submandibular lymph nodes. The central lower lip and chin drain into the submental nodes.
- **Facial vein**
  - *Deep facial branch:* this branch travels deeply and connects to the pterygoid venous plexus, which then has intracranial connections.
  - *Retromandibular:* this vessel is formed within the parotid gland at the posterior border of the ramus of the mandible by the maxillary and superficial temporal veins. Inferiorly, it has an anterior and a posterior division. The anterior division contributes to the common facial vein as does the facial vein to then enter the internal jugular vein. The posterior division joins with the posterior auricular vein to form the external jugular vein.

Nerves

Cutaneous Nerves

The cutaneous nerves of the face are primarily derived from the trigeminal nerve and branches from all three its divisions (ophthalmic, maxillary, and mandibular). These divisions are also abbreviated as V1, V2, and V3, respectively. A small area over the angle of the mandible is supplied by the branches of the cervical plexus.

- **Ophthalmic nerve (V1)**
  - *Supraorbital nerve:* this branch supplies branches to the upper eyelid and then distributes to the skin of the forehead posteriorly to the vertex of the skull.
  - *Supratrochlear nerve:* this nerve provides branches to the upper eyelid and the adjacent skin of the central forehead.
  - ***Infratrochlear nerve:*** supplies the skin of the eyelids and lateral nose.
  - *Lacrimal nerve:* after supplying the lacrimal gland, it is distributed to the upper eyelid.
  - *External nasal nerve:* an extension of the anterior ethmoidal nerve that supplies the skin over the lower half of the nose.
- **Maxillary nerve (V2)**
  - *Infraorbital nerve:* supplies the lower eyelid, the upper lip, and the lateral nose.
  - *Zygomaticofacial nerve:* supplies the skin over the prominence of the cheek.
  - *Zygomaticotemporal nerve:* supplies the anterior aspect of the temporal region (ie, lateral region of the forehead).
- **Mandibular nerve (V3)**
  - *Mental nerve:* supplies the skin over the chin and the lower lip.
  - *Buccal nerve:* supplies the skin overlying the buccinator muscle as well as the buccal gingival and adjacent mucosa.
  - *Auriculotemporal nerve:* supplies the skin of the temporal region and carries postganglionic parasympathetic "hitchhiking" fibers from the otic ganglion that leave the auriculotemporal nerve and travel to the parotid gland. Fibers are also found traveling to the anterior pinnae and the temporomandibular joint.
- **Great auricular nerve:** derived from fibers of C2 and C3 from the cervical plexus and is primarily distributed to the skin over the parotid gland and the ear lobe. In addition, some fibers supply the skin over the angle of the mandible.

Motor Nerves

Classically, all but two muscles of the face receive their innervation via the facial nerve, although the trigeminal nerve innervates the temporalis and masseter muscles found superficially on the face.

- **Facial nerve:** At the skull base, the facial nerve leaves the stylomastoid foramen and travels medially toward the face. This nerve travels through the parotid gland and forms an upper **temporofacial** and lower **cervicofacial** division. Five branches emanate from these divisions and supply the muscles of facial expression. These branches coalesce as they approach the muscles of facial expression forming the so-called **pes anserine.**

- *Temporal branches:* innervate the frontalis, orbicularis oculi, and corrugator supercilii muscles.
- *Zygomatic branches:* innervate the orbicularis oculi and zygomaticus major muscles.
- *Buccal branches:* innervate the procerus, levator labii superioris alaeque nasi, levator labii superioris, levator anguli oris, zygomaticus minor (when present), zygomaticus major, buccinator, risorius, levator anguli oris, orbicularis oris, nasalis, and depressor anguli oris.
- *Marginal mandibular branches:* cross superficially to the facial vessels over the mandible and innervate the depressor anguli oris, depressor labii inferioris, mentalis, and orbicularis oris.
- *Cervical branch:* innervates the platysma muscle.

- **Trigeminal nerve: mandibular nerve (V3)**
  - *Masseteric nerve:* supplies the masseter muscle and temporomandibular joint.
  - *Deep temporal nerves:* Two to three in number supply the overlying temporalis muscle.
- **Sympathetics**
  - *External carotid plexus:* These postganglionic sympathetic fibers derived from the superior cervical ganglion of the sympathetic trunk within the neck travel along branches of the external carotid artery that are destined for the face (eg, facial and superficial temporal arteries). These fibers are vasoconstrictive, secretory, and pilomotor in nature.

Viscera

The viscera of the face include the parotid and lacrimal glands, external aspect of the eyeball, and opening to the oral cavity.

- **Parotid gland:** This is the largest of the salivary glands and is situated anterior to the ear and inferior to the zygomatic arch and dips inferior to the level of the mandible at the retromandibular fossa. It is invested with a dense fibrous capsule, the parotid sheath. The course of the facial nerve through the parotid gland artificially divides the parotid gland into superficial and deep parts. This gland receives its innervation from postganglionic fibers derived from the glossopharyngeal nerve (ninth cranial nerve) that have synapsed in the otic ganglion and then have traveled along the auriculotemporal nerve, which is a branch of the mandibular division (V3) of the trigeminal nerve. The parotid gland contains a parotid duct (Stensen duct) that travels inferior to the zygomatic arch and then empties into the vestibule of the mouth, between the cheek and the upper second molar tooth. An accessory parotid gland (socia parotitis) may be seen extending medially along the parotid duct, which enters the oral cavity adjacent to the upper second molar tooth after piercing the buccinator muscle. Regionally, the buccal fat pad is seen and separates the masseter from the buccinator muscles. The loss of or absence of this pad results in dimpling of the skin of the cheek.
- **Lacrimal gland:** This is the tear-secreting gland of the body located in the superolateral aspect of the orbit. The superficial aspect of this gland is seen from the facial perspective. The superficial and deep portions of the lacrimal gland are separated by the tendon of the levator palpebrae superioris muscle. Innervation to the lacrimal gland is derived from the facial nerve. Postganglionic fibers leave the pterygopalatine ganglion and travel with branches of the maxillary and ophthalmic divisions of the trigeminal nerve to terminate onto the lacrimal gland.
- **Eye:** The external aspect of the eyeball is seen on the face as the cornea, sclera, and overlying bulbar conjunctiva.
- **Lips:** These extensions of the oral cavity are composed primarily of skin, muscles, mucosa, interposed vessels and nerves, and minor salivary glands. The **vermillion border** is the demarcation between the reddened vascular edge of the lips and adjacent skin.

Technique

PAROTID GLAND SALIVARY GLAND
Transverse
FIG. 11.13

Place the patient in a supine position with the neck extended over a small bolster. Turn the head of the patient to the side opposite the one being examined. Orient the probe transversely under the ear lobe. Place the anterior edge of the probe over the mandible (acoustic shadow), masseter (typical hypoechoic muscle appearance with hyperechoic connective tissue bands), and the posterior edge over the sternocleidomastoid muscle. Tilt/fan the probe for the best image of parotid gland tissue that appears as fine grain, slightly hyperechoic. Because the parotid gland tends to attenuate US energy, it is often not possible to observe its deep surface. However, the external carotid artery and the retromandibular vein can often be seen at the deep aspect of the parotid gland.

CLINICAL APPLICATIONS

US imaging of the parotid gland is mainly performed when there is a parotid gland swelling. Inflammatory diseases are the most common diseases affecting the salivary glands. In acute inflammation, salivary glands are enlarged and hypoechoic. Viral salivary gland infections are the most common in children. **Parotitis** is a viral infection (mumps) of the parotid gland, which results in glandular swelling. Glandular swelling stretches the capsule and the fascia of the parotid gland resulting in considerable pain.

Benign neoplasms such as **pleomorphic adenomas** (mixed tumor) and Warthin tumors (adenolymphoma, cystadeno lymphoma, and papillary cystadenoma lymphomatosum) are slowly growing, painless masses of the parotid gland. The most common malignant neoplasms occurring are mucoepidermoid carcinoma and adenoid cystic carcinoma. Salivary glands may also be affected by lymphoma as a painless, progressive swelling. They are usually associated with autoimmune disease, most often Sjögren syndrome. Patients who are HIV-positive often have sialolithiasis and swelling of the parotid glands.

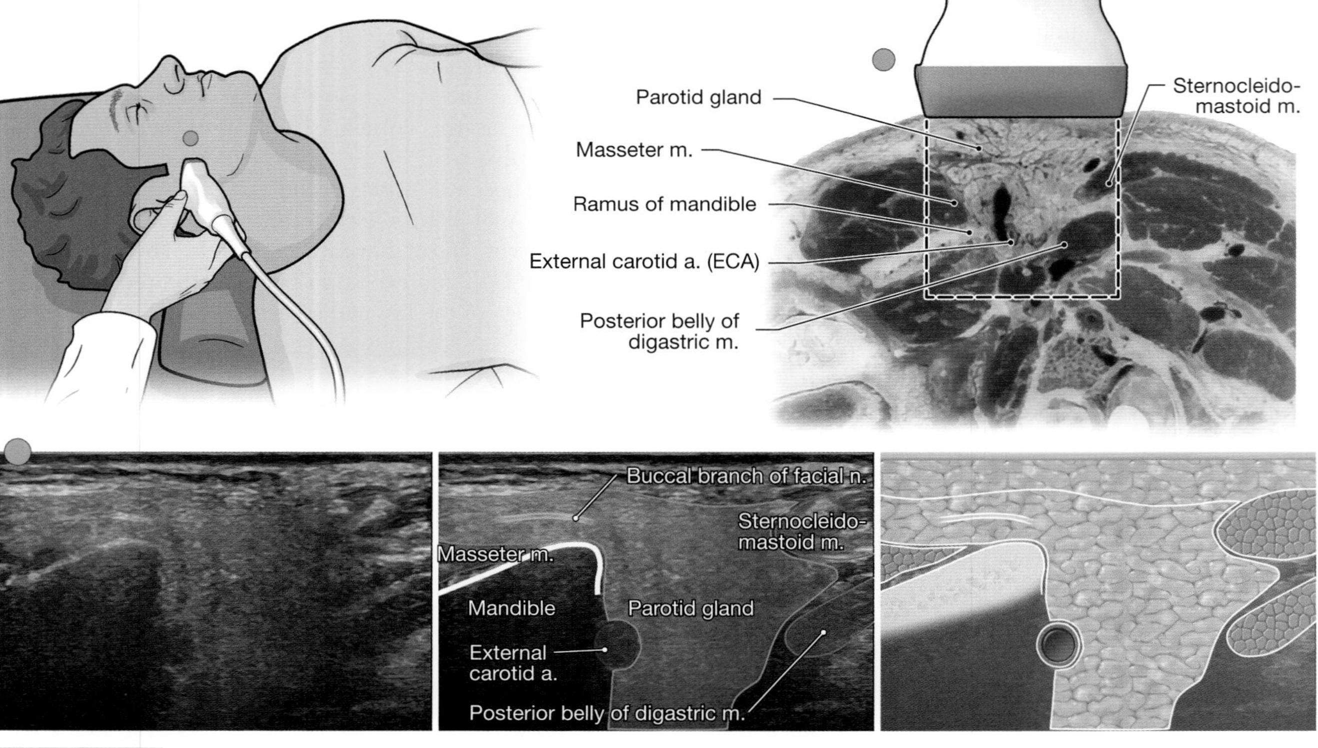

Figure 11.13 Transverse view of the parotid salivary gland, masseter, and mandible.

Eye and Orbit

Review of the Anatomy

The eyeball (globe) is located anteriorly in the bony orbit, covered anteriorly by the eyelids. Most of the remainder of the orbit is occupied by orbital fat. The numerous nerves and vessels serving the eye, eyelids, and face around the orbit, plus the extraocular muscles that move the eye, all traverse the orbital fat to reach the eye or other targets within and around the orbit.

The deep surfaces of the eyelids are covered by **conjunctiva**, which then reflects over the **sclera** (the white outer layer of the eye), and attaches along the corneoscleral junction. The conjunctiva forms a sac when the eyelids are closed, which contains a thin layer of lacrimal gland secretions.

The wall of the eyeball consists of three layers. The outer fibrous layer is made up mainly by the sclera, plus the (normally) transparent cornea anteriorly. The middle vascular layer consists of the choroid posteriorly, which is continuous with the ciliary body and iris anteriorly. The ciliary body, which extends anteriorly from the choroid, is a circumferential triangular elevation consisting of ciliary muscles, ciliary processes, and ciliary epithelium. The pigmented iris extends anteriorly from the ciliary body over the anterior surface of the lens with a central opening, the pupil. The inner layer consists of the visual (neural) retina posteriorly and the nonvisual retina anteriorly. The choroid layer is attached to the retina internally and the sclera externally.

The **lens**, a normally transparent biconvex disc, is suspended behind the iris via a circumferential system of zonular fibers attached to the lens capsule centrally and projections (ciliary processes) from the ciliary body peripherally. Collectively, the zonular fibers make up the suspensory ligament of the lens.

The interior of the eye is described as containing three chambers: the anterior chamber, the posterior chamber, and the vitreous chamber. The anterior chamber is located between the posterior (inner) surface of the cornea anteriorly and the anterior surfaces of the iris and lens posteriorly. The small posterior chamber is located between the posterior surface of the iris and the anterior surface of the lens. The anterior and posterior chambers contain aqueous humor. **Aqueous humor** is secreted from the ciliary epithelium into the posterior chamber and flows into the anterior chamber through the pupil. The vitreous chamber, occupied by the gelatinous vitreous humor, is located in the remainder of the globe between the posterior surface of the lens anteriorly and the retina posteriorly.

The central processes of the retinal ganglion cells converge at the optic disc to form the optic nerve (CN II), which exits the posteromedial aspect of the eye and traverses the orbital fat to exit the orbit posteriorly via the optic canal. The optic nerve is surrounded by a sheath consisting of all three meningeal layers: dura, subarachnoid, and pia. The subarachnoid space of the optic nerve sheath is continuous with the intracranial subarachnoid space.

Technique

EYE AND OPTIC NERVE
Transverse
FIG. 11.14

A high-resolution linear array US transducer should be selected for examination of the eye and optic nerve. The patient should be in a supine position and the examination is performed with the eyes closed. A generous amount of standard water-soluble US gel should be applied to the closed eyelids so that the probe face stands off from contact with the eyelids

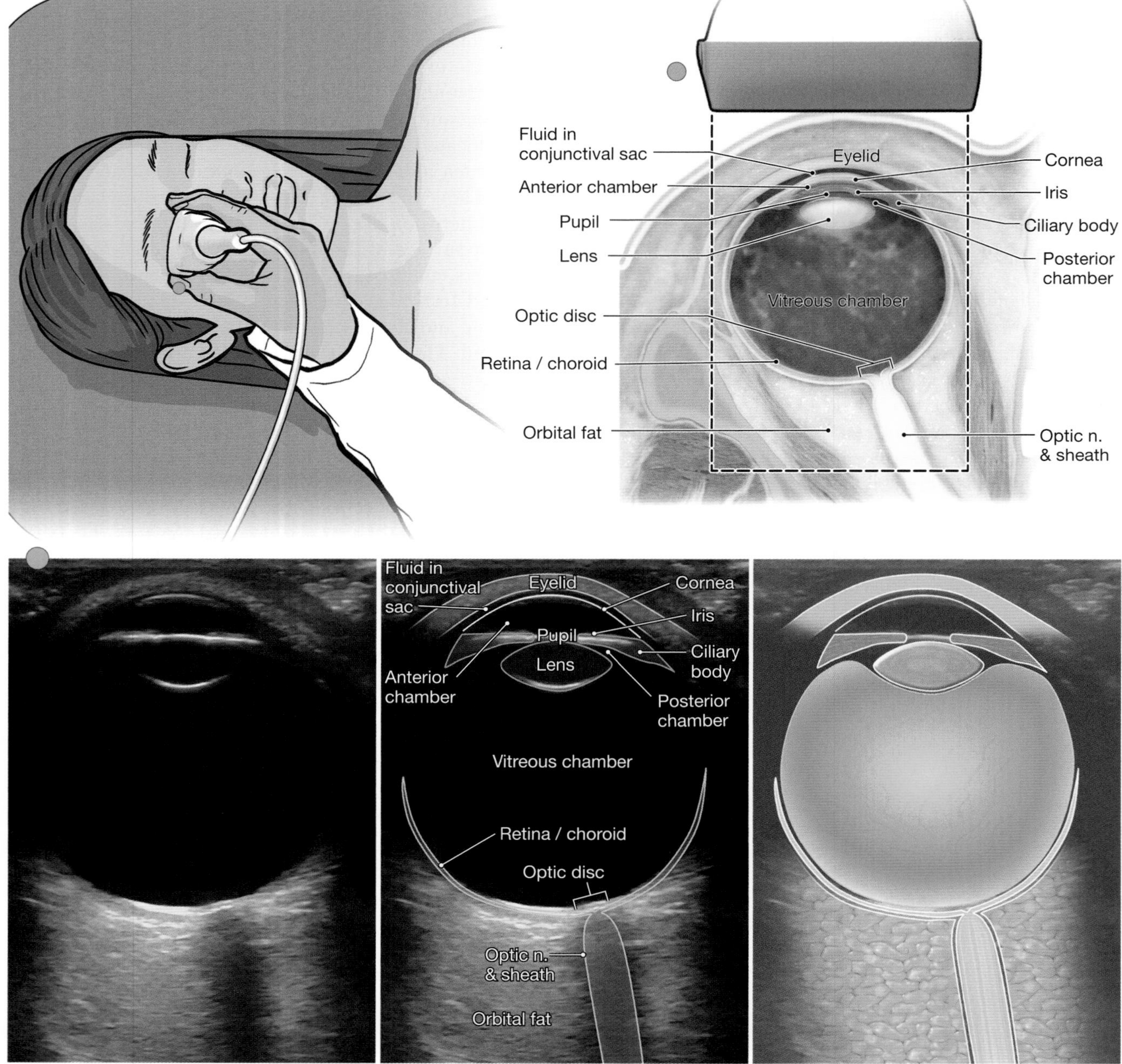

Figure 11.14 Transverse view of the orbital contents, including the eye, optic nerve, and orbital fat.

and minimal pressure is applied to the eye through the probe face. In some patients, the use of sterile US gel may be indicated (the presence of cuts or lacerations of the eyelids, for example) and additionally, a sterile occlusive dressing can be placed over the closed eyelids before applying gel.

OPTIC NERVE AND SHEATH
Transverse
FIG. 11.15

The patient's eyes should be closed. Ask the patient to look straight ahead. Place the probe transversely over the eyelids/eye with the probe marker side directed to the right. Adjust the scan depth so that the entire globe and anterior 1 to 1.5 cm of orbital fat behind the globe are visible in the image. Carefully adjust the probe position and tilt as needed (remind the patient to look straight ahead) to identify, from anterior to posterior, the eyelid, the thin anechoic stripe of fluid in the conjunctival sac, the hyperechoic curving surface of the cornea parallel to the eyelid, the iris and the pupil, the hyperechoic anterior and posterior reflections of the lens capsule (along with the normally anechoic lens between), and the ciliary body extending posteriorly from the iris. Identify the anechoic aqueous humor within the anterior and posterior chambers and the anechoic vitreous humor within the vitreous chamber. The retinal and choroid layers cannot be resolved separately with US examination, appearing as a thin hypoechoic stripe lining the interior of the globe just outside the vitreous chamber (there is often a hyperechoic line at the inner surface of the retina where it is perpendicular to the US beam). Adjust the probe position and tilt as needed until the hypoechoic optic nerve can be seen exiting the globe posteriorly.

To best visualize the optic nerve along with the optic nerve sheath, place the probe transversely over the upper eyelid of the closed eye to be examined with the probe marker directed laterally. Slide the probe up and down a

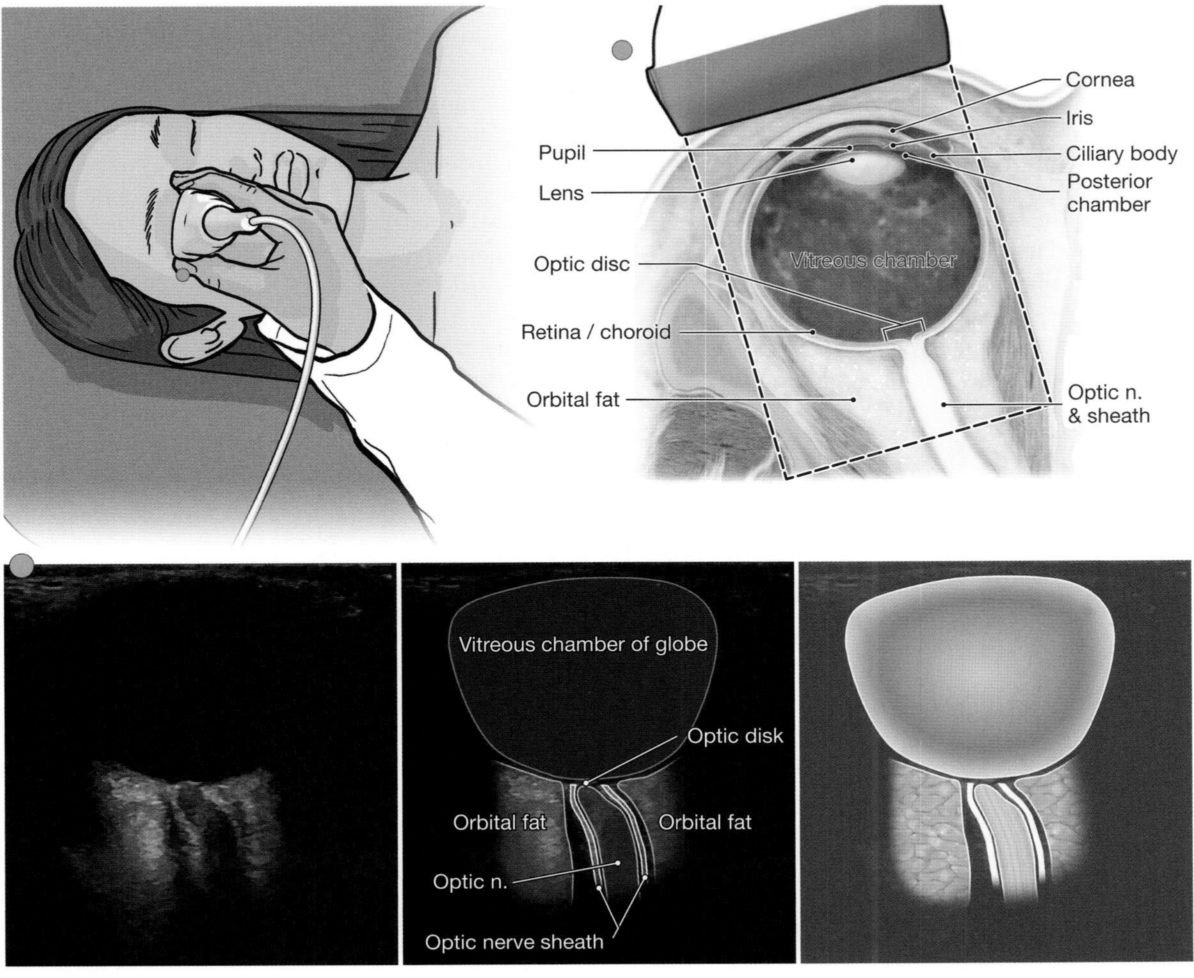

Figure 11.15 Transverse view of the optic nerve and optic nerve sheath.

very short distance until the hypoechoic optic nerve can be identified exiting the globe posteriorly. Carefully rock the probe face "heel to toe" (marker side to non-marker side) until the hyperechoic optic nerve sheath can be seen on both sides of the optic nerve at least 5 or 6 mm posterior to the optic disc. The optic nerve sheath is sometimes described as having a "stack of coins" appearance with alternating hyperechoic and hypoechoic lines. Variable hypoechoic areas are commonly seen just outside the nerve sheath—these are edge-shadowing artifacts. The optic disc most commonly appears as a small (less than 1 mm) central elevation toward the vitreous chamber where the optic nerve exits the globe. For evaluation of possible optic nerve swelling as the result of increased intracranial pressure, the optic nerve sheath diameter (ONSD) is measured 3 mm posterior to the optic disc, from the outer edge of the sheath to the outer edge of sheath.

IRIS AND PUPIL
Coronal
FIG. 11.16

To observe the consensual light reflex, place the probe against the zygomatic bone/inferior margin of the orbit with the probe face just in contact with the lower eyelid while aiming the US beam up toward the superior margin of the orbit (marker directed laterally). A generous amount of gel is often helpful in obtaining a good image. Carefully tilt/fan the probe until the iris and pupil can be well seen. While maintaining the image of the iris and pupil, ask an assistant to shine a light into the contralateral eye and look for consensual pupillary constriction.

CLINICAL APPLICATIONS

US examination of the eye is commonly used in emergency departments for examination of structures of the eye in patients with traumatic injuries involving the orbit/eye. US examination is contraindicated when rupture of the globe is clinically suspected, as any pressure applied to the ruptured eye can result in further extrusion of eye contents/humors.

US can be used to examine the eye when direct examination and funduscopy are not possible because of eyelid edema or hematoma or hemorrhage in the anterior chamber (hyphema). US examination of the eye can be used for detecting globe wall perforation, intraocular foreign bodies, lens dislocation/subluxation, cataracts, vitreous hemorrhage, retinal detachment, hyaloid/vitreous detachment, and choroidal detachments. There are also US techniques for testing the pupillary light reflex when the pupil cannot be directly examined.

US measurement of the optic nerve/ONSD is used when elevated intracranial pressure is suspected, such as in patients with head injuries, altered consciousness, or possible intracranial hemorrhage. Swelling/enlargement of the optic nerve and its sheath has been shown to develop earlier in the course of elevated intracranial pressure than swelling of the optic disc/papilledema. Papilledema can also be seen in US images as an increased prominence of the optic disc protruding toward the vitreous chamber as the disc swells. Normally, the optic disc is relatively flat with a very small central elevation of the disc toward the vitreous chamber. US examination is also used in the evaluation of the posterior wall (retinal/choroidal) or optic nerve sheath masses such as primary benign or malignant tumors or metastases.

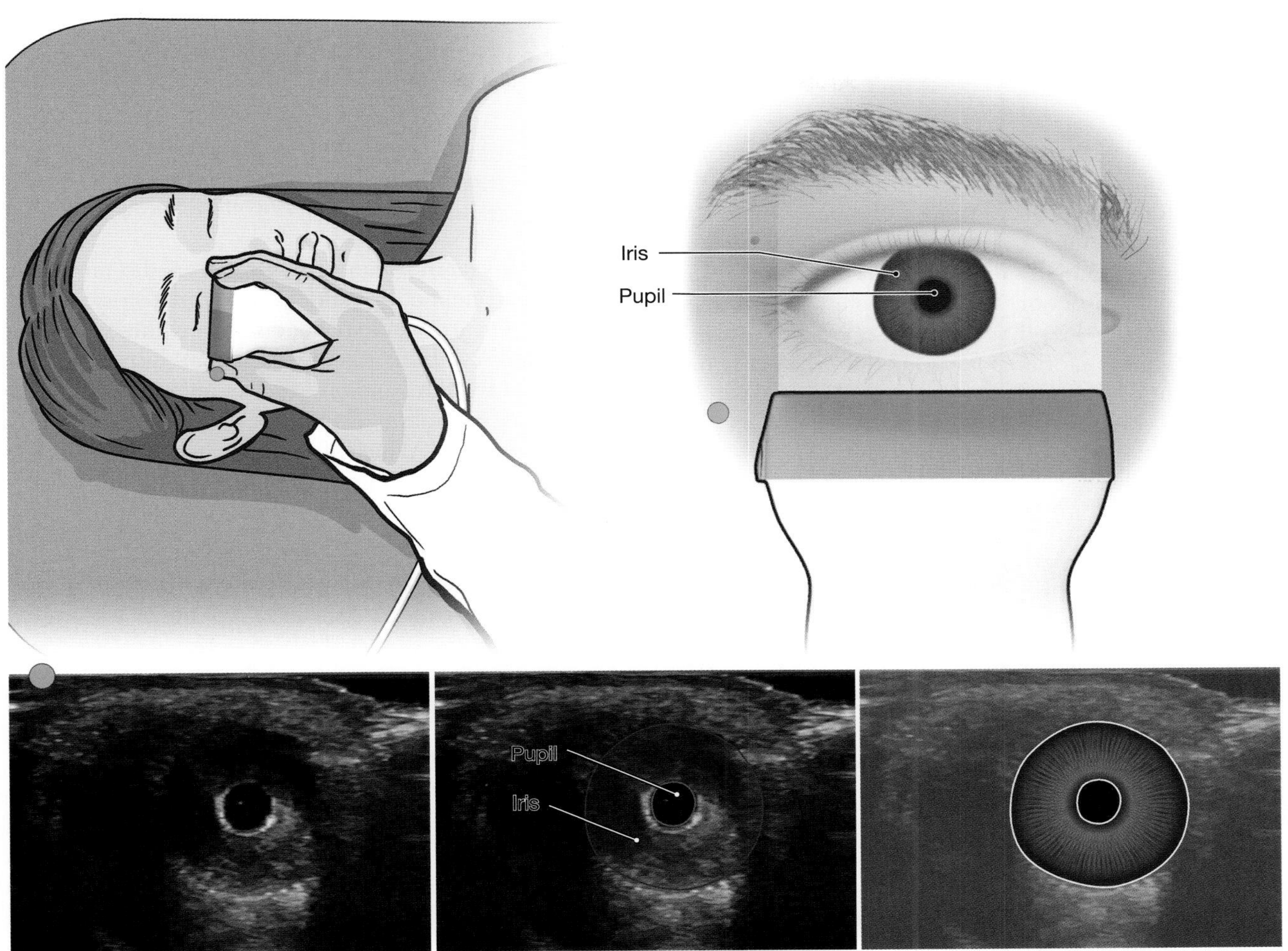

Figure 11.16 Coronal view of the iris and pupil.

11 Neck, Face, and Eye

Multiple Choice Questions

1. A 55-year-old woman comes to the physician because of a 6-month history of progressive swelling on the left side of her face. Physical examination shows a painless swelling over the parotid gland, and an ultrasound-guided needle biopsy shows a malignant parotid tumor. A parotidectomy is performed. Postoperatively, physical examination shows weakness at the inferior portion of the orbicularis oris. Which of the following nerves was most likely injured?

   A. Mandibular division of the trigeminal
   B. Marginal mandibular branch of facial
   C. Zygomatic branch of facial
   D. Buccal branch of facial
   E. Buccal nerve

2. A 45-year-old woman comes to the physician because of a 6-month history of progressive swelling of the anterior portion of her neck. Physical examination shows an enlarged thyroid gland. An ultrasound-guided needle biopsy of the thyroid gland shows a benign tumor measuring 3 × 6 cm. A partial thyroidectomy is performed. Postoperatively, physical examination shows hoarseness and difficulty breathing on exertion. Which of the following nerves was most likely injured during the thyroidectomy?

   A. Internal branch of superior laryngeal
   B. External branch of superior laryngeal
   C. Recurrent laryngeal
   D. Ansa cervicalis
   E. Vagus

3. A 68-year-old man is brought to the emergency department because of a 2-day history of feeling dizzy and falling. His pulse is 110/min, blood pressure is 190/110 mm Hg, and respirations are 21/min. Physical examination shows carotid bruits bilaterally. An ultrasound Doppler examination shows 90% occlusion in both the common carotid arteries proximal to their division into external and internal carotid arteries. A stent is placed in both the common carotid arteries, and the flow is restored bilaterally. Postoperatively, physical examination shows that his tongue is deviated to the right when he is asked to protrude it. Which of the following nerves was most likely injured during the procedure?

   A. Right lingual
   B. Right hypoglossal
   C. Left hypoglossal
   D. Right glossopharyngeal
   E. Right vagus

4. A 59-year-old man was brought to the emergency department after falling from a three-story scaffolding. On arrival, the patient is unconscious with a fractured jaw, broken teeth, facial lacerations, an open tibial fracture, and on hypovolemic shock. An emergency central venous line is inserted into the internal jugular vein. Which of the following is a reliable landmark during ultrasound guide to access this vein?

   A. The interval between the sternal and clavicular heads of the sternocleidomastoid muscle
   B. The lateral border of the sternocleidomastoid muscle
   C. Midclavicular line
   D. Parasternal line
   E. Jugular notch

5. A 45-year-old woman comes to the physician because of a 6-month history of progressive swelling of the anterior portion of her neck. Physical examination shows an enlarged thyroid gland. An ultrasound-guided needle biopsy of the thyroid gland shows a benign tumor measuring 3 × 6 cm. A partial thyroidectomy is performed. Postoperatively, physical examination shows hoarseness and difficulty breathing on exertion. Which of the following vessels accompany the nerve injured during the thyroidectomy procedure?

   A. Inferior thyroid artery
   B. Inferior and superior thyroid arteries
   C. Superior thyroid artery and vein
   D. Superior and middle thyroid veins
   E. Superior, middle, and inferior thyroid veins

6. A 55-year-old man is brought to the emergency department 45 minutes after being involved in a motor vehicle collision. He is in hypovolemic shock. Physical examination shows an unconscious man with multiple lacerations on his face and blood within the oral cavity. An emergency airway is established with a cricothyroidotomy, and a central venous line is inserted in the subclavian vein via a supraclavicular approach. An artery is injured during the cricothyroidotomy procedure, causing a delay in establishing the airway. Which of the following arteries was most likely injured?

A. Inferior thyroid
B. A branch from the costocervical trunk
C. Transverse cervical
D. Cricothyroid
E. Superior laryngeal

7. A 40-year-old man comes to the emergency department because of a 2-month history of a progressive swelling on the right side of his face underneath the mandible. Physical examination shows a hard, nontender mass in the right submandibular region. An ultrasound-guided biopsy of the mass shows a mucoepidermoid carcinoma of the submandibular gland. A submandibulectomy is performed removing the gland and its duct. Which of the following nerves need to be identified and preserved during the procedure?

A. Nerve to mylohyoid
B. Lingual
C. Inferior alveolar
D. Buccal
E. Glossopharyngeal

8. A 55-year-old man comes to the emergency department because of difficulty breathing for the past 2 hours. Physical examination shows a swollen tongue protruding from his mouth. The patient's oxygen saturation does not improve with bag-mask ventilation. Intubation is unsuccessful because of massive soft-tissue edema of his larynx. A decision is made to perform cricothyrotomy. An ultrasound is placed at the area of the neck to perform an incision. At which of the following locations will an incision be most likely made?

A. The cricothyroid membrane, which is located at the junction of the clavicle and the sternum
B. The cricothyroid membrane, which is located between the thyroid cartilage and the cricoid cartilage below
C. The thyrohyoid membrane, which is located between the thyroid cartilage (Adam's apple) and the hyoid bone above
D. The sternal notch, which is located at the junction of the clavicle and the sternum
E. The trachea, which is located below the cricoid cartilage

9. A 15-year-old boy is brought to the physician by his parents because of fever and a sore throat for the past 7 days. He has a history of a genetic immunodeficiency with recurrent tonsillitis. Physical examination shows enlarged erythematous palatine tonsils with petechiae and pus. Which of the following lymph nodes is most likely to become visibly enlarged first during ultrasound examination of this patient?

A. Submandibular
B. Parotid
C. Jugulodigastric
D. Submental
E. Retropharyngeal

10. A 65-year-old woman comes to the physician because of a scheduled biopsy of a growth she has had on her lower lip for the past 6 months. The patient has smoked 1 pack of cigarettes daily for 30 years and lost 9 kg (20 lb) over the last 2 months. A biopsy of her lower lip shows a squamous cell carcinoma. The patient is evaluated for surgical excision with lip reconstruction. If the cancer was to metastasize, which of the following lymph nodes during ultrasound examination will most likely be involved first?

A. Occipital
B. Parotid
C. Retropharyngeal
D. Jugulodigastric
E. Submental

12

Focused Assessment With Sonography for Trauma (FAST)

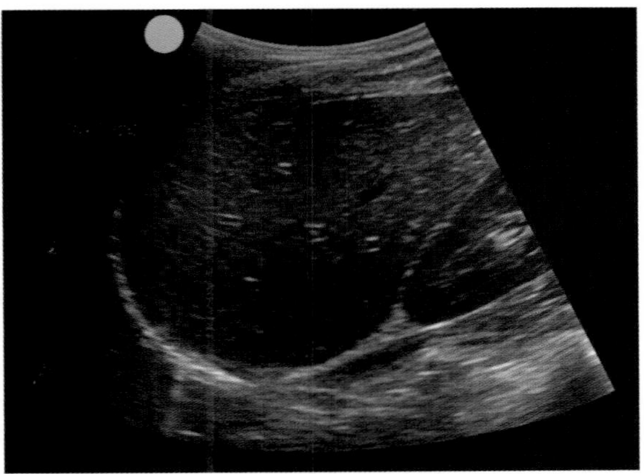

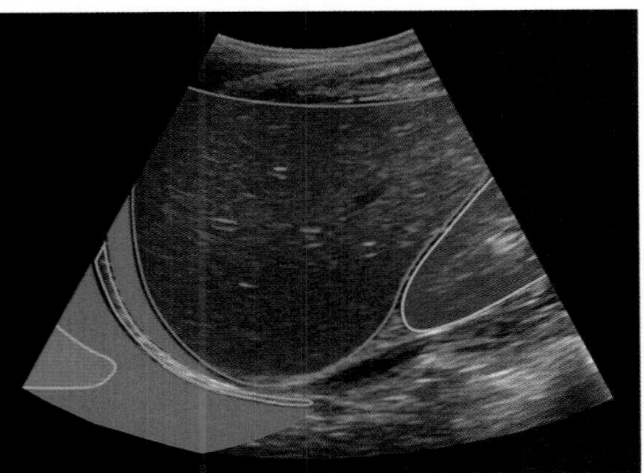

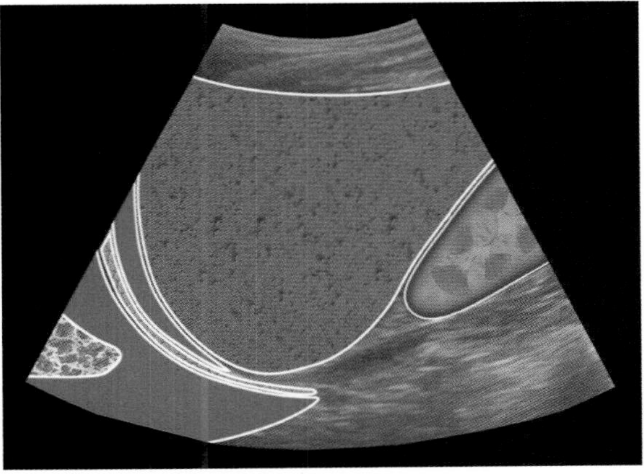

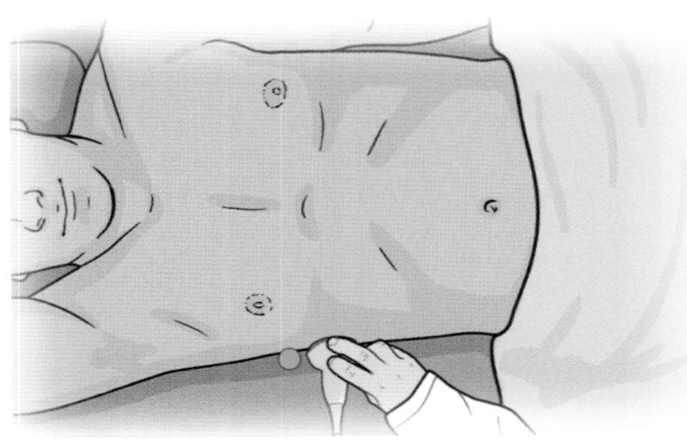

Overview of Focused Assessment With Sonography for Trauma

Focused assessment with sonography for trauma (FAST) is used in the setting of blunt or penetrating thoracoabdominal trauma to detect the presence of free fluid (presumed to be blood in trauma patients until proven otherwise) in the pericardial space, the pleural spaces, the right and left upper quadrants of the abdomen, and the pelvis. In the extended FAST (eFAST) examination, the lung fields are additionally examined for the presence of pneumothorax. The FAST (or eFAST) examination is noninvasive and performed at the bedside in the emergency department (ED). Patients can be continuously monitored and treated in the ED because their transport is not required, and negative or equivocal examinations can be repeated as patient hemodynamic status changes. Although organ injuries such as liver lacerations or splenic fractures can sometimes be seen during the FAST examination, it is neither intended for this purpose and nor is a sensitive method for detecting organ/soft tissue injury. The FAST examination is accurate and sensitive for its intended purpose that is, detecting free fluid in the previously listed anatomical locations.

Patient Positioning

In the ED, patients presenting with thoracoabdominal trauma are commonly placed in the supine position for observation, monitoring, and treatment. **Trendelenburg positioning** (tilting the bed 15-30° such that the head is lower than the feet) increases intraperitoneal fluid pooling in the upper quadrants, increasing the sensitivity of the FAST examination in these locations. Reverse Trendelenburg positioning (tilting the bed such that the feet are lower than the head) increases fluid pooling in the lower parts of the pleural spaces (**costodiaphragmatic recesses**) and in the pelvis, increasing the sensitivity of the examination in these sites.

Probe Selection

For the FAST examination, either a microconvex phased array (cardiac) probe or a curved array (abdominal) probe should be selected.

Review of the Anatomy

The anatomy and scanning techniques for the FAST examination are the same anatomy and techniques used for ultrasound (US) scanning of the heart (subxiphoid 4-chamber or parasternal long-axis views), the right and left upper quadrants of the abdomen, and suprapubic views of the pelvis. The additional knowledge and skills required for the FAST examination are the ability to recognize the appearance of free fluid (anechoic) and understanding the sites where free fluid commonly accumulates relative to the main structures in each of these locations.

Right Upper Quadrant

Technique

RIGHT UPPER QUADRANT
Longitudinal (Intercostal Oblique)
FIG. 12.1

If the patient can cooperate, the palm of the right hand should be placed behind the head, abducting the arm and helping to open up the intercostal spaces on the right. The probe should be placed along the mid-axillary line at about the horizontal level of the xiphisternal junction with the probe marker directed superiorly. The probe face should be rotated until it is parallel to the intercostal spaces (the intercostal oblique orientation), which minimizes rib shadowing over the structures of interest and brings the probe into closer alignment with the typical orientation of the right kidney. Identify the speckled appearance of the liver and the hyperechoic stripe representing the diaphragm over the curving superior surface of the liver. The probe face should be tilted posteriorly until the interface between the visceral surface of the liver and the right kidney comes into view. The potential space at the hepatorenal recess is commonly referred to as **Morison pouch**. This is the most dependent site in the peritoneal space above the transverse mesocolon and so is a common location for free fluid accumulation in the upper abdomen. The hepatorenal recess should be carefully and completely scanned for any anechoic fluid collections.

RIGHT UPPER QUADRANT
Longitudinal (Intercostal Oblique)
FIG. 12.2

Next, slide the probe superiorly (one or two intercostal spaces) until the superior surface of the liver, the diaphragm, and the lower part of the right hemithorax can be seen in the image. In the presence of normally aerated lung, the hyperechoic diaphragm creates a mirror image **artifact** over the inferior extent of the right lung such that

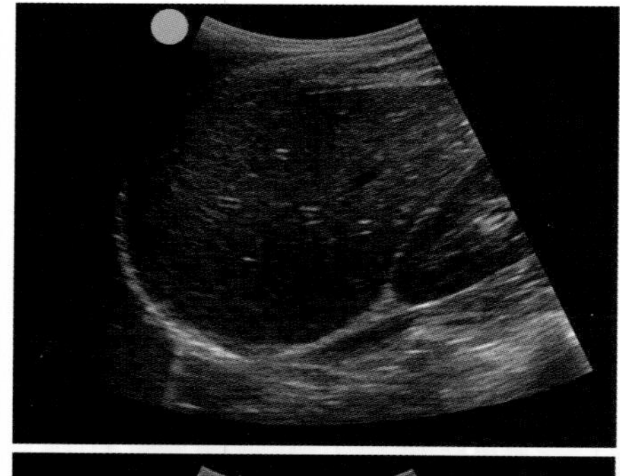

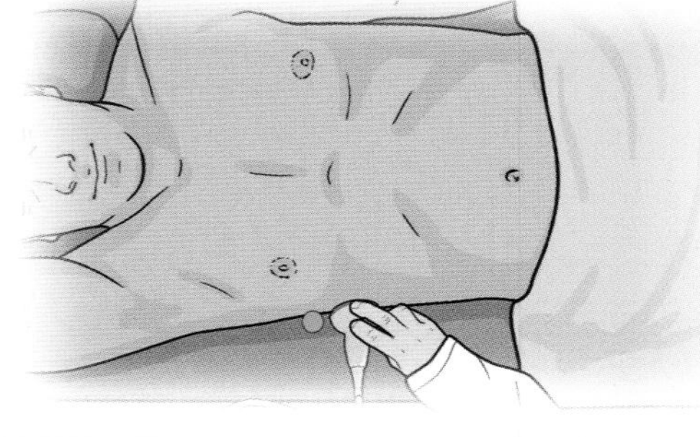

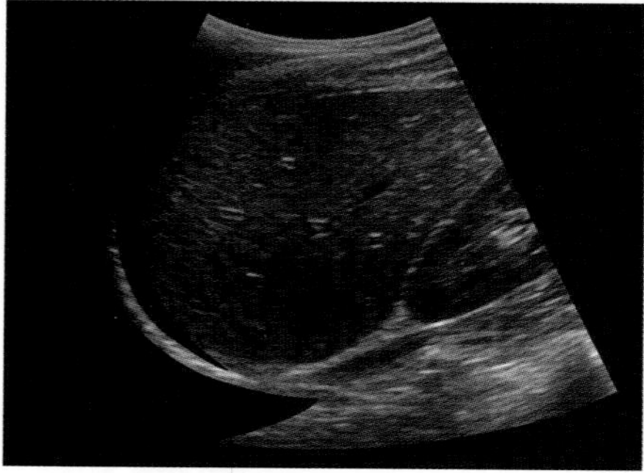

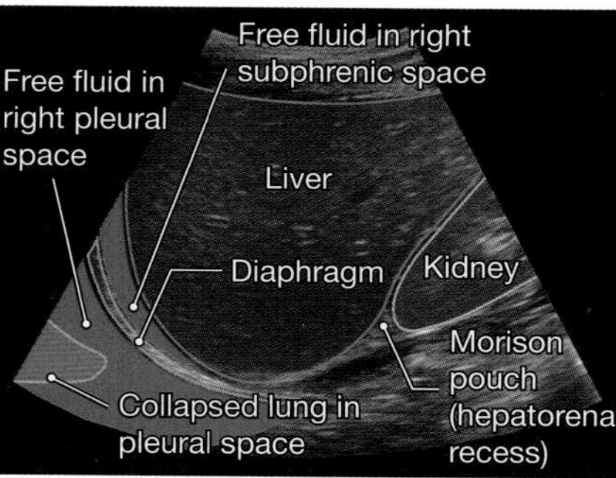

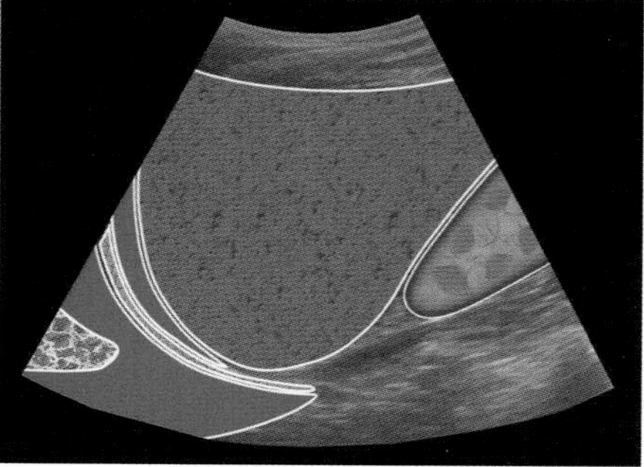

Figure 12.1 Upper panels: Normal right upper quadrant ultrasound view including most of the hepatorenal interface. Lower panels: Artist's rendering of the same view with free fluid accumulation in the potential space at the hepatorenal recess (Morison pouch).

the speckled appearance of liver is mirrored above the diaphragm in the right hemithorax. Mirror image artifacts are produced when a smooth brightly reflective surface (the diaphragm in this instance) reflects sound waves which are then reflected back toward the "mirror" as they encounter tissue reflectors (liver parenchyma and vasculature in this instance) and then once again reflected from the "mirror" back to the probe transducer. This longer sound path results in images (liver in this instance) being projected above (beyond) the diaphragm.

RIGHT UPPER QUADRANT
Longitudinal (Intercostal Oblique)
FIG. 12.3

Next, slide the probe inferiorly until the inferior edge of the liver (liver tip) and the inferior pole of the right kidney can be seen in the image. Free fluid may accumulate around the inferior edge of the liver before becoming visible in the potential space at the hepatorenal recess (Morison pouch).

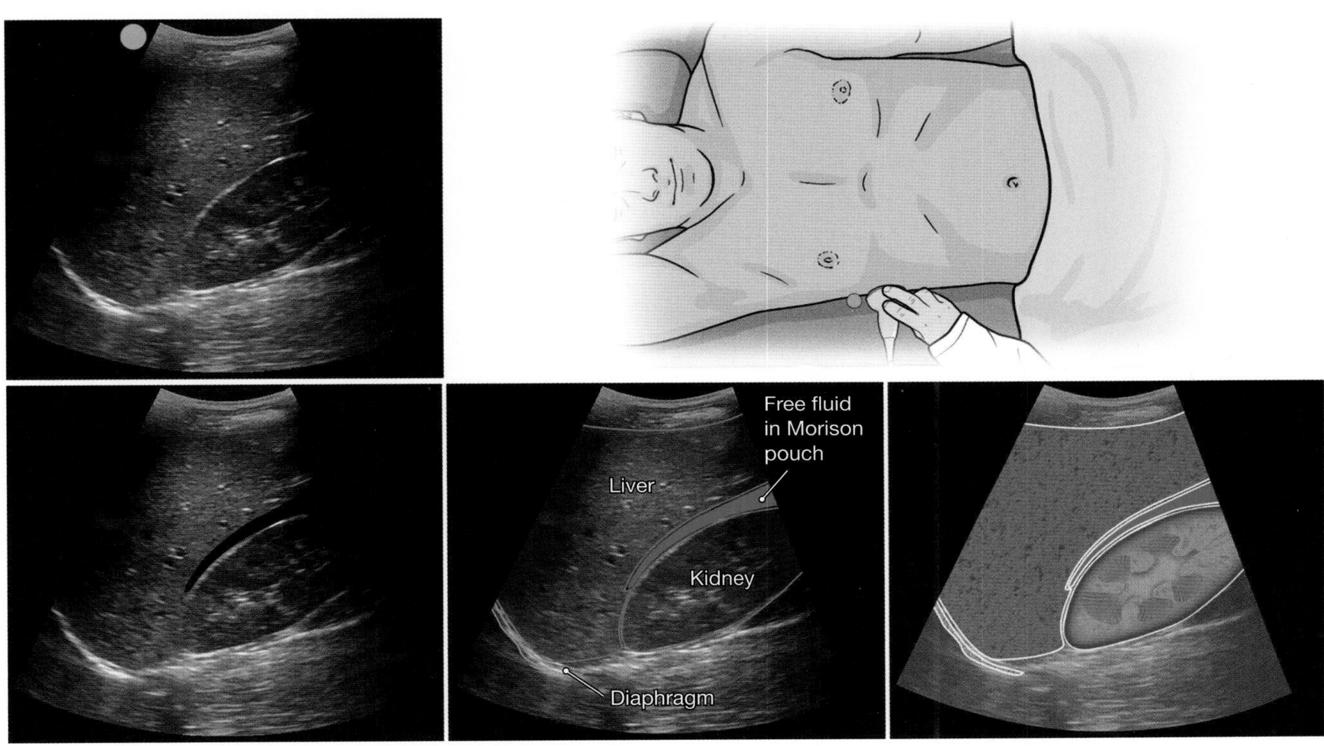

Figure 12.2 Upper panels: Normal right upper quadrant ultrasound view including the right hemithorax, diaphragm, liver, and upper part of the hepatorenal recess. Lower panels: Artist's rendering of the same view with free fluid accumulations in the right pleural and right subphrenic spaces.

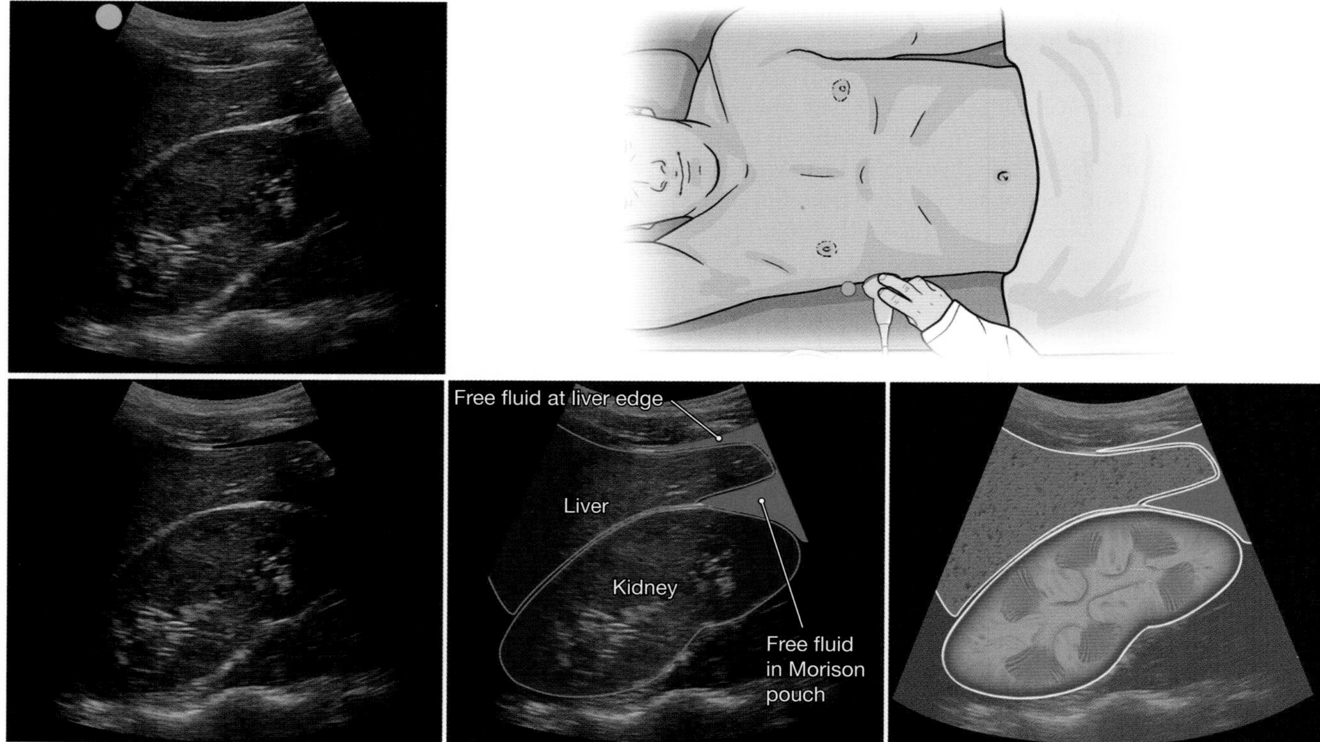

Figure 12.3 Upper panels: Normal right upper quadrant ultrasound view including the inferior edge of the liver and inferior part of the hepatorenal interface. Lower panels: Artist's rendering of the same view with free fluid accumulation at the inferior edge of the liver tracking into the inferior part of Morison pouch.

Left Upper Quadrant

Technique

LEFT UPPER QUADRANT
Longitudinal (Intercostal Oblique)
FIG. 12.4

If the patient can cooperate, the palm of the left hand should be placed behind the head, abducting the arm and helping to open up intercostal spaces on the left. The probe should be placed along the posterior axillary line one or two intercostal spaces above the level of the xiphisternal junction with the probe marker directed superiorly. Note that the left upper quadrant probe position is both more posterior and more superior than it is for the right upper quadrant views. The probe face should be rotated until it is parallel to the intercostal spaces (the intercostal oblique orientation), which minimizes rib shadowing over the spleen and left kidney. Identify the speckled appearance of the spleen and the hyperechoic stripe of the diaphragm curving over the superior surface of the spleen. Fan the probe face slightly anteriorly until the interface between the spleen and left kidney can be identified. In the left upper quadrant, free fluid most commonly accumulates in the left subphrenic space between the diaphragm and the superior surface of the spleen and to a lesser extent in the potential space at the splenorenal recess. Carefully scan the left subphrenic space and splenorenal recess for any free fluid collections.

LEFT UPPER QUADRANT
Longitudinal (Intercostal Oblique)
FIG. 12.5

Next, slide the probe superiorly (one or two intercostal spaces) until the spleen, the diaphragm, and the lower part of the left hemithorax can be seen in the image. In the presence of a

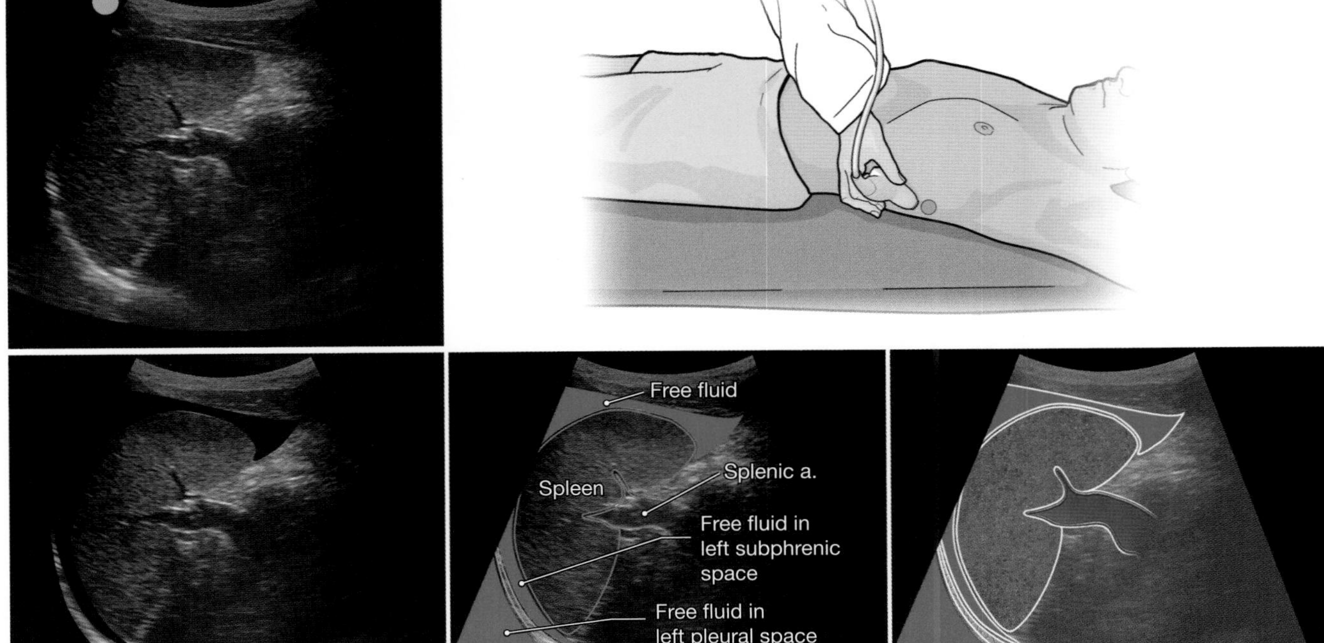

Figure 12.4 Upper panels: Normal left upper quadrant ultrasound view including the diaphragm, spleen, and left kidney. Lower panels: Artist's rendering of the same view with free fluid accumulation in the left subphrenic space and splenorenal recess.

normally aerated lung, the hyperechoic diaphragm creates a mirror image artifact over the lung fields such that the speckled appearance of the spleen is mirrored over the left hemithorax/pleural space. The presence of free fluid in the pleural space (hemothorax or **pleural effusion**) abolishes the mirror image artifact and the space above the diaphragm appears anechoic, often with atelectatic lung floating in and out of view with respiratory efforts. In this position, look again for any free fluid accumulation between the diaphragm and the spleen (left subphrenic space).

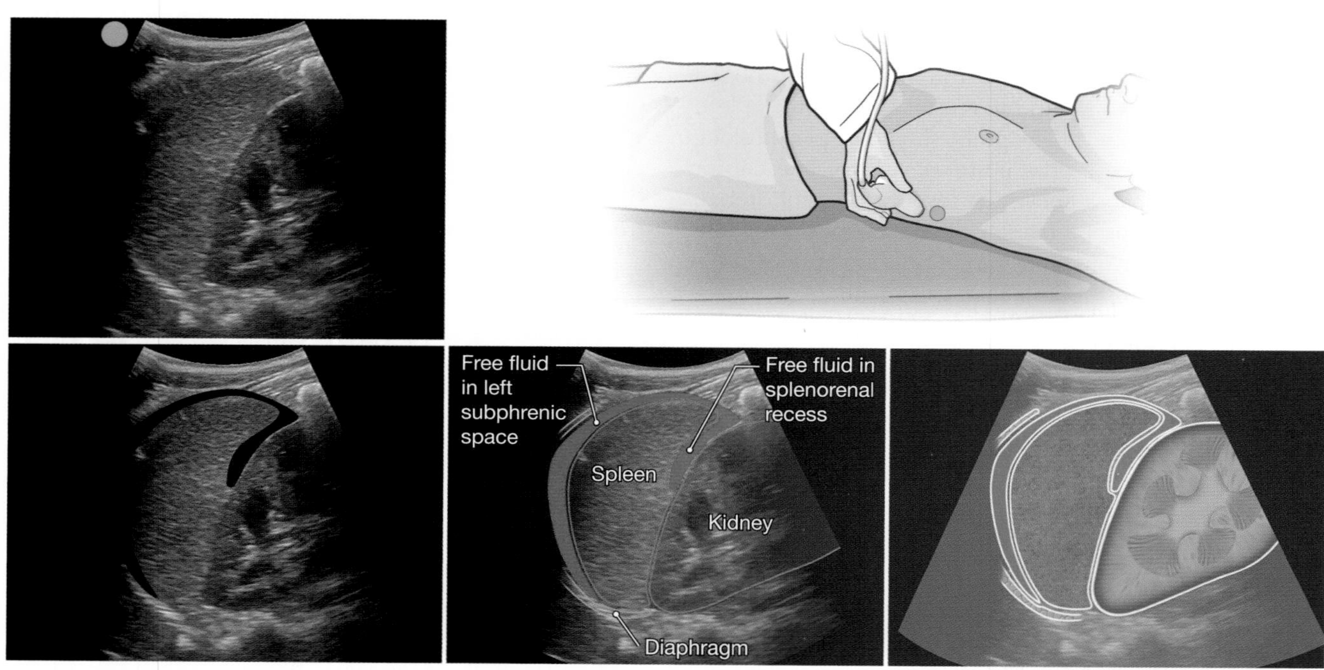

Figure 12.5 Upper panels: Normal left upper quadrant ultrasound view including the left hemithorax, diaphragm, and spleen. Lower panels: Artist's rendering of the same view with free fluid accumulations in the left pleural and subphrenic spaces.

Suprapubic Views of Abdomen/ Pelvis

Technique

SUPRAPUBIC FEMALE PELVIS
Longitudinal (Sagittal/ Parasagittal)
FIG. 12.6

At the pelvic inlet, the inferior extent of abdominal peritoneum drapes over the pelvic viscera. In females, the peritoneum covers the fundus and body of the uterus and extends laterally over the uterine tubes to the pelvic walls as the broad ligaments. The peritoneum extending anteriorly from the uterus and reflecting onto the urinary bladder forms a relatively shallow space, the vesicouterine pouch, between the anterior/inferior aspect of the uterus and the urinary bladder. The peritoneum covering the posterior/superior aspect of the uterus and uterine cervix descends to just above the posterior fornix of the vagina and then reflects onto the anterior surface of the rectum forming a deep potential space, the rectouterine pouch. The rectouterine pouch is commonly clinically referred to as the **pouch of Douglas**.

The rectouterine pouch is the most dependent part of the peritoneal space in the supine position, and so US examination in these locations is sensitive to relatively small amounts of intraperitoneal free fluid. Unfortunately,

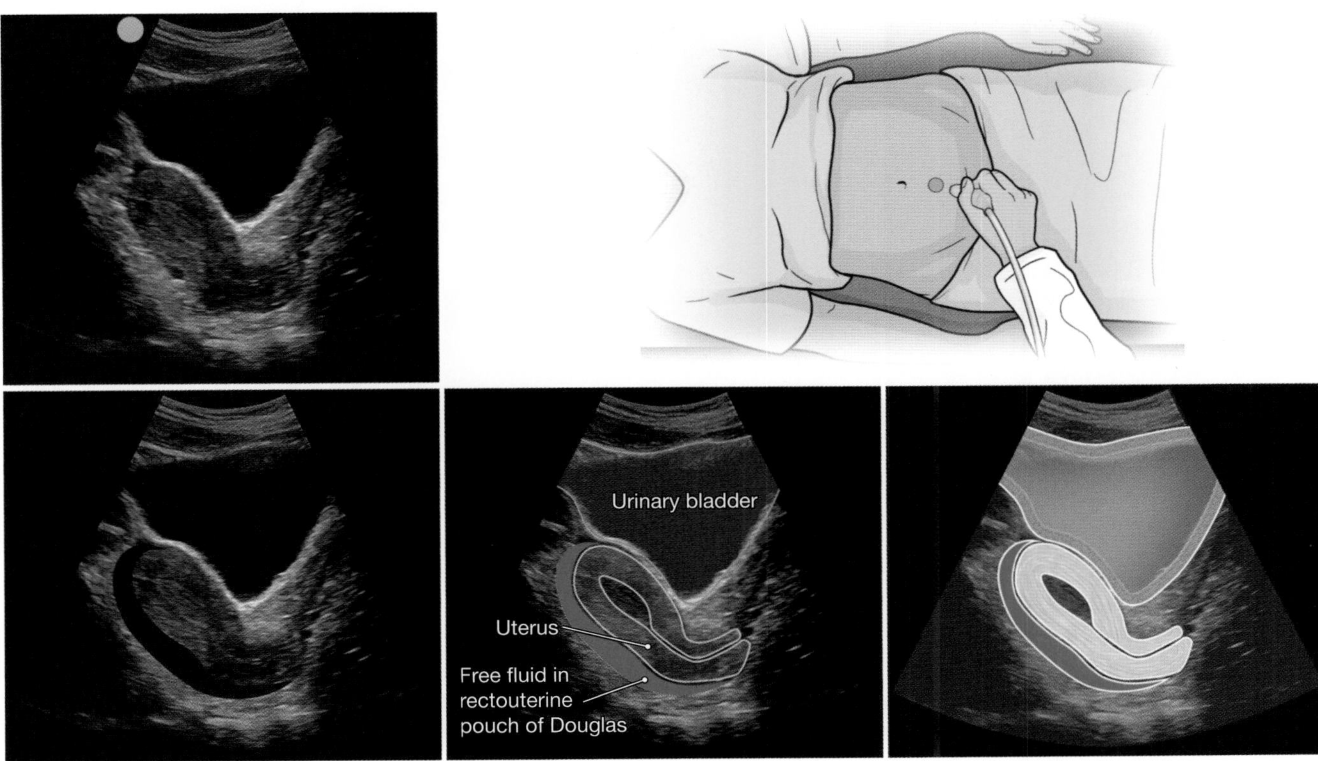

Figure 12.6 Upper panels: Normal longitudinal (sagittal/parasagittal) suprapubic view of the female pelvis. Lower panel: Artist's rendering of the same view with intraperitoneal free fluid accumulating in the rectouterine pouch of Douglas and over the fundus of the uterus toward the vesicouterine pouch.

if the urinary bladder is not at least partially full, bowel gas shadowing can interfere substantially with US examination in this area. A full urinary bladder displaces loops of bowel superiorly and provides an excellent acoustic window for US examination of pelvic structures behind the urinary bladder. Because of this, at least one FAST examination should be performed along with the initial assessment of patients presenting with thoracoabdominal trauma before placing a Foley catheter.

The heel of the probe (nonmarker side) should be placed just over (or just above) the pubic symphysis with the marker side directed toward the head. Adjust the probe position and tilt until pelvic landmarks and structures can be identified. Urine, like all fluids, appears anechoic and the urinary bladder wall appears hyperechoic. In longitudinal views, full urinary bladders are roughly triangular with the apex pointing superiorly.

Posterior to the urinary bladder, identify the fundus and body of the uterus, the hyperechoic endometrial stripe, and the cervix. Scan carefully to the left and right of the midline looking for any free fluid collections in the rectouterine and vesicouterine pouches.

SUPRAPUBIC MALE PELVIS
Longitudinal (Sagittal/ Parasagittal)
FIG. 12.7

At the pelvic inlet, the inferior extent of abdominal peritoneum drapes over pelvic viscera. In males, peritoneum draping over the urinary bladder reflects onto the anterior surface of the rectum, forming the rectovesical pouch. The superior poles of the seminal vesicles are just beneath the inferior extent of the rectovesical pouch.

The heel of the probe (nonmarker side) should be placed just over (or just above) the pubic symphysis with the marker side directed toward the head. Adjust the probe position and tilt until pelvic landmarks and structures can be identified. Identify the urinary bladder, the seminal vesicles, and the prostate gland. Scan carefully along the superior/posterior aspect of the urinary bladder for any free fluid collection in the rectovesical pouch.

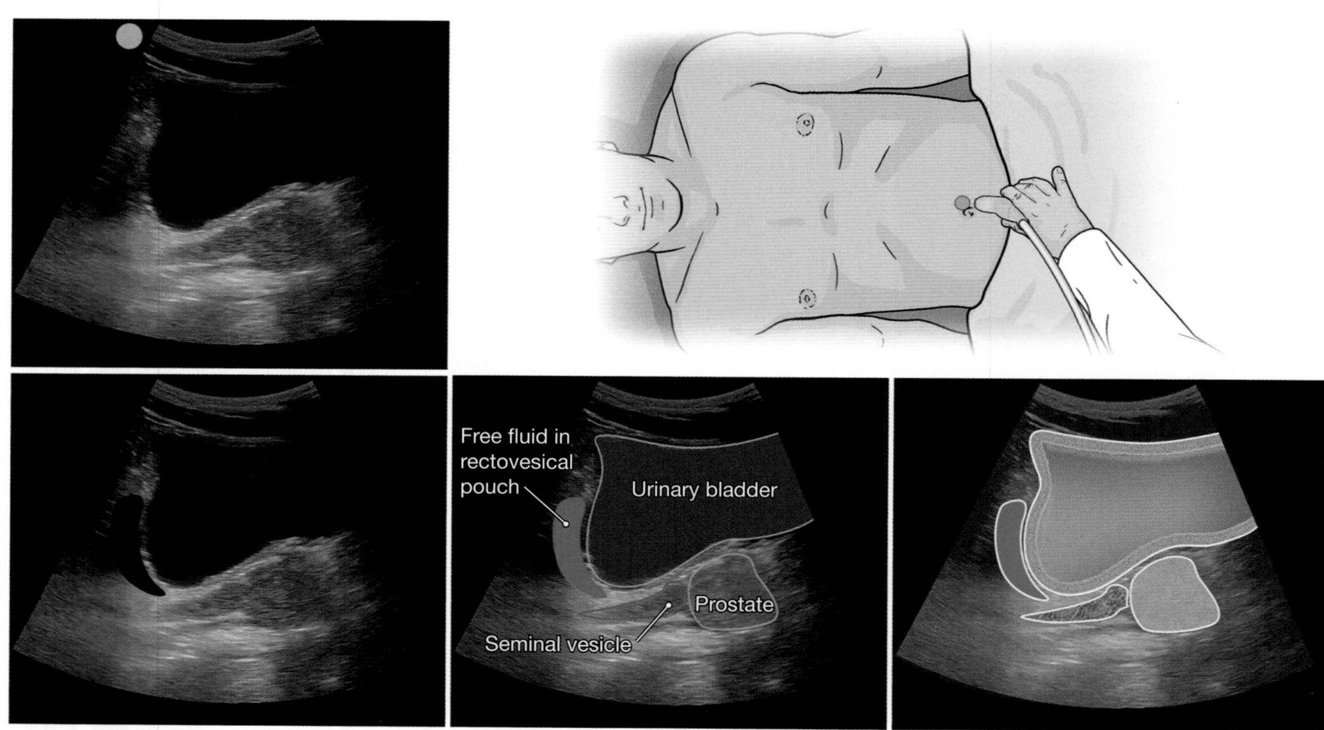

Figure 12.7 Upper panels: Normal longitudinal (sagittal/parasagittal) suprapubic view of the male pelvis. Lower panel: Artist's rendering of the same view with intraperitoneal free fluid accumulating in the rectovesical pouch.

SUPRAPUBIC FEMALE PELVIS
Transverse
FIG. 12.8

After completing the suprapubic examination of the pelvis in the longitudinal plane, rotate the probe 90° counterclockwise so that the marker side is directed to the right and position the probe face just superior to the pubic symphysis. Adjust the probe position and tilt until pelvic landmarks and structures can be identified. In transverse views, full urinary bladders are roughly rectangular.

Identify the urinary bladder, uterus, and endometrial stripe. Scan carefully superiorly and inferiorly along the uterus, looking for any free fluid collections in the rectouterine and/or vesicouterine pouches.

SUPRAPUBIC MALE PELVIS
Transverse
FIG. 12.9

After completing the suprapubic examination of the pelvis in the longitudinal plane, rotate the probe 90° counterclockwise so that the marker side is directed to the right and position the probe face just superior to the pubic symphysis. Adjust the probe position and tilt until pelvic landmarks and structures can be identified. In transverse views, full urinary bladders are roughly rectangular.

Identify the urinary bladder and the seminal vesicles. Scan carefully along the superior/posterior aspect of the urinary bladder just superior to the seminal vesicles for any free fluid collection in the rectovesical pouch.

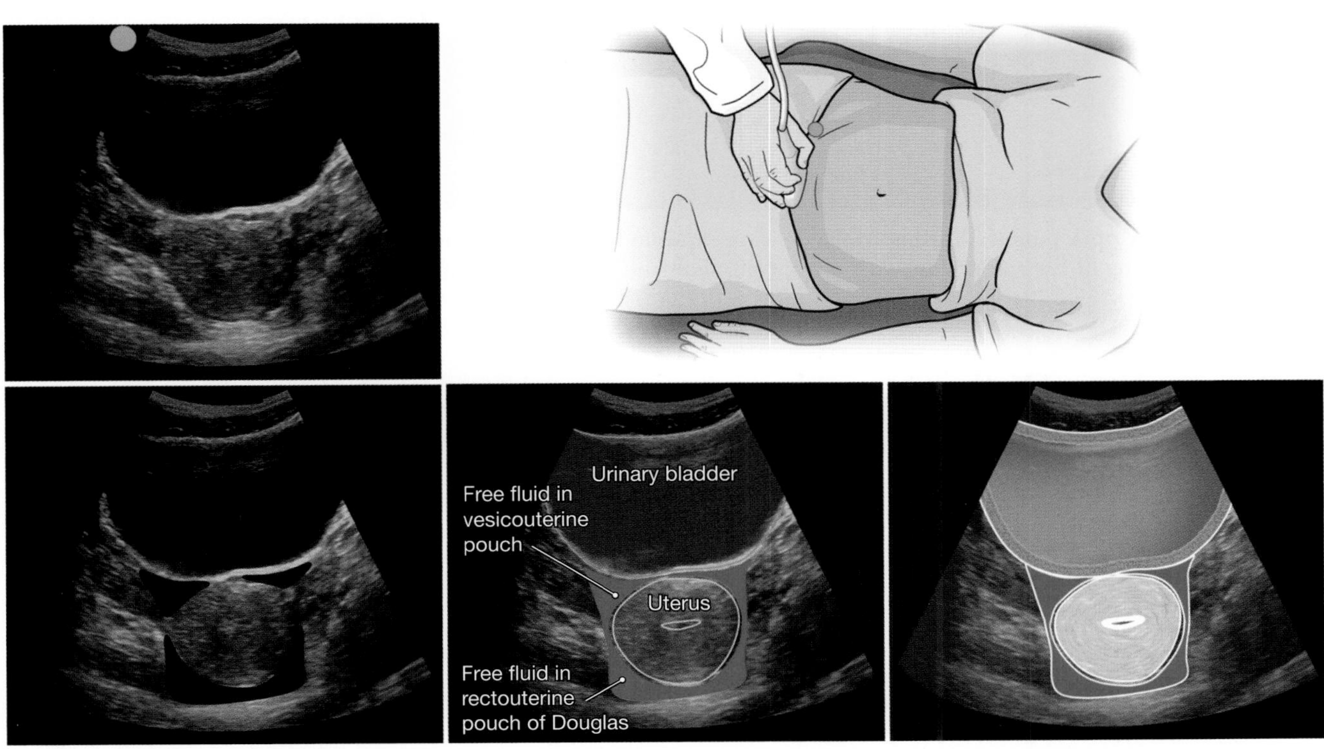

Figure 12.8 Upper panels: Normal transverse suprapubic view of the female pelvis. Lower panel: Artist's rendering of the same view with intraperitoneal free fluid accumulating in the rectouterine pouch of Douglas and the vesicouterine pouch.

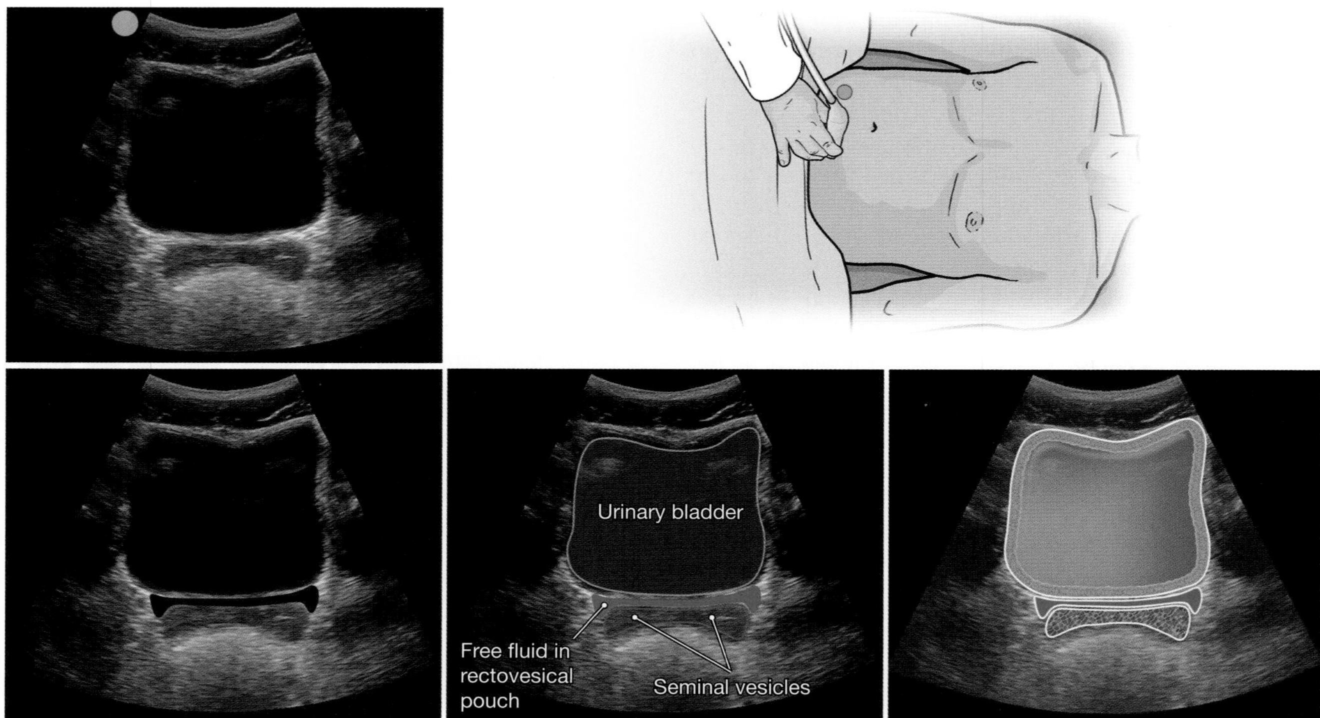

Figure 12.9 Upper panels: Normal transverse suprapubic view of the male pelvis. Lower panel: Artist's rendering of the same view with intraperitoneal free fluid accumulating in the rectovesical pouch.

Heart and Pericardial Space

SUBXIPHOID 4-CHAMBER VIEW
FIG. 12.10

The **subxiphoid 4-chamber view** uses the liver as a sonographic window to view the heart and pericardium. If the patient can cooperate, flexing the knees to 90° and placing the soles of the feet on the bed relaxes the abdominal musculature. To obtain this view, place the probe face just to the right of the midline 2 to 4 cm below the xiphoid process, depending on the width of the subcostal arch. The probe should be far enough below the xiphoid process so that the sides of the probe face are not pressing against ribs/costal cartilages. Next, exert pressure directly posteriorly, and then with a scooping motion, flatten the probe against the abdominal wall, directing the US beam upward and slightly toward the left shoulder. Adjust probe position and tilt until the liver, heart chambers, and **pericardium** can be identified. If needed, increase the depth setting until the posterior pericardium adjacent to the free wall of the left ventricle can be clearly seen in the far field. If possible, ask the patient to take a deep breath, which brings the heart closer to the probe and improves the image quality. Carefully scan along the heart and pericardium, looking for any free fluid or blood accumulating between the speckled-appearing myocardium and the hyperechoic pericardium.

Note: When a **microconvex phased array (cardiac) probe** is used, many US units automatically place the screen marker dot to the right of the screen image rather than to the left of the screen image as in all other applications. If the screen marker dot is on the left of the image as usual (as it should be when a curved array or abdominal probe is used), then the marker side of the probe should be directed toward the patient's right axilla to obtain display images as shown in Figure 12.10. If the marker dot is on the right of the screen image, then the marker side of the probe should be directed toward the patient's left flank to obtain the same image orientation on the display.

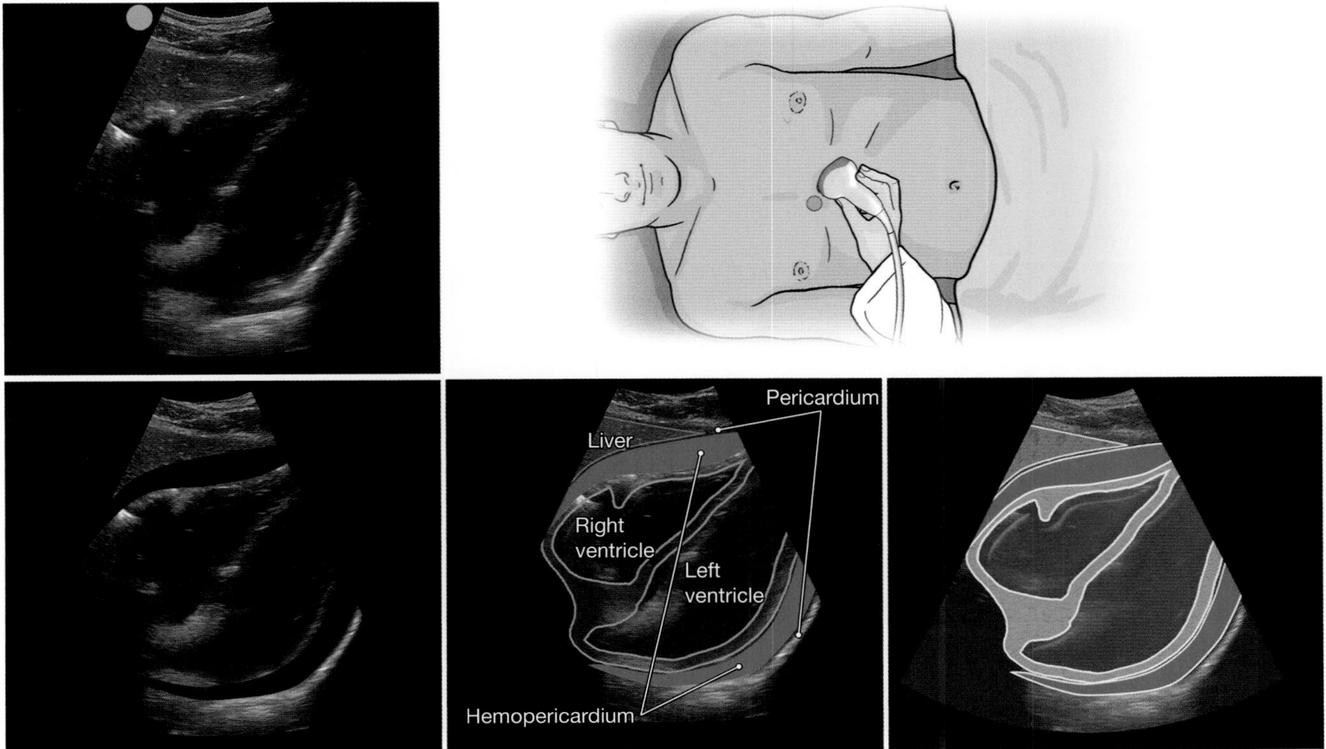

Figure 12.10 Upper panels: Normal subxiphoid 4-chamber view of the heart and the pericardium. Lower panels: Artist's rendering of the same view with free fluid in the pericardial space.

PARASTERNAL LONG-AXIS VIEW
FIG. 12.11

To obtain the parasternal long-axis view, place the probe face just to the left of the sternum in the third, fourth, or fifth intercostal space approximately along a line connecting the right shoulder and left nipple. This orients the probe/US beam along the long axis of the left ventricle. Adjust the probe position up or down 1 intercostal space at a time as needed, until an image of the heart as shown in Figure 12.11 can be best seen. The posterior free wall of the left ventricle and adjacent posterior pericardium should be identified in the far field. The left atrium, mitral valve, inflow tract of the left ventricle, outflow tract of the left ventricle, aortic valve, and ascending aorta should be identified. The interventricular septum and outflow tract of the right ventricle should be seen in the near field. The descending thoracic aorta can often be seen just posterior to the left atrium near the position of the mitral valve annulus. The apex of the left ventricle should be beyond the edge of the display image to the left. Carefully scan along the heart and the pericardium and look for any free fluid accumulating between the speckled-appearing myocardium of the left ventricle and the hyperechoic pericardium, and continue around the apex of the left ventricle and between the free wall of the right ventricle and the anterior pericardium.

Note: When a microconvex phased array (cardiac) probe is used, many US units automatically place the screen marker dot to the right of the screen image, rather than to the left of the screen image as in all other applications. If the screen marker dot is on the left of the image as usual (as it should be when a curved array or abdominal probe is used), then the marker side of the probe should be directed toward the patient's left flank to obtain display images as shown in Figure 12.11. If the marker dot is on the right of the screen image, then the marker side of the probe should be directed toward the patient's right shoulder to obtain the same image orientation on the display.

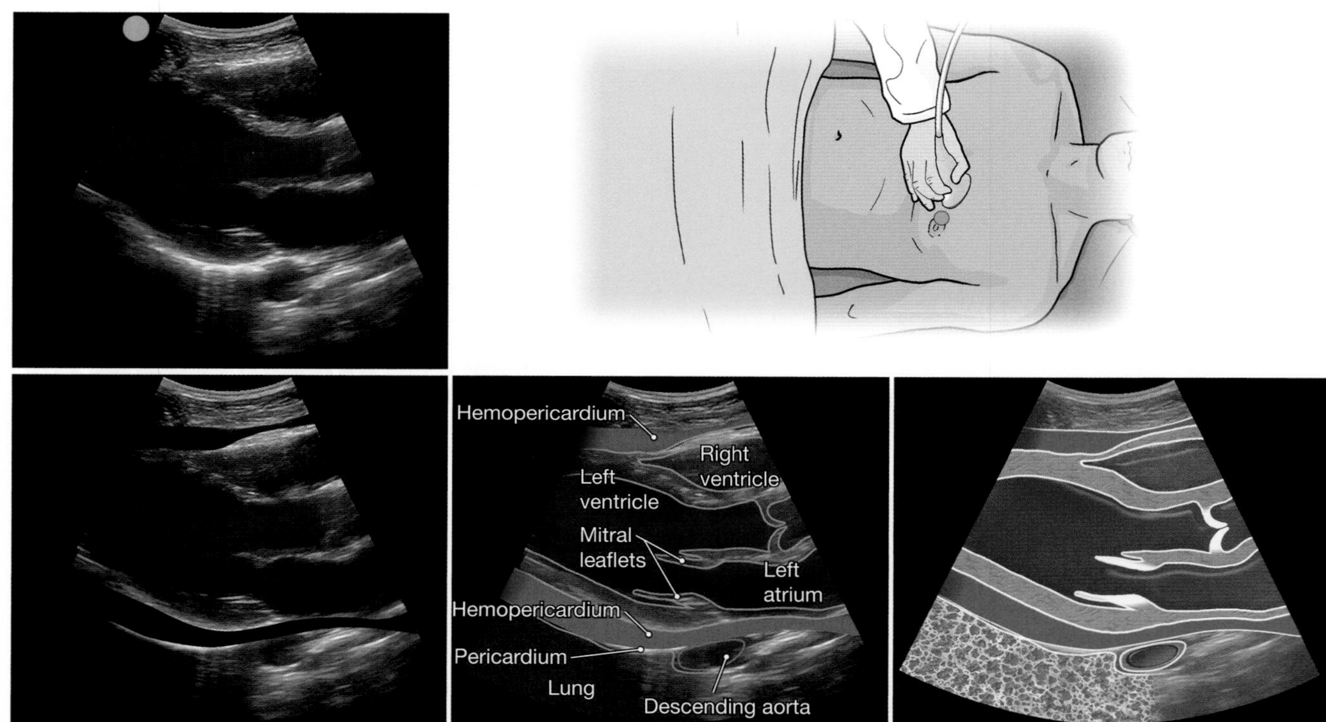

Figure 12.11 Upper panels: Normal parasternal long-axis view of the heart and the pericardium. Lower panels: Artist's rendering of the same view with free fluid in the pericardial space.

Multiple Choice Questions

1. A 63-year-old woman is brought to the emergency department because of a fall from a 3-m (10-ft)-high balcony of her apartment. She has severe chest pain, dyspnea, tachypnea, tachycardia, and cough. A radiograph of the hips and lower limbs shows multiple spiral fractures. After 2 hours, she develops signs of Beck triad. Which of the following ultrasound views will most likely identify fluid in the pericardial cavity?

A. Parasternal long axis
B. Parasternal short axis
C. Apical
D. Subcostal inferior vena cava

2. A 55-year-old woman is brought to the emergency department because of a 1-week history of progressive pain in the right side of her lower abdomen. She experienced a feeling of abdominal fullness and discomfort. She also cannot lie down easily. A focused assessment with sonography for trauma (FAST) examination and a computed tomography scan of the abdomen are performed. A diagnosis of an ovarian tumor is made. Which of the following ultrasound views will most likely identify fluid in the abdominal cavity in this patient?

A. Hepatorenal
B. Left subphrenic
C. Left splenorenal
D. Longitudinal suprapubic
E. Suprapubic transverse

3. A 55-year-old man is brought to the emergency department 45 minutes after being involved in a motor vehicle collision. Physical examination shows a wound in the neck just above the middle of the right clavicle in the first rib. A radiograph of the thorax shows collapse of the right lung and a tension pneumothorax. Which of the following is the typical ultrasonographic finding for the diagnosis of pneumothorax?

A. Absence of pleural sliding
B. Presence of A lines
C. Presence of B lines
D. Presence of E lines
E. Presence of lung pulse

4. A 35-year-old woman is admitted to the emergency department 45 minutes after being involved in a motor vehicle collision. Physical examination shows that her left lower back is bruised and swollen. She has a sharp pain during respiration. A radiograph of her chest shows a fracture of the 11th rib on the left side. Which of the following organs would most likely sustain an injury?

A. Kidney
B. Pancreas
C. Lung
D. Spleen
E. Liver

5. A 75-year-old woman is brought to the emergency department because of a 2-hour history of severe chest pain, dyspnea, tachycardia, cough, and fever. An ultrasound examination shows significant pericardial effusion. A pericardiocentesis is performed, and the needle is inserted using the subxiphoid approach. The needle passes too deeply, piercing the visceral pericardium and enters the heart. Which of the following chambers would be the first to be penetrated by the needle?

A. Left ventricle
B. Left cardiac apex
C. Right atrium
D. Right ventricle
E. Left atrium

6. A 28-year-old woman is brought to the emergency department because of a 3-hour history of sharp pain in the left lower quadrant. An ultrasound examination shows a ruptured ectopic pregnancy close to the left ovary. There is a small amount of fluid in the abdominal cavity from the bleeding from the rupture site. Which of the following locations is the fluid most likely present?

A. Rectouterine pouch (of Douglas)
B. Hepatorenal pouch (of Morison)
C. Vesicouterine pouch
D. Right subphrenic space
E. Paracolic gutters

13

Clinical Applications

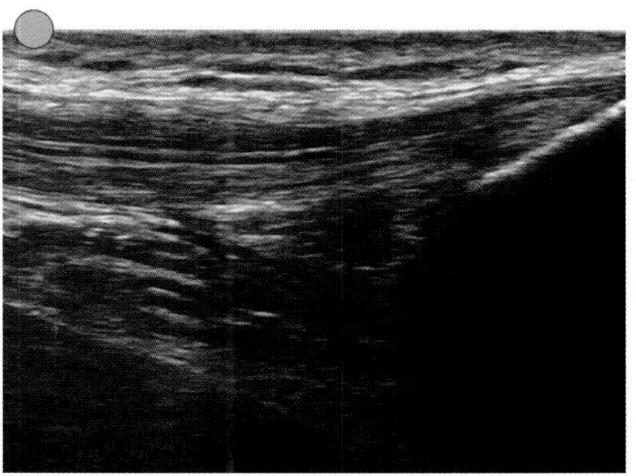

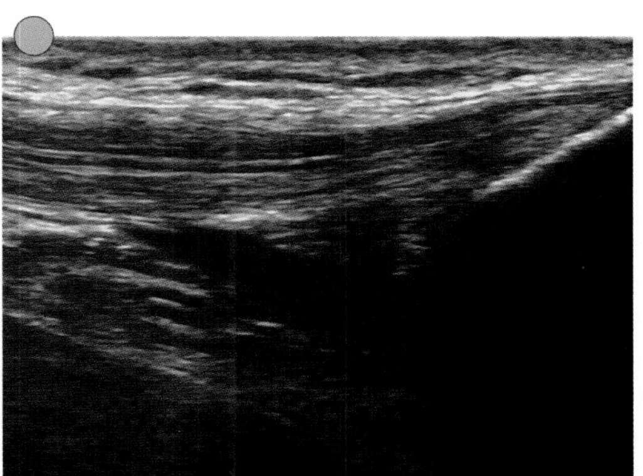

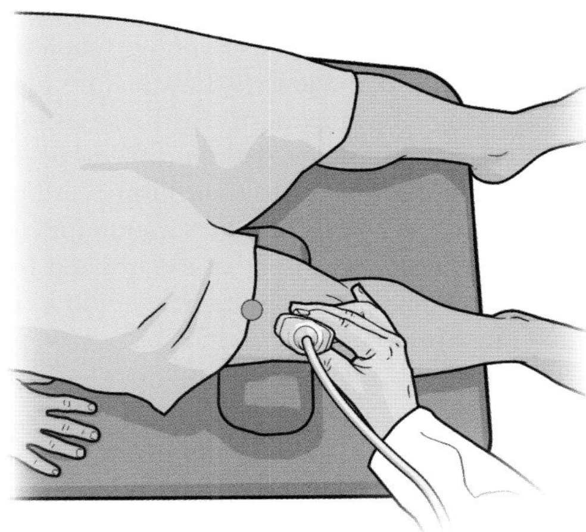

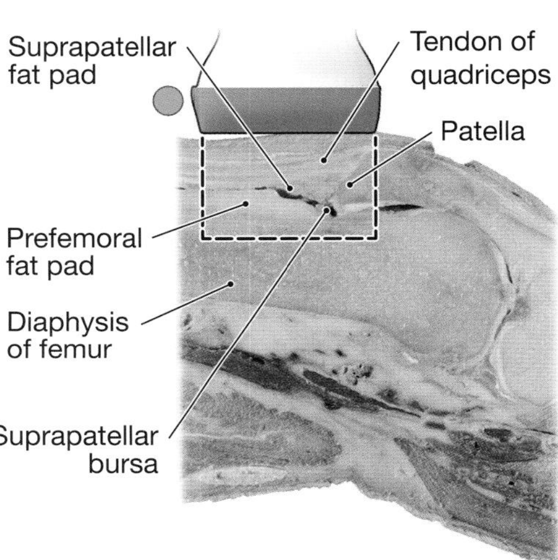

Central Venous Catheterization

Indications

In the management of critically ill patients, establishing vascular access and initiating resuscitation is crucial. Various procedures can be used for vascular access, with peripheral access being the first choice. However, if peripheral access is not possible, central venous access should be considered to ensure fluid resuscitation and enable the measurement of hemodynamic variables inassessible noninvasively. Central venous access also allows for the administration of medications and nutritional support that cannot be given through peripheral catheters.

Central venous catheterization is indicated in several clinical situations. Common reasons include monitoring central venous pressure (CVP), obtaining venous access for emergencies or routine procedures, collecting serial blood samples, administering medications, and performing invasive venous interventions such as pacemaker insertion, hemodialysis, and aggressive treatment protocols for septic shock. Furthermore, it is used for volume resuscitation in situations such as hypothermia and severe hemorrhagic shock, for patients with a history of IV substance abuse, major burns, obesity, or those in long-term care who may have difficulties with peripheral access. The use of central venous catheterization during cardiopulmonary resuscitation is controversial but offers rapid and easy administration of medications. It is also utilized for delivering medications such as vasopressors, chemotherapeutic agents, and parenteral nutrition, which can cause phlebitis when administered through peripheral lines.

Contraindications

Most contraindications to central venous catheterization are considered relative because they depend on the availability of alternative options and the urgency of central venous access. The main relative contraindications include coagulopathy, anatomical distortion, vasculitis, local cellulitis, prior long-term venous cannulation, prior injections of sclerosis agents, presence of another device, vascular injury near the insertion site, need for mobility, and antibiotic hypersensitivity (with antibiotic-impregnated catheters). Central venous catheterization can be challenging in morbidly obese patients due to obscured surface landmarks and difficulties caused by excess adipose tissue. However, the use of sonographic guidance can help overcome this limitation. Panniculitis near the site of femoral vein catheterization also poses a problem in obese patients.

Coagulopathy and thrombocytopenia are commonly considered contraindications to central venous catheterization, but the actual risk of significant bleeding is low.

Anatomy for Ultrasound Central Venous Access

Central venous access may be obtained in the subclavian, internal jugular, or femoral vein with use of a linear high-frequency probe.

Subclavian Vein

For central venous catheterization of the subclavian vein, the patient should be lying flat on their back. Although Trendelenburg positioning is not necessary, it can be used for preventing air embolism. The arm on the same side as the access site should be kept close to the body to avoid any anatomical distortion caused by the clavicle.

There are two approaches to accessing the subclavian vein: infraclavicular and supraclavicular. Anatomically, the subclavian vein is located behind the medial third of the clavicle and subclavius muscle, below the subclavian artery, in front of the scalenus anterior muscle and phrenic nerve, and above the first rib and pleura. The relationship between the medial third of the clavicle and the subclavian vein serves as a helpful landmark for catheter placement.

In the infraclavicular approach, a small sandbag or rolled towel can be placed between the shoulder blades to retract the shoulder, bringing the vein closer to the clavicle. Ultrasound guidance is used for locating the subclavian vein, and the needle is inserted with the bevel pointing inferomedially, toward the opposite clavicular head. The operator can use the suprasternal notch and the costoclavicular junction as reference points for the needle direction.

In the supraclavicular approach, the patient's head and neck are rotated away from the access site to provide better access along the lateral border of the clavicular head of the sternocleidomastoid muscle. The needle is inserted superiorly and behind the clavicle, just lateral to the clavicular head of the sternocleidomastoid muscle. It is important to insert the needle horizontally to avoid pneumothorax. Negative pressure applied with a syringe helps confirm entry into the vein by drawing dark blood. Once venous access is achieved, the needle is stabilized, and a guidewire is advanced through it.

Internal Jugular Vein

INTERNAL JUGULAR VEIN
Transverse
FIG. 13.1

Central venous catheterization is more commonly performed on the internal jugular veins. The internal jugular vein originates at the base of the skull in the posterior compartment of the jugular foramen. It collects blood from the skull, brain, and superficial areas of the face and neck. The vein runs downward in the neck alongside the carotid artery and eventually joins the subclavian vein behind the sternal edge of the clavicle to form the brachiocephalic vein.

Anatomically, the internal jugular vein is positioned anterolaterally within the carotid sheath, in comparison to the carotid artery and vagus nerve. The sternal notch, sternocleidomastoid muscle, and clavicle serve as useful landmarks for locating the vein. The internal jugular vein can be found coursing along the medial head of the sternocleidomastoid muscle, forming the apex of the anterior cervical triangle. It is often visible at the middle of the triangle, around the level of the clavicle, before its union with the subclavian vein.

The internal jugular vein may appear pulsatile due to its proximity and connection to the right atrium. However, it is important to exercise caution as the common carotid artery is in close proximity to the internal jugular vein at this level. Improper technique or confusion of pulsations can lead to arterial puncture. The use of sonographic guidance can help reduce the risk of arterial injury during internal jugular cannulation. Placing the patient in the Trendelenburg position can increase filling of the internal jugular vein, aiding in its identification during the procedure.

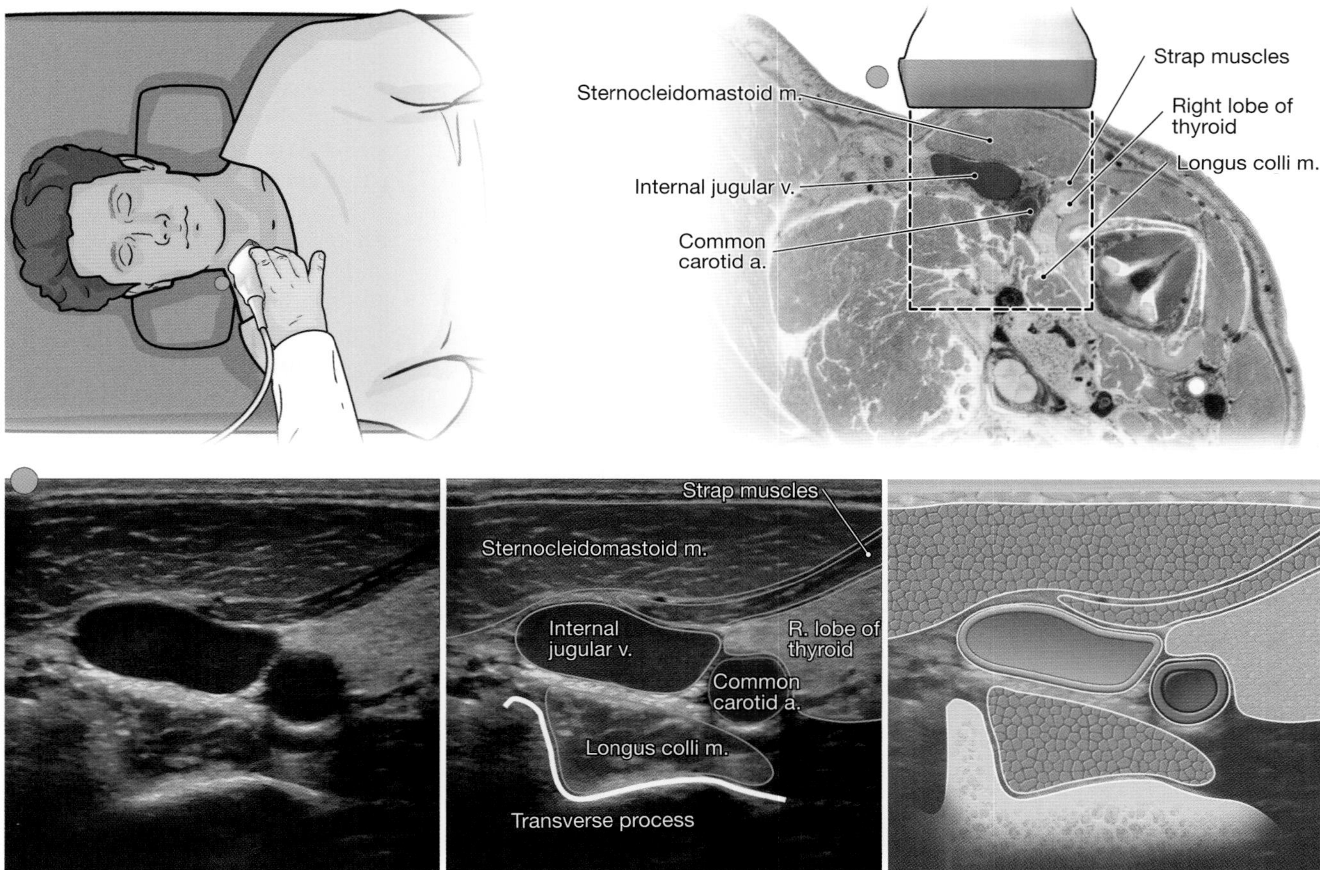

Figure 13.1 Transverse view of the internal jugular vein and common carotid artery in the inferior third of the neck.

Femoral Vein

FEMORAL VEIN
Transverse
FIG. 13.2

To perform central venous catheterization of the femoral vein, the patient is positioned supine with the targeted leg abducted and externally rotated to expose the femoral triangle. Elevating the buttock with rolled sheets or a pillow can provide better exposure during the procedure. While the reverse Trendelenburg position may be used to enhance the filling of the femoral vein from the inferior vena cava, its effectiveness may vary among patients.

The femoral vein is typically accessed near the inguinal ligament due to the close relationship between the artery and vein. As the anatomy changes distally in the thigh, the artery may assume an anterior position, making it less suitable for catheterization. The femoral pulse can be palpated to help locate the femoral vein. The needle is inserted at a 45° angle in a cephalic direction toward the umbilicus, approximately 1 cm medial to the femoral pulse. Ideally, the femoral pulse should be palpated two fingerbreadths beneath the inguinal ligament.

During palpation, pressure on the femoral vein may compress it and hinder cannulation. It is important to release digital pressure while keeping the fingers on the skin to serve as a visual reference for the underlying anatomy.

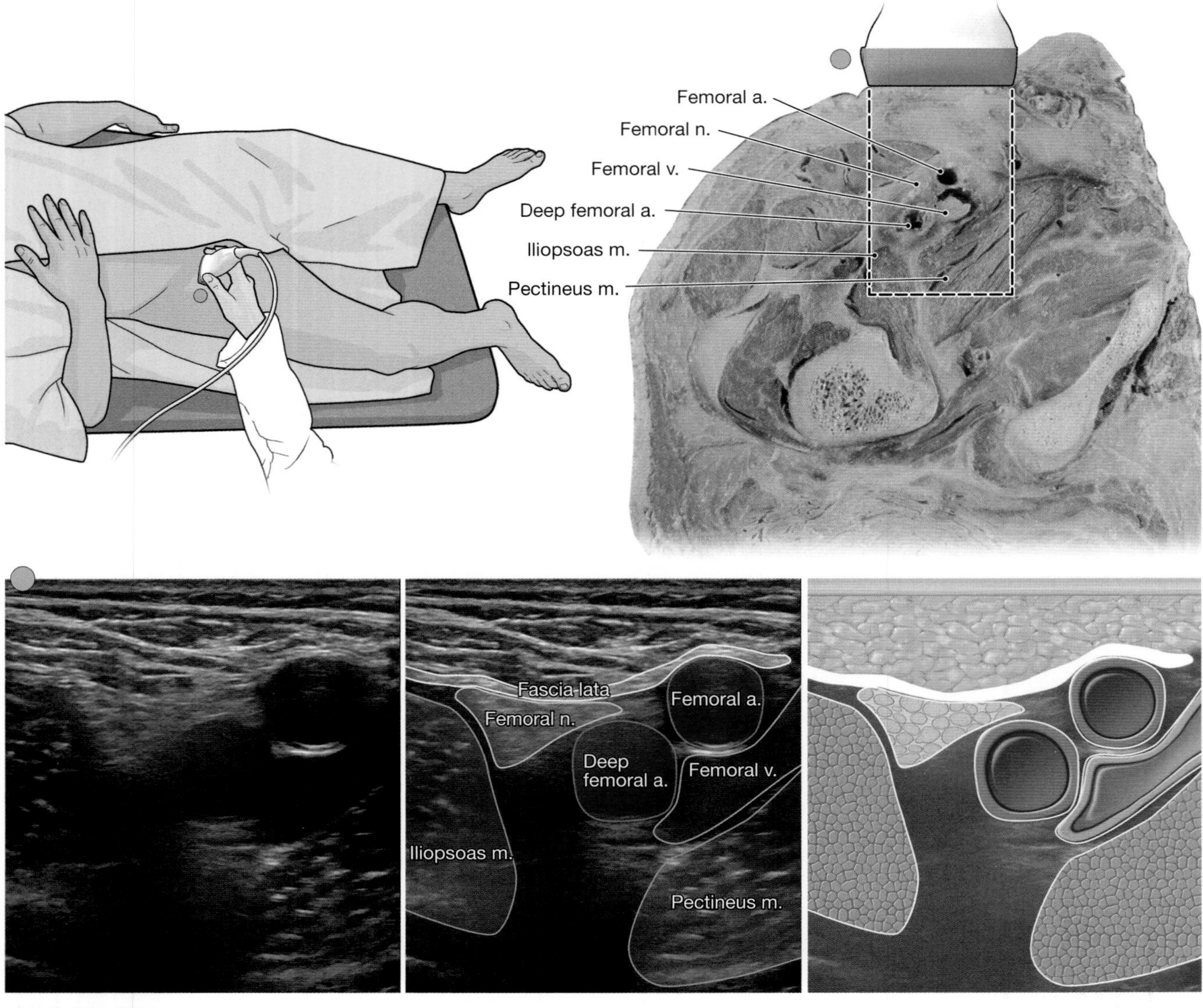

Figure 13.2 Transverse view of the femoral vein, femoral artery, deep femoral artery, and femoral nerve in the femoral triangle.

Lumbar Puncture

Introduction

The lumbar puncture procedure is a common procedure performed in emergency departments to gather crucial diagnostic and treatment information for various neurological conditions, both infectious and non-infectious. The examination of cerebrospinal fluid (CSF) obtained through lumbar puncture has proven to be immensely valuable, particularly in identifying urgent and life-threatening conditions resulting from infections. However, it is important to note that lumbar puncture itself carries potential risks, underscoring the need for a thorough neurological examination before proceeding with the procedure. It is worth mentioning that lumbar puncture alone rarely provides a definitive diagnosis, and CSF analysis should be interpreted alongside a comprehensive medical history, physical examination, and supplementary laboratory tests.

Indications

Lumbar puncture and CSF analysis are performed for both urgent and nonurgent reasons. The primary reason for conducting lumbar puncture is to investigate suspected meningitis and other central nervous system (CNS) infections. In emergency cases, lumbar puncture is also used when there is suspicion of subarachnoid hemorrhage despite a negative CT scan. Nonurgent indications for lumbar puncture include evaluating CNS conditions such as CNS syphilis, hydrocephalus, unexplained seizures, and demyelinating disorders. Additionally, lumbar puncture can be used for therapeutic purposes such as spinal anesthesia, relieving pseudotumor cerebri, intrathecal medication administration, and contrast medium injection for myelography.

In the emergency room, lumbar puncture is commonly performed for diagnosing or ruling out meningitis in patients with symptoms such as fever, headache, altered mental status, or signs of meningeal irritation. CSF examination is highly sensitive and specific in detecting bacterial and fungal meningitis, which result in a high rate of lumbar punctures in suspected cases.

The second most common indication for lumbar puncture is suspected subarachnoid hemorrhage. Although a head CT scan can provide a diagnosis, lumbar puncture is also valuable, especially when the CT scan is negative and when more than 24 hours have passed since the event. Lumbar puncture is appropriate to rule out subarachnoid hemorrhage in cases where the initial CT scan is negative.

Contraindications

Performing lumbar puncture is contraindicated in patients with tissue infection near the puncture site for preventing the injection of infectious pathogens. Additionally, there are other contraindications including elevated intracranial pressure, thrombocytopenia, and other coagulation disorders.

Elevated intracranial pressure is a contraindication because the sudden pressure change during lumbar puncture can potentially trigger or worsen brain herniation, leading to serious complications such as cardiorespiratory collapse, seizures, or sudden death. Certain indicators, including focal neurological findings, papilledema, and radiographic evidence of increased intracranial pressure, have been associated with poor outcomes in patients with elevated intracranial pressure, who deteriorated after undergoing lumbar pressure.

Procedure

INTERLAMINAR SPACE
THECAL SAC
Transverse
FIG. 13.3

To perform a lumbar puncture, the patient should be positioned in the lateral recumbent position with the hips, knees, and chin flexed toward the chest. This position maximizes the opening of the interlaminar spaces. If the patient cannot assume this position, they may be allowed to sit up and lean forward with the support of a Mayo stand to achieve optimal interlaminar space opening. The L3-L4 interspace should be located and marked on the patient. This can be done by palpating the posterior superior iliac crests and moving fingers medially toward the spine to identify the L3-L4 space. In older children and adults, lumbar puncture can be performed at the L2-L3 interspace or as low as the L5-S1 interspace. However, in children less than 12 months of age, it is recommended to perform lumbar puncture below the L2-L3 interspace due to the lower level of the conus medullaris. Once the patient is in position, place the ultrasound at the L2-L3 interspace, and stabilize the spinal needle on the index finger parallel to the ultrasound field. The needle is slowly inserted through the subcutaneous tissue using the thumbs, with a slight angle toward the umbilicus. The needle is advanced slowly and smoothly, and a popping sensation may be felt when it penetrates the ligamentum flavum (first pop) and dura mater (second pop). When fluid return is observed, the needle can be partially

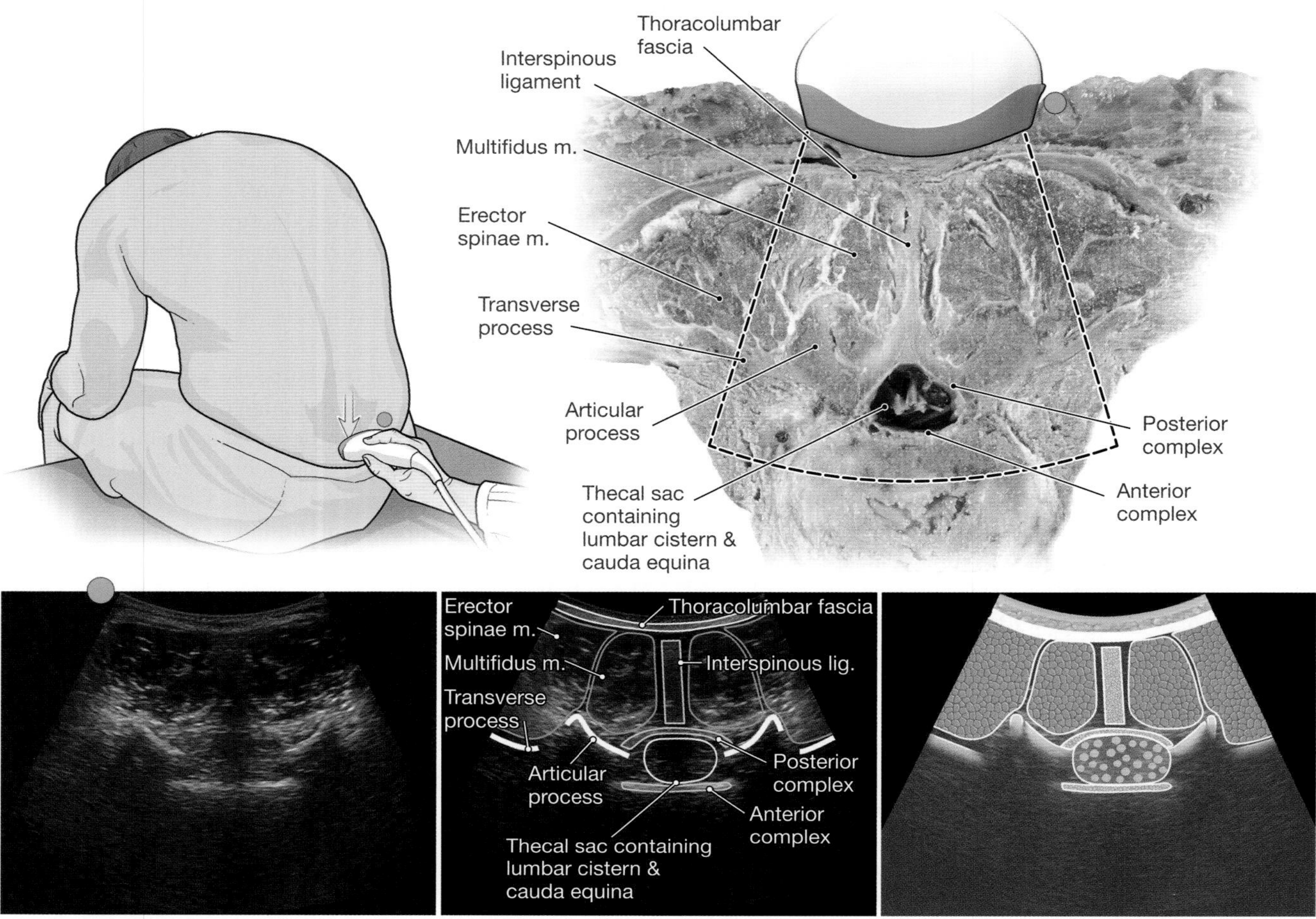

Figure 13.3 Transverse view of the interlaminar space and thecal sac containing lumbar cistern and cauda equina. Posterior complex: Ligamentum flavum, extradural fat, and posterior aspect of dura mater. Anterior complex: Anterior aspect of the dura mater, extradural fat, and posterior longitudinal ligament.

LAMINAE
INTERLAMINAR SPACES
Longitudinal
FIG. 13.4

withdrawn to allow for collection. The stylet of the needle can also be incrementally removed to check for fluid return. If no fluid return is observed, the stylet is replaced, and the needle is advanced or withdrawn slightly before rechecking for fluid return. This process is repeated until fluid return is achieved.

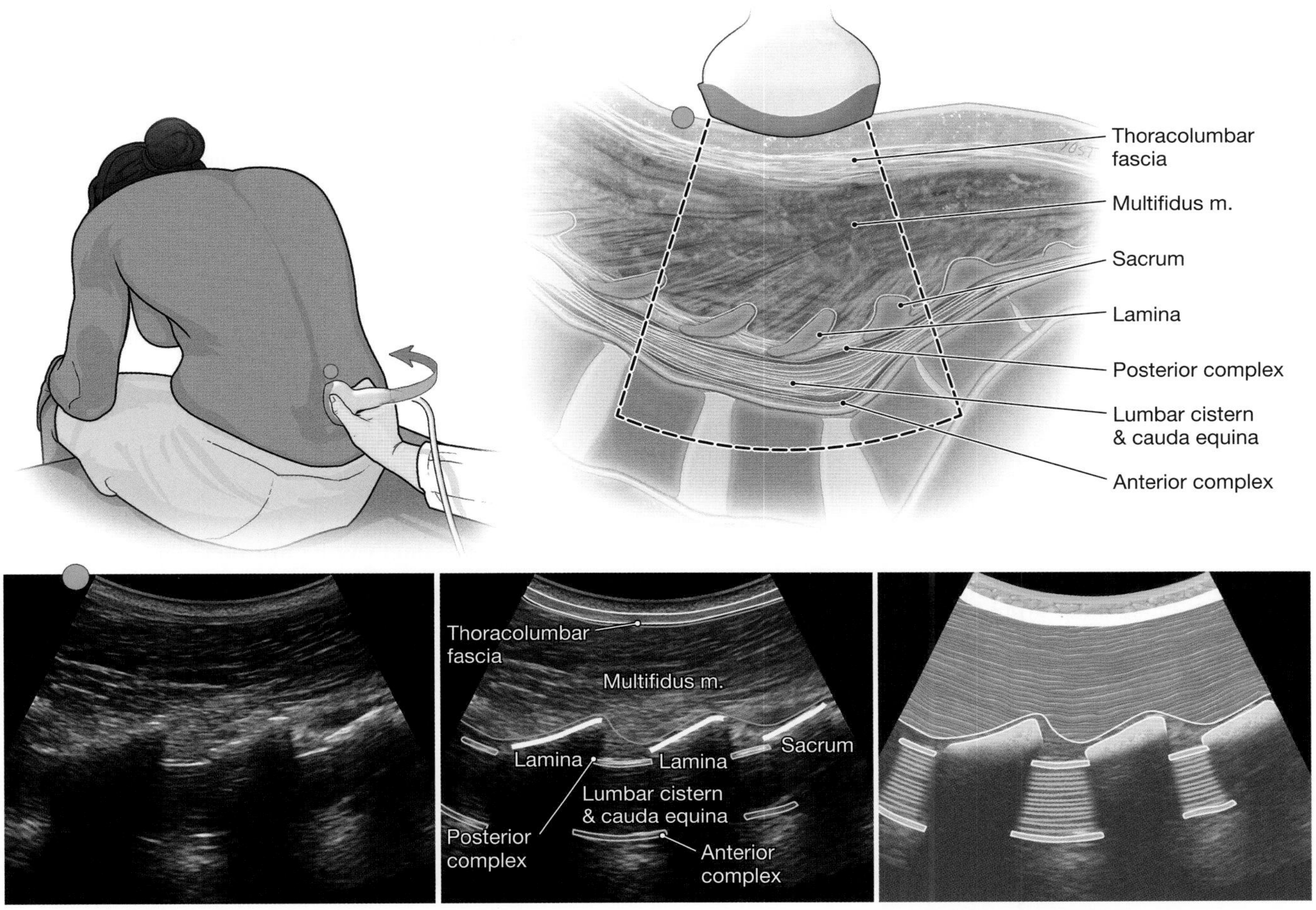

Figure 13.4 Longitudinal (parasagittal oblique) view of the laminae, interlaminar spaces, and thecal sac with overlying multifidus muscle. Posterior complex: Ligamentum flavum, extradural fat, and posterior aspect of dura mater. Anterior complex: Anterior aspect of the dura mater, extradural fat, and posterior longitudinal ligament.

Pericardiocentesis

Introduction

Pericardial tamponade is a life-threatening condition that necessitates prompt diagnosis and treatment. Pericardiocentesis is a procedure used for draining excessive fluid buildup in the pericardial space. Pericardial effusions can arise from various causes such as trauma, malignancy, infections, or myocardial rupture. When these effusions progress to cardiac tamponade, there is a significant rise in pericardial pressure, hindering the heart's expansion. Patients typically exhibit Beck triad of symptoms, including low blood pressure; distended neck veins; and distant, muffled heart sounds. Initially, compensatory mechanisms such as increased heart rate, arterial vasoconstriction, and venoconstriction help maintain cardiac output. However, when these compensatory mechanisms fail, cardiac filling and output are critically compromised, leading to shock and cardiac arrest. Even draining a small amount of fluid from the pericardial space can help stabilize hemodynamically unstable patients. Over the years, the techniques for pericardiocentesis have significantly evolved. The use of ultrasound guidance has reduced the complication rate associated with the procedure.

Indications

SUBXIPHOID 4-CHAMBER VIEW
FIG. 13.5

Pericardiocentesis can be used for both diagnostic and therapeutic purposes.

Diagnostic Pericardiocentesis

Diagnostic pericardiocentesis is a nonurgent procedure performed to extract fluid from the pericardial space for analysis. The obtained fluid can be instrumental in diagnosing various conditions, including malignancies and viral and bacterial pericarditis. Assessing the pH of the fluid can help distinguish between inflammatory and non-inflammatory processes. The fluid can also be cultured to identify bacterial infections or examined for the presence of neoplastic cells.

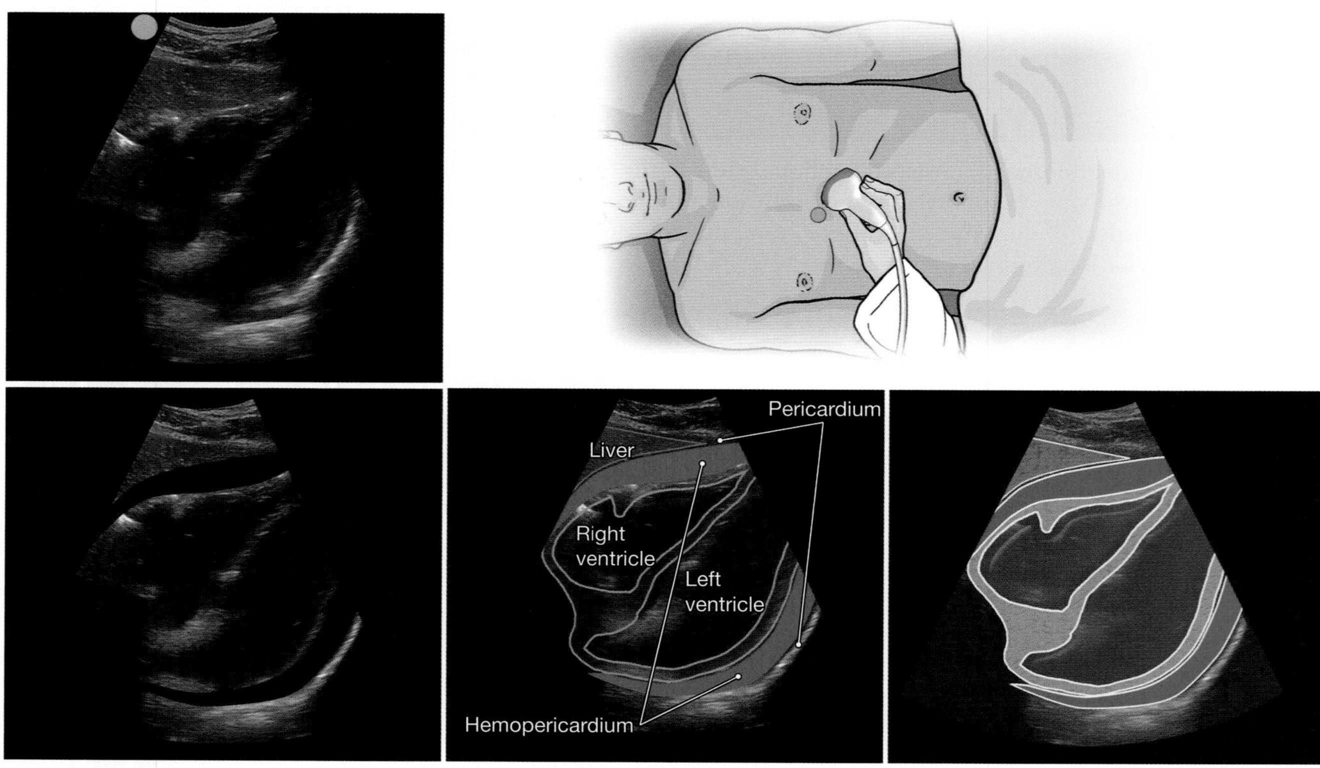

Figure 13.5 Upper panels: normal subxiphoid 4-chamber view of the heart and pericardium. Lower panels: Artist's rendering of the same view with free fluid in the pericardial space.

Therapeutic Pericardiocentesis

Therapeutic pericardiocentesis can be performed as an urgent or nonurgent procedure. In nonurgent cases, it may be used for palliative or preventive purposes. In urgent situations, where patients remain hypotensive despite fluid resuscitation, therapeutic drainage becomes necessary. Indications for therapeutic pericardiocentesis include pulseless electrical activity, non-hemorrhagic and hemorrhagic pericardial effusions. Although some experts argue that traumatic cardiac tamponade should be treated with immediate thoracotomy, pericardiocentesis can provide temporary relief and delay the need for definitive surgical intervention. Even the removal of as little as 10 to 50 mL of fluid can significantly improve the cardiac output. However, due to the rapid reaccumulation of blood in traumatic hemorrhagic tamponade, pericardiocentesis alone is not considered a definitive procedure. In cases of traumatic cardiac tamponade, pericardiocentesis should be followed immediately by a thoracotomy procedure.

Contraindications

Performing pericardiocentesis in hemodynamically unstable patients does not have contraindications. However, contraindications include thrombocytopenia, anticoagulant therapy, a recent thoracoabdominal surgery, presence of prosthetic heart valves, pacemakers, cardiac pacemakers, and inadequate facilities for cardiorespiratory resuscitation in patients with pericardial effusions that have not yet developed into tamponade.

Procedure (Parasternal Approach)

PARASTERNAL LONG-AXIS VIEW
FIG. 13.6

Ultrasound-guided pericardiocentesis using the parasternal method is considered the most stable and controlled approach. It ensures avoidance of important structures such as the diaphragm, phrenic nerve, and liver.

Place the patient in a supine position. Monitor the patient's vital signs, CVP, and electrocardiogram (ECG) throughout the procedure. Use the ultrasound transducer to identify the optimal entry site wherein the fluid collection is most prominent and closest to the transducer. For the parasternal approach, the entry site should be in the 5th intercostal space just next to the sternum. Caution should be exercised to avoid injury to the internal thoracic artery, which lies laterally to the entry site. Advance the needle over the superior border of the rib to prevent damage to the neurovascular bundle located along the inferior border. Insert the sheathed needle at the designated entry site, guiding it safely through the layers toward the fluid collection using ultrasound guidance. Aspirate during needle advancement to confirm when the fluid is reached. Once the needle reaches the fluid, advance it an additional 2 mm and then slide the sheath over the needle. The needle can be withdrawn at this point. Injecting agitated saline can be performed to confirm correct placement of the sheath in the pericardial space. If bubbles are visualized on ultrasound within the pericardial space, it indicates proper positioning of the sheath.

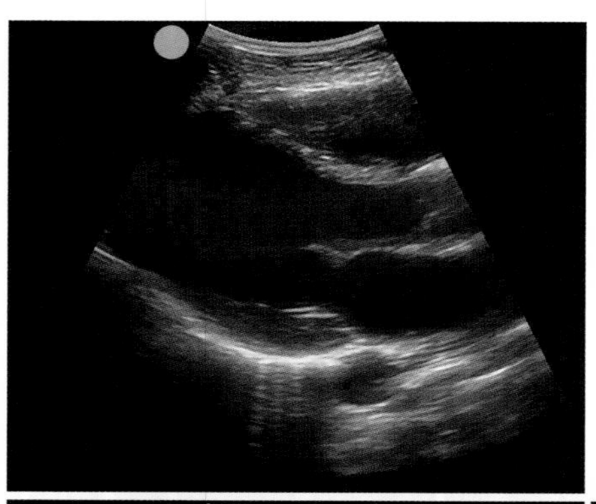

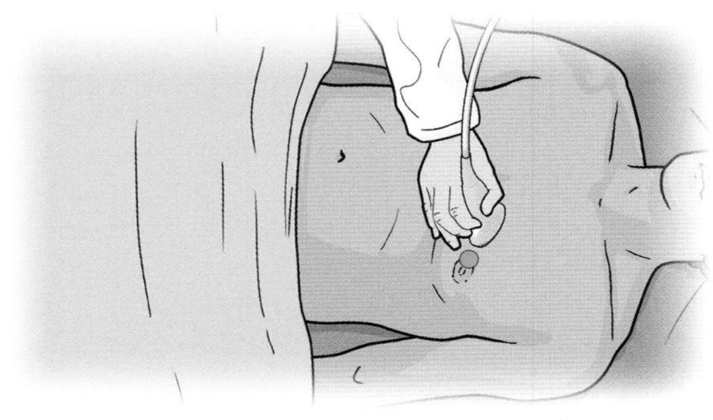

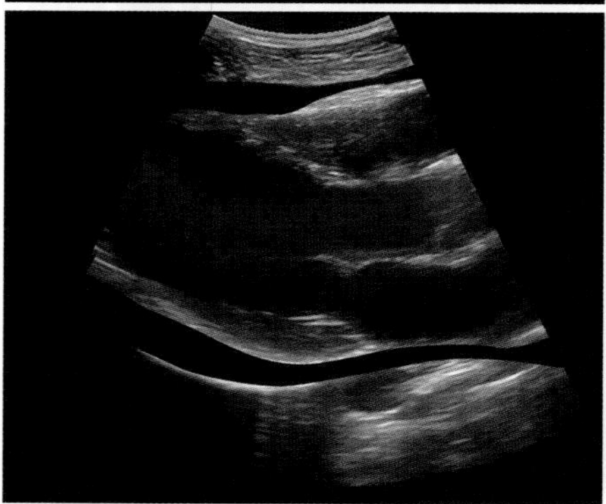

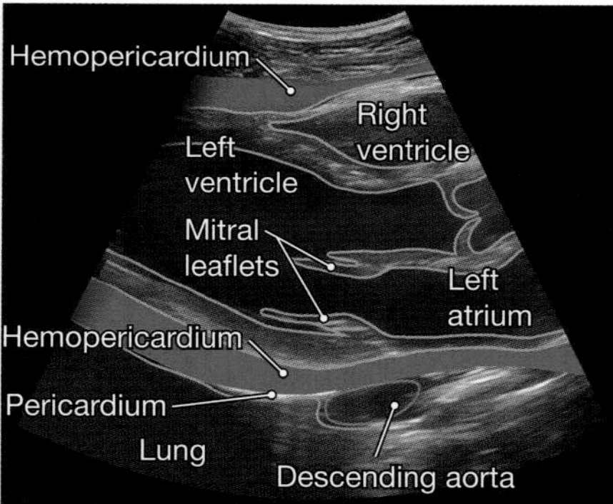

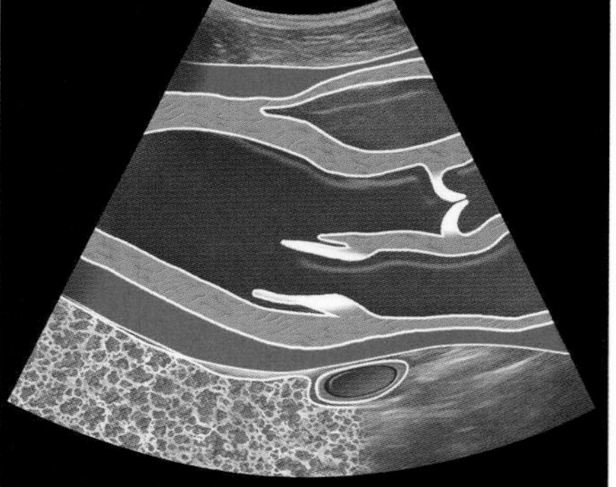

Figure 13.6 Upper panels: normal parasternal long-axis view of the heart and pericardium. Lower panels: Artist's rendering of the same view with free fluid in the pericardial space.

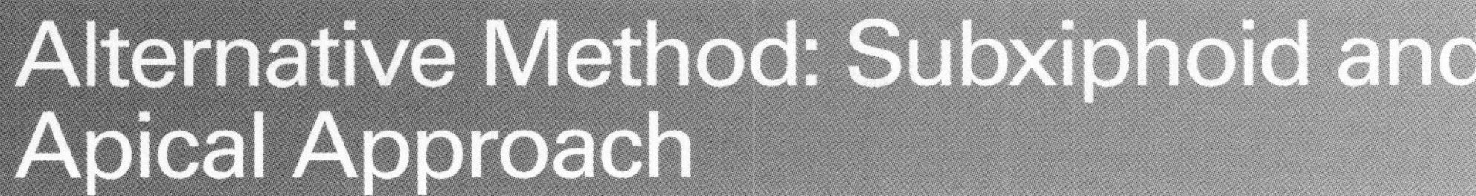

Alternative Method: Subxiphoid and Apical Approach

Subxiphoid Approach

The subxiphoid approach is recommended for pericardiocentesis when echocardiography is not readily accessible. In this approach, the needle is inserted at a 45° angle between the xiphisternum (the lower part of the sternum) and the left costal margin (the lower edge of the ribcage) in a transverse plane. The needle is directed toward the left shoulder and passed through several layers, including the skin, superficial fascia, anterior rectus sheath, left rectus abdominis muscle, posterior rectus sheath, diaphragm, and fibrous pericardium.

Apical Approach

The apical approach of pericardiocentesis is not recommended in emergencies but is utilized in nonurgent cases. In this approach, the needle is inserted within the intercostal space, about 1 cm away from the apex beat of the heart. The needle is directed toward the patient's right shoulder. This region has a superficial location of the pericardial sac and a relatively larger transverse diameter, while important structures like the pleura are absent. The apical approach offers several advantages over the parasternal and subxiphoid approaches. The pericardial sac is situated superficially, and smaller vessels are located near the apex. Additionally, compared to the right ventricle, the left ventricle has thicker walls, making it less susceptible to serious punctures.

Anatomic Pitfalls

Pericardium: The pericardial sac has the capacity to stretch and accommodate 2 to 3 L of fluid. Chronic fluid accumulation gradually increases the intrapericardial pressure, while even a small acute accumulation of around 100 mL can cause a sudden rise in the pressure. This can lead to cardiac tamponade and a rapid decrease in the cardiac output. The pericardium is extensively innervated by the phrenic nerve, which explains why touching the pericardium with a needle elicits severe pain in patients.

Liver: The left lobe of the liver is in close proximity to the xiphisternum. While performing the subxiphoid approach, it is important to insert the needle at a 45° angle relative to the horizontal plane to avoid injuring the liver. Entering at an angle lower than 45° may result in liver or stomach injury. By advancing the needle at the appropriate angle, it enters the diaphragmatic pericardium, bypassing the diaphragm and the contents of the peritoneal cavity.

Right Ventricle and Marginal Artery: During the parasternal and subxiphoid approaches, there is a risk of encountering the thin-walled right ventricle as the needle enters the pericardium at the diaphragmatic pericardium, which is in close proximity to the acute angle of the right ventricle. The marginal artery follows along the acute angle of the right ventricle. This proximity between the diaphragmatic pericardium, right ventricle, and marginal artery increases the risk of right ventricle perforation and potential injury to the marginal artery.

Knee Joint Aspiration

Introduction

Arthrocentesis refers to the procedure where the knee joint is punctured and the synovial fluid is aspirated. This technique is important for evaluating the knee joint that is causing pain, inflammation, and swelling, and it can be carried out in the emergency department of surgical theater.

Anatomy

The knee joint involves the connection between the lower end of the femur and the upper part of the tibia forming a biaxial condylar synovial joint. The synovium, a thin membrane that produces the synovial fluid, covers the femur in a saddle-like shape. It extends forward and upward on the femur behind the patella, and then descends backward and downward on the back surface of the femur. It also covers the sides of the cruciate ligaments and reaches down to the tibial articular surfaces. The synovium also provides some coverage to the proximal fibula. The front part of the synovial saddle rests on the front lower part of the femur behind the patella, curving upward toward the patella. The space between the femoral condyles and behind the patella, particularly when the knee is extended, usually allows for easier aspiration of the synovial fluid because there is a lesser chance of encountering excessive synovial tissue or contacting a bony surface.

Indications

Knee joint aspiration is performed in various situations such as the following: Diagnostic purposes for septic arthritis, arthritis caused by crystal deposits, systemic rheumatic disorders (Gout and pseudogout), and cases of unknown inflammation. For traumatic injuries such as joint effusion resulting from bone or ligament damage. Acute hemarthrosis (an inflammatory reaction can follow the bleed, resulting in the proliferation of the synovium), where knee joint aspiration is performed to relieve painful joint bleeding. For painful effusions and medication administration (intra-articular corticosteroid injections) for acute or chronic arthritis. In addition, synovial fluid obtained through knee joint aspiration holds significant diagnostic value that can provide information on viscosity, glucose levels, total protein, uric acid, lactate, cell count, rheumatoid factor, mucin clots, and crystals. The synovial fluid can undergo testing for gram stain culture, tuberculosis, and fungal cultures.

Contraindications

Knee joint aspiration is a safe invasive procedure with only absolute contraindication of overlying cellulitis or skin infection. Other relative contraindications include bleeding disorders, overlying burn, prosthetic joints, and potential spread of internal infections from superficial bacteria.

Anatomy of Knee Joint Aspiration

KNEE JOINT EFFUSION
Longitudinal
FIG. 13.7

Position the patient with their knee joint either fully extended or slightly flexed at an angle of 15° to 20°, depending on patient's comfort. Once the patient is in position, gently touch and locate with the ultrasound the superomedial part of the patella. Identify the joint space located behind the patella. Place the needle at a 45° angle on the sagittal plane, approximately 1 cm behind the identified landmark. There will be a small resistance as the needle penetrates the joint capsule. Once the needle is inside the joint space, aspiration of fluid can be performed. Similarly, instead of draining the fluid, an intra-articular medication can be administered.

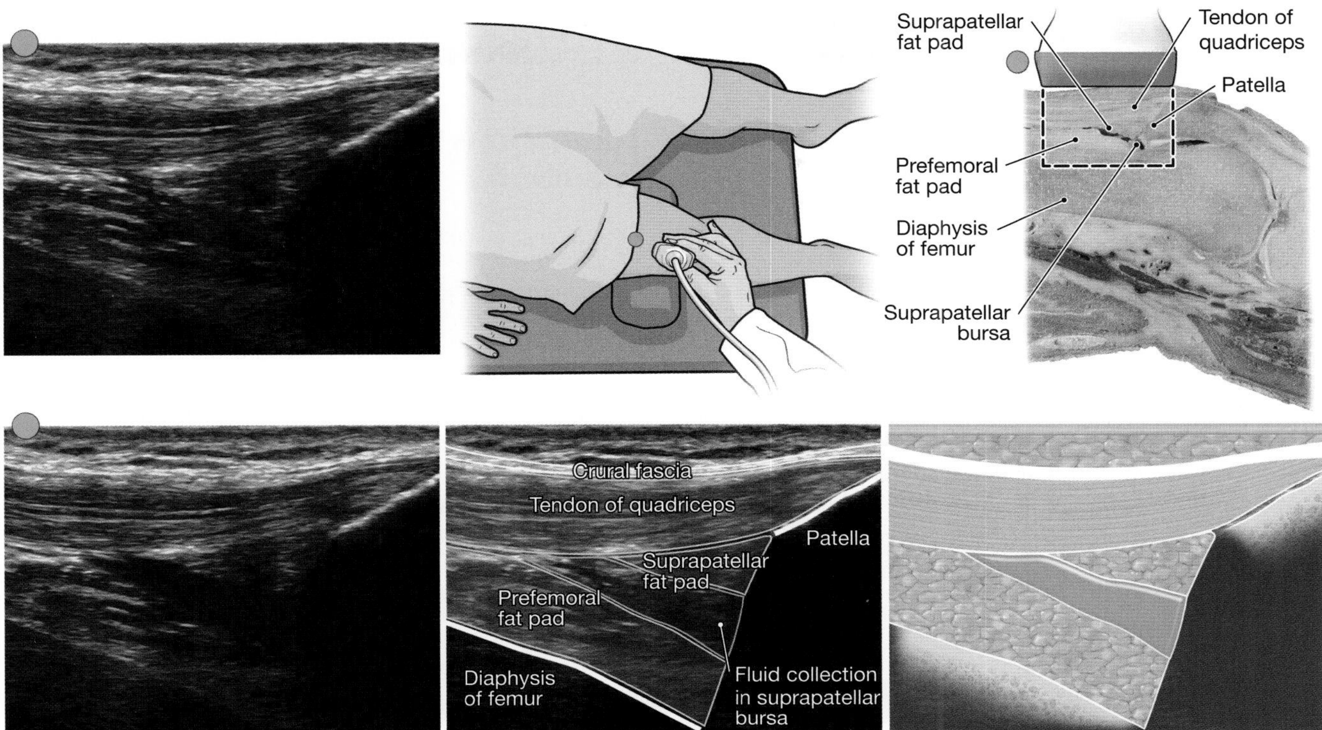

Figure 13.7 Upper panels: Normal longitudinal view of the suprapatellar knee. Lower panels: Artist's rendering of the same view with a knee joint effusion seen in the suprapatellar bursa.

Shoulder Aspiration

In the context of shoulder pathology, ultrasound has proven to be highly effective in diagnosing, injecting, and aspirating the shoulder joint. It outperforms magnetic resonance imaging (MRI) in diagnosing rotator cuff pathologies, especially full-thickness rotator cuff tears. Ultrasound-guided joint injections have shown better success rates compared to relying solely on bony landmarks, particularly in small joints. This approach minimizes complications and the associated increased morbidity resulting from incorrect injections. Ultrasound-guided aspiration of the shoulder joint, especially for conditions such as calcific tendonitis, has provided significant symptomatic relief when conservative therapy has failed.

Indications for Shoulder Aspiration/ Injection

GLENOHUMERAL JOINT EFFUSION
Transverse
FIG. 13.8

Ultrasound is highly recommended before performing any aspiration of the shoulder joint as it can detect fluid collections that may not be apparent during a clinical examination. Conditions such as obesity, inflammation, cellulitis, or pain can mask the presence of fluid, making it difficult to diagnose without imaging. Ultrasound also allows the examiner to identify areas of hypervascularity and differentiate between a solid soft-tissue mass and synovial fluid by applying compression with the ultrasound probe.

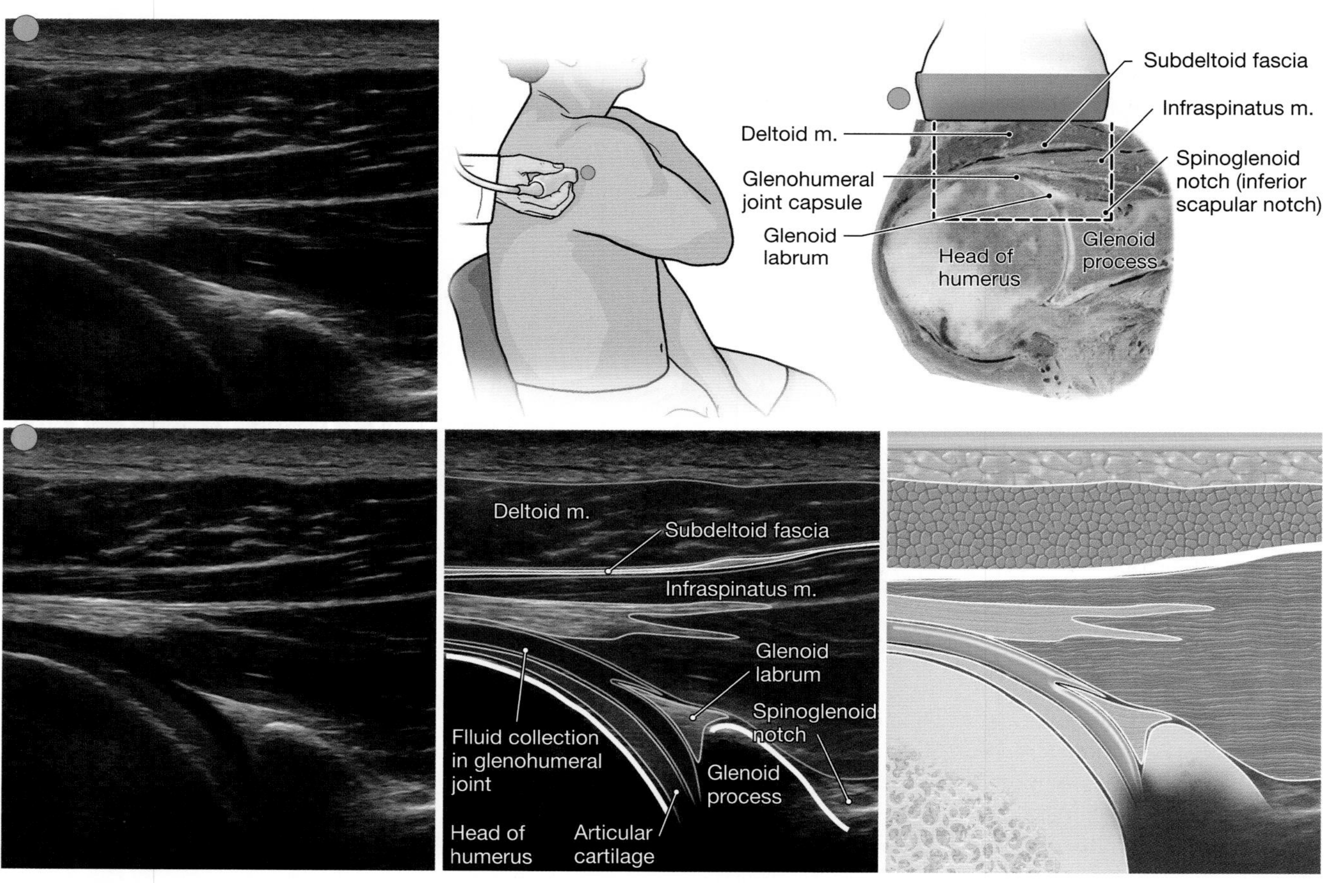

Figure 13.8 Upper panels: normal transverse view of the posterior aspect of the glenohumeral joint. Lower panels: Artist's rendering of the same view with an effusion in the glenohumeral joint.

Calcific Tendonitis

Calcific deposit formation in and around the shoulder joint is a prevalent condition, particularly affecting the rotator cuff. Its occurrence varies widely in the general population, ranging from 2.7% to 63%. Despite numerous theories, the exact cause of this condition remains unknown. The prevailing theory suggests that reduced blood supply in a critical area plays a central role in triggering calcification. Typically, individuals experience gradual and chronic shoulder pain, with a higher prevalence among women than men. The condition is more commonly observed on the right side and tends to affect individuals between the ages of 30 and 50. Symptoms can range from no apparent signs to significant discomfort, irrespective of the size, shape, or location of the calcification. A diagnosis can be easily established through clinical examination and radiographic findings. Patients often report restricted movement and experience pain during strenuous activities, particularly in the latter part of the day.

Calcification commonly occurs in the rotator cuff, with the supraspinatus muscle near its insertion being the most frequently affected, followed by the infraspinatus, teres minor, and subscapularis muscles. Conservative treatment options are typically considered initially, including the use of nonsteroidal anti-inflammatory drugs (NSAIDs) and physical therapy. If pain persists, local steroid injections may be recommended. However, the preferred treatment method nowadays is needle aspiration of the calcium deposits, which has shown positive outcomes such as pain reduction, improved range of motion, and patient satisfaction in the short term.

For accurate assessment, a high-frequency ultrasound with a frequency of 7.5 to 12 MHz is recommended. The initial setting should be at 7.5 MHz, which can be adjusted based on the patient's body habitus. It is important to examine both shoulders for comparison. It is advised to scan the normal or less-symptomatic side first to establish a baseline for comparison with the symptomatic shoulder. This approach helps identify subtle abnormalities and allows for disregarding findings that may be considered abnormal in the symptomatic shoulder if they are also present in the asymptomatic side.

The procedure for treating calcification involves more than simple aspiration and includes a lavage step. The choice of an anterior or posterior approach depends on the location of the calcification and the most convenient path to access it. In the posterior approach, the patient sits upright, and the physician punctures the joint capsule laterally to the glenohumeral joint along the medial border of the humeral head, ensuring avoidance of the suprascapular nerve and circumflex blood vessels.

For the anterior approach, the patient lies supine, and ultrasound imaging is used for guiding the needle placement laterally to the coracoid process, avoiding the cephalic vein, axillary artery, and brachial plexus.

Once the skin is numbed, a 20-gauge needle is inserted toward the center of the calcification. It is essential to avoid using a smaller needle that may be blocked by the calcification or a larger needle that could potentially damage the overlying tendon. Initially, the calcium should not be immediately aspirated, as it may clog the needle. Instead, a 1% lidocaine solution is continuously injected in strong pulses to help break down the calcification. Once fluid is observed inside the calcification, repeated aspiration and lavage are performed until no more calcification is visible in the syringe. This process usually takes around 15 to 20 minutes, depending on the size of the calcification.

Complication rates are generally low, with the most common being a mild vasovagal reaction. Therefore, caution should be exercised, and patients should be in a seated position to mitigate this potential risk.

Acromioclavicular Joint Injuries

Currently, approximately 40% of all shoulder injuries in sports are attributed to the acromioclavicular joint (ACJ), ranging from sprains to dislocations. Injuries to the ACJ typically occur due to a direct impact that causes dislocation, rendering the younger generation and males more susceptible.

The stability of the ACJ relies on various factors. The deltoid muscle plays a role in stabilizing the clavicle anteriorly, whereas the trapezius muscle stabilizes the acromion posteriorly. Ligaments surrounding the joint provide additional stability. The acromioclavicular ligaments primarily resist superior and posterior displacement, and the coracoclavicular ligaments come into play when greater force is applied, further resisting displacement. The coracoclavicular ligament specifically prevents forward and backward displacement caused by the scapula.

Ultrasound imaging of the shoulder is crucial for accurately diagnosing the severity of ACJ injuries, as treatment plans differ based on the degree of injury. The most common classification system for ACJ injuries categorizes them based on the torn ligaments and the extent of the tear. Type II injuries involve a sprain of the coracoclavicular ligaments and a tear of the acromioclavicular ligaments. Although steroid injections into the coracoclavicular ligament have been suggested to provide short-term relief, they do not have a significant effect on long-term healing.

Bursitis

The subacromial-subdeltoid (SA-SD) bursa, the largest bursa in the body, plays a crucial role in reducing friction within the highly mobile shoulder joint. Its size facilitates unrestricted movement of the rotator cuff in relation to the acromion bone and deltoid muscle. Additionally, it encloses the long head of the biceps tendon, protecting it from direct contact with bone and potential tearing. Pathological conditions affecting the bursa can be broadly classified as communicating or noncommunicating distention.

Communicating SA-SD bursitis typically involves communication between the bursa and the glenohumeral joint. In 90% of patients with this type of bursitis, a concurrent rotator cuff tear is present. This condition is characterized by fluid accumulation above the greater tuberosity and retraction of the supraspinatus tendon.

Noncommunicating bursitis occurs when the bursa itself is inflamed or distended, while maintaining its structural integrity. The most common cause is impingement syndrome or narrowing of the supraspinatus tendon. Initial treatment usually involves conservative approaches such as steroid injections to alleviate pain. If the pain becomes chronic, further consultation may be necessary. Bursitis can also result from a direct blow to the shoulder, leading to blood accumulation. This type of bursitis typically resolves on its own as the blood is broken down and reabsorbed by the body. Ultrasound imaging is vital in diagnosing this condition, and aspiration of the bursa without affecting the surrounding structures is essential.

A potential complication of the lavage therapy in the glenohumeral joint is the development of bursitis, as residual calcium deposits may travel to the bursa and cause inflammation. To mitigate this, several practitioners administer a steroid injection into the bursa following the lavage procedure.

To visualize the bursa effectively, the patient's arm is hyperextended and medially rotated. Insertion of the needle during the procedure is optimized by orienting the beveled side of the needle toward the transducer, allowing real-time visualization.

Elbow Joint Aspiration

Introduction

Arthrocentesis, also called joint aspiration, is a safe and minimally invasive procedure performed in clinical settings. It involves using a needle and syringe to extract the synovial fluid from the joint capsule. This procedure serves multiple purposes, including establishing a diagnosis, providing relief from discomfort, draining infected fluid or blood, and administering medication directly into the joint space. When used as a diagnostic aid, arthrocentesis is valuable in differentiating inflammatory arthropathies from conditions such as osteoarthritis or arthritis caused by crystals.

Recent research indicates that ultrasound-guided arthrocentesis is more effective compared to the traditional palpation-guided approach using anatomical landmarks. The utilization of ultrasonography has several advantages, including reducing procedural pain, increasing the success rate of arthrocentesis, obtaining a larger amount of synovial fluid, facilitating better joint decompression, and enhancing overall clinical outcomes. Ultrasonography enables direct visualization and guidance for needle insertion, or it indirectly aids in marking the targeted site for needle insertion and estimation of the depth and direction of placement.

Indications

Before performing arthrocentesis on the elbow joint, it is important to differentiate between periarticular entities, such as bursitis, cellulitis, contusion, and tendonitis, and articular processes. Periarticular conditions generally limit the active range of motion more than the passive range and are localized to a specific area. In contrast, articular processes affect both the active and passive ranges of motion and often cause pain and swelling throughout the joint. Elbow joint aspiration serves both diagnostic and therapeutic purposes.

Diagnostic Elbow Joint Aspiration

ELBOW JOINT EFFUSION
Longitudinal
FIG. 13.9

Elbow joint aspiration is performed to diagnose various conditions including chronic arthritis (such as rheumatoid arthritis and osteoarthritis), crystal-induced arthritis (such as gout and pseudogout), septic arthritis, unidentified joint inflammation, joint effusion, and hemarthrosis. The synovial fluid obtained from the aspiration is highly valuable for diagnosis. It can be analyzed for various parameters including viscosity, glucose levels, total protein, uric acid, lactate, cell count, rheumatoid factor, mucin clots, and presence of crystals. Additionally, the fluid sample can be analyzed for Gram stain, and culture to identify bacteria, mycobacteria, and fungi.

Therapeutic Elbow Joint Aspiration

This involves effusion of blood to relieve pain; improvement in joint mobilization; injection of medications such as corticosteroids, antibiotics, or anesthetics; and draining of septic effusions.

Procedure

Traditionally, elbow joint aspiration has been performed using external anatomical landmarks. A medial approach is generally advised against, so a needle is advanced into the joint space via a lateral approach, using the center of the anconeus triangle as a landmark. However, if available, ultrasonography can facilitate a lateral, posterior, or medial approach. The lateral approach is preferred for arthrocentesis. On ultrasound, a joint capsule effusion appears as hypoechoic or anechoic fluid collection that superficially displaces the fat pad.

Ultrasound-Guided Lateral Approach for Elbow Joint Arthrocentesis

HUMERORADIAL JOINT
Longitudinal
FIG. 13.10

Follow sterile procedures and position the patient sitting up with the affected arm abducted, resting at the patient's side, and pronated and flexed to 90°. Examine the nonaffected elbow with ultrasound, and then compare it with the examination of the joint capsule of the affected elbow. The goal is to find the landmarks that form the anconeus triangle. Place the linear, transducer of 7.5 MHz longitudinally along the proximal forearm, parallel to the long axis of the radius, and with the probe marker toward the patient's head visualize the rounded radial head, lateral epicondyle, and capitulum. The lateral radiocapitellar joint space can be assessed for effusion. The common extensor tendon is superficial to the radiocapitellar joint space and can be easily identified and avoided when seen on ultrasound. Once the effusion has been clearly visualized, ensure that the center of the probe is located at the middle of the effusion. Inject 5 mL of a local anesthetic just below the center of the transducer. Use a 5- or 10-mL syringe to enter the skin at the midpoint of the transducer and at a 90° angle to the skin. Pay attention to the depth of the joint capsule effusion during the procedure. Actively aspirate the syringe as the needle advances.

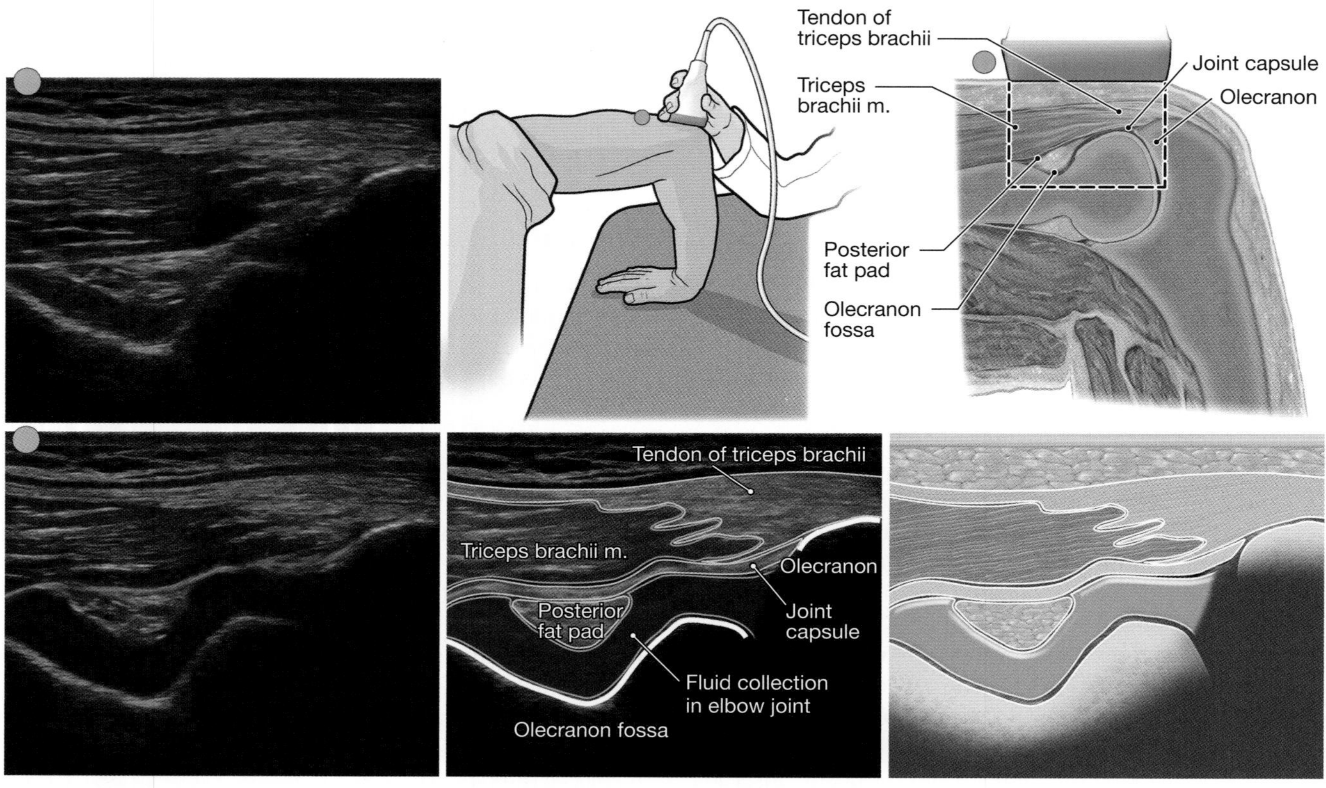

Figure 13.9 Upper panels: normal longitudinal view of the olecranon fossa and posterior fat pad at the posterior aspect of the elbow joint. Lower panels: Artist's rendering of the same view with an effusion in the elbow joint.

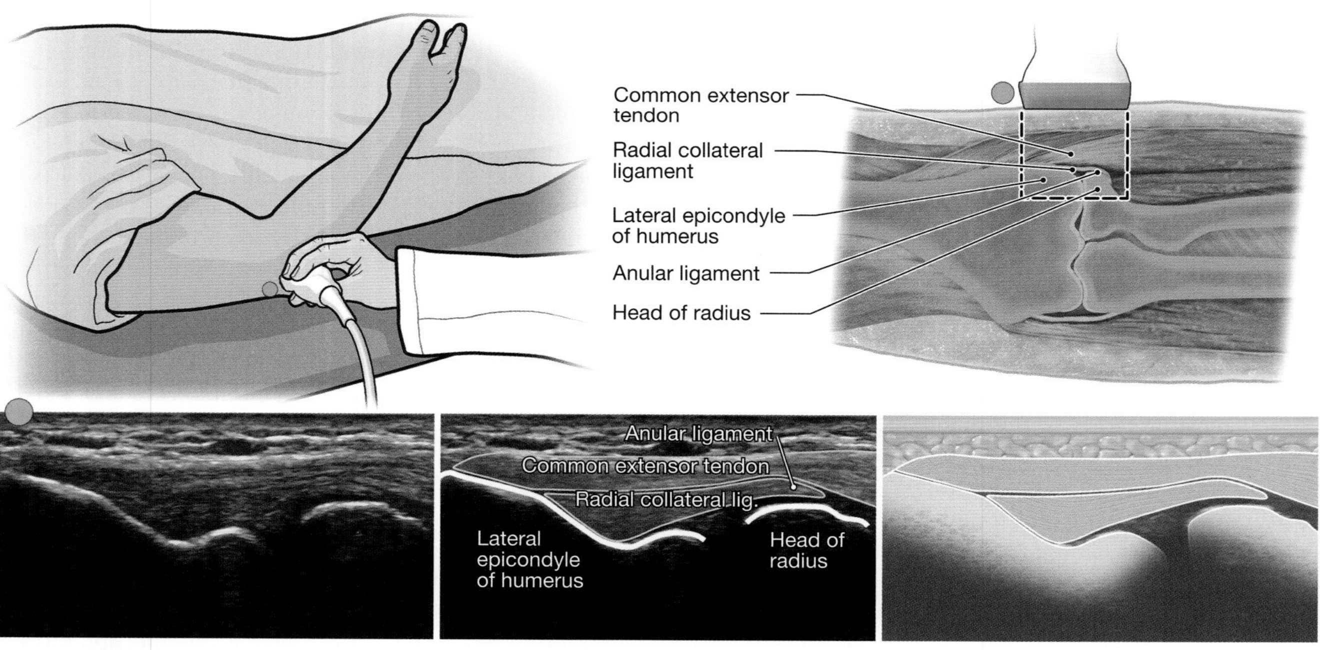

Figure 13.10 Lateral view of the humeroradial joint, common extensor tendon and radial collateral ligament.

Multiple Choice Questions

1. A 67-year-old man is brought to the emergency department because of severe chest pain. His blood pressure is 92/63 Hg, pulse is 110/min, and respirations are 25. Physical examination shows muffled heart sounds and jugular vein distention. ECG shows ST segment elevations and labs show elevated troponins confirming a myocardial infarction. Cardiac tamponade is suspected and an emergency pericardiocentesis is performed. At which of the following locations should the needle be inserted under ultrasound guidance to relieve the cardiac tamponade?

   A. Right 7th intercostal space in the midaxillary line
   B. Left 5th intercostal space at the sternal border
   C. Right 3rd intercostal space, 1 in lateral to the sternum
   D. Left 6th intercostal space in the midclavicular line
   E. At the triangle of auscultation

2. A 60-year-old woman with a history of lung cancer is scheduled to receive chemotherapy. The physician plans to insert a central venous catheter for administration of chemotherapy using an ultrasound-guided supraclavicular approach. Which of the following is the most common complication associated with this approach?

   A. Infection
   B. Pneumothorax
   C. Hematoma
   D. Atrial fibrillation
   E. Thrombosis

3. A 50-year-old woman comes to the physician because of an acute knee pain and swelling playing basketball with her friends. Her knee appears increasingly swollen, and painful to palpation. Her knee mobility is minimal. A knee joint aspiration is decided to be performed under ultrasound guidance. Into which of the following structures should the needle be inserted?

   A. Superomedial part of the patella
   B. Suprapatellar bursa
   C. Prepatellar bursa
   D. Inferolateral part of the patella
   E. Superolateral part of the patella

4. A 22-year-old woman is brought to the emergency department because of symptoms and sign of meningitis. A lumbar puncture is performed with the aid of an ultrasound to obtain cerebrospinal fluid for culture analysis. As the needle is penetrating through the tissues of the back, a first pop is felt and then a second pop. The second pop indicates that the needle is introduced into the subarachnoid space. From which of the following tissues is the first pop the result of the needle passing?

   A. Dura mater
   B. Interspinous ligament
   C. Ligamentum flavum
   D. Posterior longitudinal ligament
   E. Supraspinous ligament

5. A 60-year-old man comes to the physician because of a 2-month history of a painful right shoulder. Physical examination shows tenderness and loss of muscle mass over the rotator cuff, loss of shoulder range of motion, and stiffness of the shoulder. An ultrasound examination confirms the diagnosis of calcific tendonitis. An ultrasound-guided posterior approach involving aspiration and lavage is performed. To perform this procedure accurately under ultrasound guidance, into which of the following structures should the needle be inserted?

   A. Lateral to the glenohumeral joint
   B. Lateral to the subacromial bursa
   C. At the supraspinatus tendon
   D. Medial to the acromioclavicular joint
   E. Lateral to the infraspinatus muscle

Answers to Multiple Choice Questions

3 Back

1. **A. Arachnoid mater**
2. **C. Ligamentum flavum**
3. **E. Supraspinous**
4. **A. Between semispinalis capitis and obliquus capitis inferior, 2 cm medial to the mastoid process**

4 Upper Limb

1. **E. Ulnar collateral ligament**
2. **D. Posterior cord**
3. **D. Supraspinatus**
4. **A. Biceps brachii, long head**
5. **E. Pronator teres**
6. **D. Radial nerve**
7. **C. Median nerve**
8. **D. Guyon's canal**
9. **E. Superficial radial nerve**
10. **B. Pronator syndrome**

5 Lower Limb

1. **D. Midway between the medial malleolus and the calcaneus**
2. **A. Descending branch of the lateral circumflex femoral**
3. **E. Plantar flexion of the foot**
4. **A. Deep fibular**
5. **B. Cutaneous branch of deep fibular**
6. **A. The femoral vein lies medial to the femoral artery**

6 Thorax: Chest Wall and Pleura; Breast

1. **B. Second**
2. **D. Cupula**
3. **A. Parietal pleura**
4. **E. Between the parietal and visceral layers of the pleura**
5. **C. Superior to the upper border of the rib**
6. **A. Right tension pneumothorax**

Answers to Multiple Choice Questions

7 Heart

1. **E. Apex of the heart**
2. **D. Right second intercostal space near the lateral border of the sternum**
3. **E. Conal branch of right coronary artery**
4. **A. Right ventricle**
5. **A. Mitral**
6. **D. Azygos vein**

8 Abdomen

1. **C. Pelvic brim**
2. **B. Ilioinguinal**
3. **C. The common bile duct**
4. **C. Inferior border of the liver, cystic duct, common hepatic duct**
5. **A. Cystic artery**
6. **C. Pancreas**
7. **E. Ileum**
8. **D. Greater sac**
9. **B. Hartmann's pouch**
10. **E. Rectouterine pouch of (Douglas)**

9 Female Pelvis

1. **D. Rectouterine pouch**
2. **A. Ovarian**
3. **E. Ureter**
4. **D. Ureter**

10 Male Pelvis

1. **E. Lumbar**
2. **D. Seminal vesicles**
3. **C. General somatic efferent from pudendal**
4. **E. Superficial inguinal**

11 Neck, Face, Eye

1. **B. Marginal mandibular branch of facial**
2. **C. Recurrent laryngeal**
3. **B. Right hypoglossal**
4. **A. The interval between the sternal and clavicular heads of the sternocleidomastoid muscle**
5. **A. Inferior thyroid artery**
6. **D. Cricothyroid**
7. **B. Lingual**
8. **B. The cricothyroid membrane, which is located between the thyroid cartilage and the cricoid cartilage below**
9. **C. Jugulodigrastric**
10. **E. Submental**

12 Focused Assessment With Sonography for Trauma (FAST)

1. **A. Parasternal long axis**
2. **A. Hepatorenal**
3. **A. Absence of pleural sliding**
4. **D. Spleen**
5. **D. Right ventricle**
6. **A. Rectouterine pouch (of Douglas)**

13 Clinical Applications

1. **B. Left fifth intercostal space at the sternal border**
2. **B. Pneumothorax**
3. **A. Superomedial part of the patella**
4. **C. Ligamentum flavum**
5. **A. Lateral to the glenohumeral joint**

Glossary

Abdominal aorta: Part of the descending aorta and the largest artery in the abdomen.

Abdominal aortic aneurysm: Dilatations of the abdominal aorta of greater than 50% of its proximal normal segment (>3 cm).

Abdominal convex/curved probe: Low-to-intermediate frequency (2-5 MHz) probes with a curved face and a "footprint" of typically 4 to 6 cm (the side-to-side dimension of the probe face). Commonly used for general-purpose abdominal imaging, but also for other applications such as transabdominal pelvic imaging, obstetrical imaging, and some musculoskeletal imaging such as spine and hip joint.

Abductor pollicis brevis muscle: Located in the hand between the wrist and the base of the thumb. Main function is to abduct (move away) the thumb from the palm.

Accessary nerve (CN XI): A superficial nerve of the posterior triangle of the neck; the 11th cranial nerve. This nerve innervates only two muscles: the sternocleidomastoid and trapezius muscles.

Acoustic impedance: A property of the tissue through which sound waves are propagating related to the resistance sound encounters as it passes through that tissue.

Acromioclavicular joint: A small synovial joint between the anteromedial surface of the acromion and the lateral end of the clavicle. The joint is enclosed by a capsule, which is reinforced by a thickening along its subcutaneous superior surface, the acromioclavicular ligament.

Acute appendicitis: Acute inflammation of the appendix typically resulting from blockage of the lumen by fecalith (a hard, stony mass of feces that occurs in the intestinal tract).

Adductor muscles: Muscles that move a structure such as a limb or part of a limb toward the middle of the body.

Adductor pollicis muscle: A muscle in the hand that pulls the thumb toward the palm.

Adrenal cortex: The outer part of the adrenal gland (the inner part is the adrenal medulla), which has three separate layers. The most superficial layer is the zona glomerulosa, the middle layer is the zona fasciculata, and the deepest layer is the zona reticularis. Each layer of the adrenal cortex produces steroid hormones that are fundamental to maintaining homeostasis within the body.

Adrenal gland: Situated at the superior medial pole of the kidney, this endocrine gland is divided anatomically into a cortex and a medulla. The cortex has three separate layers, each of which produces steroid hormones that are fundamental to maintaining homeostasis within the body.

Amplitude: One measure of the intensity of sound.

Anechoic: Black on the ultrasound display. Based on the degree of echogenicity, tissues or structures are described as hyperechoic (white on the ultrasound display), hypoechoic (gray on the ultrasound display), or anechoic (black on the ultrasound display).

Ankle joint: Formed between the distal ends of the leg bones, the tibia and fibula, and the talus.

Anteflexed: Referring to when the uterine cavity is bent slightly forward relative to the cervical canal.

Anterior cervical triangle: Contains the main blood supply for the head but also many cranial nerves and viscera such as the larynx and thyroid gland. The cervical triangle includes the hyoid, thyroid cartilage, and cricoid cartilage.

Anterior compartment tendons: Tendons in the front portion of space enclosed by the deep fascia of the leg.

Anterior superior iliac spine: Bony projection of the iliac bone anterior to (in front of) the iliac crest of the pelvis.

Anterior tibiofibular ligament: This ligament is located just above the ankle, deep within the leg and holds together the tibia and fibula (the two bones of the lower leg).

Glossary

Anteverted: Referring to the uterus when the cervical canal is turned anteriorly at approximately right angles to the vaginal canal.

Aorta: Main artery that originates in the heart and carries blood away from the heart and out to the rest of the body.

Apical 4-chamber view: Ultrasound view by putting the transducer on the apex of the heart, near the apical impulse.

Aponeurosis: A flat sheetlike tendon, which anchors a muscle or connects it with the part that the muscle moves.

Aqueous humor: Fluid secreted from the ciliary epithelium into the posterior chamber of the eye, which flows into the anterior chamber through the pupil.

Artifact: Refers to anatomically incorrect or misleading elements within ultrasound images based on machine assumptions about image forming. Common examples include reverberation or mirror image artifacts on an ultrasound image.

Atrioventricular node: A collection of specialized cardiac muscle fibers that compose the conduction tissue of the heart that convey electrical signals from the atria to the ventricular musculature, resulting in its contraction. Situated within the interatrial septum adjacent to the septal leaflet of the tricuspid valve. The atrioventricular node is continuous with the common atrioventricular bundle (of His), which passes through the connective tissue separating the atria from the ventricles into the interventricular septum.

Attenuation: Progressive loss of energy as ultrasound pulses propagate through tissues, mainly due to tissue absorption of sound energy (converted to heat) plus additional energy loss due to reflection and scattering.

Axilla: Armpit or underarm, the area of the arm through which vessels and nerves of the upper limb pass after leaving the neck.

Biceps brachii muscle: The 2-headed large muscle that lies on the front of the upper arm between the shoulder and the elbow.

Bifurcation: Separation or branching of something into two parts.

Bio-effects: A biological effect or result of, in this case, ultrasound energy.

Body of pancreas: The middle part of the pancreas between the tail and the head.

Broad ligament of the uterus: Originates at the lateral border of the uterus and reaches the lateral pelvic wall. It comprises two layers of peritoneum and functions to hold the uterus in position.

Buccal artery: A branch of the maxillary artery that supplies the buccinator muscles and the skin and mucous membrane of the cheek.

Buck fascia: Deep fascia of the penis, located over the penis and extending over the pubis and perineum as the deep perineal fascia.

Bundle of His: The common atrioventricular bundle that exits inferiorly from the atrioventricular node through the central fibrous body, curving inferior to the membranous septum to reach the superior margin of the muscular interventricular septum. The bundle of His passes for a short distance on the superior aspect of the interventricular septum and then divides into a broad left branch to the left ventricle and a narrow right branch, which passes into the right ventricle.

Calcaneal tendon: In the distal (lower part of the) leg, the tendon of soleus fuses with the overlying tendon of gastrocnemius to form the calcaneal tendon, which is commonly referred to as the "Achilles tendon."

Calcaneofibular ligament: One of the three components of the fibular collateral ligament of the ankle. Other two are the anterior talofibular and posterior talofibular ligaments.

Camper fascia: A superficial fatty layer, part of the fascia of the anterior abdominal wall. (The deep membranous layer is called Scarpa fascia.) Camper fascia lies over the inguinal ligament and merges with the superficial fascia of the thigh. It continues over the pubis and perineum as the superficial layer of the superficial perineal fascia.

Cardiac tamponade: Compression of the heart that occurs when the pericardial sac, which resists sudden distention, contains excessive fluid or blood.

Cardiac veins: These include the great cardiac vein, middle cardiac vein, small cardiac vein, smallest cardiac veins, and anterior cardiac veins. Cardiac veins return deoxygenated blood that contains metabolic waste products from the myocardium to the right atrium. This blood then flows back to the lungs for reoxygenation and removal of carbon dioxide.

Cardinal ligament of Mackenrodt: The cardinal ligament is composed of fibromuscular pelvic fascia and functions to provide support to the uterus and extends from the cervix and vagina to the pelvic walls, traveling inferior to the base of the broad ligament.

Carotid sinus: The expanded upper part of the common carotid artery, just before its bifurcation into internal and external carotid arteries, that contains nerve endings sensitive to stretch (such as pressure inside the artery), which, when stimulated, results in reflex slowing down of the heart rate, dilation of the blood vessels, and lowering of blood pressure.

Carpal tunnel: Osseofibrous passage from the wrist into the hand for the median nerve and the flexor tendons, created by the carpal bones and flexor retinaculum.

Caudate lobe of the liver: In the left lobe of the liver, it is the medial superior segment.

Celiac artery: First major branch of the abdominal aorta. Supplies oxygenated blood to the stomach, liver, spleen, part of the duodenum and pancreas, and part of the esophagus that descends into the abdomen.

Coccyx: Triangular bone formed by fusion of the last few spinal vertebrae. Located in the lower back near the sacrum.

Colle fascia: The membranous layer of the fascia of the anterior abdominal wall.

Common carotid artery: The left and right common carotid arteries originate from the aorta and brachiocephalic artery, respectively, and end by dividing into the external and internal carotid arteries.

Common extensor tendon: Attached to the lateral epicondyle of the humerus, this tendon functions as the shared upper attachment for several extensor muscles in the forearm.

Common fibular nerve: Begins at the top of the popliteal fossa, where the sciatic nerve splits into the tibial and common fibular nerves.

Common flexor tendon: Attaches to the medial epicondyle of the humerus, this tendon functions as the shared upper attachment point for several flexor muscles in the forearm.

Common hepatic artery: Arises from the celiac trunk and travels toward the liver along the superior border of the pancreas.

Common hepatic branches: The common hepatic artery branches into the proper hepatic artery, the gastroduodenal artery, and occasionally the right gastric artery.

Conjunctiva: The mucous membranes lining the deep surfaces of the eyelids, then covering the sclera (the white outer layer of the eye) to attach along the corneoscleral junction. The conjunctiva forms a sac when the eyelids are closed, which contains a thin layer of lacrimal gland secretions.

Cords of the plexus: Three large fiber bundles that derive from the anterior and posterior divisions of the brachial plexus. The cords are named by their position with respect to the axillary artery: posterior cord, medial cord, and branches (lateral/superior to the artery, medial/inferior to the artery between the artery and vein, and posterior/deep to the artery).

Coronal view/orientation: In an ultrasound procedure, the probe is placed on the body surface along an imaginary plane dividing the body (or part of the body being scanned) into anterior (front) and posterior (back) parts.

Cortex: The outermost or superficial layer of an organ.

Costocervical trunk: A branch of the subclavian artery.

Costodiaphragmatic recesses: Lower parts of the pleural spaces in which the costal and diaphragmatic parts of parietal pleura are not separated by intervening lung. These are potential spaces where fluid can accumulate.

Cricoid cartilage: Ring-shaped cartilage of the larynx that lies anterior to the sixth cervical vertebrae and marks the transition from larynx to trachea and pharynx to esophagus.

Cubital fossa: Triangular depression at the anterior elbow formed by the brachioradialis muscle laterally, the pronator teres muscle medially, and a line interconnecting the humeral epicondyles superiorly.

Cubital tunnel: Space of the dorsal medial elbow that allows passage of the ulnar nerve around the elbow. It is bordered by the medial epicondyle of the humerus, the olecranon process of the ulna, and the tendinous arch joining the humeral and ulnar heads of the flexor carpi ulnaris muscle.

Deep cervical fascia: These fasciae subdivide the deeper layers of the neck. Each of these layers contributes to the column of fascia known as the carotid sheath, which envelopes the carotid artery, internal jugular vein, and vagus nerve in the neck.

Glossary

Deep cervical lymph nodes: A group of cervical lymph nodes found near the internal jugular vein.

Deep radial nerve: One of two terminal branches of the radial nerve, which courses posteriorly and enters the substance of the supinator muscle, traveling between two layers of the muscle into the posterior compartment of the forearm, emerging as the posterior interosseous nerve.

Deltoid ligament: Referred to collectively as the deltoid ligament, the medial ligament complex of the ankle has 4 named parts—the anterior tibiotalar ligament, the tibionavicular ligament, the tibiocalcaneal ligament, and the posterior tibiotalar ligament.

Diffuse reflection: When sound waves encounter elements within tissues that are irregular or "bumpy" to sound waves (irregularities that are smaller than the wavelength of the ultrasound), diffuse reflection or *scattering* occurs. The scattered sound waves interfere with one another in complex patterns, giving rise to the speckled echo-texture of tissues such as liver, spleen, kidney, and myocardium.

Distal forearm: The end toward the wrist is called the distal end of the radius, the larger of the two bones of the forearm.

Doppler ultrasound: Ultrasound methods (including power Doppler, color flow Doppler, and spectral Doppler) that use high-frequency sound waves to measure the velocity of blood flow through veins and arteries.

Dorsal nasal artery: A terminal branch of the ophthalmic artery. Supplies the lacrimal sac and dorsum of the nose.

Ductus deferens: The muscular ducts that connect the epididymis of the testes with the ducts of the seminal vesicles, forming the ejaculatory ducts, which pass through the prostate gland and open into the prostatic urethra, conveying spermatozoa from the testes and seminal fluid from the seminal vesicles to the urethra where they are combined with prostatic fluid to form semen.

Duodenum: The first part of the small intestines consisting of a C-shaped tube surrounding the head of the pancreas and a final short segment joining the duodenum to the next part of the small intestines, the jejunum. Among the other three regions, the duodenum is the shortest (25 cm long or 12 fingerbreadths in length) but widest portion of the small intestine.

Echocardiography: Ultrasound imaging of the heart.

Echogenicity: Amount of ultrasound reflection by a tissue relative to surrounding tissues.

Ectopic pregnancy: Pregnancy in which the embryo is implanted outside the normal intrauterine location, eg, fallopian tube, abdomen, ovary, uterine interstitium, prior surgical scar, and cervix. Ultrasound will show an empty uterus. Approximately 95% of all ectopic pregnancies take place within the uterine tubes. Ectopic pregnancy accounts for approximately 2% of all pregnancies in the United States.

Ejaculation: The expulsion of semen from the urethra. Ejaculation is initiated by stimulation of the glans penis, which (at orgasm) results in contractions of the bulbospongiosus muscles compressing the urethra to expel the semen.

Elbow joint: Consists of three articulations between the humerus, radius, and ulna, all within a common joint capsule and synovial space.

Endometrial cancer: Most common type of uterine cancer, which develops from the endometrium of the uterus. Symptoms are similar to endometriosis, including vaginal bleeding, pain, and pelvic cramping. An ultrasound examination can detect both endometriosis and endometrial cancer.

Endometrial stripe: Endometrium on an ultrasound or magnetic resonance imaging looks like a hyperechoic (bright) stripe. Abnormally thick stripes or irregular nodules could be a sign of cancer.

Endometriosis: Mass of endometrial tissue found in different extraendometrial locations such as uterine walls and ovaries.

Epididymis: Convoluted duct extending from the testicle to the vas (ductus) deferens. Its main purpose is to store sperm and allow for its maturation prior to its release. The epididymis is made up of a head, body and tail. It is in the head and body of the epididymis where the spermatozoa are stored and undergo maturation.

Epigastric: The epigastric region is the upper central region of the abdomen and is located between the costal margins and the subcostal plane.

Epigastric hernia: Type of hernia situated at the anterolateral abdominal wall in which extraperitoneal fat or portion of the greater omentum or portion of the small intestines protrude through a defect in the linea alba superior to the umbilicus.

Erection: Erection is a process influenced by the parasympathetic nervous system and muscular contraction. Parasympathetic fibers from the pelvic splanchnic nerves cause arterial dilation of the erectile tissue, leading to engorgement and enlargement of the corpora cavernosa and corpus spongiosum.

Extensor compartments of the wrist (I-VI): The extensor tendons are divided into six extensor compartments: I: extensor pollicis brevis, abductor pollicis longus; II: extensor carpi radialis longus, extensor carpi radialis brevis; III: extensor pollicis longus compartments II and III are divided by Lister tubercle of the distal radius; IV: extensor digitorum, extensor indicis; V: extensor digiti minimi; VI: extensor carpi ulnaris runs in the groove of the ulnar head.

Extensor digiti minimi: The extensor muscle of the forearm that acts on the little finger. Its tendon crosses the wrist through extensor compartment V.

Extensor digitorum/extensor indicis: The extensor muscles of the forearm that act on the fingers and the index finger, respectively. Their tendons cross the wrist through extensor compartment IV.

External abdominal oblique muscle: Largest, outermost of the three flat muscles of the lateral abdominal wall.

External carotid arteries: Supply multiple branches to the exterior of the head and neck. The superficial temporal artery and the maxillary are the two terminal branches of the external carotid artery.

Facial artery: Extends from the external carotid artery, through or by the submandibular gland, over the mandible just anterior to the masseter muscle where its pulse is palpable and terminates as the angular artery traveling toward the medial canthus of the orbit.

Facial vein: Is the continuation of the angular vein at the level of the lower orbital margin. It receives the infraorbital and deep facial veins. Drains either in internal jugular vein or in the anterior branch of the retromandibular vein to form the common facial vein.

Fallopian (uterine) tubes: Pair of tubes along which eggs travel from the ovaries to the uterus. Fallopian tubes project laterally from the junction of the fundus and body of the uterus and open into the peritoneal cavity adjacent to the ovaries.

Fanning: Regarding an ultrasound probe, proper rotation and tilting (toggling) of the probe face are critical to view structures of interest in their true longitudinal axis or transverse axis (and to change a view from longitudinal to transverse, or vice versa) and to produce accurate images of structures that are not parallel to the skin surface.

Fasciae: Thin fibrous tissue that encloses an organ or muscle.

Fecalith: A hard, stony mass of feces that occurs in the intestinal tract and may cause appendicitis.

Female pelvis: The body cavity immediately below the abdomen that is located between the hip bones in a female. In females, the pelvis is typically smaller in size, denser, and less thick than in males. In comparison, the female pelvic cavity has less depth and width, the pubic arch (also known as the subpubic angle) is greater in size, and the greater sciatic notch is broader.

Femoral artery: Continuation of the external iliac artery as it passes under the inguinal ligament. Lies just medial to the femoral nerve in the femoral triangle.

Femoral triangle: Anatomical region of the upper third of the thigh. The main contents of the triangle are, from lateral to medial, the femoral nerve and branches, the femoral artery and branches, the femoral vein and tributaries, and deep inguinal lymph nodes and lymphatic channels (within the femoral canal).

Femoral trochlea: Femoral articular surface for the patella. The femoral condyles, separated posteriorly and inferiorly by the intercondylar fossa, are joined anteriorly to form the femoral trochlea.

Femoral vein: The femoral vein lies just medial to the femoral artery in the femoral triangle and continues as the external iliac vein as it passes under the inguinal ligament.

Femoral vessels: Blood vessels (femoral artery and femoral vein) that pass under the inguinal ligament and through the femoral triangle and then into the adductor (subsartorial) canal down the length of the thigh until behind the knee where they become continuous with the popliteal artery and vein.

Femoral nerve: Major nerve that supplies the anterior compartment of the thigh. Branch of the lumbar plexus, which leaves the posterior abdominal wall in a groove between iliacus and psoas major below the inguinal ligament to enter the femoral triangle. The femoral nerve innervates iliacus, pectineus (usually), sartorius, and quadriceps femoris and provides the cutaneous supply to areas of the anterior thigh, medial leg, and medial aspect of the foot.

Fibromyoma (leiomyoma): Most common benign tumor of the uterus, primarily composed of smooth muscle and connective tissue. Most common cause of dysmenorrhea, pain, bleeding, and heavy menstrual cycles. Commonly identified by use of ultrasound and surgically removed.

Fibular collateral ligament: Fibular collateral ligament of the knee is a narrow-rounded cord that attaches superiorly to the lateral epicondyle of the femur just above the groove for the popliteus tendon, crosses the lateral aspect of the knee joint directed slightly posteriorly, and attaches below to the lateral surface of the fibular head, along with the biceps femoris tendon.

Fibularis brevis/longus tendons: The 2 muscles of the lateral compartment of the leg that evert (bends in an outward direction) and assist in plantarflexion at the ankle. Their tendons cross the ankle joint behind the lateral malleolus.

Flexor carpi ulnaris muscle: Muscle of the forearm that acts to flex and adduct the hand. It arises by two heads (humeral and ulnar) and is connected by a tendinous arch beneath which the ulnar nerve and artery pass.

Flexor pollicis longus muscle: A muscle of the anterior compartment of the forearm that flexes the thumb. Its tendon enters the hand through the carpal tunnel along with the tendons of flexor digitorum superficialis, flexor digitorum profundus, and the median nerve.

Flexor tendons of the digits (fingers): After emerging from the carpal tunnel, the flexor tendons of the digits cross the palm and enter fibrous sheaths, which begin just proximal to the metacarpophalangeal joints, for their course along the palmar surfaces of the digits.

Focused assessment with sonography for trauma (FAST) exam: Used in the setting of blunt or penetrating thoracoabdominal trauma to detect the presence of free fluid (presumed to be blood in trauma patients until proven otherwise) in the pericardial space, the pleural spaces, the right and left upper quadrants of the abdomen, and the pelvis.

Galea aponeurotica: This flattened tendon of the scalp connects the frontalis and occipitalis muscles and terminates on the zygomatic arch.

Gallbladder: Pear-shaped organ located under the liver, which stores and modifies bile from the liver. During digestion, the gallbladder releases bile through a tube called the common bile duct, which connects the gallbladder and liver to the small intestine. Bile is important for emulsification and subsequent digestion and absorption of dietary fat.

Gallstones (cholelithiasis): Formed because of crystallization of bile constituents and made of cholesterol crystals mixed with bile pigments and calcium. Bile crystallizes to form sand, gravel, and finally stones. Stones may ulcerate through the wall of the gallbladder into the transverse colon passing naturally through the rectum. They might also ulcerate through the wall of the body into the duodenum and get lodged at the ileocecal junction, leading to obstruction. Stones lodged in the bile duct interfere with bile flow to the duodenum, resulting in obstructive jaundice. Finally, stones lodged at the hepatopancreatic ampulla block the biliary and the pancreatic duct systems. In this case, bile may enter the pancreatic duct system, causing aseptic or noninfectious pancreatitis.

Glenohumeral joint: This is the shoulder joint, a ball-and-socket joint between the scapula and the humerus and the major joint connecting the upper limb to the trunk.

Glenoid labrum: A fibrocartilaginous collar around the glenoid fossa of the scapula, which expands the surface of the shoulder joint and serves as an attachment site for the shoulder joint capsule and the lateral glenohumeral ligament. An important passive stabilizer in the human shoulder joint.

Glossopharyngeal nerve: Cranial nerve IX, the cranial nerve of the third pharyngeal arch. In the neck, this nerve innervates the stylopharyngeus muscle and provides sensory innervation including taste to the posterior one-third of the tongue and supplies much of the pharyngeal mucosa.

Gluteal surface of ilium: External surface of the wing of the ilium marked by the anterior, posterior, and inferior gluteal lines that separate the origins of the gluteal muscles.

Gluteus maximus muscle: Large, rhomboid-shaped muscle that originates from the posterior surface of the ilium posterior to the posterior gluteal line, the posterior surface of the sacrum, and the posterior surface of the sacrotuberous ligament and inserts into the posterior edge of the iliotibial tract and the gluteal tuberosity of the proximal femur. Gluteus maximus is the largest and most superficial muscle of the gluteal region.

Gluteus medius muscle: Originates from the gluteal surface of the ilium between the posterior and anterior gluteal lines and inserts onto the lateral surface of the greater trochanter of the femur.

Gluteus minimus muscle: Lying deep to gluteus medius, gluteus minimus originates from the surface of the ilium between the anterior and inferior gluteal lines and inserts onto the anterior surface of the greater trochanter.

Great auricular nerve: This nerve, derived from C2 and C3, ascends superficial to the sternocleidomastoid muscle toward the ear and skin over the parotid region.

Greater omentum: Suspends down from the greater curvature of the stomach, draping over the transverse colon and other abdominal viscera. It transmits the right and left gastroepiploic vessels along the greater curvature of the stomach.

Guyon canal: A narrow anatomic corridor at the wrist just outside the carpal tunnel, which conveys the ulnar artery and nerve into the hand. Guyon canal is a location where the ulnar nerve is vulnerable to compressive injury. Guyon canal syndrome is a relatively rare peripheral ulnar neuropathy, which involves injury to the distal portion of the ulnar nerve as it travels through Guyon canal.

Hamstring muscles: The hamstring muscles of the posterior compartment of the thigh (biceps femoris, semitendinosus, and semimembranosus) originate from a large common tendon attached along the posterior/posterolateral surface of the ischial tuberosity.

Head of pancreas: Widest part of the pancreas, located in the right side of abdomen and framed by the C-loop of the duodenum.

Hepatic veins: The hepatic veins (left, right, and middle) are valveless veins located in the intersegmental planes of the liver. These veins drain into the inferior vena cava; however, frequently the left and middle hepatic veins often merge before joining the inferior vena cava.

High-frequency linear probes: Because of their high resonant frequencies (8-15 MHz), these probes offer the best image detail but poor depth penetration. Consequently, they are used for musculoskeletal, peripheral nerves, thyroid gland, breast, superficial vascular, and other imaging applications that require high-resolution images from relatively superficial tissues (approximately 5-6 cm maximum depth from the skin surface).

Hip joint: The head of the femur articulates with the acetabulum of the pelvic bone to form the hip joint.

Hodgkin disease: Type of malignant lymphoma with the following clinical features: painless, progressive enlargement of the lymph nodes, spleen, and other lymphoid tissue; night sweats; fever; and weight loss.

Humeroulnar joint: Part of the elbow joint. It is composed of two bones, the humerus and ulna, and is the junction between the trochlear notch of ulna and the trochlea of humerus.

Hyoid bone: U-shaped bone composed of a body and greater and lesser horns (cornu) does not articulate to surrounding bones but is rather suspended by muscles and ligaments at the C3 vertebral level. Its greater and lesser horns allow for attachment of muscles and ligaments. The hyoid bone suspends the laryngotracheal tube.

Hyperechoic: White on the ultrasound display. Based on the degree of echogenicity, tissues or structures are described as hyperechoic (white on the ultrasound display), hypoechoic (gray on the ultrasound display), or anechoic (black on the ultrasound display).

Hypoechoic: Gray on the ultrasound display. Based on the degree of echogenicity, tissues or structures are described as hyperechoic (white on the ultrasound display), hypoechoic (gray on the ultrasound display), or anechoic (black on the ultrasound display).

Hypoglossal nerve: Cranial nerve XII, which innervates muscles of the tongue. Specifically, this nerve will supply the intrinsic muscles of the tongue and 3 extrinsic muscles that include the styloglossus, hyoglossus, and genioglossus. Primarily, these muscles retract, depress, and protrude the tongue, respectively.

Iliotibial tract/tendons: Also called the iliotibial band, this courses distally along the vastus lateralis muscle, crosses the tibiofemoral joint laterally, and attaches to Gerdy tubercle at the anterolateral surface of the lateral tibial condyle. The posterior edge of the iliotibial tract near its tibial attachment lies a short distance anterior to the fibular collateral ligament. The iliotibial tract arises at its proximal end from the tendons of the tensor fasciae latae and gluteus maximus muscles.

Incisional hernia: Hernia subtype of the anterolateral abdominal wall where the abdominal viscera extend out of a defect in the abdominal wall resulting from surgery or trauma.

Inferior pole of patella: Inferior edge/surface of the patella (kneecap), which provides attachment site for the patellar ligament. Patellar tendinopathy is a common condition in sports and may occur in any location of the patellar tendon, but the most commonly affected area is the inferior pole of the patella.

Inferior vena cava: A large vein that empties into the heart. It carries blood from the legs and feet and from organs in the abdomen and pelvis.

Infraorbital artery: A branch of the maxillary artery that, on the face, supplies the skin and associated muscles in the infraorbital, lateral nasal, and superior labial regions.

Infraspinatus muscle: The infraspinatus and teres minor muscles originate from the infraspinous fossa. Their tendons pass beneath the posterior edge of the acromion and over the posterior aspect of the glenohumeral joint and humeral head to insert on the middle and inferior facets of the greater tubercle. The tendons of infraspinatus and teres minor are two of the four rotator cuff tendons.

Inguinal canal: Starts at the deep inguinal ring and continues to the superficial ring where it terminates. This canal carries the spermatic cord or the round ligament of the uterus and the genital branch of the genitofemoral nerve. Both of these structures travel through the deep inguinal ring and the inguinal canal.

Insonation window: The acoustic (insonation) window or field is the area defined by the pathway of the ultrasound beam between the transducer and the acoustic reflector. Acoustic window refers also to the optimal placing of the transducers so that the areas of interest are clearly imaged.

Intercostal arteries: The intercostal arteries travel between the ribs. Each intercostal space is typically supplied by a posterior intercostal artery and a pair of anterior intercostal arteries. The anterior intercostal arteries are branches of the internal thoracic arteries, and the posterior intercostal arteries are branches of the descending thoracic aorta.

Intercostal muscles: Three types: (1) *external intercostals* (located superficially; its fiber orientation runs medially and downward in a direction in line with the external abdominal oblique muscle of the anterior abdominal wall); (2) *internal intercostals* (deep to the external intercostal muscle, this muscle runs in a direction opposite the external intercostals downward and laterally, in line with the internal abdominal oblique muscle); and (3) *innermost intercostals* (deepest of the intercostal muscles, running in the same direction as the internal intercostals).

Intercostal space: A space between two adjacent ribs.

Intercostal veins: Run alongside the intercostal arteries and nerves. Similar to the arteries, there are posterior intercostal veins that drain to the azygos/hemiazygos venous system. The anterior intercostal veins are tributaries of the internal thoracic veins. The posterior intercostal veins of the first intercostal space drain into the right and left brachiocephalic veins. The posterior intercostal veins of the second and third intercostal spaces come together and form the superior intercostal vein. The right superior intercostal vein drains into the azygos vein, and the left superior intercostal vein drains into the left brachiocephalic vein.

Interlaminar space: In the lumbar region, large spaces between adjacent vertebral arches appear and gaps form (interlaminar spaces) in the bony covering of the spinal canal, which are filled by the ligamenta flava. The size of these gaps increases with flexion, and they provide soft-tissue windows for ultrasound imaging of the lumbar spinal canal and its contents.

Internal abdominal oblique muscle: Offers support to the abdominal wall, assists in forced respiration, aids in raising pressure in the abdominal area, and turns and rotates the trunk with help from other muscles.

Internal carotid arteries: There is one internal carotid artery on each side of the head and neck, arising from the common carotid arteries where these bifurcate into the internal and external carotid arteries at cervical vertebral level 3 or 4. Internal carotid artery supplies the brain, whereas the external carotid nourishes other portions of the head, such as face, scalp, skull, and meninges.

Internal jugular vein: The internal jugular vein is the primary venous outlet from the cranium and travels in the anterior triangle of the neck within the carotid sheath. This vessel will join with the subclavian vein to form the brachiocephalic vein.

Interosseous: Situated between bones, such as an interosseous membrane.

Intertubercular groove: A deep groove on the humerus that separates the greater tubercle from the lesser tubercle.

Jejunum: Located in the proximal two-fifths of the small intestine, and is emptier, wider, and thicker-walled when compared with the ileum. The jejunum has the valvelike tall, circular, and closely packed folds called the plicae circulares.

Lacrimal artery: A branch of the ophthalmic artery. On the face, supplies the lacrimal gland and upper eyelid.

Lacrimal gland: Tear-secreting gland of the body located in the superolateral aspect of the orbit of the eye. The superficial aspect of this gland is seen from the facial perspective. The superficial and deep portions of the lacrimal gland are separated by the tendon of the levator palpebrae superioris muscle.

Larynx: Larynx or voice box is composed of nine cartilages—three paired and three unpaired. The larger unpaired cartilages are the thyroid, cricoid, and epiglottis. The smaller paired cartilages are the arytenoids, corniculates, and cuneiforms. The larynx terminates at the sixth cervical vertebrae and becomes the trachea, which continues inferiorly in the midline just anterior to the esophagus in the neck.

Lateral compartment of the leg: The leg is separated into anterior, lateral, and posterior compartments by intermuscular septa and surrounded by the deep fascia of the leg. The lateral compartment of the leg, also known as the *peroneal compartment*, is one of the three compartments in the leg between the knee and foot. Muscles within this compartment primarily produce foot eversion at the ankle joint.

Lateral femoral condyle: One of two projections on the lower femur. The other is the medial femoral condyle. The medial condyle is larger than the lateral condyle because of more weight-bearing medial to the knee.

Lateral femoral cutaneous nerve: A branch of the lumbar plexus, which passes from the posterior abdominal wall to the lower limb, below the inguinal ligament, and medial to the anterior superior iliac spine along the superficial surface of the sartorius muscle at its origin.

Lateral malleolus: The lateral malleolus forms the lateral surface of the ankle joint and is the prominence on the outer side of ankle, formed by the lower end of the fibula.

Lateral resolution: In ultrasound, the ability to distinguish side-by-side small reflectors, lateral resolution, is best near the focal depth, where the beam is narrowest.

Lateral thyroid lobe: Left and right lobes of the thyroid gland, situated in front of the neck. The two conical lobes lying on either side of and attached to the larynx are connected by a narrow isthmus that crosses in front of the trachea.

Left atrium: Most posteriorly located structure of the heart, with thicker walls than the right atrium and an endocardium thicker than that of the right atrium because of higher pressures. The left atrium receives oxygenated blood from the lungs and communicates with the left ventricle via the left atrioventricular valve (mitral).

Left liver lobe: Divided into medial and lateral segments, each of which is subdivided into superior and inferior areas (segments). It consists of the medial superior (caudate lobe), medial inferior (quadrate lobe), lateral superior, and lateral inferior segments.

Left portal vein: The hepatic portal vein is located in the right upper quadrant of the abdomen, originating behind the neck of the pancreas. Immediately after entering the liver, the portal vein divides into right and left branches.

Left upper quadrant of the abdomen: The abdominal wall is divided into right and left upper quadrants and right and left lower quadrants via vertical and horizontal planes that form four quadrants.

Left ventricle: One of the chambers of the heart. Traditionally, the left ventricle has been divided into the aortic vestibule and the ventricle proper. The aortic vestibule contains the smooth portion of the interventricular septum, the membranous septum, the aortic semilunar valve, and the aortic root. The wall of the left ventricle is approximately three times thicker than the wall of the right ventricle because of its need to propel blood into the high-pressure systemic circulation.

Left coronary artery: Short artery that arises from the posterior (left) aortic sinus of Valsalva and runs between the pulmonary trunk and ascending aorta before bifurcating into the anterior interventricular and circumflex arteries.

Lens: Normally transparent biconvex disc that is suspended behind the iris via a circumferential system of zonular fibers attached to the lens capsule centrally and projections (ciliary processes) from the ciliary body peripherally. Collectively, the zonular fibers make up the suspensory ligament of the lens.

Lesser occipital nerve: This branch, derived from C2 and C3, ascends along the posterior border of the sternocleidomastoid toward the skin of the auricle and occiput.

Lesser omentum: Dual layer of peritoneum from the porta hepatis of the liver, which continues to the lesser curvature of the stomach and the beginning of the duodenum. The hepatogastric and hepatoduodenal ligaments compose the lesser omentum.

Levator scapulae: This muscle attaches medially to the transverse processes of the upper 4 cervical vertebrae and laterally to the superior angle of the scapula. Upon contraction, this muscle elevates and retracts the scapula.

Glossary

Linea alba: The fusion of the aponeurosis of the external abdominal oblique, internal abdominal oblique, and transversus abdominis muscles forms a midline avascular connective tissue white line known as the linea alba, which is positioned between the two rectus abdominis muscles and stretches from the xiphoid process to the pubic symphysis.

Linear probe (high-frequency): One of 3 commonly used surface probe types for most general-purpose ultrasound imaging applications. The other two are abdominal probes and cardiac probes.

Listening mode: The listening mode (as opposed to pulse mode) of the transducer is used most often during a typical ultrasound scan. Each pulse transmitted by the transducer creates a display image that is formed one scan line at a time and a pulse is transmitted along one of a thousand or so sequential scan lines from one side of the image to the other. The next pulse along the next scan line is not transmitted until all of the echoes from the previous pulse have had time (listening mode) to return to the transducer.

Long head of biceps brachii tendon: The tendon of the long head of biceps brachii occupies the intertubercular groove and is stabilized in that position by the transverse humeral ligament. Superiorly, the tendon curves over the humeral head and passes through a small interval (rotator cuff interval) between the tendons of supraspinatus and subscapularis to enter the glenohumeral joint space.

Longitudinal (intercostal oblique) view: In longitudinal views, the probe face is oriented along the long axis of the body such that the body is divided by an imaginary plane into equal/unequal right and left parts (sagittal/parasagittal, respectively) or by an imaginary plane into front and back parts (coronal). In an intercostal oblique view, the probe face is placed in and aligned with an intercostal space (which is slightly oblique to a true coronal longitudinal axis of the body).

Longitudinal (oblique) view: In longitudinal views, the probe face is oriented along the long axis of the body such that the body is divided by an imaginary plane into equal/unequal right and left parts (sagittal/parasagittal, respectively) or by an imaginary plane into front and back parts (coronal). In a longitudinal oblique view, the probe face is oblique to a true longitudinal axis of the body, commonly in order to image a structure that itself is not aligned with a true longitudinal axis.

Longitudinal (parasagittal) view: In longitudinal views, the probe face is oriented along the long axis of the body such that the body is divided by an imaginary plane into equal/unequal right and left parts (sagittal/parasagittal, respectively) or by an imaginary plane into front and back parts (coronal).

Longitudinal (sagittal/parasagittal) view: In longitudinal views, the probe face is oriented along the long axis of the body such that the body is divided by an imaginary plane into equal/unequal right and left parts (sagittal/parasagittal, respectively) or by an imaginary plane into front and back parts (coronal).

Lumbar vertebrae: The five lumbar vertebrae, similar to all typical vertebrae, consist of a body anteriorly and a vertebral arch posteriorly. The vertebral arch consists of right and left pedicles that attach the arch to the vertebral body and right and left laminae that fuse in the midline and form the bony roof of the vertebral canal.

Lymphatic vessels/nodes: Lymph nodes are normally small oval or bean-shaped collections of lymphocytes surrounded by a capsule, which filter lymphatic fluid carried from tissues via networks of lymphatic vessels. Lymph nodes and vessels are important parts of the immune system.

Lymphoma: Cancer of the lymphoid tissue.

Male pelvis: The bowl-shaped part of the body cavity below the abdomen that is located between the hip bones in a male.

Mandibular nerve (V3): One of the divisions of the trigeminal nerve from which the cutaneous nerves of the lower face are primarily derived. Includes the mental nerve (supplies the skin over the chin and lower lip); the buccal nerve (supplies the skin overlying the buccinator muscle as well as the buccal gingival and adjacent mucosa); and the auriculotemporal nerve (supplies the skin of the temporal region and also carries postganglionic parasympathetic "hitchhiking" fibers from the otic ganglion that will leave the auriculotemporal nerve and travel to the parotid gland).

Marker side: Related to orientation in ultrasound imaging, there is a display orientation marker on the screen image (by convention on the left side of the display except in cardiac imaging where the marker is on the right side) and a probe orientation marker on one end of the probe face. When the probe orientation marker is pointed toward the patient's right side, for example, structures displayed on the screen image on the side with the orientation marker are anatomically to the right of structures displayed on the nonmarker side. Structures displayed on the nonmarker side of the image, in this example, are anatomically to the left of structures seen on the orientation marker side of the image.

Maxillary nerve (V2): One of the divisions of the trigeminal nerve from which the cutaneous nerves of the midface are primarily derived. Includes the infraorbital nerve (supplies the lower eyelid, upper lip, and lateral nose); zygomaticofacial nerve (supplies skin over the prominence of the cheek); and the zygomaticotemporal nerve (supplies the anterior aspect of the temporal region, ie, lateral region of the forehead).

McBurney point: Point over the right side of the abdomen that is one-third of the distance from the anterior superior iliac spine to the umbilicus. Acute appendicitis presents as right lower quadrant pain at McBurney point.

Meckel diverticulum: Outpouching of the ileum. This tissue, usually 2 in. long, is derived from the unobliterated yolk stalk and is located 2 ft from the ileocecal junction. Meckel diverticulum can be free or connected with the umbilicus through a fistula or a fibrous cord. Complications include ulceration, perforation, bleeding, and obstruction, which can require surgical intervention.

Medial femoral condyle: One of 2 projections on the lower femur. The other is the lateral condyle. The medial condyle is larger than the lateral condyle because of more weight-bearing medial to the knee.

Medial malleolus: The bony prominence at the medial aspect of the ankle. In the leg, the expanded distal end of the tibia forms the superior and medial (medial malleolus) surfaces of the bony arch of the ankle joint, articulating with the upper surface (trochlea) of the talus.

Median nerve: Arises in the axilla from its medial and lateral roots, branches of the medial and lateral cords of the brachial plexus. The nerve leaves the axilla along the anterior surface of the axillary artery and subsequently courses through the anterior compartment of the arm immediately adjacent to the brachial artery. The median nerve has no branches in the arm but supplies most of the muscles in the anterior compartment of the forearm, plus five muscles in the hand, and supplies sensation to the palmar surfaces of the lateral (thumb side) 3½ digits (from the thumb to half of the ring finger) and adjacent palm.

Medulla: The inner part of the kidney, which contains the loops of Henle and the collecting tubules.

Mental artery: A branch of inferior alveolar artery, which is a branch of the maxillary artery. Exits the mental foramen to supply adjacent skin and soft tissues over the lower lip and chin.

Mesovarium: Each ovary is suspended by the mesovarium, which attaches the ovaries to the posterior/superior layer of the broad ligament.

Metacarpophalangeal joint: A joint of the fingers between the head of a metacarpal bone and the base of a proximal phalanx (knuckle joint). Other joints of the fingers are proximal interphalangeal (head of proximal phalanx and base of middle phalanx) and distal interphalangeal (head of middle phalanx and base of distal phalanx).

Microconvex phased array (cardiac) probe: One of three commonly used surface probe types for most general-purpose ultrasound imaging applications. Used extensively in heart ultrasound imaging (echocardiography) but well-suited for imaging any relatively large, nonsuperficial structures through narrow sonographic windows (like intercostal spaces).

Micturition: Urination.

Midhumerus: Middle region (shaft) of the humerus, a long bone in the arm.

Mitral valve (bicuspid valve): Left atrioventricular valve (mitral valve) rests between the left atrium and left ventricle. This valve is often called the *bicuspid valve*, although one may be able to distinguish an aortic (anterior) leaflet, a mural leaflet, and two smaller leaflets at the left and right ends of the valve orifice.

Morison pouch: When imaging the liver and kidney, this is the potential space at the hepatorenal recess (between the liver and the right kidney). This is the most dependent site in the peritoneal space above the transverse mesocolon, so it is a common location for free fluid accumulation in the upper abdomen.

Murphy sign: Tenderness due to acute inflammation of the gallbladder (acute cholecystitis).

Musculoskeletal structures: Bones of the skeleton, muscles, cartilage, tendons, ligaments, joints, and other connective tissue that support and bind tissues and organs together.

Myotendinous junction: In ultrasound imaging, the area where hypoechoic muscle tissue becomes continuous with hyperechoic connective tissue forming a tendon.

Neck of fibula: Connects the head of the fibula (the smaller of the two leg bones) with the shaft. The common fibular nerve crosses the neck of the fibula posterolaterally.

Neck of pancreas: Thin section between the head and the body of the pancreas.

Neurovascular structures: A neurovascular structure (bundle) is the combination of nerves, arteries, veins, and lymphatics in the body that travel together.

Nonmarker side: Related to orientation in ultrasound imaging, there is a display orientation marker on the screen image (by convention on the left side of the display except in cardiac imaging where the marker is on the right side) and a probe orientation marker on one end of the probe face. When the probe orientation marker is pointed toward the patient's right side, for example, structures displayed on the screen image on the side with the orientation marker are anatomically to the right of structures displayed on the nonmarker side. Structures displayed on the marker side of the image, in this example, are anatomically to the left of structures seen on the orientation marker side of the image.

Ophthalmic nerve (V1): One of the divisions of the trigeminal nerve from which the cutaneous nerves of the upper face are primarily derived. Includes the supraorbital nerve (supplies branches to the upper eyelid and then distributes to the skin of the forehead posteriorly to the vertex of the skull); supratrochlear nerve (provides branches to the upper eyelid and adjacent skin of the central forehead); infratrochlear nerve (supplies the skin of the eyelids and lateral nose); and lacrimal nerve (after supplying the lacrimal gland, it is distributed to the upper eyelid).

Optic nerve (CN II): The central processes of retinal ganglion cells converge at the optic disc to form the optic nerve, which exits the posteromedial aspect of the eye and traverses the orbital fat to exit the orbit posteriorly via the optic canal. The optic nerve is surrounded by a sheath consisting of all 3 meningeal layers: dura, subarachnoid, and pia.

Os coxae: Hip bones (two bones of the pelvis). Other bones of the pelvis are the sacrum and coccyx.

Ovaries: Female reproductive organs covered by germinal epithelial, which is closely related to embryologic peritoneum.

Pancreas: The pancreas is both a digestive exocrine gland and a hormone-producing endocrine gland located in the retroperitoneal space of the abdomen.

Pancreatitis: Inflammation of the pancreas caused by gallstones or alcohol consumption. Symptoms include severe and constant epigastric pain radiating to the back.

Parasternal long-axis view: One of several standard echocardiography views in which the probe face is placed near the left side of the sternum in the third or fourth intercostal space and oriented along the long axis of the left ventricle (along an imaginary line connecting the right shoulder and left nipple.

Parasternal short-axis view: One of several standard echocardiography views in which the probe face is placed near the left side of the sternum in the third or fourth intercostal space and oriented perpendicular to the long axis of the left ventricle, by rotating the probe face 90° clockwise from the parasternal long axis position.

Parathyroid glands: Normally located on the posterior aspect of the thyroid gland, the parathyroids are divided into two superior and two inferior glands. These structures maintain serum calcium levels and are derived from the fourth and third pharyngeal arches, respectively. The inferior parathyroids may sometimes be found in the thorax.

Paraumbilical veins: These veins, nested in the falciform ligament, connect the left branch of the portal vein with small periumbilical subcutaneous veins. The periumbilical subcutaneous veins are radicles of the superior epigastric, inferior epigastric, thoracoepigastric, and superficial epigastric veins. The paraumbilical veins are almost always closed but can become patent and dilated in portal hypertension.

Parotid gland: The largest of the salivary glands, located on either side of the mouth and in front of both ears.

Parotitis: Viral infection (mumps) of the parotid gland, which results in glandular swelling. Glandular swelling stretches the capsule and the fascia of the parotid gland resulting in considerable pain.

Patellar ligament: Sometimes called the patellar tendon, this is an extension of the quadriceps tendon and extends from the patella (kneecap) to the anterior surface of the tibia.

Pectineus muscle: Originates from the pectineal line of the superior pubic ramus, just above the inguinal ligament, enters the thigh deep to the inguinal ligament forming the medial half of the floor of the femoral triangle, and inserts on the body of the femur immediately below the lesser trochanter.

Pectoral muscles: Pectoralis major and minor, four paired muscles that cover the front of the rib cage and act on the upper limb.

Pelvic diaphragm: The musculature of the pelvic floor, composed mainly of the right and left levator ani muscles and completed posteriorly by the coccygeus muscles and their perineal fascia. The pelvic diaphragm acts to support all the pelvic viscera, flexes the anorectal junction to maintain fecal continence (its relaxation allows for defecation), and helps in voluntary micturition (urination).

Penis: External male reproductive organ, also used for urination.

Pericardiocentesis: Removal of fluid from the pericardial sac so as to relieve the problem of tamponade. Although pericardiocentesis can be performed using landmarks alone, ultrasound-guided pericardiocentesis allows for visualization of the effusion, as well as the needle path and guide wire during the procedure, and has been shown to reduce clinical errors such as pneumothorax.

Pericardium: Fibroserous sac that encloses the entire heart and a portion of the great vessels and is composed of two layers, one fibrous and one serous.

Peyer patches: Small collections of lymphoid tissue found throughout the ileum region of the small intestine. Function is to monitor intestinal bacteria and prevent growth of intestinal pathogenic bacteria.

Phalanx: One of the small bones of the fingers or toes (plural phalanges).

Pharynx: Thin, skeletal muscle semicylinder begins at the base of the skull and descends to the sixth cervical vertebrae, where it becomes the narrowed esophagus posteriorly and opens into the larynx (voice box) anteriorly. The pharynx is divided into a naso, oro, and laryngo (hypo) pharynx as it passes posterior to these regions.

Phrenic nerve: In the neck, the phrenic nerve (C3, C4, and C5), which supplies the diaphragm, descends almost vertically along the superficial surface of the anterior scalene muscle to travel between the subclavian artery and vein. Injury to this nerve may impair respiration. Irritation of this nerve results in spasm of the ipsilateral diaphragm (eg, hiccups).

Piezoelectric crystals: An ultrasound transducer probe generates and receives sound waves using a principle called the piezoelectric (pressure electricity) effect. In the probe, there are many piezoelectric crystals.

Plantar aponeurosis: Distinct, thickened band of deep fascia that attaches posteriorly to the periosteum of the medial process of the calcaneal tubercle and extends anteriorly along the central part of the sole of the foot, over the superficial surface of flexor digitorum brevis muscle. At about midfoot the aponeurosis begins to expand medially and laterally, dividing into separate bands for each of the toes that attach to the metatarsophalangeal joint capsules and associated ligaments.

Pleomorphic adenomas: Benign neoplasms (mixed tumors), slowly growing, painless masses of the parotid gland.

Pleura: Thin, serous membrane composed of mesothelial cells that produce small amounts of serous fluid, which facilitates movements of the lungs. Pleura envelopes each lung and consists of parietal and visceral layers.

Pleural space: A potential space located between the parietal and visceral pleurae. During normal respiration, the lungs are not fully expanded and, as result, the parietal pleura is not in contact with the visceral pleura. The areas in which the parietal pleura is not in direct contact with the lung parenchyma are termed recesses, of which there are two.

Pleural effusion: The presence of free fluid in the pleural space (hemothorax or pleural effusion). Pleural effusion abolishes the mirror image artifact and the space above the diaphragm appears anechoic, often with an atelectatic lung floating in and out of view with respiratory effort.

Popliteal artery: The femoral artery becomes the popliteal artery as it leaves the subsartorial canal and enters the popliteal fossa through the adductor hiatus of adductor magnus.

Popliteal fossa: Diamond-shaped space posterior to the knee joint, formed by the muscles of the posterior compartments of the thigh and leg, through which major neurovascular structures cross between the thigh and the leg.

Popliteus muscle: Thin, flat, triangular-shaped muscle in the floor of the popliteal fossa and proximal part of the posterior compartment of the leg.

Portal triad: The vessels that branch and travel together within the liver: branches of the proper hepatic artery, branches of the portal vein, and branches of the hepatic (bile) duct, together commonly known as the portal triad.

Portal vein: The portal vein is formed by the splenic vein and the superior mesenteric vein posterior to the neck of the pancreas. The portal vein is about 8 cm (3.2 in.) long and collects venous blood from the gastrointestinal tract, spleen, pancreas, and gallbladder.

Posterior cervical triangle: A region of the neck, the posterior cervical triangle is bounded interiorly by the posterior edge of the sternocleidomastoid, posteriorly by the anterior edge of the upper trapezius, and inferiorly by the middle third of the clavicle.

Posterior compartment: In the thigh, the posterior compartment muscles are the hamstrings: biceps femoris, semitendinosus, and semimembranosus.

Pouch of Douglas: The rectouterine pouch, also known as the pouch of Douglas, is a potential space created by the peritoneal fold reflecting from the posterior surface of the uterus onto the anterior surface of the rectum. The pouch of Douglas is the lowest point in the peritoneal cavity in the supine position and so a place where free fluid (such as blood) commonly accumulates.

Probe transducers: Part of the ultrasound equipment, which converts electricity into sound producing the pulse that is directed into tissues and converts sound (echoes reflected back to the probe from the tissues) into electrical signals that are then filtered and amplified to form an anatomical image of the slice being examined.

Prostate: Located immediately inferior to the bladder, posterior to the pubic symphysis, and anterior to the rectum, the prostate gland is anatomically divided into five lobes: the anterior, middle, posterior, and the right and left lateral lobes. It has a base at the bladder neck where the urethra exits the bladder and enters the prostate, and an apex resting on the pelvic floor.

Prostate-specific antigen (PSA): A protein produced by normal, as well as malignant, cells of the prostate gland. The PSA test measures the level of PSA in a man's blood. For this test, a blood sample is sent to a laboratory for analysis. The results are usually reported as nanograms of PSA per milliliter (ng/mL) of blood. The blood level of PSA is often elevated in men with prostate cancer. In addition to prostate cancer, a number of benign conditions can cause a man's PSA level to rise, eg, prostatitis (inflammation of the prostate) and benign prostatic hyperplasia (BPH) (enlargement of the prostate).

Proximal: Situated nearer to the point of attachment of a limb or the beginning of a vessel or nerve.

Pubic arch: Part of the pelvis, the subpubic angle or the pubic arch, is formed by the convergence of the inferior rami of the ischium and pubis on either side, below the pubic symphysis. The angle at which they converge is known as the subpubic angle.

Pubocervical ligament: Composed of bands of connective tissue and connects the posterior border of the pubis to the cervix of the uterus.

Pulse mode: The transducer is in pulse mode less than 1% of the time. The display image is formed one scan line at a time and a pulse is transmitted along one of a thousand or so sequential scan lines from one side of the image to the other. The next pulse along the next scan line is not transmitted until all of the echoes from the previous pulse have had time to return to the transducer (during this period, the probe is said to be in "listening mode").

Purkinje fibers: One of the major specialized cardiac conduction muscle fibers, the sinoatrial and atrioventricular nodes as well as the bundles of His being the others. Purkinje fibers are in a subendocardial network of specialized cardiac muscle cells, which arise from the left and right bundle branches. This network conveys the excitatory impulse from the branches of the common bundle (of His) to the myocardium of the ventricles.

Quadratus femoris muscle: Paired muscle of the gluteal region, deep to gluteus maximus, which acts to externally rotate the thigh. The sciatic courses over quadratus femoris just before entering the posterior compartment of the thigh.

Quadriceps femoris tendon: A thick, strong tendon formed by contributions from the rectus femoris and the vastus muscles. The quadriceps femoris tendon is commonly described as trilaminar with a superficial layer formed by rectus femoris, an intermediate layer formed by vastus lateralis and medialis, and a deep layer formed by vastus intermedius. The quadriceps femoris tendon attaches to the superior surface of the patella, which is in turn attached to the tibial tuberosity via the patellar ligament.

Radial nerve: The radial nerve begins in the axilla as the largest branch of the posterior cord of the brachial plexus and ends near the elbow joint by dividing into its terminal branches, the deep and superficial radial nerves.

Radiocapitellar joint: Ball-and-socket joint that is composed of the radial head and humeral capitulum and that is lateral to the ulnohumeral joint. The radiocapitellar joint allows for forearm supination and pronation.

Rectouterine ligament: Maintains the anatomical position of the cervix upward and posteriorly.

Rectus abdominis muscles: These are the anterior abdominal muscles ("abs" or "six-pack"), a paired muscle running vertically on each side of the anterior wall of the abdomen.

Rectus femoris and vastus muscles: The rectus femoris muscle is one of the fourquadriceps muscles. The others are the vastus medialis, the vastus intermedius (deep to the rectus femoris), and the vastus lateralis. All four parts of the quadriceps muscle attach to the patella via the quadriceps tendon.

Rectus sheath: Formed by the fusion of the aponeuroses of the external abdominal oblique, internal abdominal oblique, and transversus abdominis muscles, which surrounds the rectus abdominis muscle (and the pyramidalis muscle, when present).

Renal artery: Each kidney is supplied by a renal artery, which branches from the abdominal aorta, and is drained by a renal vein, which opens into the inferior vena cava.

Renal calculi: Kidney stones or nephroliths are formed of high levels of calcium and, as a result, are easily detectable with ultrasound when patients are suspected of nephrolithiasis because of renal colic. Based on the size and shape of kidney stones, severe colicky pain may be produced at the renal calyx or while traveling down through the ureter. In addition, hydronephrosis or obstruction of the ureters by a stone can be a surgical emergency. Urolithiasis is the condition in which renal calculi may present at any part of the urinary tract. Another type of kidney stone is the staghorn calculi or coral calculi. These stones fill every part of the renal pelvis and calyces. Their composition is of magnesium ammonium phosphate known as struvite or calcium carbonate apatite. They are formed most commonly in women because of recurrent infections. The clinical symptoms include fever, pain, hematuria, and abscess formation.

Reverberation artifact: Common ultrasound artifact that occurs when a sound pulse reverberates back and forth between two strong parallel reflectors, resulting in display of a "ring-down" or "comet tail" artifact in the image.

Right atrium: One of the four chambers of the heart, with the thinnest wall. Divided into two parts, the sinus venarum and the right atrium proper, the right atrium receives mixed venous (deoxygenated) blood returning from body tissues. The external surface of the right atrium is broad, triangular, and pyramidal in shape. Within the right atrium there are two large orifices for the superior and inferior vena cavae.

Right coronary artery: Arises from the anterior (right) aortic sinus of Valsalva. The artery passes between the pulmonary trunk and the edge of the right auricle and descends in the right coronary sulcus.

Right upper quadrant ultrasound: Right upper quadrant is one of the four quadrants of the abdomen. A right upper quadrant ultrasound examines the liver, right kidney, and gallbladder, as well as the diaphragm over the superior surface of the liver and lower part of the right hemithorax.

Right ventricle: One of the 4 chambers of the heart, the right ventricle is the most anterior of all the heart chambers and is almost in contact with the sternum. The right ventricle has thin walls and is separated into two parts, the inflow and outflow parts. The inflow portion contains the tricuspid valve, papillary muscles, interventricular septum, and trabeculae carneae. The outflow portion (conus arteriosus) opens across the pulmonary valve into the pulmonary artery.

Root of the neck: The root of the neck (thoracocervical region) is the junction between the thorax and neck. It includes the superior thoracic aperture through which pass all the structures going from the head/neck to the thorax, and the opening from the neck into the upper limb through which pass the vessels and nerves from the neck to the upper limb.

Rotator cuff: Group of tendons of four muscles that reinforce the shoulder joint capsule and help stabilize the shoulder joint, especially during forceful rotations. The rotator cuff consists of the tendons of supraspinatus, subscapularis, infraspinatus, and teres minor muscles.

Round ligament of the uterus: Runs within the (anterior/superior) layer of the broad ligament and serves to hold the uterus anteverted and anteflexed by supporting the fundus of the uterus forward. The ligament attaches to the uterus anteriorly below the fallopian tubes. The round ligament passes through the inguinal canal at the deep inguinal ring and exits at the superficial inguinal ring into the labium majus.

Rugae: Longitudinal folds of mucous membrane, created as the stomach experiences contraction. The gastric canal, a grooved channel along the lesser curvature formed by the rugae, directs fluids toward the pylorus.

Sacrum: One of the bones of the pelvis, formed by the fusion of five sacral vertebrae. The others are the os coxae (two hip bones) and coccyx. The posterior wall of the pelvic cavity is parallel to the curvature of the sacrum.

Salivary stones: Most often located in the submandibular gland (60%-90% of cases) and may be multiple, causing sialolithiasis, which can cause partial or total obstruction of the salivary duct. Salivary stones (sialoliths) when present in the distal part of the submandibular duct (Wharton duct) may be palpable in the floor of the mouth.

Saphenous nerve: A branch of the femoral nerve. The saphenous nerve continues through the thigh along the deep surface of sartorius, emerges between sartorius and the tendon of gracilis just above the knee joint, and then pierces the deep fascia to provide cutaneous supply to the medial surface of the leg from the knee joint to the medial aspect of the foot.

Sartorius muscle: Originates from the medial aspect of the anterior superior iliac spine, crosses the thigh from lateral to medial, and inserts along with gracilis and semitendinosus on the medial aspect of the proximal tibia.

Scalene interval: Also known as the scalene hiatus, the interval between scalene anterior and scalene medius through which the roots and trunks of the brachial plexus emerge.

Scalene muscles: The scalene muscles are located deep in relation to the sternocleidomastoid muscle, lateral to the cervical spine, connecting the vertebrae to the first two ribs. The deep fascia or prevertebral fascia envelopes the scalene muscles. These muscles arise from the cervical vertebrae and descend to attach to the first and second ribs. Functionally, the scalene muscles (anterior, middle, and posterior) are used to elevate the first and second ribs as is seen in forced inspiration.

Scarpa fascia: Deep membranous layer of the fascia of the anterior abdominal wall; Scarpa fascia joins with the membranous superficial layer of perineal fascia (Colle fascia) inferiorly, and medially with the superficial fascia of the penis and over the scrotum (tunica dartos).

Sciatic nerve: Largest branch of the lumbosacral plexus with nerve fibers from L4 to S3. The sciatic nerve is a major source of innervation in the lower limb and leaves the pelvis through the greater sciatic foramen inferior to piriformis and descends through the gluteal region immediately deep to the gluteus maximus and coursing over the gemellus superior, the tendon of obturator internus, inferior gemellus, and finally, the quadratus femoris.

Semimembranosus tendon: Strong, fibrous connective tissue cord located at the back of the thigh in the popliteal fossa, which attaches the semimembranosus muscle to the tibia. It crosses behind the medial condyle in contact with the fibrous joint capsule of the knee and is separated from the tendinous edge of medial gastrocnemius by a (normally) thin bursa communicating with the knee joint.

Seminal fluid: Secreted by the seminal vesicles and contributes to the quality of the semen. Seminal fluid is rich in fructose, choline, and other proteins that provide nutrients to the spermatozoa.

Seminal vesicles: Consist of lobulated glandular structures, which originate from the diverticula of the ductus deferens. They are found inferolateral to the ductus deferens ampullae. The seminal vesicles, which extend superiorly from the prostate gland between the bladder and the rectum, join the ductus deferens near their end, forming the ejaculatory ducts.

Semispinalis capitis: This muscle attaches superiorly between the superior and inferior nuchal lines and inferiorly from the transverse and articular processes and associated ligaments of the lower cervical and upper thoracic vertebrae.

Semitendinosus tendon: Semitendinosus muscle tapers to a long thin tendon just beyond midthigh. The semitendinosus tendon continues distally along the superficial surface of semimembranosus and crosses the knee joint posteromedially accompanying the tendons of gracilis and sartorius to insert on the anteromedial surface of the body of the tibia near the inferior end of the tibial collateral ligament.

Serratus anterior: This muscle arises typically from the upper 8 ribs and inserts onto the vertebral border of the scapula.

Sinoatrial node: The normal pacemaker of the heart; one of the specialized cardiac conduction muscle fibers that compose the conduction tissue of the heart that sends electrical signals to the cardiac musculature, resulting in its contraction. The sinoatrial node is located at the junction of the base of the superior vena cava with the right auricle.

Sialolithiasis: The condition of stone formation in a salivary gland and/or its duct. Salivary stones are most often located in the submandibular gland (60%-90% of cases) and may be multiple, causing sialolithiasis, which can cause partial or total obstruction of the salivary duct. Salivary stones or sialoliths when present in the distal part of the submandibular duct (Wharton duct) may be palpable in the floor of the mouth.

Sjogren syndrome: An autoimmune disease that most commonly affects women over 40 years of age and is characterized by intense lymphocytic and plasma cell infiltration and destruction of salivary and lacrimal glands, resulting in dry mouth and eyes.

Sound waves: Mechanical waves of alternating pressures that propagate through media (such as tissues) as a series of compressions as the wave pressure rises, and rarefactions as the wave pressure falls, of the molecules in the medium.

Spatial resolution: The ability to distinguish and display small objects that are close together as separate in space. Small objects are displayed as the width of the beam at the depth they are located (lateral smearing artifact).

Specular reflection: Specular reflection occurs when sound waves encounter a smooth surface or a smooth interface between two tissues with different acoustic properties. This type of reflection is responsible for the hyperechoic edges/interfaces seen in ultrasound images and for the bright appearance of fibrous structures such as tendons, ligaments, and organ capsules. Specular reflection is best for image forming when the surface or interface is perpendicular to the path of the sound pulses.

Spigelian hernia: Spigelian hernia (lateral ventral hernia) is a type of hernia of the anterolateral abdominal wall situated at the semilunar line. The diagnosis of a Spigelian hernia is confirmed with ultrasound or computed tomography scan.

Spinal canal: The spinal cord, including the conus medullaris, cauda equina, and the surrounding spinal meninges, is housed within the vertebral (spinal) canal, which is formed by the aligned vertebral foramina and associated soft tissues including the ligamenta flava, intervertebral disks, and the posterior longitudinal ligament.

Spinous process: Bony prominence that projects posteriorly in the midline from the junction of the right and left laminae from the back of each vertebra.

Spleen: A vascular lymphatic organ located below the diaphragm at 9th to 11th ribs in the left hypochondriac region superiorly to upper pole of the left kidney and the tail of the pancreas. The spleen is supported by the splenorenal and splenogastric ligaments and is covered by the peritoneum, except at the hilum.

Splenic artery: A large, tortuous vessel that courses over the superior surface of the pancreas before entering the splenorenal ligament to enter the hilum of the spleen. This artery is the largest branch of the celiac trunk and usually has numerous terminal branches that include the short gastric arteries, the left gastroepiploic (gastro-omental) artery, and pancreatic branches.

Splenic artery aneurysm: Most common aneurysm of the viscera, more common in women. However, rupture is more common in males. These focal dilatations of the splenic artery can be saccular or true aneurysms. Their discovery is typically incidental, but they are most commonly associated with atherosclerosis, different types of vasculitis, fibromuscular dysplasia, portal hypertension, and cirrhosis. The most common complication of splenic aneurysm is rupture (5% of cases), which presents with left upper quadrant pain.

Splenic vein: The splenic vein originates from the merging of venous sinusoids in the spleen. The splenic vein also receives venous drainage from the short gastric, left gastroepiploic, and pancreatic veins. The splenic vein typically joins the superior mesenteric vein behind the neck of the pancreas to form the portal vein.

Splenius capitis: This muscle originates from the spinous processes and associated ligaments of the cervical and upper thoracic spinous processes and travels superiorly to insert onto the mastoid process and superior nuchal line. Bilateral contraction results in extension of the neck.

Steatosis: Fatty liver disease (alcoholic or nonalcoholic), with triglyceride accumulation. In addition, viral hepatitis and certain medications can also cause steatosis. If steatosis is pronounced and chronic, it may lead to fibrosis and eventually liver cirrhosis. Recent studies place the prevalence of liver steatosis to approximately 15% of the general population. Ultrasound can diagnose liver steatosis by identifying poor demarcation of intrahepatic architecture, revealing the loss of diaphragmatic demarcation, and showing that liver echogenicity is higher than of renal cortex and spleen.

Sternal angle of Louis: A palpable clinical landmark in surface anatomy, it is also known as the manubriosternal junction and is the synarthrotic joint formed by the articulation of the manubrium and the body of the sternum. The costal cartilages of the second ribs articulate with the sternum at the sternal angle.

Sternocleidomastoid muscle: This long strap-shaped neck muscle arises from the manubrium of the sternum and medial aspect of the clavicle, and then ascends to attach to the mastoid process of the temporal bone. It acts to turn the face to the opposite side.

Subcostal nerve: The ventral ramus of the 12th thoracic nerve that supplies innervation to the muscles of the anterior abdominal wall.

Sublingual gland: Located at the floor of the mouth covered by the oral mucosa (small ducts opens at the base of the sublingual fold) between the geniohyoid, intrinsic muscles of the tongue, hyoglossus muscle (medially), and the mylohyoid muscle. Its medial side is wrapped around the terminal part of the submandibular duct. It receives postganglionic parasympathetic fibers from the submandibular ganglion.

Submandibular gland: Second largest salivary gland located overlying the posterior belly of the digastric and stylohyoid muscles at the inferior (superficial) surface of mylohyoid muscle. A smaller and deeper portion is also found on the superior surface of the mylohyoid muscle. The duct of the submandibular gland (Wharton duct) runs from its deep aspect or glandular hilum at the level of the mylohyoid muscle toward the medial aspect of the sublingual gland. The facial artery usually grooves or traverses the superficial portion of this gland on its way to the face. The lingual artery and vein run at its medial side. Autonomically, the submandibular gland receives its innervation via a branch of the facial nerve, cranial nerve VII.

Subscapularis muscle: This muscle originates from the anterior surface of the scapula. Its tendon passes through the subcoracoid space inferior to the coracoid process and deep to the coracobrachialis and short head of biceps brachii muscles, then over the anteromedial aspect of the glenohumeral joint and humeral head to insert on the lesser tubercle. The subscapularis tendon is one of the four rotator cuff tendons.

Subxiphoid 4-chamber view: One of standard transthoracic approaches used in ultrasound examinations of the heart (echocardiography), also including apical and parasternal long-and-short axis. The subxiphoid 4-chamber view uses the liver as a sonographic window to view the heart and pericardium. This is one of the views used in the eFAST examination to determine if there is free fluid accumulating in the pericardial space (hemopericardium or pericardial effusion).

Superficial radial nerve: One of the two terminal branches of the radial nerve, it joins the radial artery and continues distally in the forearm under the brachioradialis muscle, winding across its distal tendon to supply the skin over the anatomical snuffbox, dorsal aspect of the hand, thumb, and proximal index and middle fingers.

Superficial temporal artery: One of two terminal branches of the external carotid artery that provides small branches to the parotid gland, anterior ear, and then courses into the scalp as terminal frontal and parietal branches. Larger branches prior to this termination include the transverse facial branch, which travels superficial to the masseter superior to the zygomatic arch and supplies the parotid gland and masseter muscle, and the zygomaticoorbital branch, which travels to the lateral angle of the orbit and supplies the orbicularis oculi muscle.

Superior mesenteric artery: Arises from the abdominal aorta posterior to the neck of the pancreas. It descends across the third part of the duodenum and left renal vein and enters the root of the mesentery posterior to the transverse colon and continues into the right iliac fossa. The superior mesenteric artery gives rise to numerous intestinal (jejunal and ileal) arteries, the inferior pancreaticoduodenal artery, the middle colic artery, the right colic artery, and the ileocolic artery.

Superior pole of patella: The superior surface/edge of the patella (kneecap) provides the attachment area for the quadriceps tendon.

Supraclavicular nerve: This nerve, derived from C3 and C4, travels inferiorly and terminates as 3 branches that cross the medial, middle, and lateral aspects of the clavicle to supply regional skin.

Supraorbital artery: A branch of the ophthalmic artery. On the face, supplies regional muscles and anastomoses with the angular artery and frontal branch of the superficial temporal arteries.

Suprapubic view: Transabdominal views of lower abdomen/pelvis with the probe positioned just at/above the body/symphysis of the pubic bone.

Supraspinatus: In the upper limb, the supraspinatus muscle originates from the supraspinous fossa and its tendon passes through the subacromial space to insert on the superior facet of the greater tubercle of the humerus. The tendon of supraspinatus is one of the four rotator cuff tendons.

Supratrochlear artery: A terminal branch of the ophthalmic artery. Supplies skin of the medial orbital region.

Sympathetics: The external carotid plexus, postganglionic sympathetic fibers derived from the superior cervical ganglion of the sympathetic trunk within the neck, travel along branches of the external carotid artery that are destined for the face (eg, facial and superficial temporal arteries). These fibers are vasoconstrictive, secretory, and pilomotor in nature.

Tarsal tunnel: Related to the posterior compartment of the leg, the tarsal tunnel transmits the tendons of the deep posterior compartment muscles along with the tibial nerve and the posterior tibial vessels from the leg into the plantar aspect of the foot. It is a fibro-osseous tunnel consisting of a shallow depression along the posterior surface of the medial malleolus, the medial surface of the posterior process and body of the talus, and the medial surface of calcaneus, spanned by the flexor retinaculum.

Tendon of flexor carpi radialis: Tendon that crosses into the hand along the medial surface of the scaphoid just outside the carpal tunnel, between 2 layers of the transverse carpal ligament.

Tendon of popliteus: Also known as the popliteal tendon, it is part of the posterolateral corner of the knee, a stabilizing structure in knee rotation. The tendon of popliteus approaches and attaches to the lateral femoral condyle just deep to the femoral (proximal) attachment of the fibular collateral ligament of the knee.

Tendons of extensor pollicis muscles: In the hand and just distal to the extensor retinaculum, the tendon of extensor pollicis longus forms the medial/posterior boundary of the anatomical "snuffbox," and the tendons of extensor pollicis brevis and abductor pollicis longus form its lateral/anterior boundary.

Tensor fasciae latae muscle: This muscle originates along a line that begins at the lateral aspect of the anterior superior iliac spine and extends a few centimeters posteriorly along the iliac crest as far as the tubercle of the crest, and inserts via the iliotibial tract, a thickened band of the fascia lata, onto the proximal tibia.

Testes: Male reproductive organs responsible for the production of spermatozoa and sex hormones. They are covered by a membranous structure known as the tunica albuginea, which is located under a visceral layer called the tunica vaginalis. Their development occurs in the retroperitoneum, after which they descend into the scrotum.

Thenar muscles: Muscles in the palm of the hand at the base of the thumb. The three thenar muscles are the abductor pollicis brevis, flexor pollicis brevis, and opponens pollicis.

Thoracic duct: Primary lymphatic channel in the body, which drains the entire body with the exception of the upper right half of the thorax, right upper limb, and right half of the head. Begins in the abdomen and courses primarily in the thorax. Its termination is into the junction of the left subclavian vein and left internal jugular vein (venous angle); therefore, a portion of this structure is found in the left neck. In the neck, at approximately the seventh cervical vertebrae, the thoracic duct takes an outward curve between the carotid and vertebral arteries prior to emptying into the venous angle.

Thorax: Part of the body that occupies the space between the neck and abdomen. The bony cage of the thorax is conical in shape, and has a narrow apex superiorly (the superior thoracic aperture, leading to the root of the neck) and a wide base inferiorly (the inferior thoracic aperture guarded by the diaphragm).

Thrombus: Blood clot.

Thyroid cartilage: One of the nine cartilages of the larynx and the largest of these. This structure sits anterior to the C4 and C5 vertebrae. The thyroid cartilage is connected superiorly to the hyoid bone via the thyrohyoid membrane and inferiorly to the cricoid cartilage by the cricothyroid ligament.

Thyroid gland: This endocrine gland is contained in its own fibrous capsule and is composed of left and right lateral lobes that are united across the midline by the isthmus that overlies the second through fourth tracheal rings. The thyroid gland regulates the rate of metabolism in the body by secreting thyroid hormones (thyroxine and triiodothyronine) and affects calcium balance through the hormone calcitonin (secreted by thyroid parafollicular or C-cells).

Thyroid lateral lobes: The thyroid gland is divided into two lateral (on each side) lobes that are connected by the isthmus, which crosses the midline of the upper trachea at the second and third tracheal rings. The normal thyroid gland has lateral lobes that are symmetrical with a well-marked centrally located isthmus.

Tibial collateral ligament: The tibial collateral ligament of the knee is a long (8-10 cm) flattened band attached superiorly to the medial epicondyle of the femur. The ligament passes across the medial surface of the knee joint and attaches distally to the anteromedial surface of the body of the tibia 4 to 5 cm below the tibiofemoral joint line. The ligament is described as having superficial and deep layers.

Tibial nerve: Nerve in the leg that, along with the popliteal vessels, passes between the medial and lateral heads of gastrocnemius and under the tendinous arch of soleus to enter the posterior compartment of the leg at the inferior extent of the popliteal fossa, passing superficial to popliteus muscle and deep to triceps surae.

Tibial tuberosity: The large and primary weight-bearing bone of the leg.

Tibiocalcaneal ligament: In the leg, the nearly vertical tibiocalcaneal ligament spans between the inferior edge of the medial malleolus and the sustentaculum tali of calcaneus. One of the four named parts of the deltoid ligament of the ankle joint.

Toggling: Regarding an ultrasound probe, proper rotation and tilting (fanning) of the probe face are critical to view structures of interest in their true longitudinal axis or transverse axis (and to change a view from longitudinal to transverse, or vice versa) and to produce accurate images of structures that are not parallel to the skin surface.

Trachea: The large airway conveying air to and from the pharynx/larynx and lungs. The larynx ends at the sixth cervical vertebrae and becomes continuous with the trachea, which continues inferiorly in the midline just anterior to the esophagus in the neck, and then enters the thorax where it ends by dividing into the right and left main bronchi.

Transduction: In ultrasound imaging, conversion of a mechanical force (such as sound) to electricity by deforming a piezoelectric crystal. Returning echoes deform piezoelectric crystals, resulting in a net charge across the crystal, which results in current to be amplified, filtered, and processed to form an image. The ultrasound pulse that is transmitted into tissues is produced by "reverse piezoelectric effect" wherein alternating current is transduced by the crystals into sound waves.

Transverse processes: In the spine, the transverse processes project laterally from the junction of the pedicles and laminae, and immediately posterior to this point, articular processes project superiorly and inferiorly.

Transverse cervical nerve: This nerve, derived from C2 and C3, travels anteriorly and superficial to the sternocleidomastoid toward the midline of the neck providing regional cutaneous innervation.

Transversus abdominis muscles: Muscle layer of the anterior and lateral (front and side) abdominal wall that is deep to (layered below) the internal oblique muscle.

Transversus abdominis plane block (TAPB): Ultrasound-guided block used typically to block T9-T10 nerves. Used to accurately guide the needle bevel into a plane between internal abdominal oblique and transversus abdominis muscles in order to provide local anesthetic for abdominal wall incisions medial to the block.

Trapezius muscle: Trapezius muscle, which supports the arm and moves the scapula, is a large paired muscle that extends lengthwise from the occipital bone to the lower thoracic vertebrae of the spine and laterally to the spine of the scapula.

Trendelenburg position: A patient bed position in which the bed is tilted 15° to 30° such that the head is lower than the feet. This increases intraperitoneal fluid pooling in the upper quadrants, increasing the sensitivity of the FAST exam in these locations.

Triceps brachii: In the arm, the main muscle of the posterior compartment of the arm is the triceps brachii, which is formed from 3 heads: the long head, the medial head, and the lateral head. The three heads join and form the triceps tendon, which crosses the elbow to insert on the olecranon process of the ulna.

Trigeminal nerve (CN V): The trigeminal nerve has three divisions: the ophthalmic nerve (V1), the maxillary nerve (V2), and the mandibular nerve (V3). Through its divisions the trigeminal nerve supplies sensation to the face and motor innervation to the muscles of mastication (chewing).

Tubercles: Greater and lesser tubercles serve as attachment sites for the tendons of the rotator cuff muscles and are situated at the anterior aspect of the proximal humerus, separated by the intertubercular groove.

Ulnar artery: Artery in the arm that, accompanied by the ulnar nerve, travels through the anterior compartment of the forearm and crosses the wrist through Guyon canal, between the pisiform bone and the hook of the hamate bone. The brachial artery divides into its terminal branches, the radial and ulnar arteries, in the cubital fossa. The ulnar artery passes deep to the pronator teres muscle and joins the ulnar nerve between flexor carpi ulnaris and flexor digitorum profundus for the remainder of its course in the forearm and then through Guyon canal into the hand.

Ulnar collateral ligament: Ligament in the arm, located at the medial aspect of the elbow uniting the distal aspect of the humerus to the proximal aspect of the ulna.

Ulnar nerve: This nerve in the arm arises in the axilla from the medial cord of the brachial plexus, travels through the arm posterior to the median nerve, crosses the elbow joint through the cubital tunnel, travels through the anterior compartment of the forearm accompanied by the ulnar artery, and crosses the wrist into the hand through Guyon canal.

Uncinate process of the pancreas: Lower part of the head of the pancreas located to the left posterior to the superior mesenteric vessels.

Ureter: Retroperitoneal muscular organ that joins the kidney to the urinary bladder. It courses along the psoas major muscle and transverse processes of the lumbar vertebrae and crosses anterior to the bifurcation of the common iliac artery to descend into the pelvis.

Urethral crest: Located on the posterior aspect of the prostatic urethra with several openings bilaterally to receive seminal fluid from the prostatic ducts. The seminal colliculus, also referred to as the verumontanum, is an enlargement of the urethral crest that serves as an opening for the ejaculatory ducts and the prostatic utricle.

Urinary bladder: A muscular sac located in the midline of the pelvis anteriorly (the rectum occupies the midline of the pelvis posteriorly). The urinary bladder is made up of bundles of smooth muscles known as the detrusor muscle and is located inferior to the peritoneum. As the bladder fills, it extends toward the pelvic brim.

Urolithiasis: Condition in which renal calculi may present at any part of the urinary tract. About 70% to 80% of kidney stones (renal calculi or nephroliths) are formed of high levels of calcium and, as a result, are easily detectable with ultrasound examination when patients are suspected of nephrolithiasis because of renal colic. Based on the size and shape of kidney stones, severe colicky pain may be produced at the renal calyx or while traveling down through the ureter. In addition, hydronephrosis or obstruction of the ureters by a stone can be a surgical emergency.

Uterus: Fibromuscular female reproductive organ lined by endometrium in which a fertilized ovum may develop into an embryo and then fetus, during the course of a pregnancy. It is supported and kept in place by numerous ligaments such as the round, broad, and cardinal ligaments, as well as the rectouterine, pubocervical, and uterosacral ligaments. The uterus occupies the space between the bladder and rectum at the level of the pelvic midline.

Vagina: The pathway that serves to excrete menstrual products and receives the penis and ejaculate during intercourse. The vaginal canal extends inferiorly from the cervix and terminates at the vaginal vestibule in the perineum. The vagina receives its blood supply from the vaginal branches of the uterine and internal iliac arteries. It is supported in the pelvis by the levator ani, the urogenital diaphragm, and the perineal body.

Vagus nerve (CN X): In the neck, the vagus nerve has several branches, including a pharyngeal nerve that supplies all muscles of the pharynx and soft palate and a superior laryngeal nerve that divides into an internal and external branch. Other branches of the vagus nerve in the neck include usually two cardiac nerves destined for the thorax. The vagus nerve descends through the thorax giving branches to the airways and thoracic esophagus and then enters the abdomen where it provides parasympathetic supply to the gastrointestinal tract as far as the left colic flexure.

Vastus lateralis muscle: Part of the quadriceps femoris muscle, which also consists of rectus femoris, vastus intermedius, and vastus medialis. Vastus lateralis originates from the distal inferior surface of the greater trochanter of the femur, from the superolateral part of the intertrochanteric line, and from a line along the lateral lip of the linea aspera.

Vermillion border: Demarcation between the reddened vascular edge of the lips and adjacent skin.

Vertebral artery: The first branch of the subclavian artery. These vessels supply approximately one-third of the blood to the brain and supply branches to the cervical spinal cord and adjacent muscles. The paired vertebral arteries enter the transverse foramina of the sixth cervical vertebrae and then travel through the transverse foramina of the remaining cervical vertebrae to turn posteriorly and enter the cranial vault through foramen magnum.

Warthin tumors: Benign neoplasm (adenolymphoma, cystadenolymphoma, papillary cystadenoma lymphomatosum), slowly growing, painless masses of the parotid gland.

Whipple procedure: This surgery is also known as pancreaticoduodenectomy, surgical resection done in some cases for pancreatic cancer.

Index

Note: Page number followed by f indicates figures and t indicates tables.

A

Abdomen
- abdominal wall. *See* Abdominal wall
- adrenal gland, 216–217
- gallbladder. *See* Gallbladder
- gastrointestinal viscera. *See* Gastrointestinal viscera
- kidneys, 216
  - left kidney, 218, 218f–219f
  - right kidney and right liver lobe, 221f
- liver. *See* Liver
- pancreas. *See* Pancreas
- peritoneum. *See* Peritoneum
- spleen, 216
  - intercostal oblique, 219f
- ureters, 216
- vessels, 228f
  - abdominal aortic aneurysm, 231
  - aorta and inferior vena cava, 232f
  - bifurcation of, 233f
  - celiac artery, 229f
  - hepatic veins, 227
  - inferior mesenteric artery, 226
  - inferior mesenteric vein, 226
  - inferior vena cava posterior, 234f
  - left gastric (coronary) vein, 226
  - paraumbilical veins, 227
  - portal vein, 226
  - splenic artery aneurysm, 231
  - splenic vein, 226
  - superior mesenteric artery, 225–226, 230f–231f
  - superior mesenteric vein, 226, 230f–231f

Abdominal aortic aneurysm, 231

Abdominal (convex/curved array) probes, 2–3

Abdominal wall
- anatomy
  - anterior, 194
  - iliohypogastric nerve, 195
  - inguinal canal, 194
  - inguinal (Hesselbach) triangle, 194
  - lymphatic drainage, 195
  - subcostal nerve, 195
  - thoracoabdominal nerves, 195
  - vasculature, 195
- clinical applications, 198
- technique
  - external abdominal oblique muscle, 196–197, 197f
  - internal abdominal oblique muscle, 196–197
  - rectus abdominis and rectus sheath, 196, 196f
  - transversus abdominis muscle, 196–197, 197f

A/B lines, lungs, 169

Accessory nerve, 259, 261

Acoustic impedance, 10, 12f

Acromioclavicular (AC) joint
- anatomy, 38
- technique, 43, 47f

Acromioclavicular joint (ACJ) injuries, 321

Acute appendicitis, 207

Adductor canal
- thigh
  - anatomy, 111
  - technique, 112–113, 112f

Adrenal gland, 216–217

Amplitude, 18, 19f

Anal canal, 201

Ankle and foot
- anatomy
  - ankle joint, 147–148
  - anterior compartment muscles, 148
  - anterior compartment tendons, 148
  - deep fibular nerve, 149
  - deep layer, 149–150
  - deltoid ligament, 148
  - dorsalis pedis artery, 148–149
  - fibular collateral ligament complex, 148
  - Kager fat pad, 149
  - lateral compartment muscles, 149
  - lateral compartment tendons, 149
  - metatarsals, 147
  - plantar aponeurosis, 150
  - posterior compartment, 149
  - posterior tibial artery, 150
  - subtendinous calcaneal (retrocalcaneal) bursa, 149
  - superficial fibular nerve, 149
  - superficial layer, 149
  - tarsal bones, 147
  - tarsal tunnel, 150
  - tendons and insertions, 150
  - tibial collateral ligament complex, 148
  - tibial nerve, 150
  - tibiofibular ligaments, 148
- clinical applications, 157
- technique
  - anterior compartment tendons, 151, 151f
  - anterior talofibular ligament, 152, 153f
  - anterior tibiofibular ligament, 152, 152f
  - calcaneal tendon insertion, 156–157, 161f
  - calcaneofibular ligament, 153, 155f
  - fibularis brevis tendon, 153–154, 156f
  - fibularis longus and brevis tendons, 153, 154f
  - fibularis longus tendon, 154, 158f
  - plantar aponeurosis, 157, 162f
  - tarsal tunnel and contents, 155, 159f
  - tibiocalcaneal ligament, 155–156, 160f

Ankle joint, 147–148

Anterior abdominal wall, 194

Anterior cardiac vein, 180

Anterior cervical triangle, neck
- accessory nerve, 261
- ansa cervicalis, 260
- anterior jugular vein, 262
- C2 and C3, 260
- cervical plexus, 260
- common carotid artery, 261–262
- costocervical trunk, 262
- cricoid cartilage, 260
- dorsal scapular artery, 262–263
- facial nerve, 260
- glossopharyngeal nerve, 261
- hyoid bone, 259–260
- hypoglossal nerve, 261
- internal jugular vein, 262
- internal thoracic artery, 262
- internal thoracic veins, 166, 171
- lymphatics, 263
- prevertebral muscles, 260

Index

Anterior cervical triangle, neck (*Continued*)
- scalene muscle, 260
- subclavian artery, 262
- suprahyoid muscles, 260
- sympathetic trunk, 261
- thyrocervical trunk, 262
- thyroid cartilage, 260
- vagus nerve, 260–261
- vertebral artery, 262

Anterior compartment muscles
- ankle and foot, 148
- arms, 53
- leg, 136

Anterior compartment tendons, 148, 151, 151f
Anterior gluteal region, 105, 105f–106f
Anterior superior iliac spine, 95–96, 95f
Anterior talofibular ligament, 152, 153f
Anterior tibial artery, 138
Anterior tibiofibular ligament, 152, 152f
Anterolateral abdominal wall, 195
Aortic sinuses of Valsalva, 181
Aponeuroses, 194
Appendix, 201
Aqueous humor, 283
Arms
- anterior compartment muscles, 53
- axillary artery, 55
- brachial artery, 56–57, 56f–57f
- clinical application, 59
- median and ulnar nerves midhumerus, 57, 57f
- median nerve, 53, 55–56, 56f
- musculocutaneous nerve, 54, 55–56, 56f
- posterior compartment muscles, 53
- radial nerve, 53, 55–58, 56f, 59f–60f
- ulnar nerve, 53, 55–56, 56f

Arthrocentesis, 318, 323
Articular processes, 28, 30f
Ascending aorta, 187f
Ascending pharyngeal artery, 261
Aspiration
- elbow joint, 323, 324f
- knee joint, 318, 319f
- shoulder, 320–322

Attenuation
- air, 13
- bone, 13
- clean acoustic shadowing, 14f
- definition, 13
- fluids, 13

Axillary artery, 48, 55

B

Back
- cervical spine/greater occipital nerve, 32–33, 34f
- lumbar spine. *See* Lumbar spine

Biceps brachii, 40, 40f–41f
Bioeffects, 24
Bladder, 241
- thickening, 255

Blood vessels, 7
Bones, 7
- gluteal region, 103
- knee, 123
- leg, 136
- proximal thigh and inguinal region, 92
- shoulder, 38
- thigh, 110
- thoracic wall, 166–167

Brachial artery, 56–57, 56f, 57f
Brachial plexus, 259
- anatomy
  - axillary artery, 48
  - pectoralis muscles, 48
- technique
  - cords, 50–51, 52f
  - roots/trunks and divisions, 49, 49f–50f

Brachiocephalic artery, 187f
Breasts
- anatomy, 173
- clinical applications, 176
- technique
  - intercostal space, 174, 174f
  - nipple and areola, 175, 175f
  - pectoral muscles ribs, 174, 174f
  - pleural line, 174, 174f

Buck fascia, 194
Bundle of His, 183
Bursitis, 321–322

C

Calcaneal tendon insertion, 156–157, 161f
Calcaneofibular ligament, 153, 155f
Calcific tendonitis, 321
Camper fascia, 194
Cardiac borders, 180
Cardiac (sector array) probes, 3
Cardiac tamponade, 191
Cardiac ultrasound (US), 184
Cardiac valves, 182
Cardiac veins, 182
Cardinal ligament (of Mackenrodt), 239
Cecum, 201
Central nervous system (CNS), 311
Central venous catheterization
- anatomy
  - femoral vein, 310, 310f
  - internal jugular vein, 309, 309f
  - subclavian vein, 308
- contraindications, 308
- indications, 308

Cervical vertebrae, 32
Chest wall, 166–167
- pleural line, 168–170
- structures, 168–170

Chordae tendineae, 181
Clavicle, 38
Coccyx, 246
Colle fascia, 194
Colon, 201
Common carotid artery, 261–262
Common extensor tendon, 67, 71f
Common fibular nerve, 138
Common flexor tendon, 67, 70f
Conduction tissue, heart, 182–183
Conjunctiva, 283
Coronary arteries
- left, 182
- right, 182

Coronary ligament, 200
Cortex, 216
Costocervical trunk, 262
Costodiaphragmatic recess, 167
Cricoid cartilage, 260
Crystal arrays, 15–16, 16f
Cubital fossa, 61, 63, 63f–64f
Cutaneous nerves, 259, 280
Cystic artery, 212
Cystic duct, 212

D

Deep back muscles, 26, 32
Deep cervical fascia, 258, 278
Deep fibular nerve
- ankle and foot, 149
- leg, 138

Deep group of muscles, 103
Deep inguinal lymph node, 97–98, 101f
Deep layer
- ankle and foot, 149–150
- leg, 137

Deltoid ligament, 148
Deltoid muscles, 38
Diagnostic elbow joint aspiration, 323, 324f
Diagnostic pericardiocentesis, 314
Diffuse reflection, 20–21, 20f–21f, 23f
Display orientation markers, 4
Doppler ultrasound, internal thoracic artery, 172
Dorsalis pedis artery, 148–149
Dorsal scapular nerve, 259, 262–263
Ductus deferens, 247
Duodenum
- ascending (fourth) part, 200
- descending (second) part, 200
- superior (first) part, 200
- transverse (third) part, 200

E
Echocardiography, 184, 191
Ectopic pregnancy, 242
Ejaculation, 249
Elbow
  anatomy
    cubital fossa, 61
    elbow joint, 61
    median nerve, 61
    muscles, 61
    radial nerve, 61
    ulnar nerve, 62
  clinical application, 68
  technique
    common extensor tendon, 67, 71f
    common flexor tendon, 67, 70f
    cubital fossa, 63, 63f–64f
    cubital tunnel, ulnar nerve in, 65–66, 68f
    elbow joint, 64–65, 66f–67f
    radial collateral ligament, 67, 71f
    superficial/deep radial nerves, 64, 65f
    triceps brachii muscle/tendon, 66, 69f–70f
    ulnar collateral ligament, 67, 70f
Elbow joint aspiration
  indications
    diagnostic, 323, 324f
    therapeutic, 323
  procedure, 323, 324f
Endocardium, 180
Endometrial cancer, 242
Endometrial stripe, 241
Endometriosis, 242
Epididymis, 247
Epigastric hernia, 198
Epiploic appendages, 201
Erection, 249
Esophagus, 271
Extended focused assessment with sonography for trauma (eFAST) examination, 191, 292
Extensor digitorum longus, 136
Extensor hallucis longus, 136
External abdominal oblique muscle, 196–197, 197f
External intercostal muscle, 166
Eye and orbit
  aqueous humor, 283
  clinical applications, 286
  conjunctiva, 283
  iris and pupil, 287f
  lens, 283
  optic nerve and optic nerve sheath, 285f
  orbital contents, 284f
  sclera, 283

F
Face
  buccal artery, 280
  cutaneous nerves, 280
  deep cervical fascia, 278
  dorsal nasal artery, 280
  facial artery, 278
  facial vein, 280
  galea aponeurotica, 278
  infraorbital artery, 280
  lacrimal artery, 280
  lacrimal gland, 281
  lymphatic vessels/nodes, 280
  mental artery, 280
  motor nerves, 280–281
  muscles, 278, 279t
  parotid gland, 281
  parotitis, 282
  pleomorphic adenomas, 282
  superficial temporal artery, 278
  supraorbital artery, 278
  supratrochlear artery, 280
  technique, 282, 282f
Facial artery, 261, 278
Falciform ligament, 199
Fallopian tubes, 239
Fasciae, 258
Fascia lata, 103
Fatty liver, 207
Female pelvis
  anatomy
    fallopian tubes, 239
    ovaries, 239
    pubic arch, 238
    uterus, 238–239
    vagina, 239
  clinical applications, 242
  suprapubic views, abdomen/pelvis, 299, 299f, 301f
  technique
    fundus, 240
    myometrium, 240
    sagittal/parasagittal, 240, 240f
    suprapubic view, 241, 241f
Femoral artery, 111
Femoral nerve, 93
Femoral triangle, 93, 96–97, 100f
Femoral vein, 310, 310f
Femoral vessels, 93
Fibroglandular tissue, 174–175
Fibromyomas, 242
Fibroserous sac, 180
Fibula, 136
Fibular collateral ligament complex, 148
Fibularis brevis, 137
Fibularis brevis tendon, 153–154, 156f
Fibularis longus, 137
  brevis tendons, 153, 154f
Fibularis longus tendon, 154, 158f
Fibularis tertius, 136
Focused assessment with sonography for trauma (FAST) examination, 292
  anatomy, 293
  costodiaphragmatic recesses, 292
  left upper quadrant, 297–298, 297f–298f
  probe selection, 292
  right upper quadrant, 294–295, 294f–296f
  suprapubic views, abdomen/pelvis
    female pelvis, 299, 299f, 301f
    male pelvis, 300, 300f, 302f
    parasternal long-axis view, 304f
    pouch of Douglas, 299
    subxiphoid 4-chamber view, 303f
  Trendelenburg positioning, 292
Forearm
  anterior compartment tendons, 72
  carpal tunnel, 72
  clinical application, 80
  distal, 75, 76f–77f
  extensor retinaculum, 72–73
  median nerve, 72
  posterior compartment muscles, 72–73
  proximal, 74–75, 74f–75f
  radial arteries, 72
  tendons, 72–73
  ulnar arteries, 72
Fundus, 200, 240

G
Galea aponeurotica, 278
Gallbladder
  clinical applications, 213
  cystic artery, 212
  cystic duct, 212
  functions, 212
  Hartmann pouch, 212
  insonation window, 213
  intercostal view of, 213, 214f
  Murphy sign, 212
  subcostal view of, 213, 215f
Gallstones (cholelithiasis), 213
Gastrocnemius, 137
Gastrointestinal viscera
  large intestine, 201
  small intestine, 200–201
  stomach, 200
Glenohumeral joint, 38, 43, 47f
Glenoid labrum, 43, 47f
Glossopharyngeal nerve, 261
Gluteal maximus, 103

Index

Gluteal region
  anatomy
    bones, 103
    deep group of muscles, 103
    fascia lata, 103
    gluteal maximus, 103
    gluteus medius, 103
    gluteus minimus, 103
    greater/lesser sciatic foramina, 103
    hamstring origin, 104
    iliotibial tract, 103
    lumbosacral plexus, 104
    sciatic nerve, 104
    superior/inferior gluteal arteries, 104
    tensor fasciae latae, 103
  technique
    anterior gluteal region, 105, 105f–106f
    clinical applications, 108
    gluteus medius, 106–107, 107f–108f
    gluteus minimus, 106–107, 107f–108f
    greater trochanter, 106–107, 107f
    sciatic nerve, 107–108, 109f
Gluteus medius, 103, 106–107, 107f–108f
Gluteus medius and minimus, 93
Gluteus minimus, 103, 106–107, 107f–108f
Great auricular nerve, 259
Greater occipital nerve, 32–33, 33f
Greater omentum, 199

H

Hamstring muscles, 113–115, 117f–122f
Hand
  carpal tunnel, 72
  clinical application, 80
  digits/digital flexor tendons, 73
  digits, flexor tendons of, 79–80, 84f–87f
  intrinsic muscles, 73
  median nerve, 72
  radial arteries, 72
  thenar eminence, 78–79, 83f
  ulnar arteries, 72
Hartmann pouch, 212
Haustra, 201
Heart
  anatomy
    cardiac borders, 180
    cardiac valves, 182
    cardiac veins, 182
    conduction tissue, 182–183
    coronary arteries, 182
    left atrium, 181
    left ventricle, 181–182
    pericardium, 180
    right atrium, 180–181
    right ventricle, 181
  apical 4-chamber view of, 184f
  apical 5-chamber view of, 185f
  clinical applications, 190
  technique
    apical views, 184–185, 184f–185f
    inferior vena cava view, 185, 186f
    parasternal long-axis (PLAX) view, 186, 188f
    parasternal short-axis (PSAX) view, 186–190, 188f–189f
    subxiphoid view, 190–191, 190f
    suprasternal view, 185, 187f
Hepatic veins, 227
Hernias
  epigastric, 198
  incisional, 198
  Spigelian, 198
High-frequency linear probe, 33
Hip joint, 96, 99f
Hip joint capsule, 92
Hodgkin disease, 220
Hyoid bone, 259–260
Hypoglossal nerve, 261

I

Ileum, 201
Iliacus muscles, 93
Iliofemoral ligament, 96, 99f
Iliohypogastric nerve, 195
Iliopsoas, 96, 99f
Iliotibial tract, 103, 113, 115f
Image producing, 18–19, 18f–19f
Incisional hernia, 198
Inferior mesenteric artery, 226
Inferior mesenteric vein, 226
Inferior vena cava (IVC), 180, 186f
  fissures for, 202
Infraspinatus muscles, 39
Infraspinatus tendon, 42, 46f
Inguinal canal, 194
Inguinal (Hesselbach) triangle, 194
Innermost intercostal muscle, 166
Insonation window, 213
Intercostal arteries, 166
Intercostal muscles
  external, 166
  innermost, 166
Intercostal nerves, 166
Intercostal veins, 166
Interlaminar space thecal sac, 27, 28f
Internal abdominal oblique muscle, 196–197
Internal jugular vein, 309, 309f
Isthmus, 238

J

Jejunum, 200–201

K

Kager fat pad
  ankle and foot, 149
  leg, 137
Kidneys, 216
  left kidney, 218, 218f–219f
  right kidney and right liver lobe, 221f
Knee
  anatomy
    articular surfaces, 123
    bones, 123
    common fibular nerve, 125
    fibular collateral ligament, 124
    gastrocnemius, 124–125
    hamstring tendons, 124
    iliotibial tract, 124
    joint capsule, 123
    knee joint, 123
    leg posterior compartment, 124
    menisci, 123
    popliteal fossa, 125
    popliteal vessels, 125
    popliteus, 125
    quadriceps femoris, 124
    sciatic nerve, 125
    soleus, 125
    tibial collateral ligament, 123–124
    tibial nerve, 125
  clinical applications, 133
  technique
    collateral ligaments, 127–129, 130f–131f
    infrapatellar knee, 127, 128f–129f
    popliteal fossa, 129–133, 131f, 134f–135f
    suprapatellar knee, 126–127, 126f–127f
Knee joint aspiration
  anatomy, 318
  anatomy of, 318, 319f
  contraindications, 318
  indications, 318
Knobology and image optimization, 7–8
  depth, 7
  focal points, 8
  gain, 8
  tissue harmonics imaging, 8

L

Lacrimal gland, 281
Laminae interlaminar spaces, 29, 31f
Large intestine, 201
Larynx, 271
Lateral compartment muscles
  ankle and foot, 149
  leg, 137

Lateral compartment tendons, 149
Lateral femoral cutaneous nerve, 93, 96, 98f
Leaflets, 181, 183, 185, 187, 190
Left anterior descending (LAD) artery, 182
Left atrium, 181
Left coronary artery, 182
Left gastric (coronary) vein, 226
Left ventricle, 181–182
Leg
  anatomy
    anterior compartment muscles, 136
    anterior tibial artery, 138
    bones, 136
    common fibular nerve, 138
    deep fibular nerve, 138
    deep layer, 137
    extensor digitorum longus, 136
    extensor hallucis longus, 136
    fibula, 136
    fibularis brevis, 137
    fibularis longus, 137
    fibularis tertius, 136
    gastrocnemius, 137
    Kager fat pad, 137
    lateral compartment muscles, 137
    plantaris, 137
    popliteal vessels, 138
    posterior compartment muscles, 137
    posterior tibial artery, 138
    sciatic nerve, 138
    soleus, 137
    superficial fibular nerve, 138
    superficial layer, 137
    sural nerve, 138
    tibia, 136
    tibialis anterior, 136
    tibial nerve, 138
  clinical application, 144
  technique
    anterior compartment, 139–140, 139f–140f
    lateral compartment, 140–141, 141f–143f
    posterior compartment, 142–143, 144f–146f
Leiomyomas, 242
Lens, 283
Lesser occipital nerve, 259
Lesser omentum, 199
Levator scapulae, 258
Ligamentum venosum, 200
Linea alba, 194
Linear (linear array) probes, 3
Lingual artery, 261
Liver
  biopsy, 207
  caudate lobe, 203f, 205f
  cirrhosis, 207
  clinical applications, 207
  diaphragm, 211f
  fatty, 207
  fissures and ligaments, 202
  hemithorax, 211f
  inferior vena cava (IVC), 203f, 210f
    middle and left hepatic veins, 204f
  left lobe, 203f, 205f
  left portal vein and branches, 203f
  ligamentum venosum, 203f
  lobes of
    left lobe, 202
    right lobe, 201
  Morison pouch, 211f
  portal triad, 201, 206f
  portal vein, 208f–209f
  right lobe of, 211f
  superior mesenteric vein, 205f
Long thoracic nerve, 259
Lower limb
  ankle and foot. *See* Ankle and foot
  gluteal region. *See* Gluteal Region
  knee, 123–133, 126f–132f, 134f–135f
  leg, 136–144, 139f–146f
  proximal thigh and inguinal region, 92–99, 95f–102f
  thigh. *See* Thigh
Lumbar puncture, 311
  contraindications, 311
  indications, 311
  procedure, 311–312, 312f–313f
Lumbar spine
  articular processes, 28, 30f
  clinical applications, 30
  deep back muscles, 26
  interlaminar space thecal sac, 27, 28f
  laminae interlaminar spaces, 29, 31f
  spinal canal, 26
  spinous process laminae, 27, 27f
  transverse processes, 28, 29f
  vertebrae, 26
Lumbosacral plexus, 104
Lung point, 169
Lymphatic drainage, 195
Lymphatics, 259
  thoracic duct, 263
Lymphoma, 220

M

Male pelvis
  anatomy
    bones of, 246
    ductus deferens, 247
    epididymis, 247
    micturition process, 247
    pelvic diaphragm, 246
    pelvic inlet and outlet, 246
    penis, 248
    prostate, 248
    prostate-specific antigen, 248
    sacrococcygeal joint, 246
    seminal fluid, 247
    seminal vesicles, 247
    testes, 247
    ureters, 246–247
    urethral crest, 248
    urinary bladder, 246–247
  ejaculation, 249
  erection, 249
  suprapubic views, abdomen/pelvis, 300, 300f, 302f
  technique
    penis, 251, 252f–253f
    scrotum and testes, 252, 254f
    transabdominal (suprapubic) view, 250–251, 250f–251f
Mammary glands, 173
Manubrium, 166
Masseteric fascia, 278
Maxillary artery, 262
McBurney point, 201, 207
Meckel diverticulum, 207
Medial compartment muscles, 93
Median nerve
  arms, 53, 55–56, 56f, 57
  elbow, 61
Medulla, 216
Mercedes Benz sign, 190
Mesometrium, 238
Mesovarium, 238–239
Metatarsals, 147
Micturition process, 247
Morison pouch, 294
Motor nerves, 280–281
Murphy sign, 212
Muscles, 61
Musculocutaneous nerve, 54–56, 56f
Myocardium, 180
Myometrium, 240

N

Neck
  anatomy
    anterior cervical triangle, 259–263
    fasciae, 258
    posterior cervical triangle, 258–259
  clinical applications, 269
  technique
    carotid sinus, 264, 265f, 267f
    common carotid artery, 264, 264f–265f, 267f, 269f
    deep cervical lymph node, 269f
    external carotid arteries, 266f–267f, 270f
    internal carotid artery, 264, 265f–267f, 270f

Index

Neck (*Continued*)
internal jugular vein, 264, 264f, 269f–270f
jugulodigastric lymph node, 270f
posterior belly of digastric muscle, 270f
sternocleidomastoid muscle, 270f
thyroid gland, 264, 264f
vertebral artery, 268f
viscera of, 274f–277f
clinical applications, 276
larynx/trachea, 271
parathyroid glands, 272
pharynx/esophagus, 271
salivary stones, 276
Sjögren syndrome, 276
sublingual gland, 271
submandibular duct, 273f
submandibular salivary gland, 273f
thyroid gland, 271–272
thyroid nodules, 276
Nerves, 7
Noncommunicating bursitis, 322

O
Occipital artery, 261
Optic nerve, 285f
sheath, 285f
Os coxae, 246
Ovaries, 239

P
Pancreas
abdominal aorta, 223, 223f
blood supply, 222
cancer, 224
ducts, 222
pancreatitis, 224
uncinate process, 222, 224f
Pancreatitis, 224
Panniculitis, 308
Parasternal approach, 316, 316f
Parasternal long-axis (PLAX) view, 186, 188f
Parasternal short-axis (PSAX) view, 186–190, 188f–189f
Parathyroid glands, 272
Paraumbilical veins, 227
Parietal pleurae, 167
Parotid fascia, 278
Parotid gland, 281
Parotitis, 282
Pectinate muscles, 180
Pectineus/adductor muscles, 98–99, 102f
Pectoralis major muscle, 175
Pectoralis muscles, 48
Penis, 248, 251, 252f–253f, 255
Pericardial sac, 180
Pericardiocentesis, 191, 314
anatomic pitfalls, 317
apical approach, 317
contraindications, 315
indications, 314f
diagnostic, 314
therapeutic, 315
subxiphoid approach, 317
Pericardium, 303
parasternal long-axis view of, 188f
serous, 180
subxiphoid 4-chamber view of, 190f
visceral, 180
Peritoneal cavity, 199–200
Peritoneum
coronary ligament, 200
greater omentum, 199
lesser omentum, 199
ligamentum venosum, 200
parietal and visceral, 199
transverse mesocolon, 199
Peyer patches, 200
Pharynx, 271
Phrenic nerve, 259
Phrenicocolic ligament, 199
Piezoelectric effect, 15, 16f
Plantar aponeurosis, 150, 157, 162f
Plantaris, 137
Pleomorphic adenomas, 282
Pleura, 166–167
Pneumothorax, 172
Point-source sound waves, 17
Popliteal vessels, 138
Portal triad, 201, 206f
Portal vein, 226
Posterior auricular artery, 261
Posterior cervical triangle, neck, 258–259
lymphatics, 259
muscles, 258–259
nerves, 259
vessels, 259
Posterior compartment, 149
Posterior compartment muscles
arms, 53
leg, 137
Posterior tibial artery
ankle and foot, 150
leg, 138
Pouch of Douglas, 299
Prevertebral fascia, 258
Probe orientation markers, 4
Probe patency of the foramen ovale, 181
Probe transducers, 15–16
Prostate, 248
Prostate-specific antigen, 248
Proximal humerus, 38
Proximal thigh and inguinal region
anatomy
femoral nerve, 93
femoral triangle, 93
femoral vessels, 93
femur, 92
gluteus medius and minimus, 93
hip joint capsule, 92
iliacus muscles, 93
lateral femoral cutaneous nerve, 93
medial compartment muscles, 93
nerves and vessels, 93–94
pelvic bones, 92
psoas major muscles, 93
rectus femoris, 93
sartorius, 93
tensor fasciae latae, 93
technique
anterior superior iliac spine, 95–96, 95f
clinical application, 99
deep inguinal lymph node, 97–98, 101f
femoral triangle, 96–97, 100f
hip joint, 96, 99f
iliofemoral ligament, 96, 99f
iliopsoas, 96, 99f
lateral femoral cutaneous nerve, 96, 98f
pectineus/adductor muscles, 98–99, 102f
rectus femoris, 96, 97f
sartorius, 96, 97f
tensor fasciae latae, 96, 97f
Psoas major muscles, 93
Pubic arch, 238
Pubocervical ligament, 239
Pulmonary semilunar valve, 181
Purkinje fibers, 183
Pylorus, 200

Q
Quadriceps femoris, 113, 114f

R
Radial collateral ligament, 67, 71f
Radial nerve
arms, 53, 55–58, 56f, 59f–60f
elbow, 61
Rectum, 201
Rectus abdominis muscles, 196, 196f
Rectus femoris, 93, 96, 97f
Rectus sheath, 194, 196, 196f
Renal artery, 216
Renal calculi, 216
Right atrium, 180–181
Right coronary artery, 182
Right ventricle, 181
Rugae, 200
Ruptured urinary bladder, 255

S

Sacculations, 201
Sacrococcygeal joint, 246
Sacrum, 246
Salivary stones, 276
Sartorius, 93, 96, 97f
Scalenes, 258
Scapula, 38
Scarpa fascia, 194
Sciatic nerve
  gluteal region, 104, 107–108, 109f
  leg, 138
  thigh, 113–115, 117f–122f
Sclera, 283
Scrotum, 252, 254f
Seminal fluid, 247
Seminal vesicles, 247
Semispinalis capitis, 258
Serous pericardium, 180
Serratus anterior, 259
Shoulder
  anatomy
    acromioclavicular joint, 38
    clavicle, 38
    deltoid muscles, 38
    glenohumeral joint, 38
    infraspinatus muscles, 39
    proximal humerus, 38
    scapula, 38
    subscapularis, 39
    supraspinatus muscles, 38–39
    teres minor muscles, 39
  aspiration, 320
    acromioclavicular joint (ACJ) injuries, 321
    bursitis, 321–322
    calcific tendonitis, 321
    indications, 320, 320f
  clinical applications, 43
  technique
    acromioclavicular (AC) joint, 43, 47f
    biceps brachii, 40, 40f–41f
    glenohumeral joint, 43, 47f
    glenoid labrum, 43, 47f
    infraspinatus tendon, 42, 46f
    subscapularis, 41, 42f–43f
    supraspinatus tendon, 41–42, 44f–45f
Sialolithiasis, 276
Sibson fascia (suprapleural membrane), 167
Sinoatrial node, 183
Sinus venarum, 180
Sjögren syndrome, 276
Skeletal muscle, 7
Skin, 7
Small intestine, 200–201
Soleus, 137
Sonographic Murphy sign, 213
Sound waves, 10–12
  acoustic impedance, 10, 12f
  bone and air, 10
  definition, 10
  diffuse reflection, 20–21, 23f
  point-source sound waves, 17
  propagation, 10
  reflection and through-transmission, 10, 11f
  specular reflection, 20–21, 20f–21f
Spatial resolution, 18, 19f
Specular reflection, 20–21, 20f–21f
Spigelian hernia, 198
Spinal canal, 26
Spinous process laminae, 27, 27f
Spleen, 216, 219f
Splenic artery aneurysm, 231
Splenic vein, 226
Splenius capitis, 258
Splenomegaly, 220
Steatosis, 207
Sternal angle (of Louis), 166
Sternocleidomastoid, 258
Sternum, 166
Stomach, 200
Subacromial-subdeltoid (SA-SD) bursa, 321–322
Subclavian vein, 308
Subcostal nerve, 195
Sublingual gland, 271
Submandibular gland, 271
Subscapularis, 39, 41, 42f–43f
Subtendinous calcaneal (retrocalcaneal) bursa, 149
Sulcus terminalis, 180
Superficial cervical fascia, 258
Superficial/deep radial nerves, 64, 65f
Superficial fibular nerve
  ankle and foot, 149
  leg, 138
Superficial investing fascia, 258
Superficial layer
  ankle and foot, 149
  leg, 137
Superficial temporal artery, 262, 278
Superior/inferior gluteal arteries, 104
Superior mesenteric artery, 225–226, 230f–231f
Superior mesenteric vein, 226, 230f–231f
Superior thyroid artery, 261
Superior vena cava, 180
Supraclavicular nerve, 259
Suprahyoid muscles, 260
Supraorbital artery, 278
Suprapubic catheter placement, 255
Supraspinatus muscles, 38–39
Supraspinatus tendon, 41–42, 44f–45f
Supraventricular crest, 181
Sural nerve, 138
Sympathetic trunk, 261

T

TAPB. *See* Transversus abdominis plane block (TAPB)
Tarsal bones, 147
Tarsal tunnel, 150, 155, 159f
Tendons, 7
Teniae coli, 201
Tensor fasciae latae, 93, 96, 97f, 103
Teres minor muscles, 39
Testes, 247, 252, 254f, 255
Therapeutic elbow joint aspiration, 323
Therapeutic pericardiocentesis, 315
Thermal bioeffects, 24
Thigh
  anatomy
    adductor canal, 111
    anterior compartment, 110
    bones, 110
    femoral artery, 111
    posterior compartment, 110
  clinical applications, 116
  technique
    adductor canal, 112–113, 112f
    hamstring muscles, 113–115, 117f–122f
    iliotibial tract, 113, 115f
    quadriceps femoris, 113, 114f
    sciatic nerve, 113–115, 117f–122f
Third occipital nerve, 32–33
Thoracoabdominal nerves, 195
Thoracoabdominal trauma, 172
Thorax
  clinical applications, 172
  costal cartilages and pleural line, 170, 170f
  internal thoracic vessels, 170–171, 171f–172f
  pleura, 167
  wall
    intercostal arteries, 166
    intercostal muscles, 166
    intercostal nerves, 166
    intercostal space and pleural line, 168f–169f
    intercostal veins, 166
Thrombus, 180
Thyrocervical trunk, 262
Thyroid cartilage, 260
Thyroid gland, 271–272
Thyroid nodules, 276
Tibia, 136
Tibial collateral ligament complex, 148
Tibialis anterior, 136

Index

Tibial nerve
ankle and foot, 150
leg, 138
Tibiocalcaneal ligament, 155–156, 160f
Tibiofibular ligaments, 148
Tissues appearance, 5–7, 6f
blood vessels, 7
bone, 7
nerves, 7
skeletal muscle, 7
skin, 7
tendons, 7
Trachea, 271
Transverse cervical nerve, 259
Transverse mesocolon, 199
Transverse processes, 28, 29f
Transversus abdominis muscle, 196–197, 197f
Transversus abdominis plane block (TAPB), 198
Trapezius, 258
Triceps brachii muscle/tendon, 66, 69f–70f

U

Ulnar collateral ligament, 67, 70f
Ulnar nerves
arms, 53, 55–56, 56f, 57, 57f
elbow, 62, 65–66, 68f
Ultrasound (US)
breast, 176
cardiac, 184
central venous access, 308–310
ectopic pregnancy, 242
elbow joint arthrocentesis, 323
endometrial cancer, 242
endometriosis, 242
eye, 286
gel, 3–4
penis, 255
pleura, 172
Spigelian hernia, 198
testes, 255
transversus abdominis plane block (TAPB), 198
Ultrasound (US) probes
abdominal (convex/curved array) probes, 2–3
applications, 2–3
cardiac (sector array) probes, 3
controlling/manipulating, 3–4
crystal arrays, 15–16, 16f
display orientation markers, 4
image producing, 18–19, 18f–19f
knobology and image optimization, 7–8
depth, 7
focal points, 8
gain, 8
tissue harmonics imaging, 8
linear (linear array) probes, 3
piezoelectric effect, 15, 16f
point-source sound waves, 17
probe orientation markers, 4
probe transducers, 15–16
sound waves, 10–12
tissues appearance, 5–7, 6f
blood vessels, 7
bone, 7
nerves, 7
skeletal muscle, 7
skin, 7
tendons, 7
Upper limb
arms, 53–59, 56f–57f, 59f–60f
brachial plexus, 48–51, 49f–50f, 52f
forearm. *See* Forearm
hand. *See* Hand
shoulder, 38–43, 40f–47f
wrist. *See* Wrist
Ureters, 216, 246–247
Urethral crest, 248
Urinary bladder, 246–247
Urolithiasis, 220
Uterine tubes, 239
Uterosacral ligament, 239
Uterus
anteverted and anteflexed, 238
broad ligament, 238
cardinal ligament, 239
isthmus, 238
pubocervical ligament, 239
round ligament, 238
uterosacral ligament, 239

V

Vagina, 239
Vasculature, 195
Vertebrae, 26
Visceral pericardium, 180
Visceral pleurae, 167

W

Wrist
carpal tunnel, 76–77
clinical application, 80
extensor retinaculum compartments, 77–78, 81f–82f
Guyon canal, 76–77
median nerve, 72
radial arteries, 72
ulnar arteries, 72